IRENE HOFFERT

D1450103

IRENE HOFFERT

NUTRITION:
Principles and Application in Health Promotion

J. B. LIPPINCOTT COMPANY

Philadelphia / Toronto

NUTRITION:
Principles and Application in Health Promotion

CAROL WEST SUITOR, M.S., R.D.

Clinical Nutritionist, Frances Stern Nutrition Center,
New England Medical Center Hospital, Boston;
Education Specialist, Massachusetts Nutrition Resource Center.
Formerly Nutrition Instructor, St. Elizabeth's Hospital
School of Nursing, Boston

MERRILY FORBES HUNTER, R.N., B.A.

Course Chairperson, Advanced Clinical Nursing,
St. Elizabeth's Hospital School of Nursing, Boston

ISBN 0-397-54256-9

Library of Congress Catalog Card Number 79-22569

Printed in the United States of America

3   5   7   9   8   6   4   2

Library of Congress Cataloging in Publication Data

Suitor, Carol West.
   Nutrition, principles and application in health
promotion.
   Bibliography: p.
   Includes index.
   1. Nutrition. I. Hunter, Merrily Forbes, joint
author. II. Title
QP141.S84   613.2   79-22569
ISBN 0-397-54256-9

Dedication

To my loving parents,
Kathlyn Case West and Robert Knowlton West

Carol West Suitor

To my son, Sam, who makes life a joy
and **to my grandmothers,**
Mary McKenzie Forbes and Mabel Elizabeth Waters,
who gave me love and inspiration

Merrily Forbes Hunter

Preface

The authors believe that achieving and/or maintaining optimal nutritional status is an essential component of health promotion. Our teaching and clinical experiences have impressed us with the need for a practical nutrition text—one which presents a broad base of knowledge and guides the reader in using facts and principles to provide high quality nutritional care. This text is designed to help students and health professionals to acquire relevant information about nutrition which they can use professionally and personally. It is our hope that readers will adopt the nonjudgmental, client-centered approach taken in the text.

The arrangement of content in this text merits special attention since it differs from the usual. We have found this arrangement of content to be useful, but it is not critical to successful use of the text. For example, material in Section Two could be understood without having read Section One. The content has been developed with flexibility in mind. The text can be used when nutrition and diet therapy are taught as separate courses, when nutrition is integrated into other courses, or when a nutrition source book is needed.

There are four major sections: Promoting Normal Nutrition, Relationship of Nutrients to Normal Body Function, Providing Nutritional Care, and Diet Changes for Meeting Special Needs. As the names of the sections imply, each one has a special focus. Topics in Section One are oriented toward practical aspects of normal nutrition. Students are encouraged to find out how various dietary patterns can meet the body's need for nutrients and energy. Eating "prudently" and controlling weight are described as examples of ways to promote health. Roles which religion, culture, and behavior play in food behaviors are introduced in Section One in a manner which stimulates further inquiry. Section One emphasizes ways to promote sound eating habits throughout the life cycle and includes practical guidelines for planning, purchasing, and safely storing and preparing nutritious food.

Section Two focuses on the physiological contributions nutrients make to body structure and function. The interrelated role of nutrients in maintaining a state of dynamic equilibrium is emphasized. We have found this approach to be more meaningful to students than studying nutrients one by one. At the end of Section Two, facts and principles useful for evaluating nutrition information are presented in detail, preparing the student to deal more effectively with new fads and nutrition messages in the media.

Section Three guides the student in developing skills for providing nutritional care. The format of this section parallels the clinical care process, presenting tools for assessment, planning, and providing nutritional care. Since nutritional care often involves influencing behavior, there is strong emphasis on application of concepts from the behavioral sciences. Effective means for providing nutrition education are explored.

In Section Four diet therapy is discussed from a physiological perspective. Common stressors and ways in which they interfere with optimal nutritional status are presented. The focus is on interrelationships among physiological changes, diet modifications, and roles of the health professional in providing nutritional care. Students will find several features to be especially useful, namely: (1) general concepts which are applicable to a number of situations, (2) concrete examples of ways to use the clinical care process to assist clients to modify their food-related behaviors, and (3) practical suggestions to adapt diets to individual needs.

Throughout the text the authors have referred to persons who are recipients of health care services as "clients." We have chosen this term since we feel that it suggests that the health care recipient should have the opportunity to participate in his care-related decisions and should be a responsible participant in his health care program.

To decrease confusion the pronoun "he" has been used when reference is made to the client. (Exceptions are made when the client is definitely a pregnant woman or a mother.) When referring to a health professional of any type, the pronoun "she" has been used. The use of these pronouns is not meant to denote the person's gender.

The authors have worked to assure the accuracy of content. We welcome comments concerning errors, omissions, and/or strengths of the text. Since new developments are reported frequently, we encourage the reader to supplement the text with current reliable publications.

Carol West Suitor
Merrily Forbes Hunter

Acknowledgments

We wish to express our thanks to the many persons who provided us with support and assistance in the writing of this text. We are especially grateful to each of the following people: Joanne Malenock, R.D., M.S., Assistant Professor of Nutrition, School of Nursing, University of Pittsburgh, reviewed the entire manuscript and gave us many constructive suggestions. James M. Rabb, M.D., Clinical Associate in Medicine, Harvard Medical School, Associate Clinical Professor of Medicine, Tufts Medical School at St. Elizabeth's Hospital, formerly Head, Nutrition Support Clinic, University of Chicago Hospital and Clinics, reviewed and commented helpfully on Chapters 20, 21, 32, and 33. Helen Fagan, Director of St. Elizabeth's Hospital School of Nursing, provided encouragement and support from the start of the project. Linda Sleeper typed the entire manuscript and somehow managed to have everything completed on time. Bernice Heller, Editor, and Eleanor Faven, Production Editor, J. B. Lippincott Co., provided frequent encouragement and technical assistance.

We are also appreciative of the assistance Kathy Boyd, Librarian, gave us and of the ideas Lovie Condrick, R.N., provided at the onset of the project. We thank our students for asking so many thought-provoking questions.

We are especially pleased to have families and friends who not only were supportive but also were understanding and patient during the writing of the text.

Contents

PART TWO | Relationship of Nutrients to Normal Body Function 139

PART THREE | Providing Nutritional Care 209

Appendices

5 | Modified diets 443

PART ONE

Promoting Normal Nutrition

1
Overview of nutrition and nutritional concerns

There can be no question about the place of prevention among the various priorities for a future health care system: it belongs at the very top. Indeed, it is so desirable a goal, from every point of view, that there are mounting pressures within and outside the medical profession to expand the role of preventative medicine now . . .[1] (Report of the President's Biomedical Research Panel)

The focus of this book is the fundamental role of nutrition in the promotion of health, in the prevention of illness, and in the restoration of health following illness or injury. Attention is directed toward ways in which health professionals can be instrumental in *preventing* problems related to nutrition. It is time for health workers to stop being content just to clean up the stove while the pot continues to boil over.

INTRODUCTION

You are what you eat.

Your nutrition can determine how you look, act, and feel; whether you are grouchy or cheerful, homely or beautiful, physiologically and even psychologically young or old; whether you think clearly or are confused, enjoy your work or make it a drudgery, increase your earning power or stay in an economic rut.[2]

Nutrition messages like these bombard the consumer from all sides. Doctor, nurse, dietitian, quack, neighbor, in-law, and actor all speak with the voice of authority. The thrust of their messages is the same—good nutrition promotes good health—but the advice they give may differ greatly.

Unfortunately, conflicting nutrition messages leave many a consumer shrugging "What's the use?" rather than changing his eating behavior. On the other hand, another consumer may try to take positive action.

Because this individual feels that what he eats is important, he takes a vitamin pill as he gulps down his coffee in the morning. A donut gives him energy on his break. A "natural" granola bar replaces lunch. It is supplemented by "ice cream without guilt"—a sweetened yogurt cone from a nearby shop. This series of contradictions continues through the day. The consumer fits his version of good nutrition into his lifestyle with a minimum of thought and effort. He often ends up no better off than the person who does not try to change.

Health professionals have an important role in promoting health by assisting consumers in making informed food choices. An essential element for improving the situation is guided study of nutrition and tools for effecting change.

There are numerous obstacles to promoting desirable changes in eating habits. The interplay between an individual's mind and body often results in eating behaviors contrary to what is known to be beneficial. Emotions, culture, lifestyle, capabilities, and resources all influence food habits. If health workers can take a broad view of nutrition, they may learn to be more effective promoters of health.

NUTRITION AND HUMAN NEEDS

Effective health promotion requires an understanding of the numerous ways in which nutrition relates to human needs. An examination of Figure 1.1 shows that food or nutrition can be related to many types of needs.

Nutritive needs Nutrition has been simply defined as "the food you eat and how your body uses it." The physiological need for food is actually the need for

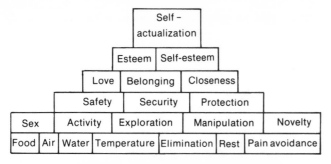

FIGURE 1.1. Maslow's hierarchy of needs, as adapted by Kalish. (From *The Psychology of Human Behavior* by R. A. Kalish. Copyright © 1966 by Wadsworth, Inc. Reprinted by permission of the publisher, Brooks/Cole Publishing Company, Monterey, California)

nutrients. Nutrients are the chemicals necessary for the proper functioning of the body. Each nutrient has one or more of the following functions: (1) providing energy for body processes and exercise; (2) providing structural material, as for the bones and muscles; and (3) regulating body processes.

Some of the nutrients (chemicals) are simple elements such as iron. Other nutrients (still chemicals) are large complex molecules such as proteins. Since there are more than 50 different nutrients, similar ones are grouped together. Broad nutrient categories include carbohydrate, fat, protein, vitamins, minerals, and water. Table 1.1 categorizes components of food which are of importance to nutrition. It should be noted that the term *micronutrients* is sometimes used to refer to both vitamins and minerals. Minerals needed in very small amounts are called *trace elements* or *trace minerals*. Those trace elements more commonly known as metals (e.g., iron, zinc, copper) are sometimes called *trace metals*. *Fiber* is not considered

to be a nutrient since it is not absorbed; however, fiber plays important roles in the diet.

The most basic nutrient need is for water, the most abundant chemical in the body. Water is so vital to all body processes that thirst impels us to drink long before our "water level" becomes dangerously low.

Usually the next nutritional priority is for fuel or energy. Every body cell requires a continuous supply of fuel. Hunger drives us to eat and is satisfied only by nutrients providing energy. Carbohydrate, fat, and protein are the nutrient groups which provide energy. The term *caloric value* refers to the amount of energy or kilocalories a nutrient or food can supply to the body. Different foods which supply the same number of calories also supply the same amount of enegry for body processes and exercise.

There are no known clear-cut physiological signals which lead an individual to ingest particular vitamins, minerals, fats, or proteins. The lack of clear signals does not mean that these nutrients are not required.

TABLE 1.1 *Components of food of importance* to nutrition*

CARBOHYDRATES	LIPIDS (FATS)	MICRONUTRIENTS	
		VITAMINS	MINERALS
*Poly*saccharides	Triglycerides (fat)	Fat soluble	Major minerals (needed by the
Starch	Fatty acids	A (retinol)	body in relatively large
Cellulose (see also	Saturated	D (calciferol)	quantity)
under fiber)	Monounsaturated	E (tocopherol)	Calcium (Ca)
*Di*saccharides	Polyunsaturated, includ-	K (phytylmenaquinone)	Chloride (Cl)
Sucrose	ing linoleic acid	Water soluble	Magnesium (Mg)
Maltose	Cholesterol	C (ascorbic acid)	Phosphorus (P)
Lactose	Phospholipids	B complex:	Potassium (K)
*Mono*saccharides	Lecithin	B_1 (thiamine)	Sodium (Na)
Glucose		B_2 (riboflavin)	Trace minerals or trace elements
Fructose		B_6 (pyridoxine,	Cadmium‡ (Cd)
Galactose	*PROTEIN*	pyridoxal, or	Chromium‡ (Cr)
Sugar alcohols	Types of protein:	pyridoxamine)	Copper‡ (Cu)
Sorbitol	Complete	B_{12} (cyanocobalamine)	Fluoride (F)
Mannitol	Partially complete	Biotin	Iodide (I)
Xylitol	Incomplete	Folic acid (folacin)	Iron‡ (Fe)
	Types of amino acids:	Niacin (nicotinic	Manganese‡ (Mn)
	Essential: histidine,	acid or niacinamide)	Molybdenum‡ (Mo)
WATER	isoleucine, leucine,	Pantothenic acid	Nickel‡ (Ni)
	lysine, methionine,	Choline	Selenium‡ (Se)
FIBER	phenylalanine, threonine,		Silicon† (Si)
Cellulose	tryptophan, and valine		Tin‡ (Sn)
Hemicellulose	Nonessential: alanine,		Vanadium‡ (V)
Lignin	arginine, aspartic acid,		Zinc‡ (Zn)
Pectin	cysteine, cystine,† glutamic		
Other indigestible	acid, glycine, hydroxylysine,		
substances from	hydroxyproline, proline,		
plant foods	serine, tyrosine†		

* Not all of the substances listed are required in the diet
† Semiessential
‡ Also called trace metals

4

Proteins, certain fats, vitamins, and minerals are needed for structural and regulatory functions vital to the normal operation of the body.

Food is the usual vehicle for meeting the need for nutrients. Foods usually differ in their nutrient content. No one food can be depended upon to provide all of the nutrients necessary for normal growth and health. *Nutritive value* refers to the nutrient content of a specific amount of food.

Non-nutritive needs Food may be used as a vehicle for meeting other needs identified in Figure 1.1. Chewing food helps meet the need for activity. Cooking and tasting new foods provides opportunities to meet the need for manipulation and exploration. Storing food may help satisfy the need for security. Following traditional cultural food habits gives many individuals a sense of belonging. Eating at an expensive restaurant may give an individual a sense of esteem. Creating a new casserole or dessert can provide an opportunity to meet the need for self-actualization (sometimes referred to as self-fulfillment or self-realization).

Influences on nutritional status

Nutritional status refers to both the types and amounts of nutrients available in the body and the body's utilization of nutrients. Good nutritional status is necessary, but not sufficient, for optimal health.

Nutritional status is influenced by many factors. Nutrient intake is affected by psychological, sociocultural, and physiological influences. The form of food eaten may influence the bioavailability of certain nutrients, i.e., whether they can be used by the body. Once inside the body, nutrients work together in physiological processes. Physiological processes can be influenced by thoughts and emotions. Interactions of nutrients with each other and with the individual are exceedingly important.

Nutritional status can be likened to a performance by an orchestra. In both cases a harmonious, pleasing result is influenced by similar types of things. This is illustrated in Table 1.2.

When nutritional status is good, the harmonious

TABLE 1.2 *Comparison of factors influencing orchestral performance and nutritional status*

FACTORS INFLUENCING ORCHESTRAL PERFORMANCE	FACTORS INFLUENCING NUTRITIONAL STATUS
Contribution of each instrument	Contribution of each nutrient
Balance of instruments	Balance of nutrients
Musical score	Genetic plan
Skill of musicians	Functioning of body parts such as the intestinal tract, heart, lungs, muscles
Conductor	Controls provided by the brain (nervous system) and glands (endocrine system)

result is indicated by the characteristics usually associated with good health. A few of these characteristics are (1) a good supply of energy for performing the usual activities of the day; (2) maintenance of healthy skin, muscles, and other body tissues; and (3) normal healing of injuries and recovery from illness. It is important to realize that if an individual develops symptoms of illness, his nutritional status is not necessarily poor. On the other hand, it is not possible to have optimal health when malnutrition (poor nutritional status) is present.

The complexity of our society sometimes complicates the achievement of optimal nutritional status. An example is provided by a look at food options available to Americans. We are presented with a myriad of choices in the supermarkets. In contrast, very limited selections are available at fast food chains or vending machines. This is significant since there is a growing trend toward food consumption away from home. The consumer with too many or two few food choices faces a real challenge in achieving an optimal intake of required nutrients, using foods in forms which suit his taste and lifestyle.

NUTRITIONAL STATUS AND CONCERNS IN THE U.S.

How well have Americans been able to meet the challenge of achieving good nutritional status? Government-sponsored nutrition studies provide information about nutritional status of populations in the U.S. One of these, the Ten State Nutrition Survey in 1968 to 1970, included a large proportion of poor families, with children heavily represented.[3] Although the data cannot be considered representative of the total population of the U.S., they do indicate that malnutrition exists. Significant numbers of individuals were identified as having low intakes of one or more essential nutrients or having a problem of obesity.

Another survey, the Health and Nutrition Examination Survey (HANES), an ongoing study, indicates generally good mean (average) intakes of all nutrients except iron.[4] Averages can be misleading, however, for HANES reported that substantial numbers of individuals consumed less than standard amounts of nutrients such as calcium (a mineral) and vitamins A and C.

The findings of nutrition surveys do not necessarily reflect all of the health concerns of Americans related to food and nutrition. Following is a brief look at a few of the nutritional concerns of Americans.

IS OUR FOOD SAFE TO EAT?

Not until 1906 was concern over the safety of the food supply great enough to stimulate enactment of laws for governmental control at the national level. The Food, Drug and Cosmetic Act of 1906 authorized formation of the Food and Drug Administration (FDA).

Despite many actions taken by the FDA since then to eliminate adulteration of foods and to prevent the use of harmful amounts of food additives, consumers still question whether our food is really safe to eat.

Concern centers primarily on food additives. Additives can be grouped into two categories: (1) intentional food additives, substances which are used to improve the food in some way, and (2) unintentional food additives such as pesticides and other agricultural chemicals.

In the past decade the banning of some commonly used additives sparked growing doubts regarding the safety of our food. The linking of these additives with cancer and birth defects was a cause for alarm. This association was made for cyclamates, a very popular artificial sweetener, banned by the FDA in 1969. Cyclamates had been on the market since the early 1950s. The safety of saccharin has been the subject of heated controversy also. Consumer concern grew when DES (a hormone called diethylstilbestrol, used to stimulate growth in animals) was also linked with cancer and was banned in 1972. Numerous widely used dyes have been banned recently, all of them linked with cancer.

Besides banning additives, the FDA developed plans to review the safety of substances on the GRAS (Generally Recognized as Safe) list of food additives. The GRAS list includes salt, spices, natural flavorings, and many other fairly common additives. The review is still in progress; therefore questions regarding safety persist. Many consumers have switched to "natural" and "organic" foods sold in health food stores, believing that these are the safest foods to eat. In the midst of the controversy, what stand should the health professional take?

SHOULD I CHANGE THE TYPE OF FOOD I EAT TO PREVENT DISEASE?

Many typical eating habits have been blamed for shortening the lives of Americans. The prime targets of criticism have been overconsumption of fats, cholesterol, and sugar and underconsumption of fiber. The major diseases related to food intake are cardiovascular disease (heart disease, stroke, high blood pressure), diabetes, cancer of the breast, and cancer of the gastrointestinal tract. Myocardial infarction (heart attack) was estimated to be the cause of death for 646,073 Americans in 1976.[5] Many other persons have survived a heart attack or stroke to find their activites significantly restricted. The number of diabetics in the U.S. is estimated to be about 10 million; many of these people may not even know they have the disease.[6] Although the types of cancer which may have a relationship with food intake are much less prevalent than is heart disease, they still are major causes of illness and death.

Fats and cholesterol Americans are advised by the American Heart Association and other groups to cut down on intake of calories, eggs (a major source of cholesterol), and fat to reduce the risk of developing cardiovascular disease. They are encouraged to use more polyunsaturated oils (most types of vegetable oil) than saturated fats (mainly animal fats). Some manufacturers reinforce these suggestions for diet change by promoting products as "high in polyunsaturates" or "low in cholesterol." Numerous cookbooks give directions for "cooking for a healthy heart." Women have been advised that reduction in their fat intake may also be helpful by decreasing the risk of cancer of the breast.

The scientific community is not in total agreement over the relationship of diet to the incidence of these diseases. Conflicting ideas about the value of dietary changes have been put forward by individuals and organizations. Americans are left scratching their heads, trying to decide if it is really worthwhile to give up the ice cream cones (high in animal fat and cholesterol) they enjoy so much.

Fiber Recently Americans have been told that if they increase their intake of fiber, it may save their lives. These are among the types of diet changes that have been suggested:

1. Follow a high roughage diet, substituting whole grain products and unprocessed or lightly processed fruits, vegetables, nuts, and seeds for all refined and highly processed foods such as sugar, white bread, peeled cooked fruits.

or

2. Supplement the usual highly processed American diet with unprocessed bran three times daily. Use an amount of bran which produces a daily (or more frequent) bowel movement which is large, formed, and easy to pass.

Food producers, particularly in the cereal industry, quickly latched on to the interest in fiber. Statements referring to food fiber now appear in advertisements and on cereal boxes. Sales of bran cereals have soared.

For those who think of bran as "so much sawdust," such advice is hard to swallow. They may be delighted when they learn that not all researchers agree. Still, the prospect of preventing the above-named diseases is attractive and Americans may again be troubled by controversy. Should they change their eating habits or not?

HOW CAN I LOSE WEIGHT AND THEN KEEP THE WEIGHT OFF?

A large percentage of Americans weigh more than they think they should. Many of these individuals are concerned primarily about their appearance. They recognize that a trim figure or physique may be necessary to achieve high social standing in America. Other individuals are concerned, with reason, about the health risks associated with the extra fat they carry. One result of this concern is the expenditure of large sums of money to deal with the problem of overweight.

Money is spent on exercise clubs, weight-reducing machines, pills, books, injections, and doctors. The money is often spent to no avail. If weight is lost, the "success" is usually followed by a return to the original or a higher weight. The noted nutritionist Jean Mayer describes this type of dieting as "the rhythm method of girth control."[7]

Despite the numerous "easy solutions" offered in magazines and books, excess weight is a growing health problem in America. The afflicted continue to look for easy answers. If they realize that there are only difficult solutions, they may ask if the benefits of weight loss are really worth the pain required to achieve it.

HOW CAN I GET MY FAMILY TO EAT RIGHT?

Changing lifestyles have diluted the influence that parents have on children. TV commercials, for example, may have considerable impact on children's attitudes toward certain foods. In the case of mothers working outside the home, the individual who is providing child care usually exerts a major influence on the child's developing food habits. Parents may dislike the eating behaviors their children learn but be unaware of methods of promoting desirable changes.

The concern over the eating habits of senior citizens is also related to changing lifestyle. The problem lies primarily with those who are living alone. Even if older persons have the financial resources to purchase a well-balanced diet, they often have little interest in cooking and eating by themselves. Limited facilities, mobility, energy, and fixed income compound the problem. The sons and daughters of these senior citizens may want to help but find that there are many obstacles to success.

HOW CAN WE HELP THE POOR TO OBTAIN THE FOOD THEY NEED?

The United States   The Ten State Nutrition Survey clearly showed that the poor have lower nutritional status than the rest of the population. There have been some improvements and changes in programs designed to assist the poor. Nevertheless, the poor remain at greater risk than the general population of developing nutritional deficiencies and certain other nutrition-related health problems. Americans are concerned for financial as well as for humanitarian reasons. They want the tax dollars that are spent for assistance programs to produce good results. They want to know what will *really* help.

The world   The growing concern about the poor and hungry has expanded to include the world population. The global food problem overwhelms our comprehen-

sion (Fig. 1.2). Jean Mayer estimates "it would seem reasonable to set the number of people *suffering* [our italics] from malnutrition at 400 million and to add to that another billion who would benefit from a more varied diet.[8]

The world map in Figure 1.3 indicates the prevalence of food deficits in developing countries. Forty-three nations have been designated as "food priority countries" by the United Nations because they have very low incomes, inadequate diets, and the expectation of continuing cereal-grain deficits. The consequences of the hunger which results from these food deficits is a global problem. Food becomes a political issue, an economic exchange medium, and a tool for international coercion. Sterling Wortman states that without economic development and social progress in the world "there can be no long-term assurance of increased well-being or of peace anywhere in the world."[9] Many Americans hope to ease world tensions by alleviating the hunger problem.

Not all of the foregoing questions have definitive answers. This text explores these issues and others in the course of discussing normal nutrition and methods of promoting it. It also presents much information regarding assisting persons to avoid or cope with nutritional problems associated with ill health.

(Text continues on p. 10.)

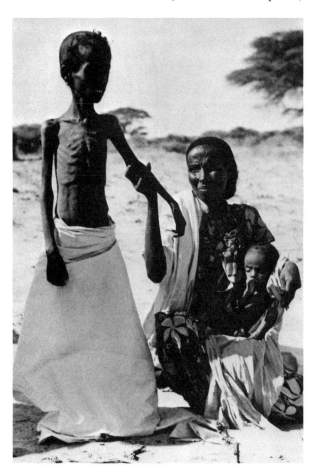

FIGURE 1.2. Successive years of drought have left thousands of nomadic people suffering from severe malnutrition, like the children of this Somalian woman. Courtesy WHO

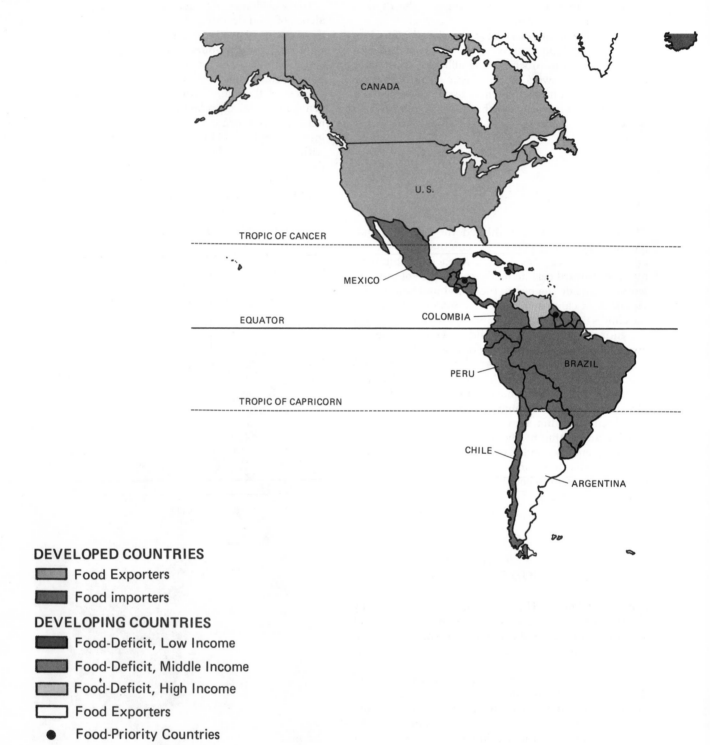

DEVELOPED COUNTRIES

Food Exporters

Food importers

DEVELOPING COUNTRIES

Food-Deficit, Low Income

Food-Deficit, Middle Income

Food-Deficit, High Income

Food Exporters

● Food-Priority Countries

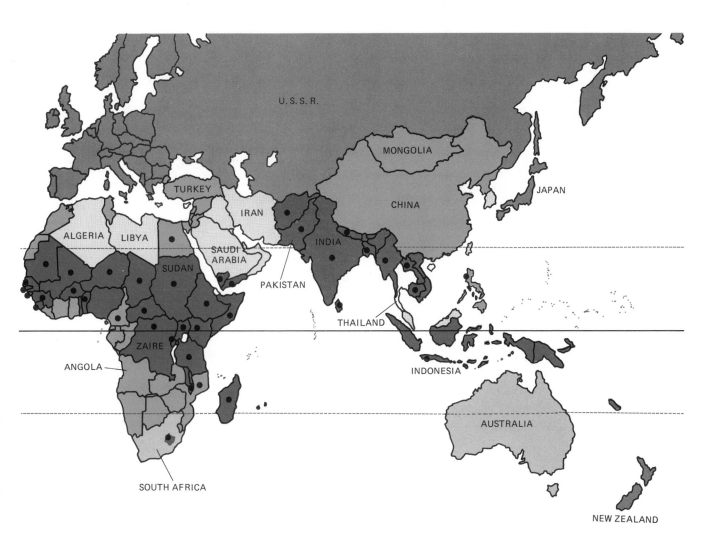

FIGURE 1.3. Impact of food deficits and poverty is concentrated in the broad band of developing nations, as is shown on this map based on categories established by the International Food Policy Research Institute (IFPRI). A few developed countries are major exporters of food; the rest have net food deficits but can pay to import food. Almost all developing countries have a food deficit and only those in the relatively high-income category have the foreign exchange with which to buy food without constraint. The United Nations has identified 43 "food-priority countries" (black disks) with especially low incomes, inadequate diets, and large projected cereal-grain deficits. (Used with permission from *Food and Agriculture* by Sterling Wortman. Copyright © 1976 by Scientific American, Inc. All rights reserved)

STUDY QUESTIONS

1. Use Table 1.1 to identify the category of nutrients to which each of the following belongs: pyridoxine, linoleic acid, lactose, lysine, manganese, folacin, chromium.
2. List several examples of ways in which food helps meet non-nutritive needs. (Use examples which are different from those given in the text.)
3. Visit a bookstore to find out what types of nutrition books are available and which, if any, are prominently displayed. From the titles, does it appear that the books deal with current nutritional concerns? Discuss.

References

1. The Overview Cluster. A general appraisal of the place of biomedical science in medicine: the Overview Cluster's observations. *Nutr. Today* 11(1):26, 1976.

2. Davis, A.: *Let's Eat Right to Keep Fit.* New York: Harcourt, Brace and World, Inc., 1954.

3. Highlights from the Ten-State Nutrition Survey. *Nutr. Today,* 7(4):4, 1972.

4. National Center for Health Statistics. *Dietary Intake Findings United States, 1971–1974.* DHEW Publ. No. (HRA) 77-1647. Washington DC: U.S. Govt. Printing Office, 1977.

5. *Heart Facts 1979.* Dallas TX: The American Heart Association, July 1978.

6. Public Inquiries and Reports Branch, OPEC, National Heart, Lung, and Blood Institute. *Fact Sheet, Diabetes and Cardiovascular Disease.* DHEW Publ. No. (NIH) 77-1212. Washington DC: U.S. Govt. Printing Office, 1977.

*7. Mayer, J.: *A Diet for Living.* New York: David McKay Co., 1975, p. 73.

8. Mayer, J.: The dimensions of human hunger. *Sci. Amer.* 235:40, 1976.

9. Wortman, S.: Food and agriculture. *Sci. Amer.* 235:39, 1976.

* Recommended reading.

2

Meeting nutrient needs by following a "Daily Food Guide"

Nutrient Needs of Family Members

Nutrients promote health by making possible the normal operation and maintenance of the body. No matter how different people are in size, appearance, activity, race, or age, they all need the *same* nutrients: protein, fat, carbohydrate, vitamins, minerals, and water. Calcium, for example, is a well-known mineral which is essential for the growth of bones and teeth, but it is needed even after growth is complete in order to keep the bones strong and to sustain life itself.

Family members may differ considerably in the *amount* of nutrients they need. Nutrient needs of healthy individuals vary for the following reasons:

1. Body size. The bigger the body, the more energy is required to move it and the more nutrients are required to repair and maintain it.
2. Physical activity. When two individuals of the same size and age are compared, the greater the level of physical activity the higher the energy requirement.
3. Growth. When growth spurts occur, nutrient requirements increase. Growth increases the need for structural materials such as protein and minerals, calories (since energy is needed to build body tissues), and nutrients which help to regulate body processes. If essential nutrients are not present in adequate amounts, growth cannot take place.
4. Substances lost from the body. Normal blood loss associated with menstruation results in loss of the mineral iron from the body. Therefore women need more iron than do men, despite the smaller size of women. Heavy perspiration increases the need for water and for certain minerals. Lactation (breast

feeding) increases the mother's need for most nutrients.
5. Metabolic rate. Chemical reactions occurring in the body (metabolism) can be speeded up (high metabolic rate) or slowed down (low metabolic rate) under certain circumstances. When the metabolic rate is increased, as when shivering in cold weather, there is increased need for specific nutrients and for energy. A low metabolic rate, as when sleeping, reduces certain nutrient requirements.
6. Age. Most of the effects of age are related to differences in the five characteristics listed above. The result of aging is primarily a tendency toward a decreasing requirement for calories throughout the adult years.

Since all of the preceding factors are acting at the same time in a given individual, a wide variation in total nutrient needs for each family member is possible. Fortunately there are some general concepts about nutrient needs and how these needs can be met which apply to most families.

1. The likelihood of meeting nutrient requirements is increased if a wide *variety* of foods that have undergone minimal processing* is used.
2. Nutrients known to be essential are available in food. For most individuals multivitamin preparations are of little, if any, benefit. Specific nutritional supplements may be recommended for healthy individuals in certain age groups and during pregnancy and lactation.
3. Infants and children require more nutrients per kilogram of body weight than do adults. In the case

* Foods which have undergone minimal processing are whole foods which have been washed, trimmed, and cooked only as necessary, such as cooked oatmeal, fresh fruit, baked potato, milk, broiled chicken.

of calcium and a few other nutrients, the total recommended intake for a child is actually *more* than that for the much larger adult. Since the total energy needs of children are usually smaller than those of adults, the foods children eat should be carefully chosen to provide optimal nutrient intake without exceeding energy requirements.

4. Women in the childbearing years have high iron requirements compared to the amount of iron in the typical diet. Pregnancy increases the need for iron even more. Women should be encouraged to select iron-rich or iron-fortified foods each day.

5. Pregnancy, a time of growth and increased body size, is a period when nutrient requirements sharply increase. Selection of adequate amounts of nutritious foods is of paramount importance to both the mother and the developing baby.

6. Senior citizens have about the same nutrient needs as do younger adults of comparable size, but their need for calories is usually less. Careful selection of food is desirable to assure adequate nutrient intake without excessive caloric intake.

Desirable characteristics of diets

There are a number of points to consider when planning diets for optimal nutrition:

1. If the diet is to promote health, it must provide all essential nutrients in adequate amounts for daily needs. The amounts of nutrients which should allow *healthy* Americans to achieve their full growth and health potential are set forth in a nutrient guide called Recommended Dietary Allowances (RDA) (see inside back cover). Actually the RDA was intended as a guide for groups of healthy persons rather than for individual application. The RDA is not the same as minimum requirements. Instead it incorporates a fairly generous safety margin to cover individual differences and normal stresses of daily living. Not all essential nutrients are listed in the Recommended Dietary Allowances. It is *assumed* that if the listed nutrients are provided in recommended amounts by a *varied* diet, the other

TABLE 2.1 *Guide to good eating—a recommended daily pattern**

FOOD GROUP	RECOMMENDED NUMBER OF SERVINGS†				
	CHILD	TEENAGER	ADULT	PREGNANT WOMAN	LACTATING WOMAN

MILK
1 cup milk, yogurt, OR
Calcium Equivalent:
  1½ slices (1½ oz) cheddar
    cheese‡
  1 cup pudding
  1¾ cups ice cream
  2 cups cottage cheese‡
	3	4	2	4	4

MEAT
2 ounces cooked, lean meat,
fish, poultry, OR
Protein Equivalent:
  2 eggs
  2 slices (2 oz) cheddar
    cheese‡
  1 cup dried beans, peas
  4 tbsp peanut butter
	2	2	2	3	2

FRUIT-VEGETABLE
  ½ cup cooked or juice
  1 cup raw
  Portion commonly served
  such as a medium-size
  apple or banana
	4	4	4	4	4

GRAIN, whole grain,
fortified, enriched
  1 slice bread
  1 cup ready-to-eat cereal
  ½ cup cooked cereal,
  pasta, grits
	4	4	4	4	4

Courtesy of National Dairy Council, Rosemont IL 60018. Copyright © 1977. All rights reserved.
* The recommended daily pattern provides the foundation for a nutritious, healthful diet.
† The recommended servings from the Four Food Groups for adults supply about 1200 Calories. The chart above gives recommendations for the number and size of servings for several categories of people.
‡ Count cheese as serving of milk OR meat, not both simultaneously.
"Others" complement but do not replace foods from the Four Food Groups. Amounts should be determined by individual caloric needs.

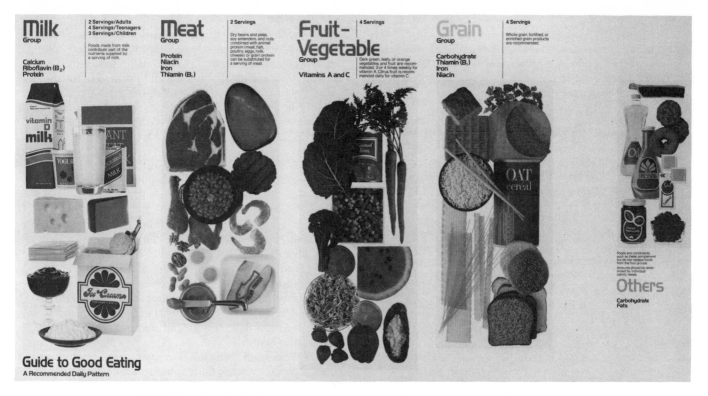

Guide to Good Eating
A Recommended Daily Pattern

FIGURE 2.1. A Guide to Good Eating. Foods in the milk group are pictured in descending order of calcium content (best sources of calcium are at the top.) Foods in the meat and grain groups are shown in descending order of iron content. (Differences in iron content of grains depend mainly on levels of fortification.) Fruits and vegetables are arranged in descending order of vitamin A value (carotene content). "Others" are low in vitamins, minerals, and proteins. "Others" should not take the place of foods in the Four Food groups. (Courtesy of National Dairy Council)

essential nutrients will also be present in adequate amounts.

2. Diets should provide enough fuel (calories) to meet the energy needs of the body. An excess or an inadequate intake of fuel can have adverse physiological and psychological effects.

3. The diet should include some foods which are good sources of fiber (the cell walls of plants). Although fiber is not considered to be a nutrient because it is not absorbed into the body, it provides the bulk which stimulates normal elimination of fecal material. Fiber also promotes a sense of satiety (feeling of being satisfied) when moderate amounts of food are eaten.

4. The diet should promote health and prevent disposing the individual to disease at any stage of life.

5. The diet must be one acceptable to the individual (family). Fortunately well-balanced diets can be planned with many kinds and combinations of foods. There is not any one food which is essential to sound nutrition.

6. A diet pattern can be chosen which is compatible with optimum performance of activities of daily living—one which avoids sluggishness from overeating as well as irritability and reduced efficiency due to lack of fuel foods (a common consequence of skipping breakfast).

The health professional should remember that when people eat, their major interest is in food, not nutrients or health. A simple guide which directs attention to making wise food selections for good tasting meals from a wide variety of choices can be a useful tool in promoting sound nutrition.

A DAILY FOOD GUIDE— THE BASIC FOUR

A food guide with the purpose of promoting good nutrition has been developed by the United States Department of Agriculture (USDA). The "Daily Food Guide" was designed to provide a flexible framework or foundation for making food selections to meet the nutrient needs specified in the Recommended Dietary Allowances. The National Dairy Council has developed a popular version called a "Guide to Good Eating" (Fig. 2.1). To help adapt the guide for differing needs of family members, some adjustments are indicated for portion sizes and/or number of portions recommended each day (Table 2.1).

The Daily Food Guide is intended to be easy to use, easy to remember, and adaptable—to increase the chance that sound nutrition can be achieved by all Americans. The guide does not name specific foods which should be eaten. Instead it combines foods which make similar nutritional contributions into four large groups: grain, fruit and vegetable, meat, and milk. It is obvious why the Daily Food Guide is frequently called the Basic Four.

To use the food guide effectively, an individual is encouraged to choose foods he likes and can afford from each group. The suggested number of servings from each food group is based on age range and the special needs of pregnancy and lactation.

POINTS OF EMPHASIS
A daily food guide

• The guide (A Guide to Good Eating) does not *apply* to infant feeding.
• Each food group makes an important, distinctive nutritional contribution.
• Each food group lacks at least one essential nutrient.
• No one food or food group, taken alone, provides adequate amounts of all of the essential nutrients.
• There is no one food which is essential to good nutrition.
• Use of a variety of foods from each group helps assure desirable intake of nutrients.

The types of foods included in each food group are summarized in Table 2.1 along with portion sizes and recommended number of servings per day. It is beneficial for health professionals to be able to correctly classify foods and to identify significant nutrient contributions of each food group. It is also helpful to be able to distinguish foods within a group which differ markedly in nutrient content from other foods in the same group.

GRAINS

In the U.S. the grain group is often underrated as a source of nutrients. Use of foods from this group has been steadily declining, with the common complaint that starchy foods are "fattening." Actually breads, cereals, and other forms of grain are lower in calories than are many of the foods which have replaced them, such as meat. Grains are also a dependable source of certain vitamins, minerals, and protein. For most of the world's population the grain group makes up the bulk of the diet and is an indispensable source of nutrients.

All grain products are included in this group if they are whole grain or if they are made from refined grains which have been enriched or fortified. Examples of foods in this group include brown rice, oatmeal, enriched spaghetti, rye bread, enriched cornmeal,* and enriched farina. (The label of the product must indicate if it is enriched or fortified, except in the case of locally produced items such as those found in bakery shops.) Although the Daily Food Guide does not distin-

---

* Corn which has been dried and ground into a meal or flour is included in the grain group, whereas fresh, frozen, and canned corn is usually classed as a vegetable.

---

guish between whole grain products and refined products to which nutrients have been added, differences exist which may have some relationship to health. The health professional should be well informed of the differences and similarities since this is an issue about which the public tends to be confused.

Whole grains of any type have three parts which differ in their food value. These parts, shown in Table 2.2, are the germ, endosperm, and bran. Refining grain removes most of the germ and bran and therefore the nutrients and other substances which those parts contain. Nutritional changes resulting from this separation are summarized in Table 2.2. The FDA has set standards for the enrichment of flour, farina, and cornmeal, which are reflected in this Table. The only nutrients added in enrichment are iron, thiamine, riboflavin, and niacin. The enrichment program has practically eliminated the deficiency diseases which used to be common because of inadequate intake of these three B complex vitamins. From this standpoint the enrichment program has been judged successful in promoting public health.

It is clear from Table 2.2, however, that enrichment does not make refined flour equal to whole wheat flour in nutritive value, except in its content of iron and the three B vitamins. For example, whole grain products always provide more of many essential *trace minerals* than do enriched products. Grain products never provide any vitamin A, C, D, or B_{12} unless these nutrients have been added during fortification. The fiber content of whole grains is also much higher than that of refined grain products. Nevertheless, many consumers prefer refined grains because of their flavor, texture, and cooking properties.

Fortified cereal products contain much higher amounts of certain nutrients than do enriched or whole grain cereals and therefore may appear to be the best choice from a nutritional point of view. However, very high amounts of nutrients are not necessarily valuable. Intake of many of the vitamins and minerals in excess of need results in their increased excretion and therefore does not benefit healthy people.

At least 4 servings daily from the grain group are recommended. Four servings provide only about 10 to 20 percent of the calories needed in a day.

FRUIT AND VEGETABLE GROUP

The fruit and vegetable group is sometimes considered to be a group of "protective foods" since it is a good source of many vitamins and minerals. In general, this group can be depended upon to provide fiber, minerals, vitamins A, C, E, and K, and B complex vitamins with the exception of vitamin B_{12}. (Vitamin B_{12} is found only in animal products.)

The fruit and vegetable group is the *only* food group which ordinarily provides significant amounts of vitamin C (ascorbic acid). Since this vitamin is essential for maintaining normal connective tissue and for

TABLE 2.2 *Selected nutrient content of whole and separated grain products per 100 gm*

Whole grain. May be eaten as is (e.g., brown rice) or may be flaked into whole grain cereal (e.g., oatmeal) or ground into whole grain cereal or flour

Endosperm. (Refined white grains contain little else) Mainly starch and protein.

Germ. High in vitamin E, many B vitamins, minerals, protein; a source of poly-unsaturated fat

Bran. High in fiber, many B vitamins, minerals

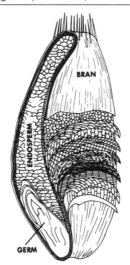

	WHOLE WHEAT FLOUR	UNENRICHED REFINED FLOUR	ENRICHED REFINED FLOUR	WHEAT GERM, CRUDE	BRAN, CRUDE
Starch (gm)	69	76	76	44	53
Protein (gm)	13	11	11	27	16
Fiber (gm)	2	—	—	3	9
B vitamins					
Thiamin (mg)	0.55	0.06	0.44*	2.01	0.72
Riboflavin (mg)	0.12	0.05	0.26*	0.68	0.35
Niacin (mg)	4.3	0.9	3.5*	4.2	21
Pyridoxine (μg)	340	60	60	1150	?
Folacin (total) (μg)	54	21	21	328	258
Minerals					
Iron (mg)	3.3	0.8	2.9*	9.4	14.9
Magnesium (mg)	183	28	28	268	490
Potassium (mg)	370	95	95	827	1120
Zinc (mg)	2.4	0.7	0.7	14.3	9.8

* Based on minimum levels of enrichment

Values for grains taken from the following sources:
Watt, B. K., and Merrill, A. L.: *Composition of Foods Raw, Processed, Prepared.* Agriculture Research Service. Agriculture Handbook No. 8. Washington DC: Superintendent of Documents, rev. 1963.
Schroeder, H. A.: Losses of vitamins and trace minerals resulting from processing and preservation of foods. *Am. J. Clin. Nutr.* 24:562, 1971.
Murphy, E. W., Willis, B. W., and Watt, B. K.: Provisional tables on the zinc content of foods. *J. Am. Diet. Assoc.* 66:345, 1975.
Perloff, B. P., and Butrum, R. R.: Folacin in selected foods. *J. Am. Diet. Assoc.* 70:161, 1977.
Orr, M. L.: Pantothenic acid, vitamin B-6 and vitamin B-12 in foods.'' Home Economics Research Report No. 36. ARS, USDA, Washington DC, 1969.

wound healing, dietary planning should not overlook it. Fruits and vegetables vary greatly in their content of vitamin C. Use of one excellent or two good sources of ascorbic acid daily assures intake of the recommended amount of vitamin C. Orange and grapefruit, both citrus fruits, are outstanding as sources of vitamin C. Just 120 ml. (½ c.) of either of these juices provides three-fourths of the RDA of vitamin C for adults. Cabbage and potatoes, if prepared in a manner which retains nutrients, are examples of good sources of vitamin C. Table 2.3 indicates several selections which would result in a comparable intake of ascorbic acid. Since some individuals choose to exclude citrus fruits from the diet, the health professional should be able to recommend suitable alternatives.

A limited number of fruits and vegetables are outstanding sources of vitamin A. They do not actually contain vitamin A itself but, rather, the substance *caro-tene* which can be converted to vitamin A by the body. Thus carotene is a *precursor* of vitamin A and has vitamin A value. Vitamin A is essential for a wide variety of body processes, including formation of normal epithelial tissue (skin and mucous membranes). The best plant sources of vitamin A are dark-green leafy vegetables, such as spinach and kale, and bright orange vegetables, such as winter squash and carrots. A few of the orange colored fruits—namely cantaloupe, apricots, papaya, and persimmon—are good sources. All light-colored vegetables, such as iceberg lettuce (commonly used in salads), are poor sources of vitamin A. Green beans, peas, corn, and oranges are quite low in vitamin A, despite their bright color. Table 2.4 illustrates the wide range of vitamin A value of selected fruits and vegetables. Use of an *excellent* source of vitamin A at least every other day or a good source each day helps provide for adequate intake of this nutrient.

TABLE 2.3 *Examples of foods and food combinations providing about 45 mg vitamin C (three-fourths of the RDA for adults)*

FOOD	PORTION SIZE	ASCORBIC ACID CONTENT MG
Orange	1 small (100 gm)	50
Strawberries	7 to 8 large (75 gm)	45
Cauliflower	180 ml (60 gm or ¾ c)	45
Green pepper, cooked	½ (50 gm)	48 (higher if raw)
Mustard greens, cooked	120 ml (100 gm or ½ c)	48
Combinations:		
Tomato juice, canned	120 ml (½ c)	16 ⎫
Leaf lettuce	100 gm	19 ⎬ 45
Banana	1 small (100 gm)	10 ⎭
Potato, mashed	120 ml (½ c)	9 ⎫
Apple, raw	1 small (100 gm)	4 ⎪
Carrot, raw	1 large	8 ⎬ 45
Pear, raw	1 7.6 cm x 6.4 cm (200 gm or 3 x 2½″)	8 ⎪
Peas, frozen	100 gm	13 ⎪
Mushrooms, raw	4 large (100 gm)	3 ⎭

Source: Church, C. F., and Church, H. N.: *Food Values of Portions Commonly Used*, ed. 12. Philadelphia: J. B. Lippincott Co., 1975.

There is no need to be concerned about the "other" day, since vitamin A is stored in the liver.

A few vegetables and fruits are reliable sources of both vitamins A and C. They include broccoli, cantaloupe, and papaya.

The contribution fruits and vegetables make to the intake of minerals and of vitamins other than A and C should not be overlooked. For this reason powdered instant breakfast drinks and fruit drinks (about 10 percent fruit juice with added water, sugar, and vitamin C) are not nutritionally sound substitutes for fruit juice. Fruits and vegetables provide folic acid (a B complex vitamin) and trace elements including iron. Folic acid and iron are especially important nutrients to consider because many Americans have low or marginal intakes of them compared to recommended

TABLE 2.4 *Vitamin A value of 100 gm portions of selected fruits and vegetables*

FOOD	PORTION SIZE	VITAMIN A IN I.U. PER 100 GM PORTION
*ABOUT TWO TIMES THE RDA FOR AN ADULT**		
Carrots, cooked, drained	180 ml (¾ c)	10,500
Sweet potato, baked	1 small	8,100
Spinach, frozen	120 ml (½ c)	7,900
ABOUT ONE HALF TO ONE TIMES THE RDA FOR AN ADULT		
Winter squash, cooked	120 ml (½ c)	3,700
Cantaloupe (bright orange variety)	¼ melon, 127 cm (5″) diameter	3,400
Apricots, raw	2 to 3 medium	2,710
Broccoli	1 stalk, 13 cm (5½″) long	2,500
10 TO 25 PERCENT OF THE RDA		
Iceberg lettuce	1/5 head	970
Tomato fresh	1 small	900
Peas, frozen cooked	160 ml (⅔ c)	600
Green beans, fresh cooked	180 ml	540
Watermelon	120 ml (½ c) much smaller than the usual portion	590
Corn on the cob, yellow variety, cooked	10.2 cm (4″) long ear	400
LESS THAN 7 PERCENT OF THE RDA		
Celery, green varieties	2 large outer stalks	270
Orange, 1 small	1 small	200
Apple, raw	1 small, 5 cm (2″) diameter	90

Source: Church, C. F., and Church, H. N.: *Food Values of Portions Commonly Used*, ed. 12. Philadelphia: J. B. Lippincott Co., 1975.
* RDA is 5000 IU for an adult male, 4000 IU for an adult female.

levels. Four or more servings per day from the fruit and vegetable group provide a significant fraction of the daily need for many micronutrients. All of the foods in this group provide some calories, but many, vegetables in particular, are low in energy value. Except for avocados and olives, all fresh fruits and vegetables are very low in fat.

POINTS OF EMPHASIS
Choice of fruits and vegetables

• *Have a total of at least four servings daily, using a variety of types.*
• *Choose at least one excellent or two good sources of vitamin C daily.*
• *Choose at least one excellent source of vitamin A every other day or a good source daily.*
• *Choose real fruits and vegetables to get the benefits of a wide variety of nutrients and of fiber.*

MILK GROUP

The milk group provides a large proportion of the daily need for many but not all of the nutrients. Milk and cheese products are significant sources of calcium, phosphorus, protein, riboflavin, and vitamin A. Vitamin B_{12} and a number of other vitamins and minerals are also present in milk. *Fortified* milk products are important dietary sources of vitamin D, the vitamin which promotes absorption and utilization of calcium. Many of the substitutions for milk, such as cheese and yogurt, do *not* provide vitamin D in significant amounts. Milk is definitely *not* a perfect food. In particular, all foods in the milk group are exceedingly *low* in vitamin C, iron, and copper.

The milk group excludes certain dairy products, namely butter and cream, because these high fat foods are low in most of the nutrients the milk group is supposed to provide. It should be noted that eggs are *not* included in the milk group. In order for eggs to be a good source of calcium, the shells would have to be eaten!

The recommended number of servings is given in terms of milliliters (cups) of fluid milk. Other milk products, such as cottage cheese, nonfat dry milk powder, evaporated milk, and ice cream may be used to replace part of the milk. If this is done, attention should be given to the serving size that is equivalent to 240 ml. (1 c.) of milk (Table 2.1). These substitutions are based primarily on calcium content since the milk group is the principal dietary source of this mineral.

Milk used in cooking can provide a large portion of the recommended milk intake. Cream soup, for example, is usually half milk by volume, and the total volume of milk-based puddings can be counted as milk. The recommended number of servings from the milk group varies with age groups, pregnancy, and lactation. The recommendation for adults is 500 ml. (2 c.) daily.

MEAT GROUP

The meat group is an excellent source of protein, B complex vitamins, and most minerals. It differs in nutritional value from the milk group in that it is a very important source of iron but provides very little calcium.

The meat group includes both animal and plant foods. The flesh foods (beef, pork, veal, poultry, fish, shellfish) are the most obvious members of this group. Other animal products such as eggs and organ meats (liver, kidney, heart, tripe, sweetbreads and brains) are also included. The plant foods belonging to the meat group are all high in protein. Examples include dried peas and beans, lentils, and nuts. All types of *dried* beans (kidney, pea, pinto, soy, black, fava, lima) and *dried* peas (split peas and garbanzos or chick peas) are called *legumes*. Peanuts are actually legumes, not nuts. New high protein meat substitutes which resemble meat in appearance, taste, and protein content are on the market. These products are made from soybeans and/or wheat protein. They are called meat analogs or textured vegetable protein (TVP). The most familiar example is imitation bacon bits. Textured vegetable protein, lentils, or any of the legumes can be used as alternatives to meat—a common practice in children's lunches with the popular peanut butter sandwich. Nuts are somewhat less valuable than other meat alternates because nuts are extremely high in calories owing to their high fat content.

High protein plant foods should be distinguished nutritionally from animal products in the meat group. Plant foods contain *no* vitamin B_{12} whereas all of the animal products in this group are good sources of this essential vitamin. The protein in plant foods is of lower quality than that in animal foods, but serves its purpose well when combined with other protein sources. Legumes, lentils, and nuts provide cellulose and other fibers; animal foods do not. Legumes are a fair source of calcium. Most legumes and lentils provide less fat than meat does, while nuts are exceedingly high in fat.

Cheese was purposely not listed in the meat group because of its very low iron content. It can be used in place of meat as a source of protein (as in macaroni and cheese), but this results in a lower iron intake.

"OTHER" FOODS

A large number of available foods do not belong in any of the four food groups. These foods have sugar, fat, starch, and/or unenriched refined cereal products as their principal ingredients. Examples include butter and margarine, salad dressing, vegetable oil and shortening, jelly, carbonated beverages, gelatin desserts, candy, bacon, and salt pork. Because the main nutritional contribution of most of these foods is fuel (calories), they are commonly described as high in "empty calories." However butter and margarine are good sources of vitamin A, and oils are good sources of vitamin E. Some sweets, such as molasses and fig bars, provide significant amounts of some nutrients but at a high calorie cost.

"Other" foods are commonly regarded as desirable for reasons of palatability. The Daily Food Guide recommends that vegetable oil be used as part of the fat. Alcoholic beverages are grouped with "other" foods because they are high in calorie value but contribute few, if any, essential nutrients.

Use of the Daily Food Guide

The Daily Food Guide places emphasis on choosing a variety of foods from each food group, using at least the recommended number of servings of the specified size. An optimum number of meals is not indicated by the guide, although consumption of a "good breakfast" is urged in the government publication *Family Fare,*[1] a booklet explaining the Daily Food Guide. The "bonus of breakfast" is described as increased alertness and productivity in the morning and decreased fatigue during the day. *Family Fare* suggests including a high protein food (such as milk, meat, or eggs) with each meal. Other suggestions in the booklet involve palatability factors.

COMPARISON WITH CANADA'S FOOD GUIDE

Many nations have food guides similar to the guide developed by the USDA. Differences in attitude regarding recommended nutrient intake, differences in activity of the population involved, and differences in the food supply account for some of the variations in food guides.

Canada's Food Guide differs from the U.S. Daily Food Guide in the following ways:

1. Fruits and vegetables are grouped together, but it is specified that *at least two* of the 4 to 5 servings should be *vegetables.*
2. A *range* of 3 to 5 servings from the bread and cereal group is indicated. *Whole grain products* are recommended.
3. *Variety* is stressed, "Eat a variety of foods from each group every day."
4. Supplementation with vitamin D is specifically recommended for people who consume nonfortified milk products (or no milk at all).

Nutrition educators in the U.S. tend to emphasize these same points.

Recognizing that there are differences in food guides for similar nations, health professionals would do well to maintain flexibility when using any guide as a teaching tool.[2]

Limitations of the Daily Food Guide

The Daily Food Guide can be a useful tool in meal planning, but it does have a number of drawbacks of which the health professional should be aware. Many of the drawbacks are common to any food guide.

DIFFICULTY IN CLASSIFYING COMMONLY USED FOODS

A food guide should show a reasonable degree of conformity to customary ways of meeting nutrient needs.[3] With the rising use of convenience and take-out foods, discrepancies between the Daily Food Guide and typical eating patterns of Americans are growing. Consumers may be under the impression that popular foods are not nutritious since they do not clearly fit into a food group. Attempts to use the Basic Four Food Groups in meal planning may be abandoned when many convenience foods are used. If they do try to use the food guide, consumers may ask if potato chips can be counted as a serving of vegetable or if a shake from a fast food chain can be counted as a serving from the milk group. How, they ask, is a slice of pizza classified? The cheese rather obviously fits in the milk group, but is the crust enriched and is there enough tomato to count as a vegetable serving? Specific information about the nutritional value of foods is needed to answer questions like these. This information is obtainable from tables of food composition such as in Appendix 3C and from nutritional labeling when it is used on food products.

INAPPROPRIATE SUBSTITUTIONS

The Daily Food Guide states that all enriched or whole grain baked goods can be counted in the bread and cereal group. Cookies made with enriched flour could then be considered to be the nutritional equivalent of bread. No consideration is given to portion sizes which would be equivalent or to disadvantages of this type of substitution, such as likelihood of excessive caloric intake. The Guide to Good Eating places desserts made with grains in the "Other" group.

LACK OF ADAPTATION FOR INDIVIDUAL DIFFERENCES

The Daily Food Guide in its simple form does not clearly identify desirable adaptations, other than those in the milk group, for providing the nutrient needs of differing age groups, pregnancy, and lactation. Additional guidance is desirable, such as that provided in Chapters 7 through 9.

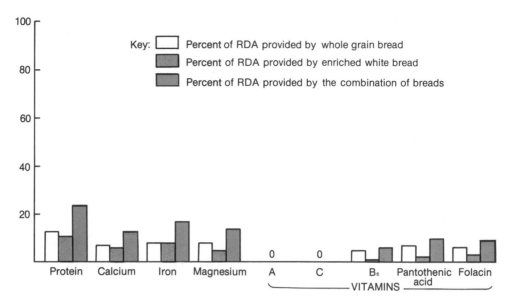

FIGURE 2.2. Percent of the RDA for an adult female provided by 4 servings from the grain group (specifically, 2 slices whole wheat bread and 2 slices enriched white bread). (Values for Figures 2.2, 2.3, 2.5, and 2.6 taken from the following sources:

Adams, C. F.: *Nutritive Value of American Foods.* Agriculture Research Service, USDA, Agriculture Handbook No. 456. Washington DC, 1975.

Pennington, J. A.: *Dietary Nutrient Guide.* Westport CT: Avi Publishing Co., 1976.

Perloff, B. P., and Butrum, R. R.: Folacin in selected foods. *J. Am. Diet. Assoc.* 70:161, 1977)

LACK OF ATTENTION TO CALORIES

Consumers in this country are very apt to be concerned about the caloric value of foods. The Daily Food Guide by itself provides no helpful information related to this concern. Most consumers are unaware that the Basic Four recommendations can be used as the foundation for a sound reducing diet. They may not realize that foods within a given food group can vary markedly in energy value. Indeed the guide does not even urge achievement and maintenance of ideal body weight.

INADEQUACY WITH RESPECT TO SELECTED NUTRIENTS

Another limitation of the Daily Food Guide is related to its effectiveness in planning for recommended nutrient intake. The standard guide (Fig. 2.1) provides for meeting Recommended Dietary Allowances of most but not all nutrients. However, since the RDA includes a generous margin of safety for most healthy individuals, consuming less than the RDA does not neces-

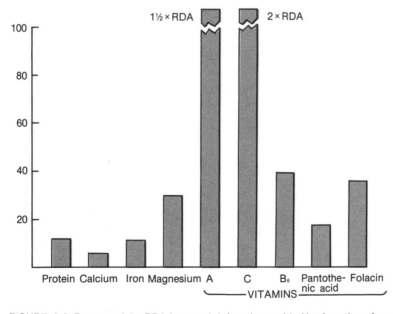

FIGURE 2.3. Percent of the RDA for an adult female provided by 4 servings from the fruit and vegetable group (specifically, 120 ml. orange juice, 150 gm. [1 medium] baked potato, 81 gm. [1 small] raw carrot, and 150 gm. [1 medium banana]. Based on 1974 RDA.

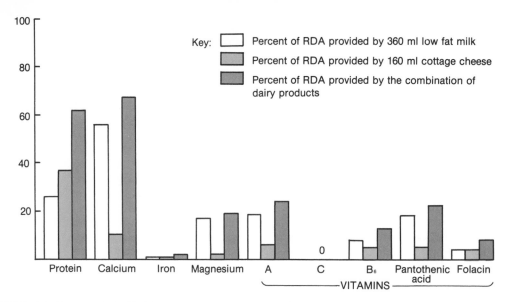

FIGURE 2.4. Percent of the RDA for an adult female provided by 2 servings from the milk group (specifically, 360 ml. [1½ c.] low fat milk and 160 m. [⅔ c.] cottage cheese). (Values for Fig. 2.4 taken from: Consumer and Food Economics Institute. *Composition of Foods, Dairy and Egg Products, Raw, Processed, Prepared.* Agriculture Research Service, USDA. Agriculture Handbook No. 8-1. Washington DC, Rev. 1976)

sarily mean that a person will develop a nutritional deficiency.

Figures 2.2 through 2.6 show the *approximate* percent of the RDA for an adult female* that is provided by the suggested number of servings from each of the four food groups, using specified foods. The individual contribution of each food is also indicated. These

tables show that foods within each food group vary in nutritive value and that each of the four food groups makes important contributions to overall nutrient intake.

Most of the nutrients included in the graphs in Figures 2.2 to 2.6 are those identified by Pennington[4] as being the best indicators of overall adequacy of a diet: calcium, iron, magnesium, and vitamins A, B_6, pantothenic acid, and folacin. She refers to these seven nutrients as *index nutrients*. Protein and vitamin C were added to the graphs because of widespread consumer interest in those nutrients.

* An adult female is used for reference because she requires more iron than does a male and because her caloric requirement and food intake are apt to be less than those of a male.

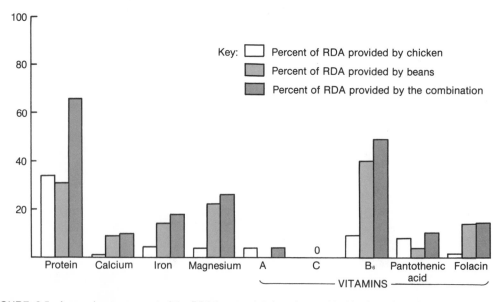

FIGURE 2.5. Approximate percent of the RDA for an adult female provided by 2 servings from the meat group (specifically, 60 gm. [2 oz.] dark chicken meat and 240 ml. [1 c.] cooked kidney beans). *Note:* amount of iron would be higher if red meat had been used instead of poultry, lower if fish had been used. Bioavailability of iron is much higher in chicken than in beans.

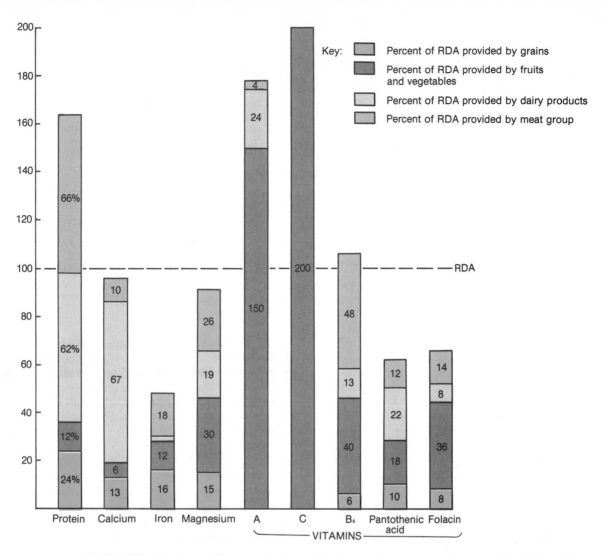

FIGURE 2.6. Selected nutritive contributions of the four basic food groups. Percent of the RDA which is contributed by meeting Basic Four guidelines for an adult female, using the following foods: 2 slices whole wheat bread, 2 slices enriched white bread, 120 ml. orange juice, 1 small carrot, 1 medium potato, 1 medium banana, 360 ml. low-fat milk, 160 ml. cottage cheese, 60 gm. chicken dark meat, and 240 ml. cooked kidney beans. Based on 1974 RDA.

TABLE 2.5 *Iron content of selected foods*

FOOD	PORTION SIZE	IRON CONTENT IN MG	
Liver, beef, fried	85 gm (3 oz)	7.5	⎫ 30–60% of the RDA for
Oysters, raw	120 gm (½ c)	6.6	⎬ a female in the
Beans, white mature, cooked	240 ml (1 c)	5.4*	⎭ childbearing years
Beef, hamburger, cooked	85 gm (3 oz)	2.7	⎫
Pork, roast, medium fat	85 gm (3 oz)	2.5	⎬
Wheat germ, crude	30 gm (1 oz)	2.6*	
Liverwurst	30 gm (1 slice)	1.6	⎬ 8–15% of the RDA
Spinach, frozen cooked	85 gm (½ c)	1.8*	
Lamb, roast, cooked	85 gm (3 oz)	1.5	⎭
Chicken, fried, including skin	85 gm (3 oz)	1.5	

30 gm raisins,* 1 egg,* 60 gm peanut butter,* 20 gm (1 Tbsp) molasses,* and 85 gm fish each provide about 6 to 7% of the RDA for an adult woman. These and many other foods make important contributions to daily iron intake.

Source: Pennington, J. A.: *Dietary Nutrient Guide.* Westport CT: Avi Publishing Co., 1976.
* Bioavailability of iron in these foods is lower than it is for meats, fish, poultry.

TABLE 2.6 *A few good food sources of folacin*

FOOD	PORTION SIZE	MG FOLACIN	
Brewer's yeast	8 gm (1 Tbsp.)	313	50–75% of RDA for adult male or female
Chicken liver	85 gm (3 oz)	204	
Toasted wheat germ	28 gm (1 oz)	118	
Romaine	240 ml (1 c)	98	20–30% of RDA for adult male or female
Cantaloupe	½	82	
Spinach	90 gm	82	
Orange juice, frozen, reconstituted	120 ml (½ c)	68	
Red kidney beans, cooked	240 ml (1 c)	68	
Beets	120 ml (½ c)	67	11–17% of RDA for adult male or female
Avocado	½	59	
Tomato	1 medium	59	
Broccoli, cooked	90 gm	50	
Asparagus	120 ml (½ c)	43	

Source: Perloff, B. P., and Butrum, R. R.: Folacin in selected foods. *J. Am. Diet. Assoc.* 70:161, 1977.

Since women in the childbearing years commonly consume less than recommended amounts of iron, it is desirable for them to include a number of iron-rich foods in their daily diet and/or use some iron-fortified foods. Consuming a source of vitamin C with a meal promotes absorption of iron. A few foods which are good sources of iron are listed in Table 2.5.

Careful food selection helps assure adequate intake of folic acid. A few good sources are listed in Table 2.6. Unfortunately many of the best sources of folic acid (liver, kidney, yeast, wheat germ) are often considered to be unappetizing. Therefore it is helpful to promote increased use of more popular foods which are fair to good sources of this vitamin. Orange juice, bananas, green beans, salad greens, and whole grains are in this category.

Eating a variety of lightly processed foods helps to assure adequate intake of almost all of the essential micronutrients. However special attention should be directed to intake of vitamin D, iodine, and fluoride and to the non-nutritive substance called fiber.

Vitamin D The recommended intake of 400 IU for children and pregnant and lactating women will not necessarily be met by following the guide. Adequate exposure to sunshine could provide the vitamin D requirement.[4]

Iodine The iodine content of food varies greatly. The *average* amount of iodine in the food supply is many times the RDA, largely because much of the milk and bread produced is high in iodine. Nevertheless, in some regions of the U.S., diets planned according to the Basic Four may be deficient in iodine. There is at present no practical way to tell. Iodine is essential for normal functioning of the thyroid gland and prevention of the deficiency disease called goiter (Fig. 2.7). Therefore, in goitrous regions, use of iodized salt (ordinary table salt to which a small amount of potassium iodide has been added by the manufacturer) is recommended. In nongoitrous regions there is no need for iodized salt.[5]

Fluoride The diet does not provide children with recommended levels of fluoride unless the water supply contains the proper amount, either naturally or by fluoridation. This mineral has only recently been recognized as a dietary essential, although its beneficial effects in strengthening of tooth enamel have been known for many years.

Fiber It is possible to follow Basic Four recommendations and select a diet which is very low in fiber or even essentially fiber-free. An increased intake of fiber

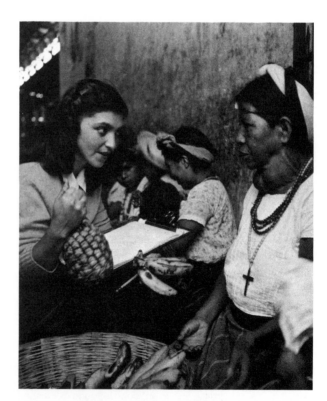

FIGURE 2.7. INCAP nurse visits the local market at Amatitlan to study prices. The villager with the swollen neck is suffering from goiter, a nutrition-deficiency disease that affects millions of people in the Americas. Courtesy WHO

rich foods daily (such as whole grains and raw fruits and vegetables) might greatly reduce use of laxatives and other aids for the elimination of fecal wastes.

> **POINTS OF EMPHASIS**
> *Suggestions for supplementing a "daily food guide"*
>
> • *Women and children can meet recommended intake of iron by including several iron-rich foods or an iron-fortified food in the daily diet.*
> • *Rounding out meals by using some extra servings from the four food groups (rather than "other" foods) helps meet nutrient needs.*
> • *Children and pregnant and lactating women should ingest 400 IU vitamin D from fortified milk or from a vitamin D supplement, especially if they have little exposure to sunshine.*
> • *Individuals living in goitrous regions should substitute iodized salt for plain salt.*
> • *Children under 12 to 18 years of age benefit from fluoride in their drinking water or as a supplement.*
> • *Use of some whole grains and raw fruits and vegetables provides fiber.*

A NUTRIENT APPROACH

Many nutritionists suggest a "nutrient approach" to meal planning and nutrition education.[6-8] The emphasis is on choosing foods because they are good sources of nutrients needed for health. To use this approach the individual needs to know the nutrient content of foods and how much of each nutrient is needed daily. To keep the approach relatively simple, attention may be focused on a few key nutrients—ones which have been found to be lacking in the diets of significant numbers of Americans. Vitamins A and C and the minerals calcium and iron are often singled out as key nutrients. However, Pennington has documented why the *seven* index nutrients previously named should all be considered in meal planning.[4]

Supporters of the nutrient approach suggest that it allows greater flexibility in food selection while assuring adequate nutritional value. Health professionals should be aware of possible limitations of the nutrient approach:

1. Some consumers require much detailed teaching before they can effectively use a nutrient approach. Many are unreceptive if arithmetic is involved.
2. Concentration on just a few nutrients may be insufficient for meeting all nutrient needs, especially if many highly processed and fortified foods are being used. Directing attention to intake of one specific nutrient at a time can lead to imbalances.

Although the nutrient approach is not emphasized in this text to the exclusion of use of food guides, several tables have been included to aid in recognizing foods which are especially good sources of specific nutrients. With either the food group or the nutrient approach, emphasis should be placed on a *varied* diet.

STUDY QUESTIONS

1. Distinguish between the RDA and the Basic Four food guide.
2. If a vitamin or mineral is not included in the RDA, does this mean that the nutrient is not essential? Explain.
3. How is flexibility incorporated into "A Guide to Good Eating?"
4. Record the foods eaten by an individual during one day. Identify the food group of the Basic Four to which each food belongs, if possible. What foods are good sources of nutrients but do not clearly fit into any classification?
5. Some books state that white enriched bread is just as nutritious as whole wheat bread. In what way is this true? In what way is this false?
6. List several ways a person who cannot tolerate citrus fruit can meet his RDA for vitamin C.
7. Name several examples of fruits and vegetables which are not very good sources of vitamin A even though they are bright green or orange in color.
8. Both meat and cheese are good sources of protein. Why is it advantageous to include cheese in the milk rather than in the meat group of the Basic Four?
9. Give some guidelines to accompany "A Daily Food Guide" to help assure that intake of micronutrients and fiber is adequate.
10. What seven nutrients have been identified as the best indicators of overall adequacy of a diet? Which of these are most commonly listed in tables of food composition and on nutritional labels on processed food?

References

*1. USDA, Agricultural Research Service, Consumer and Food Economics Institute. *Family Fare, A Guide to Good Nutrition.* Home and Garden Bull. No. 1. Washington DC: U.S. Govt. Printing Office, 1974.
2. Ahlstrom, A., and Rasanen, L.: Review of food grouping systems in nutrition education. *J. Nutr. Ed.* 5:12, 1973.
3. McClinton, P., Milne, H., and Beaton, G.: An evaluation of food habits and nutrient intakes in Canada: Design of effective food guides. *Can. J. Public Health* 62:139, 1971.
4. Pennington, J. A.: *Dietary Nutrient Guide.* Westport CT: Avi Publishing Co., 1976.
5. Cullen, R. W., and Oace, S. M.: Iodine: Current status. *J. Nutr. Ed.* 8:101, 1976.
6. Fry, B.: *Yardsticks for nutrition.* Cooperative Extension, Division of Nutritional Sciences, NY State College of Agriculture and Life Sciences at the NY State College of Human Ecology at Cornell University, Ithaca NY, 1974.
7. Poultoon, M. A.: Predicting application of nutrition education. *J. Nutr. Ed.* 4:110, 1972.
8. Meyers, L. D., and Jansen, G. R.: A nutrient approach in the fifth grade. *J. Nutr. Ed.* 9:127, 1977.

* Recommended reading

3

Meeting nutrient needs by means of vegetarian diets

In this land of affluence, where the steak dinner has long been a status symbol, there is a growing trend toward vegetarianism. The trend has been particularly evident among young adults, but does include individuals of a wide range of ages, occupations, and lifestyles.

There are two large classes of vegetarians: *lacto-ovo-vegetarians*, who use dairy products and eggs in addition to plant foods; and *vegans*, pure, strict, or total vegetarians, who use only plant foods.

Other types of "vegetarians" include (1) those who avoid red meat (beef, pork, and lamb); these individuals eat fish and/or poultry (no specific name has been widely used for this group). (2) *Lacto-vegetarians*, who use only dairy products in addition to plant foods. (3) *Fruitarians*, who usually limit their diet to fresh (raw) fruits, juices, and nuts. This latter type of diet is *dangerously* low in many essential nutrients.

REASONS FOR A VEGETARIAN EATING PATTERN

The many types of vegetarian diets reflect differences in reasons for becoming vegetarians. In the U.S. there are so many obstacles to vegetarianism that few individuals adhere to this type of diet without being firmly convinced of its value. Generally vegetarians need to spend more time preparing food than do their flesh-eating neighbors; they also have more difficulty getting a well-balanced meal when they eat away from home. They may be pressured by family and friends to give up their "eccentric" diet. Why then are the vegetarian ranks growing? Most fall into one or more of the following categories: religious, respect for all living beings; health; ethical-ecological; economic.

Each of these will be considered in more detail because vegetarianism is not just a passing fad but often is a major aspect of a different way of living and of looking at the world. It can have either a positive or negative relation to health.

Religious beliefs

SEVENTH-DAY ADVENTIST

In the U.S., the Seventh-Day Adventist Church is the largest religious group advocating a vegetarian diet. A literal interpretation of Old Testament biblical passages provides a basis for their adoption of vegetarianism. The spiritual importance of avoiding flesh foods was emphasized and explained by the Seventh-Day Adventist prophetess Ellen White in her writings. She affirmed that the body is the temple of God and that "Those who await the second coming will not include meat." According to Ellen White, meat-eating indulges the appetite with diseased, unhealthful food, which destroys the body and is therefore counter to the religion.

Some Seventh-Day Adventists are strict adherents (pure vegetarians); about half are lacto-ovo-vegetarians. Nearly all avoid pork products and shellfish since the Old Testament of the *Bible* specifically states that those foods are unclean.

EASTERN RELIGIOUS INFLUENCES AND RESPECT FOR ALL LIVING BEINGS

". . . every meal we eat spares a fellow creature, gives the gift of life."[1]

Young adults who become involved with one of the

24

Eastern religious philosophies or sects, as is common in many college communities and large cities, frequently adopt vegetarian eating patterns. Often diet considerations are the focal point of their living habits.[2] Specific diet prohibitions, such as avoidance of meat, may be closely entwined with their spiritual life. This may be completely compatible with nutritional adequacy and good health. However, in some cases, the vegetarian diets followed prohibit so many foods in addition to animal products that nutritional adequacy is impossible to achieve. This can cause serious health problems, especially for individuals with special needs such as children and pregnant or lactating women. The health professional will be able to assist these individuals effectively only if she can gain the trust and credibility of individuals who hold different beliefs and have different lifestyles from her own. She will be better equipped to do this if she knows a variety of ways for making vegetarian diets compatible with health.

Some individuals feel a moral obligation, quite apart from the specific teachings of their religion, to refrain from eating meat. They may have such strong convictions against the exploitation of animals that they avoid using animal products of any kind, including nonfood items such as wool, leather, sheepskin, gelatin capsules, and certain other pharmaceutical products.[3] Some children decide to become vegetarians, at least for a limited period of time, because of their concern for animals.

Health motives

Health reasons for vegetarianism are often closely interwoven with religious reasons, as is the case for Seventh-Day Adventists. The relationship between vegetarianism and health has been and is being studied by a number of investigators. Work to date indicates:

1. Lacto-ovo-vegetarian diets can be planned to meet all nutritional needs, laying the foundation for good health. Studies of the nutritional adequacy of freely chosen lacto-ovo-vegetarian diets have indicated that the nutrient content often exceeds Recommended Dietary Allowances.[4]
2. Vegetarians, especially vegans, tend to be lighter in weight (closer to desirable weight) than are meat eaters.[5-8]
3. The greater the degree of adherence to vegetarianism (as in vegans), the lower the blood cholesterol level tends to be.[7-11] This may reduce the risk of heart disease.
4. Seventh-Day Adventists have a lower mortality rate than the general population for heart disease and cancer. Although their longer life can be partially explained by their abstinence from tobacco and alcohol, their vegetarian eating habits also appear to be a factor.[12]
5. Since only animal foods contain vitamin B_{12}, pure vegetarians who fail to supplement their diet with this vitamin are likely to develop a serious, partially irreversible vitamin B_{12} deficiency disease.

Perceptible physical and psychological benefits resulting from a change to vegetarianism have been claimed by adherents. There is no scientific evidence available to confirm most of the benefits which were frequently noted by "new vegetarians" in a recent study.[13] Claimed benefits included physical and psychological changes such as more positive state of mind, weight loss, less frequent colds and sore throats, and more pleasing body odor.

Ethical and ecological reasons

"Every pound of beef on our table represents sixteen pounds of grain and legumes removed from the total available to a hungry world."[1]

Eating low on the food chain is often a well-thought-out change in eating pattern which is based on valuing conservation of the world's resources. Some persons avoid meat or at least greatly decrease their meat consumption because of their sense of responsibility as citizens of the world.

A diet which includes a fairly large proportion of food of animal origin places a drain on important natural resources, namely fuel, water, and land. A vegetarian diet has a favorable ecological effect because a much smaller quantity of grain and legumes is required for feeding people directly than for feeding animals. This has the following effects: (1) less land needs to be cultivated; (2) less fuel is required for making fuel-based fertilizers, operating agricultural machinery, and transporting and storing food; and (3) less water is required since it is not needed for maintaining livestock and less is needed for the crops. Clearly it would be possible to feed many more people a vegetarian rather than a meat-based diet.

Some persons who change their eating habits for ecological reasons justify use of certain flesh foods because of the more favorable efficiency with which "feed" is converted to "food." Sometimes fish is used in moderation by these individuals since fish eating is considered to have little detrimental ecological effect as long as overfishing is avoided.

It should be no surprise to find that individuals who become vegetarians for ecological reasons often choose foods which have been subjected to a minimum of processing and therefore have required the use of minimal amounts of fuel. Homegrown foods may be preferred.

Economic grounds

The sharp rise in meat prices in 1972 resulted in a meat boycott by thousands of Americans and a surge of interest in vegetarian cookery. Most participants were hopeful that meat prices would decrease; they definitely were not dedicated to vegetarianism. Many knew little about meat alternatives and how to cook them. Many discovered for the first time that vegetarian meals could be tasty, nutritious, and economical. As a result some families now avoid meat at least one day a week.

In the U.S., a vegetarian diet offers less economical advantage than it should, considering the lower cost of producing most meat alternatives. In many other countries the cost of meat is prohibitive and may be a major reason for minimizing its use.

PRINCIPLES OF MEAL PLANNING

Protein

Contrary to widespread belief, vegetarian diets can easily provide for protein needs of adults and children if they are properly planned. Many Americans eat more than twice as much protein as is necessary for optimal health, much of it in the form of meat. Parents of "new vegetarians" usually express more concern about the diet's protein content than about any other nutrient. However, vegetarians in America have access to an abundant supply of suitable food; it can more than meet their protein needs if food choices reflect application of some principles of protein nutrition.

PROTEIN QUALITY

Proteins from different food sources differ in their ability to support growth, maintenance, and repair of body tissues. Those most usable for these purposes are called high quality protein, complete protein, or protein of high biological value. The terms are synonomous. The *protein efficiency ratio* (PER) also indicates protein quality. A high PER (≥ 2.5) is assigned to proteins which are efficient at promoting growth. Protein of high biological value (high PER) is found in eggs, milk and milk products, and flesh foods of all types.

Those proteins which can support life but not growth, when eaten as the only protein source, are intermediate in biological value. They may be called partially complete proteins. Their PER falls below 2.5, but goes no lower than 0.5. This is the type of protein found in legumes, lentils, nuts, and cereal products. Plant proteins typically have somewhat lower biological value (lower PER) than do most animal proteins. There is some overlapping of protein quality among plant and animal foods.

Proteins which cannot even support life are low in biological value and are sometimes called incomplete proteins. The best example of this type of protein is gelatin. If animals are fed gelatin as their only source of protein, they will die. (Gelatin is an animal protein made from bones and cartilage.)

AMINO ACID CONTENT OF PROTEIN

Proteins differ because of differences in their chemical composition. All proteins are made up of chemicals called amino acids. There are about twenty different amino acids (Table 1.1, p. 4). Children have specific dietary requirements for at least nine of these amino acids. Each one of the nine must be present in the diet; one cannot be substituted for another. Adults require at least eight; recent evidence suggests that the ninth one (histidine) may also be required for optimal health of adults.[14]

The amino acids for which there are specific *dietary* requirements are called essential amino acids or indispensable amino acids. Two amino acids are called semiessential. The need for these two amino acids depends on the supply of the essential amino acids from which they are made. For health it is essential for a person to consume adequate amounts of each of the essential amino acids. Essential amino acids, from plant or animal foods, can be used by the body as long as *all of them are available at the same time.*

The amino acids not essential in the *diet* are called nonessential amino acids. They are not essential in the diet because they can be synthesized in the body. As long as the total amino acid (protein) intake is adequate, it does not matter which, if any, of the nonessential amino acids are obtained from the food. Low intake of nonessential amino acids is an unlikely event, because food proteins normally contain generous amounts of them.

Proteins differ in the kinds and proportions of amino acids they contain. Proteins are high in biological value if they contain desirable amounts of each of the essential amino acids. Put another way, protein with a high PER (high biological value) is a good source of each of the essential amino acids. However, if even one essential amino acid is lacking, the biological value of a protein will be low. Protein cannot be made in the body if any of the essential amino acids is missing.

Plant proteins are of intermediate rather than high biological value despite the fact that they contain each of the essential amino acids. This is explained by the less favorable proportions of the essential amino acids

---

POINTS OF EMPHASIS
Amino acid requirements

• *Children: at least nine amino acids are dietary essentials to allow both growth and maintenance of body tissue.*

• *Adults: eight or nine amino acids must be provided by the diet.*

• *To be used by the body, all of the essential amino acids must be present at the same time.*

• *Essential amino acids are used at the level of the "limiting" amino acid. Therefore the proportion of essential amino acids in a protein affects usefulness or biological value.*

found in plant proteins. All plant proteins contain less than desirable amounts of at least one essential amino acid. The essential amino acid which is present in the smallest amount relative to need is called the limiting amino acid. The limiting amino acid limits the value of the protein.

Complementing protein

Food proteins can have amino acid strengths and weaknesses. When the use of animal protein is restricted, as in vegetarian diets, combinations of foods can be used to achieve a desirable proportion of each of the essential amino acids. *Complementing* or supplementing proteins is the term used for combining foods having opposite strengths and weaknesses in essential amino acid content. Complementing proteins helps to assure adequate protein nutrition when much of the protein is supplied by plant foods. The following example illustrates the principle of complementing proteins.

Baked beans in tomato sauce might be used as a main dish by a vegetarian. The protein content of this entree is satisfactory in quantity but not in quality (biological value). The beans are low in methionine, an essential amino acid. Bringing the methionine content up to the desired level by eating more beans would require a much larger serving than most people would care to eat. To correct this situation, the meal could be planned to include another food source of protein—one which is high in the amino acid methionine. The protein contained in cereal products, particularly whole grains, would provide the needed methionine. Therefore whole wheat bread might be eaten to improve the protein quality of the meal. The beans are rich in lysine, which is the limiting amino acid in bread.

It would be less satisfactory to have the beans alone at dinner and the bread alone at lunch. Effective supplementation occurs only if all essential amino acids are provided *at the same time.* Legumes and grains, as in this example, make a very good complementary pair since the essential amino acid weakness of each is the strength of the other. Table 3.1 depicts the principle of complementing proteins. Complementing proteins can also be achieved by

including a small amount of a milk product or egg in a meal containing plant proteins. The protein in a muffin, for example, has a higher biological value than that in a slice of French bread because the muffin contains a small amount of milk and eggs. The dry milk used in making some sandwich breads improves the biological value of the protein in the bread. Milk added to a bowl of oatmeal complements the cereal protein. Lacto-ovo-vegetarians and lacto-vegetarians often complement plant proteins using eggs, milk, yogurt, or cheese. Individuals who are decreasing their use of flesh foods for ecological or economic reasons may apply the same principle in meal planning. They have the option of using small amounts of meat to complement the plant proteins they use. Including just a small amount of pork with the baked beans greatly improves the essential amino acid content of the meal.

Two foods cannot supplement each other if they are very similar in their content of essential amino acids. This is true of two different foods of the same type. Peanuts and chick peas do not supplement each other; they are both legumes.

Most nuts and seeds are similar to grains in their amino acid patterns. The protein in nuts and seeds complements legume protein only if the nuts and seeds are ground or *thoroughly* chewed.

The quantity of protein in a food also affects its ability to supplement another protein source. Although the quality of the protein in butter is good, the amount that is present is so tiny that it cannot supplement plant protein.

It should be emphasized that appropriate mixtures

POINTS OF EMPHASIS
Obtaining adequate protein without meat

• *Animal protein sources such as eggs and milk are excellent sources of all of the essential amino acids. Eggs and milk are higher in biological value than is meat.*
• *Eating a variety of plant proteins with mutually complementary amino acid patterns can provide all of the essential amino acids in adequate amounts.*

TABLE 3.1 *Complementing proteins—combining proteins so that their amino acid strengths and weaknesses balance out, resulting in a mixture of foods with good biological value*

FOOD CATEGORY	EXAMPLES		RELATIVE AMINO ACID CONTENT	
			LYSINE	METHIONINE
Legumes	Peanut butter	Chili beans	+ to ++	—
Grains	Whole wheat bread	Corn bread	—	+
	Combination		Adequate	Adequate
Grains	Rye bread	Puffed rice	—	+
Milk	Cheese	Milk	++	+
	Combination		Good	Very good

+ The protein contains more of the amino acid than does a high quality protein.
++ The protein is very high in the amino acid in comparison to a high quality protein.
— The protein is low in the amino acid in comparison to a high quality protein.

Four Food Groups for a Meatless Diet: A Daily Guide

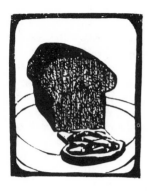

Grains, Legumes, Nuts, & Seeds

Six servings or more. Include several slices of yeast-raised, whole-grain bread, a serving of beans, and a few nuts or seeds.

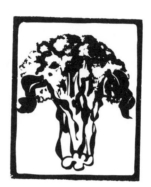

Vegetables

Three servings or more. Include one or more servings of dark leafy greens, like romaine, spinach, or chard.

Fruit

One to four pieces. Include a raw source of vitamin C, like citrus fruits, strawberries, or cantaloupe.

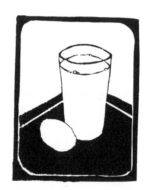

Milk & Eggs

Two or more glasses of fresh milk for adults, three or more for children. (Children under nine use smaller glasses.) Other dairy products or an egg may be used to meet part of the milk requirement. Eggs are optional—up to four per week.

FIGURE 3.1. A reliable, easy-to-use guide to balanced vegetarian meals. (Reprinted by permission from *Laurel's Kitchen: A Handbook for Vegetarian Cookery and Nutrition,* by Laurel Robertson, Carol Flinders, and Bronwen Godfrey, copyright 1976 by Nilgiri Press, Petaluma CA)

TABLE 3.2 *A sample menu for a lacto-ovo-vegetarian*

BREAKFAST	LUNCH	DINNER
Whole grain toast with peanut butter	Homemade bean soup	Meatless lasagna made with whole grain pasta
Yogurt with fresh fruit and nuts	Corn sticks	Sauteed zucchini
Herb tea	Romaine and tomato salad with cheese dressing	Spinach and Mushroom salad
		Milk

A Seventh-Day Adventist might substitute a meat analog such as vegetarian weiners, turkey-like loaf, or breakfast slices for one of the main dishes.

of plant foods can provide growing children with all of the amino acids they need. In fact special vegetable protein mixtures such as INCAPARINA have been successfully used in developing nations to treat children with protein-energy malnutrition.

GUIDELINES FOR PLANNING VEGETARIAN DIETS

Lacto-ovo-vegetarian

In the case of lacto-ovo-vegetarians and of lacto-vegetarians the Basic Four Groups can be used as a sound guide for meal planning. The number of foods that can be used is large. Palatability can easily be achieved, especially with the help of a good cookbook. (Recommended cookbooks are listed at the end of Part One.) A few adaptations in the Daily Food Guide are necessary to be sure that all nutrient needs are met:

1. Have whole grain become the basic food of the diet, especially in the form of *yeast*-leavened bread. This involves increasing the number of servings from the grain group. Vary the types of grains used. Nuts and seeds are grouped with grains.
2. Be sure to use the recommended number of servings of milk or milk equivalents for the age group. Fortified skim milk and fortified low-fat milk products are recommended. Milk products will be the only source of vitamin B_{12} unless eggs are eaten.
3. Use a serving of legumes, lentils, meat analogs, eggs, or an additional milk product daily. Vary the choice.
4. Use a wide variety of vegetables and fruits, including at least one serving of a dark green leafy vegetable daily.

5. Severely limit use of foods which are primarily a source of empty calories.

Several food guides that incorporate the adaptations listed above have been developed for lacto-ovo-vegetarians.[1,15-17] An advantage of a plan specifically designed for vegetarians is elimination of the term "meat group" with its negative connotations for those who avoid meat. A plan which is easy to follow, flexible, and based on sound nutrition is shown in Figure 3.1. The basic principles of sound nutrition which accompany this plan are:

Variety. As emphasized previously for meat eaters as well.

Whole foods. (Foods which have undergone relatively little processing). To provide a balance between calories and nutrients.

Moderation. With regard to the total amount of food eaten and the use of individual foods.

An example of well-balanced meals for a day which might be eaten by a lacto-ovo-vegetarian is given in Table 3.2.

Pure vegetarian (vegan)

When all animal foods are omitted from the diet, much more careful planning is required to achieve nutritional adequacy. Attention must be given to protein balance,[1] caloric adequacy, and intake of vitamins and minerals (especially vitamin B_{12}, vitamin D, riboflavin, and calcium). Failure to obtain a source of vitamin B_{12} may have serious consequences. A severe deficiency of vitamin B_{12} has been reported in a vegan's breastfed baby.[18]

Adequate riboflavin intake may require use of brewer's yeast, wheat germ, or another especially good riboflavin source (Table 3.3) in addition to use of dark-green leafy vegetables.

TABLE 3.3 *Plant sources of riboflavin (vitamin B_2)*

FOOD	PORTION SIZE	AMOUNT OF B_2 IN MG (RDA RANGE FOR ADULTS 1.1 TO 1.8 MG)	
Collard greens, cooked	240 ml (190 gm or 1 c)	0.38 (almost as much as is in 1 c milk)	22–32% of RDA for adult woman
Broccoli, cooked	1 medium stalk, 180 gm	0.36	
Brewer's yeast	8 gm (1 Tbsp)	0.34	
Mushrooms, raw	70 gm (1 c)	0.32	
Okra, cooked	100 gm (1 c)	0.29	
Winter squash, mashed, cooked	240 ml (1 c)	0.27	
Asparagus, cooked	145 gm (1 c)	0.26	
Wild rice	40 gm raw (makes 240 ml cooked)	0.25	9–21% of RDA for adult woman
Avocado	½ (125 gm)	0.23	
Chard, brussels sprouts, beet greens, spinach	240 ml (1 c)	0.19 to 0.25	
Wheat germ	30 gm (¼ c)	0.20	
Zucchini	210 gm (1 c diced)	0.17	
Dried peas and beans, cooked	240 ml (1 c)	0.11 to 0.18	

Source: Adams, C. F.: *Nutritive Value of American Foods in Common Units.* Agriculture Research Service, USDA, Agriculture Handbook No. 456. Washington DC: U.S. Govt. Printing Office, 1975.

TABLE 3.4 *Daily requirements of the four food groups for the adult vegan**

GRAINS	LEGUMES	VEGETABLES	FRUIT	EXTRAS NECESSARY FOR ADEQUATE NUTRITION
4 slices of whole grain yeast-leavened bread and 3 to 5 servings of grain (number based on normal body size) and 1 serving of nuts or seeds (ground or thoroughly chewed) (This provides a total of approx. 30 gm grain protein for men, 28 gm for women)	2 c fortified soybean milk and ⅓ c cooked dried peas or beans or 1¼ c cooked dried peas or beans and Other sources of vitamin B₁₂, calcium, and riboflavin	4 or more servings including 2 LARGE servings of dark-green leafy vegetables Mustard, turnip and collards, kale, broccoli, bok choy, and romaine and other dark loose-leaf lettuce provide calcium in usable form 2 additional servings, emphasizing variety	1 to 4 servings, according to caloric needs Include a source of vitamin C	Supplemental vitamin B₁₂, unless enough fortified soy milk is used to provide 2 to 3 μg daily Supplemental calcium, unless soy milk fortified with this mineral or 1½ cups (cooked) of calcium rich vegetables are used Riboflavin, as from 1 Tbsp. brewer's yeast or the equivalent (Table 3.3) Supplemental vitamin D for children and pregnant and lactating women.

Adapted from Robertson, L., Flinders, C., and Godfrey, B.: *Laurel's Kitchen: A Handbook for Vegetarian Cookery and Nutrition*. Petaluma CA: Nilgiri Press, 1977, p. 322.
*Pregnant and lactating women need more good nutrient sources to meet their higher RDAs.

A food guide for adult vegans is given in Table 3.4. Adequate nutrient intake is possible for vegans, but it requires considerable thought and effort.

STUDY QUESTIONS

1. Why is it often helpful to recognize the reasons a person has for being a vegetarian?
2. What are possible health advantages and risks associated with vegetarian eating patterns?
3. Why is vegetarianism sometimes described as "eating low on the food chain"?
4. What determines whether a protein is of high or low biological value?
5. What is meant by "complementing proteins?" Why is this a particularly desirable practice for vegans? Give some examples of complementing proteins which would be suitable for vegans.
6. What are reasons for the adaptations of "A Daily Food Guide" which have been listed for lacto- or lacto-ovo-vegetarians?

References

1. Robertson, L., Flinders, C., and Godfrey, B.: *Laurel's Kitchen*. Petaluma CA: Nilgiri Press, 1977.
2. Erdhard, D.: Nutrition education for the "now generation." *J. Nutr. Ed.* 3:135, 1971.
3. Altman, N.: *Eating for Life, A Book About Vegetarianism*. Wheaten IL: The Theosophical Publishing House, 1973.
4. Hardinge, M. G., and Stare, F. J.: Nutritional studies of vegetarians. 1. Nutritional, physiological and laboratory studies. *J. Clin. Nutr.* 2:73, 1954.
5. Ellis, F. R., and Mumford, P.: The nutritional status of vegans and vegetarians. *Symposium Proceedings* 26:205, 1967.
6. Brown, P. T., and Bergan, J. G.: The dietary status of "new" vegetarians. *J. Am. Diet. Assoc.* 67:455, 1975.
7. Sacks, F., et al.: Plasma lipids and lipoproteins in vegetarians and controls. *N. Engl. J. Med.* 292:1148, 1975.
8. Sanders, B., Ellis, F. R., and Dickerson, J. W. T.: Studies of vegans: The fatty acid composition of plasma choline phosphoglycerides, erythrocytes, adipose tissue, and breast milk, and some indicators of susceptibility to ischemic heart disease in vegans and omnivore controls. *Am. J. Clin. Nutr.* 31:805, 1978.
9. West, R. O., and Hayes, O. B.: Diet and serum cholesterol levels, a comparison between vegetarians and non-vegetarians in a Seventh-Day Adventist Group. *Am. J. Clin. Nutr.* 21:853, 1968.
10. Hardinge, M. G., and Stare, F. J.: Nutritional studies of vegetarians. 2. Dietary and serum levels of cholesterol. *J. Clin. Nutr.* 2:83, 1954.
11. Simons, L. A., et al.: The influence of a wide range of absorbed cholesterol on plasma cholesterol levels in man. *Am. J. Clin. Nutr.* 31:1334, 1978.
12. Phillips, R. L.: Role of life-style and dietary habits in risk of cancer among Seventh-Day Adventists. *Cancer Res.* 35:3513, 1975.
13. Dwyer, J. T., et al.: The "new" vegetarians. Group affiliation and dietary strictures related to attitudes and life-style. *J. Am. Diet. Assoc.* 64:376, 1974.
14. Swenseid, M. E.: Histidine, the ninth essential amino acid for adult humans. Presentation at the 60th Annual Meeting of the American Dietetic Association, Los Angeles CA, Oct. 13, 1977.
15. Register, U. D., and Sonnenberg, L. M.: The vegetarian diet. *J. Am. Diet. Assoc.* 62:253, 1973.
16. Macmillan, J. B., and Smith, E. B.: Development of a lacto-ovo-vegetarian food guide. *J. Can. Diet. Assoc.* 36:110, 1975.
*17. Vyheister, I. B., Register, U. D., and Sonnenberg, L. M.: Safe vegetarian diets for children. *Ped. Clin. North Amer.* 24:203, 1977.
18. Higginbottom, M. Sweetman, L., and Nyhan, W.: A syndrome of methylmalonicaciduria, homocystinuria, megaloblastic anemia and neurologic abnormalities in a vitamin B12-deficient breast-fed infant of a strict vegan. *N. Engl. J. Med.* 299:317, 1978.

* Recommended reading.

4

Promoting energy balance

Whether an individual gains, loses, or maintains weight is determined by his state of energy balance. For weight maintenance to occur, energy intake from food must equal energy expended for maintaining and moving the body. One of the biggest thrusts in health promotion should be directed toward maintenance of normal weight. When a person can keep weight in proper proportion to height and type of frame, he helps optimize his productive potential and reduces certain health risks. The positive effects are physiological, psychological, social, and economic. Doors closed to the very thin or to the heavy individual may be open to the person of normal weight. In our society normal weight is an asset often unrecognized by those who have it.

As weight increases above desirable levels, health risks increase. Those who carry excessive fat have a higher incidence of diabetes mellitus, gallbladder disease, and cardiovascular diseases than do lean individuals. Overfatness may aggravate the symptoms or progression of a number of diseases, such as arthritis. Extreme overfatness can cause life-threatening interference with respiration. Overfatness may decrease overall life expectancy.[1] It may also decrease the quality of life since prejudice is often directed toward the obese.[2] In severe underweight there is generally loss of muscle as well as of fat. Severe underweight has adverse effects on mortality which are related to decreased resistance to infection.

WEIGHT CLASSIFICATIONS

Normal weight is not clearly defined. Weight for a given height varies with the amount of muscle, bone, fluid, and fat. Tables such as the one adapted from Metropolitan Life Insurance Height-Weight Tables are used to estimate desirable weight for adults (Appendix 4A). This table gives the weight ranges associated with the lowest mortality rates for a given sex, height, and frame.

There is no one specific weight defined as "best." Individuals who weigh 10 to 20 percent more than the range specified in the chart are termed overweight. However, a very muscular, heavy-boned person may be at his "ideal" weight even though he is overweight according to the chart. "Overweight" is not necessarily synonomous with "overfat."

When weight exceeds the desirable range by 20 percent or more, the condition is termed obesity. The prejudicial terms "morbid," "massive," and "gross" obesity usually refer to the condition in which weight is two or more times higher than desirable weight.

If weight is below the desirable range by more than 10 percent, an individual is described as underweight. Severe underweight, in America, occurs most often in women who associate excessive thinness with beauty, in individuals with mental problems, in individuals who have certain long term illnesses such as cancer, and in individuals who require a prolonged stay in a health care facility (e.g., elderly residing in nursing homes, individuals who have undergone repeated major surgical operations).

TRENDS

The most serious nutritional problem in the U. S. and in most other technologically developed countries is overnutrition or obesity. Despite the fact that millions of dollars are spent yearly in the U.S. for treating overweight, the incidence and degree of overweight is increasing.[3] Treatment of obesity has been largely unsuccessful and is almost always unpleasant for the person losing weight. The most reasonable means of reversing the trend is to place emphasis on *prevention* of overfatness. Efforts should begin in infancy and continue throughout the entire life span. By preventing overfatness in childhood, the likelihood of becoming obese in the adult years may be greatly reduced.[4] Adults of normal weight can also benefit from health care which promotes weight maintenance. Adults in affluent societies often experience insidious weight gain. Data from the Build and Blood Pressure Study indicate that women gain an average of 12 kg. (27 lb.) between the ages of 20 and 59, all of which is probably fat.[5] Men show a similar pattern of weight gain, but the total amount gained is somewhat less than for women. The fact that undesirable weight gain is common does not mean that it is inevitable.

HEREDITARY INFLUENCES

There is some evidence that heredity has an influence on the development of overfatness. Garn and Clark[6] have reported that, at 17 years of age, children of two obese parents are, on the average, *three times* as fat as are children of two lean parents. This does not prove that heredity plays a part, since the environment in the homes may be different. However, hereditary factors are clearly implicated by the finding that if children are adopted, even from birth, the above correlation is less likely to hold true.

Even if there is a family history of obesity, children are not doomed to become obese. A person gets fat if he takes in more energy from food than he actually expends. Heredity may influence his energy expenditure and/or his appetite, thus affecting the ease with which

weight is gained. Nonetheless, individuals can take action to control their state of energy balance and to assist other family members in doing so as well. Health professionals need to foster and support this effort.

ENERGY AND ENERGY BALANCE

CALORIES

Energy is expressed in nutrition in terms of kilocalories (kcal), which are units of heat energy. One kilocalorie is the amount of heat required to raise the temperature of 1 kg. of water one degree Celsius (at room temperature). For simplicity the shorter but inaccurate term "calorie" is usually used to mean kilocalorie in nutrition. A different unit, the *kilojoule* (kJ.), is used in the metric system for expressing energy values.*

Much of the food we eat is used for fuel. The body's use of fuel might be compared to wood burning in a fireplace to produce heat. A good supply of oxygen is required if the wood is to burn. Within the body, fuel (carbohydrate, fat, and protein) is likewise combined with oxygen, but the reaction (oxidation) is slow and controlled. The oxidation of body fuels provides the heat or mechanical and chemical energy needed for body processes and for activity.

* One kJ. is equivalent to 4.184 kcal. Kilojoules have not been given in this text, but they can be determined by multiplying kcal. by 4.184.

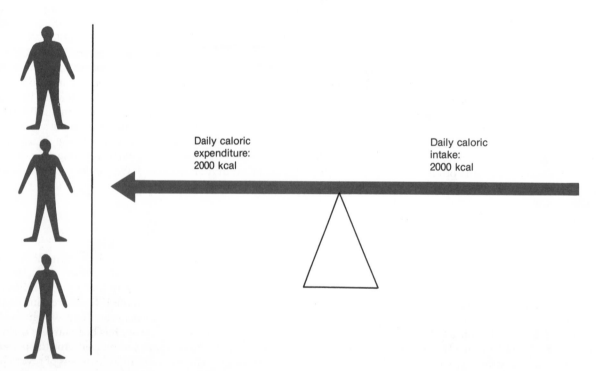

Daily caloric expenditure: 2000 kcal

Daily caloric intake: 2000 kcal

FIGURE 4.1. Energy balance.

Types of energy balance

A state of energy balance characterized by a balance between caloric input and expenditure is illustrated in Figure 4.1. If an adult takes in more fuel than he uses (is in positive caloric balance), his fat stores will increase even if the extra fuel was in the form of carbohydrate or protein (Fig. 4.2). If an individual of any age takes in less of the energy nutrients than he requires (is in negative caloric balance), his body must have some source of fuel in order to survive. During a state of negative energy balance, the body oxidizes stored fat and carbohydrate and the protein in muscle tissue to meet energy needs (Fig. 4.3).

More simply stated, an individual will become fatter *only* if he takes in more calories than his body requires. He will become thinner *only* if he takes in fewer calories than his body requires. Contrary to the statements of some popular diets, *calories do count*.

An excess intake of 3500 kcal. over a period of days,

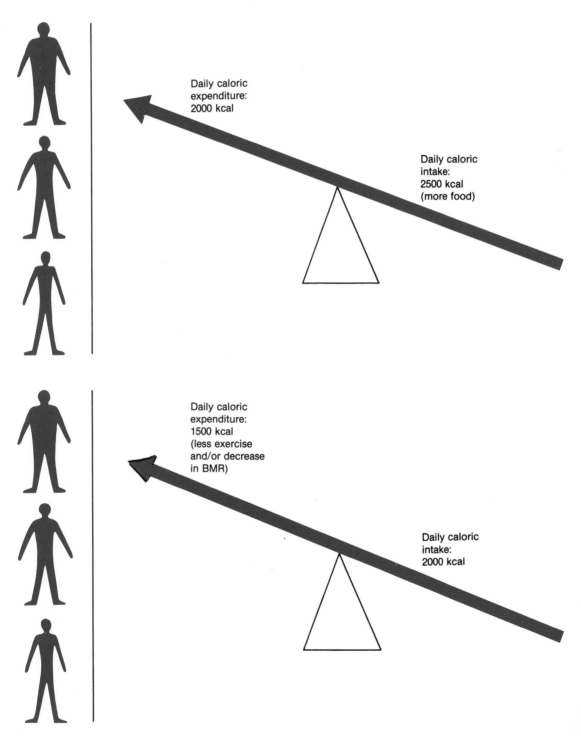

Daily caloric expenditure: 2000 kcal

Daily caloric intake: 2500 kcal (more food)

Daily caloric expenditure: 1500 kcal (less exercise and/or decrease in BMR)

Daily caloric intake: 2000 kcal

FIGURE 4.2. Positive energy balance.

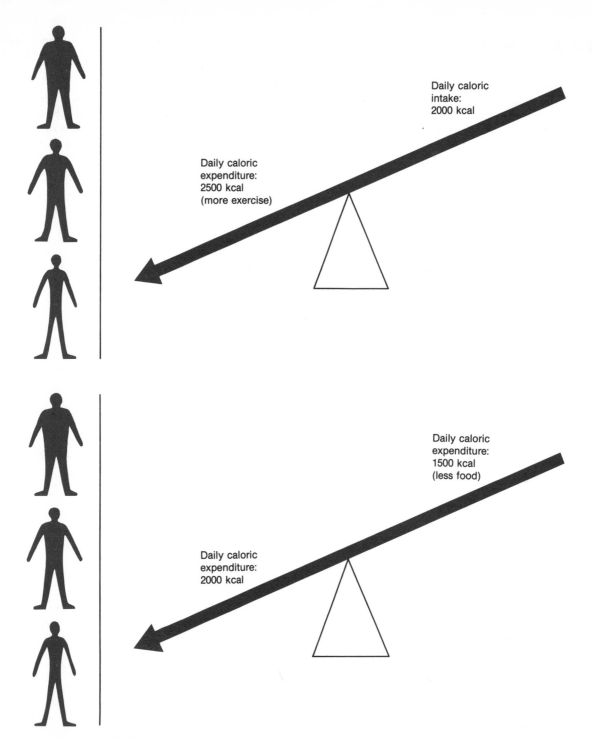

Daily caloric
intake:
2000 kcal

Daily caloric
expenditure:
2500 kcal
(more exercise)

Daily caloric
expenditure:
1500 kcal
(less food)

Daily caloric
expenditure:
2000 kcal

FIGURE 4.3. Negative energy balance.

weeks, or months generally results in a gain of about 0.45 kg. (1 lb.) of body fat.* Conversely, a caloric deficit of 3500 kcal. usually results in loss of about 0.45 kg. of body fat.[8] Caloric balance, or lack of it, is not always obvious when viewed over a short time span. It can be difficult to estimate accurately and it can be change-

* The efficiency of fat production varies among individuals. Some individuals who consume extra calories appear to use part of the energy to produce extra *heat* rather than fat.[7] Others are very efficient at producing fat. Utilization of body fat for energy varies as well.

able from day to day. Body weight fluctuates independently of the state of energy balance because of changes in water balance. Even though an individual is in negative caloric balance and is losing body fat, body weight will stay the same for awhile if the fluid content of the body is temporarily increased. Alternatively, body weight can be lost for a short time (via fluid loss) even though an individual is in caloric balance. Therefore the bathroom scale may not accurately reflect the changes in fat stores actually taking place over a short time.

Factors influencing energy balance

The major influences on energy expenditure are basal metabolism and physical activity.

BASAL METABOLISM

Basal metabolism refers to the chemical reactions occurring when the body is *at rest*. These reactions are necessary to provide energy for maintenance of normal body temperature, breathing, heartbeat, muscle tone, and the other essential activities of the cells and tissues of the resting body. The basal metabolic rate is an expression of the amount of calories expended hourly in relation to the surface area of the body (calories/meter²/hour).

More heat is lost when the surface area of the body is greater. An individual who is tall and thin has a greater surface area and normally requires more energy to keep warm than does another person of the same weight who is shorter. Their metabolic *rates* may be similar although total basal energy *requirement* is quite different.

The metabolic rate of the individual at rest rarely is basal. This is because a variety of factors can alter the metabolic rate, as indicated here:

1. Environmental temperature. The metabolic rate increases when the environmental temperature is cool in order to maintain normal body warmth. At high temperatures the metabolic rate may decrease to lower heat production by the body.
2. Fever. The metabolic rate increases by about 12.6 percent for each increase in body temperature of 1°C.
3. Recent eating. For about 12 hours following a meal the metabolic rate is slightly increased because energy is required to digest food, absorb nutrients, and alter them following their absorption.
4. Body position. Changing the posture to a more erect state, such as sitting, increases the metabolic rate above what it would be under basal conditions (lying flat).
5. Emotional states. Elation, anger, fear, and other strong emotions can increase the metabolic rate. Depression tends to decrease it.
6. Recent exercise. Following a period of exercise the metabolic rate remains elevated for a period of time. The length of time depends upon the type and duration of the exercise and whether the individual is accustomed to the exercise.
7. Sleep. Sleep slows body processes, resulting in a decrease in energy expenditure to below basal level.

The basal metabolic rate of a healthy individual is his metabolic rate when he is lying down quietly, awake and relaxed, at an environmental temperature which is comfortable for him (approximately 21 to 23°C.) having had no food in the preceding 12 hours or significant recent exercise.

The basal metabolism of a given individual is not constant throughout life. Predictable changes are the following:

1. Basal metabolic rate normally decreases slowly after an individual is about 5-years old (Fig. 4.4). During spurts of growth, as in adolescence and throughout pregnancy, the basal metabolic rate increases, since growth requires extra energy.
2. Total basal energy requirements normally increase with age until adult size is reached. A larger body cell mass normally requires more energy for its maintenance. Excess fat increases total basal metabolism but not as much as might be expected. Fat cells are less active metabolically than are muscle cells. The metabolic rate of women is usually less than that of men (Fig. 4.4), partially because women normally have a lower percentage of muscle tissue.
3. Basal metabolic rate and total energy requirement normally decrease when food intake is limited for a period of time—as during a famine or a reducing diet. This is an adaptive response of the body in an attempt to conserve the limited supply of nutrients.
4. Lactation increases the basal energy requirement since energy is required to "manufacture" the milk which is secreted.
5. The menstrual cycle in women is associated with small fluctuations in basal metabolism.

To roughly estimate the amount of energy required for the basal metabolism of an adult, the following method may be used:

1. Find ideal weight for height and frame from Appendix 4A.
2. Convert weight to kilograms (weight in pounds divided by 2.2).
3. Multiply 1 × weight in kg. × 24 hours (basal energy requirement is about 1 kcal/kg./hr.).

The result is an approximation of the number of calories needed daily just to maintain the body at rest.

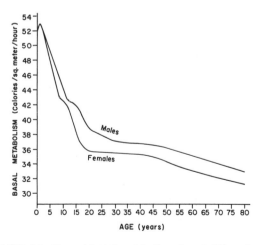

FIGURE 4.4. Normal basal metabolic rates at different ages for each sex. (From Guyton, A. C.: *Textbook of Medical Physiology*, ed. 5. Philadelphia: W. B. Saunders Co., 1976, with permission)

Multiplying 10 times ideal body weight in pounds is another easy method of estimating daily basal energy requirement for adults.

The second major component of energy expenditure is physical activity. Any movement of the whole body, or even a small part of it, expends energy. The greater the movement the greater the energy requirement. For the majority of Americans who are sedentary, exercise makes a relatively small contribution to total energy expenditure, as shown in Figure 4.5. Individuals who have strenuous occupations in terms of physical exertion and those who exercise hard for extended periods, as in sports, have high caloric requirements (Fig. 4.5).

If movement of a large part or all of the body is re-

quired, as in walking, an individual's weight influences the amount of energy expended. Anyone who has walked or climbed a long distance with a heavy pack on his back realizes that extra weight can increase energy expenditure.

An easy way to take weight into consideration when estimating energy expenditure is to use a table which gives "Met" values for specific activities (Appendix 4F). (Mets are multiples of the resting energy requirement.) The following example shows how to calculate the amount of energy a 50 kg. woman would expend if she rode a bicycle at 8 mph for half an hour:
1. Determine resting energy requirement per hour:
    Body weight in kg × 1 kcal = 50 kcal/hr
2. Multiply resting energy requirement by the number of Mets required for the activity (Appendix 4F):
    50 kcal/hr × 4.5 Mets = 225 kcal/hr
3. Multiply number of kcal/hr by the number of hours spent at the activity:
    $$\frac{225 \text{ kcal}}{\text{hr}} \times \frac{1}{2} \text{ hr} = 112 \text{ kcal energy expended}$$

For any given type of physical activity, the caloric expenditure is also affected by the individual's "training" and the form with which the exercise is carried out. Practice at vigorous exercise increases the efficiency of the heart and lungs, for example, so that less energy is needed to perform the same task. Form influences the efficiency of muscular movement; therefore good form can reduce the amount of energy expended. If physical activity is used as a means of losing weight, it can greatly increase energy expenditure, especially when the individual is heavy and "out of condition."

CONTROLLING FOOD INTAKE

The role of eating habits

When ample food is available, the amount of food eaten is usually governed by the individual. How an individual controls his food intake is influenced by physiological processes and by external factors which may be unrelated to his need for food.

PHYSIOLOGICAL CUES TO EAT

If a person is truly *hungry*, physiological changes in his body produce a state of discomfort which motivates him to obtain and eat food, even if it doesn't taste very good. Uncomfortable contractions of the stomach and a shaky, anxious, weak feeling associated with a decrease in the amount of sugar in the blood are physiological cues for eating. *Appetite* is a more pleasurable sensation involving a desire for food or drink. Appetite is apt to be greatly influenced by a person's perception of the palatability of food.

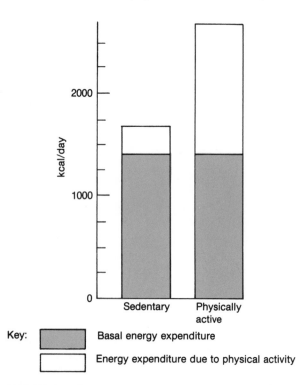

Key: ▨ Basal energy expenditure
☐ Energy expenditure due to physical activity

FIGURE 4.5. Effect of a marked change in physical activity on total energy expenditure of a man or woman who weighs about 58 kg. (126 lb.).

The hypothalamus is the part of the forebrain which participates in regulation of the body's internal environment. It is the principal organ involved in the physiological regulation of eating. When the hypothalamus is functioning properly, one portion (the feeding center or lateral nucleus) sends out signals which impel eating in order to supply the body with needed fuel. Another portion of the hypothalamus (the satiety center or ventromedial hypothalamus) acts as a brake on eating behavior by "telling" a person that he is full. People who respond to these internal cues maintain normal weight with little thought or effort. If an imbalance between caloric expenditure and intake occurs for a day or more, the messages from the hypothalamus tend to correct for imbalance on succeeding days. Thus weight lost during illness is usually regained during recovery and then normal weight is maintained.

USE OF FOOD FOR NON-NUTRITIVE PURPOSES

Even if the hypothalamus is functioning properly, individuals may choose to ignore the internal cues which ordinarily tend to regulate energy balance. People may respond instead to external cues and use food for non-nutritive purposes. Some people overeat as a means of dealing with stresses of daily living. Some people may not clearly perceive internal cues relating to hunger and satiety and thus are more likely to base their eating on external food cues. Eating behaviors may be governed more by social pressures, emotions, habits, and taste of food than by the physiological cues designed to control appetite. When external food cues are the principal determinants of eating behavior, weight changes are likely.

PROMOTING HEALTHY EATING BEHAVIORS

Specific eating behaviors are learned. Family and culture have direct impact on eating behaviors. Promotion of weight maintenance involves creating an environment which will foster the establishment of healthy eating behaviors. A number of approaches can be useful, namely:

1. Have regular mealtimes with well-balanced meals. Skipping breakfast often leads to snacking on high calorie foods and overeating at night.
2. Serve (or order) just enough food to meet the needs of the family or individual.
3. Avoid preparing or purchasing snack foods and desserts with a high sugar or fat content.
4. Express love and reward desired behavior without the use of foods high in empty calories.
5. Encourage all family members to *participate* in a variety of activities.
6. Learn constructive methods of coping with problems (stresses) of daily living.

The role of diet

NUTRIENT DENSITY AND THE CALORIC DENSITY OF FOODS

Individuals who have low caloric requirements because of sedentary lifestyle often benefit from altering food choices based on knowledge of the caloric value of foods. In order to do this safely they need to be sure that intake of essential nutrients is adequate to meet their needs. The Daily Food Guide can be used as a foundation for a diet which is reduced in calories yet provides for nutritional needs. The same number of servings of foods from each of the food groups can still be used; however, when choosing foods, more attention needs to be given to the caloric density and the nutrient density of the foods.

Caloric density refers to the number of kilocalories per unit weight of food. A large amount of a food with a low caloric density provides few calories. Foods with low caloric density are filling, at least temporarily, but do not tend to lead to overweight. Celery is an example of a food with low caloric density since two outer stalks (100 gm.) provide only 17 kcal.

Nutrient density refers to the content of specific nutrients in relation to kilocalories. It can be calculated by using this formula.[9]

$$\text{Index of Nutritional Quality (INQ or Nutrient Density)} = \frac{\text{Percent of recommended nutrient intake provided by the food}}{\text{Percent of energy requirement provided by the food}}$$

Table 4.1 gives a few examples. If the INQ for a particular nutrient is at least 0.9, Wittwer suggests describing the food as an adequate source of that nutrient. Even if the INQ of a food is not known, it is possible to select foods which provide a favorable ratio of nutrients to calories if some general characteristics of foods are known.

Fats and oils Fats and oils have the highest caloric density of any foods and are relatively low in essential nutrients. Decreasing the use of fat and of foods having a high fat content can greatly decrease caloric intake. This involves decreasing consumption of foods such as pastries, fried foods, most gravies, salad dressing, but-

TABLE 4.1 *Index of nutritional quality (INQ) for thiamine in selected foods*

FOOD	INQ*	WORD RATING†
Spinach, cooked frozen	6.0	Excellent
Pork roast, medium fat	2.6	Good
Peach, fresh	1.0	Adequate
Beef round, broiled	0.55	Fair
Dill pickles	0.0	Poor

* Calculated using the formula:
$$\frac{\text{Mg } B_1 \text{ in 100 gm food} \div 1.2 \text{ mg (RDA for } B_1)}{\text{Kcal in 100 gm food} \div 2300 \text{ kcal (RDA for kcal)}}$$
using values from Pennington.[10]
† Adjectives suggested by Wittwer, et al.[9] for these INQ ratings.

ter, and margarine. There is no *caloric* advantage in using margarine in place of butter since the two spreads are equivalent in energy value. Many other foods are high in fat and, therefore, in calories.

Alcoholic beverages Alcoholic beverages are high in caloric value and provide few, if any, essential nutrients. Alcohol itself provides most of the calories in alcoholic beverages; carbohydrate provides some of the calories contained in beer, wine, and liqueurs.

Sweeteners and sweets Sweeteners are characterized as nutritive if they provide calories. Sugar, honey, corn syrup solids, fructose, and sorbitol are all nutritive sweeteners. Their caloric value averages about 20 kcal. per teaspoon. Honey is *not* lower in calories than is sugar. In fact, when equal volumes are compared, honey provides about one-and-a-third times as many kcal. as does table sugar. All sweeteners are either very low in or completely devoid of protein, fat, vitamins, and minerals. Molasses provides some iron, but its high caloric value limits its usefulness as an iron source. Decreasing the use of table sugar and of foods containing a significant amount of nutritive sweeteners can significantly decrease caloric intake without sacrificing nutrient intake.

The nutritive sweetener fructose is sweeter than regular sugar; therefore less needs to be used to produce the same sweetening effect in foods. The small difference in caloric value which results from substituting fructose for table sugar probably has little effect on weight control.

Some sugarless candy and gum and other sugar-free dietetic foods are made with the calorie-rich nutritive sweetener *sorbitol*. Foods made with sorbitol are not significantly lower in calories than comparable foods made with sugar. "Sugar free" does not necessarily mean low in calories.

Vegetables Vegetables vary greatly in caloric density. Since vegetables have good nutrient density, all types (even potatoes and corn) are recommended for use in low-calorie diets. Potatoes are actually lower in caloric density than is meat. When trying to control weight, it can be beneficial to consume large servings of the vegetables which are lowest in calories. Low-calorie vegetables are also very high in water content. Table 4.2 names parts of plants, examples of each, and their relative caloric density.

Fruits Fruits have a surprisingly large range of caloric density because different types of fruit show wide variation in sugar and water content. Lemons and cranberries are high in water, low in sugar, and sour; they can be used as desired when trying to curb caloric intake—as long as no nutritive sweeteners are added to them. At the other extreme are dates, which are about 75 percent as high as sugar in caloric density. The sweeter a fruit tastes, the higher its caloric density is apt to be. Grapefruit, it should be noted, has about the same caloric density as do oranges, even though grapefruit doesn't taste as sweet. Although olives and avocados are classed as fruits, their high caloric density results from high fat rather than high sugar content.

Grains Grain products are remarkably similar in caloric density. Variation in caloric value per unit weight is affected primarily by added fat. When compared on a dry weight basis, servings of plain grain

---

TABLE 4.2 *Caloric density of vegetables*

VERY LOW CALORIC DENSITY (17–30 kcal/100 gm)

Stems and stalks	*Leaves*	*Shoots and sprouts*
Celery	Lettuce	Asparagus
Rhubarb	Spinach	Bean sprouts

Flowers	*Pods and "fruits"*
Cauliflower	(exceptions: pumpkin and winter squash)
Broccoli	Tomatoes
	Summer squash
	Snap beans

MODERATE CALORIC DENSITY (70–140 kcal/100 gm)
Starchy vegetables

Tubers	*Seeds* (fresh, not dried)
Potatoes	Lima beans
Sweet potatoes and yams	Peas
	Corn

WIDE RANGE OF CALORIC DENSITY
Roots
 Radishes—very low
 Beets, carrots, onions, turnips—fairly low (30–45 kcal/100 gm)
 Parsnips—moderate

products such as bread and unsweetened cereals differ significantly in caloric value only if the weight of the servings differs. This accounts for the large caloric difference between ¾ c. (9 gm.) of puffed rice (35 kcal.) and ¾ c. (84 gm.) of Grapenuts (330 kcal.). Some "diet" bread is lower in calories than ordinary loaf bread primarily because it is more thinly sliced. Other "diet" breads are actually lower in calories per unit weight because cellulose (non-nutritive fiber derived from wood pulp) is used to replace part of the flour. This substitution reduces the bread's content of certain nutrients as well as its caloric value.

Moderate use of grain products is compatible with weight control. Four servings of plain bread, cereal, pasta, or other grain products (of the size indicated in the Daily Food Guide) provide less than 300 kcal. Many individuals can eat more than four servings from this group and still keep their weight in line.

Milk products Dairy products differ greatly in caloric density because of differences in fat and water content. Those low in fat, such as skim milk and cottage cheese, contribute essential nutrients without an excessive number of calories.

Yogurt and cottage cheese are often promoted as low calorie foods. This promotion can be quite misleading. Commercially flavored yogurts, including the fruit varieties, are highly sweetened and therefore are much higher in calories than is an equivalent amount of skim milk. Although cottage cheese has high nutritive value, it also has a higher caloric density than does skim milk. Therefore, if large portions of cottage cheese are eaten in addition to the usual diet, weight gain could result. Table 4.3 shows how different forms of yogurt and cottage cheese compare to milk with regard to caloric density and content of energy nutrients.

Meat group Animal products in the meat group are a major source of calories in the diets of Americans. Those lowest in caloric density are those low in fat, such as fish, turkey, and veal. Different cuts of beef, pork, and lamb vary widely in fat content and therefore in caloric value. Hot dogs, bologna, and similar processed meat products tend to be especially high in

calories relative to their content of essential nutrients. Peanut butter and nuts are high in fat and therefore in caloric density.

No one food is accurately described by the term "fattening." Food is fattening only if eaten in excess of caloric requirement. With careful planning and with appropriate adjustment of portion sizes, any food could be included in a diet for weight maintenance. Moderation and control are required.

POINTS OF EMPHASIS
Controlling food intake

• *Pay attention to internal cues for eating, especially those which indicate fullness.*
• *Alter the environment when possible to reduce cues which lead to use of food for non-nutritive purposes.*
• *Learn to respond to external food cues by an activity which does not involve eating.*
• *Use the Daily Food Guide as a foundation diet, avoiding excessive use of fats, sugars, alcohol, and other foods of high caloric and low nutritive density.*

EXERCISING FOR MAINTENANCE

ENERGY EXPENDITURE

Increasing physical activity can be a very constructive, healthful means of promoting energy balance. Even small changes in physical activity can have large effects on body weight over a period of time. This is reflected in the following example.

Bob has been a few kilograms overweight for the past several years. He decides to increase his energy expenditure by going up and down stairs instead of tak-

TABLE 4.3 *Energy value and selected nutrient content of some dairy products*

| FOOD | KCAL | AMOUNT IN 100 GM PORTION* | | |
		PROTEIN GM	FAT GM	CARBOHYDRATE GM
Skim milk	35	3	—	5
Lowfat milk, 1% fat with nonfat milk solids added	43	4	1	5
Whole milk	61	3	3	5
Lowfat yogurt, plain	63	5	2	7
Fruit-flavored yogurt	99–105	4–5	1	19
Lowfat cottage cheese	90	14	2	4
Creamed cottage cheese	103	13	5	3

* 100 gm of any of these foods has a volume of approximately 100 ml or slightly less than ½ cup.

ing the elevator at work. He makes quite a few trips in the course of the day and his energy expenditure goes up by 100 kcal. per day, 5 days a week. He does not change his food intake. At the end of a week he has an energy deficit of 500 kcal., which is not enough to show up on the scale. However, at the end of 7 weeks he has a deficit of 3500 kcal, the equivalent of 0.41 kg. (1 lb.) of body fat. At the end of the year he is pleased to find that he has lost about 3.2 kg. (7 lb.) without having to diet.

Unfortunately, many individuals find themselves in the opposite situation. Because they are gradually decreasing their level of physical activity without also decreasing their caloric intake, their body weight increases. Omitting only 100 kcal. worth of exercise daily results in gain of approximately 4.5 kg. (10 lb.) per year. America's problem of overweight is, to a significant extent, one of underexercising rather than of overeating. Compared to Americans 50 years ago, today's average American eats *less*. Today's average American is fatter not because of gluttony, but because caloric expenditure has decreased more than has caloric intake.

Physical exercise of certain types can produce dramatic changes in energy balance. Jogging, walking briskly, jumping rope, riding a bicycle, and other relatively vigorous activities can result in the expenditure of a significant amount of energy in a relatively short time, as indicated in the example of Bob.

EFFECTS OF EXERCISE ON APPETITE

Many people think of exercise as self-defeating when trying to control weight because they associate increase in exercise with increase in appetite. This does not always hold true. Animals confined to small pens so that they cannot exercise overeat and "fatten for the slaughter." Their appetite is no longer regulated to their caloric requirements. People who have a sedentary lifestyle experience a similar problem. If these same people incorporate a moderate amount of physical exercise into their daily routine, appetite will generally increase or decrease according to the need for fuel. If they exercise to the point of exhaustion, they will probably experience a decrease in appetite.

EFFECTS OF EXERCISE ON EATING BEHAVIORS

There are some additional reasons why food intake is apt to be under better control when relatively vigorous exercise is part of the daily routine. The individual who feels a commitment to exercise avoids eating very much for at least an hour or two prior to the activity. (No one wants to jog or play handball on a full stomach!) As an extra bonus, the appetite is curbed for a while following the exercise because of a temporary decrease in the blood supply to the gastrointestinal tract. Competitive individuals may also become moti-

vated to eat less and lose excess fat in hopes that their performance will improve.

Exercise provides a healthful way of releasing tension. When exercise makes an individual feel more relaxed and able to cope with problems, use of food for non-nutritive purposes may decrease. The overall effect of exercise on eating behavior is often curtailment of the amount of food eaten and avoidance of eating at inappropriate times.

POINTS OF EMPHASIS
Beneficial effects of exercise in weight control

• *Energy expenditure is increased by exercise.*
• *Physiological control of appetite is apt to correspond closely to actual caloric need.*
• *Eating is a less attractive option before, during, and immediately after the exercise period.*
• *Tension is released, leaving an individual better able to cope with problems.*
• *Muscles are firmed, contributing to a better appearance.*

# of Cal for body at rest

STUDY QUESTIONS

1. Is a calorie (kcal.) a nutrient? Explain.
2. A person has been maintaining his weight by eating 2400 kcal. daily. If his food intake remains the same but he increases his energy expenditure by 200 kcal. per day, how much change in body fat can be anticipated after one month?
3. Distinguish between nutrient density and caloric density of dark-green leafy vegetables.
4. What is meant by the phrase "high in empty calories"?
5. From the standpoint of weight control, is it helpful to substitute molasses or honey for sugar? Explain.
6. When trying to keep from gaining weight, is it advisable to eat unlimited amounts of fruits? Explain.
7. Why is it inaccurate to say that potatoes and bread are fattening?
8. Many people think that exercise does not help control weight because it takes prolonged, very-strenuous physical activity to lose a measurable amount of weight. What significant facts are they overlooking?

References

1. Bray, G. A.: The risks and disadvantages of obesity. In L. H. Smith (ed.): *Major Problems in Internal Medicine*, Vol. 9. *The Obese Patient*. Philadelphia: W. B. Saunders Co., 1976, p. 306.
*2. Crowley, A.: The stigma and cost of obesity. *Diet. Currents* 3:24, 1976.
3. Hathaway, M. L., and Foard, E. D.: *Heights and Weights of Adults in the United States*. USDA Agriculture Research Service, Home Economics Research

Report #10. Washington DC: U.S. Gov. Printing Office, 1960.

4. U.S. Senate, Select Committee on Nutrition and Human Needs. Statement of Dr. Johanna Dwyer, New England Medical Center, Boston, MA. *Diet Related to Killer Diseases, II. Obesity.* Washington DC: U.S. Govt. Printing Office, 1977, p. 70.

5. U.S. Senate, Select Committee on Nutrition and Human Needs. Statement of Dr. Theodore van Itallie, St. Luke's Hospital Center, New York. *Diet Related to Killer Diseases, II. Obesity.* Washington DC: U.S. Govt. Printing Office, 1977, p. 44.

6. Garn, S., and Clark, D.: Trends in fatness and the origins of obesity. *Pediatrics* 57:443, 1976.

7. Sims, E. A. H.: Experimental obesity, dietary induced thermogenesis, and their clinical implications. *Clin. Endocrin. Metab.* 5:377, 1976.

*8. Bray, G. A.: Treatment of the obese patient: Use of diet and exercise. In L. H. Smith (ed.): *Major Problems in Internal Medicine,* Vol. 9: *The Obese Patient.* Philadelphia: W. B. Saunders Co., 1976.

9. Wittwer, A. J., et al.: Nutrient density—Evaluation of nutritional attributes of foods. *J. Nutr. Ed.* 9:26, 1977.

10. Pennington, J. A.: *Dietary Nutrient Guide.* Westport CT: Avi Publishing Co., 1976.

* Recommended reading

5

Meeting nutrient needs by means of a prudent diet

The role of nutrition in preventive health care encompasses more than prevention of obesity and nutrient deficiencies. Evidence is accumulating that an "overabundant" diet contributes substantially to the high incidence of six of the ten leading causes of death in the U.S., namely, heart disease, cancer, stroke and hypertension, diabetes mellitus, arteriosclerosis, and cirrhosis of the liver. Because these diseases have been related to diet and other aspects of current lifestyle in technologically advanced nations, they are sometimes called "diseases of overabundance." These diseases account for a large percentage of disability and premature death in the American population. Some less serious but very widespread diseases such as dental caries (tooth decay) and diverticulosis (a disorder of the large intestine) have also been related to diets typical of technologically developed nations.

All of the diseases of overabundance have serious impact not only on individuals and their families but also on the population as a whole. They affect the economy in general and the cost of health care in particular. Prevention if it can be achieved is potentially the least costly method and the best scientific strategy in the control of these diseases. Diet may play a large part in the preventive approach.

During a series of hearings,[1-5] the Senate Select Committee on Nutrition and Human Needs* focused attention on nutrition as an aspect of preventive health care. In testimony before this committee, experts from

---

* This committee has been disbanded. Its activities are being continued by a subcommittee of the Senate Agriculture Committee.

the health field stated that the major nutritional problems of Americans are related to overnutrition (excessive intake of certain types of nutrients and of calories) rather than to nutrient deficiency. Some of them expressed concern about the increased proportion of calories which sugar and fat contribute to Americans' diets. The decline in consumption of starch, as in potatoes and grains, was also noted as probably undesirable. Brewster and Jacobsen[6] summarize many trends in American eating habits.

A number of doctors and nutritionists recommended to the Senate Select Committee that Americans make "prudent" changes in their diet such as decreasing intake of fat, sugar, and salt. They based their recommendations on evidence suggesting that such changes may reduce risk of developing "diseases of overabundance." They pointed out that one cannot say, "If you make prudent changes in your diet, you will not develop heart disease or cancer or. . . ." Nonetheless the committee's consultants stated that the benefits of making certain dietary changes are likely to be numerous and there are no known risks for older children and adults. (A few of the suggested diet changes are not recommended for young children.)

TYPES OF EVIDENCE LINKING DIET WITH DISEASE

Controversies surround the relationships of diet with disease; therefore health professionals should be aware of the types of studies upon which conclusions are based.

RETROSPECTIVE STUDIES

The available evidence which indicts diet as a major contributor to disease is primarily epidemiological. (Epidemiology is the study of how often and in which individuals diseases occur in a population.) Epidemiologists conduct retrospective studies to try to find out if a population affected by a specific disease is different in some way from the general population. In retrospective studies they compile statistics of existing data and look for clues as to what the causative agent *might* be.

An example can illustrate the process. Suppose that populations typically consuming a high sugar diet have a much higher incidence of dental caries than populations typically consuming little or no sugar (Fig. 5.1). The information shown in Figure 5.1 would be accurately interpreted by saying that eating sugar is highly or positively correlated with the incidence of dental caries.

Does correlation mean causation? Not necessarily. The two could appear together as a result of coincidence. It could be that something else is causing both dental caries and high sugar intake as illustrated in Figure 5.2. Although correlation does not necessarily mean causation, if positive correlation is not present causation is highly unlikely.

PROSPECTIVE STUDIES

Since epidemiologists recognize the limitations of retrospective studies, they may design prospective studies to further test a *hypothesis* (an idea that has been proposed regarding a relationship between two things). A prospective study to test the hypothesis that sugar causes dental caries might be set up along the following lines:

1. Select a population of "sugar eaters" to be studied over a period of time.
2. Select a population of "sugar avoiders" to serve as a control.*
3. At predetermined intervals collect data regarding the number of caries and sugar intake.
4. Compare the incidence of dental caries with the actual sugar intake of individuals over a period of time.

If the statistics show a very high correlation between sugar intake and incidence of dental caries, causation has still not been proven but the information is more definitive. If the sugar-eating habits of the two groups were reversed (sugar avoiders begin eating sugar and

---

* A control group is necessary because it is possible that other factors influence the number of caries. According to the hypothesis it would be expected that there would be no change in the number of caries in sugar avoiders. A significant increase in caries in this control group would indicate the need to look for additional variables.

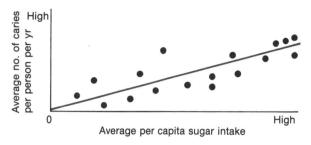

FIGURE 5.1. Hypothetical relationship between sugar intake and incidence of dental caries.

vice versa) and the same relationship between sugar intake and caries were obtained, the data would be very convincing indeed.

METABOLIC STUDIES

One of the advantages of prospective studies is that *metabolic* studies may be conducted simultaneously on the same populations to try to determine *why* a certain type of diet or dietary factor is positively correlated with a given disease. In metabolic studies, measurements are made to determine whether or not physical, physiological, or microbiological changes are occurring in living subjects. Using the example of sugar and tooth decay once again, the debris on the teeth of the individuals in a metabolic study might be examined for a substance which could dissolve tooth enamel. If such a substance were found on the teeth of the sugar eaters but not on the teeth of the sugar avoiders, the evidence supporting sugar as a causative factor in the production of tooth decay would have a logical explanation.

The possibility that another unrecognized factor is the real causative agent of tooth decay would not have been ruled out by the previously mentioned metabolic study. If feasible, the hypothesis would be further tested in carefully controlled human metabolic studies in which the only variable was sugar content of the diet. If the results of these studies supported the previous work, controversy surrounding the relationship between the diet and the disease would fade.

Metabolic studies can sometimes reveal if a physiological or microbiological response to a particular diet can explain the correlation between diet and a disease, but results must be interpreted with caution. Because many experimental difficulties occur when working with humans, laboratory animals are often used for metabolic studies instead. In some cases these animals differ from humans in very significant physiological

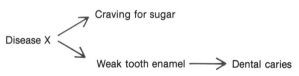

FIGURE 5.2. Conceivable relationship between dental caries and sugar intake.

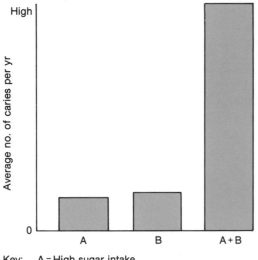

Key: A = High sugar intake

        B = Genetic defect resulting in weak tooth enamel

FIGURE 5.3. Hypothetical relationship between risk factors and the incidence of dental caries showing multifactorial effect.

ways. Thus it is difficult, if not impossible, to *prove* that diet Y is a causative agent for disease Z. One can only try to draw valid inferences from the data and use these as a basis for deciding whether to modify behavior or not.

Risk factors

It can be inferred from many epidemiological and metabolic studies that diet may be a *risk factor* in the development of certain types of cardiovascular disease

and cancer, diabetes mellitus, cirrhosis of the liver, and dental caries. Risk factors for a disease increase the odds that a person will develop that condition.

Multifactorial risk factors are risk factors appearing to interact in the individual. As a result, the chance of developing a particular disease is greatly increased when two or more of the multifactorial risk factors are present. This is illustrated in Figure 5.3.

Dietary practices which have been identified as risk factors for diseases of overabundance are indicated in Figure 5.4. Brief summaries of evidence supporting some of these correlations follow.

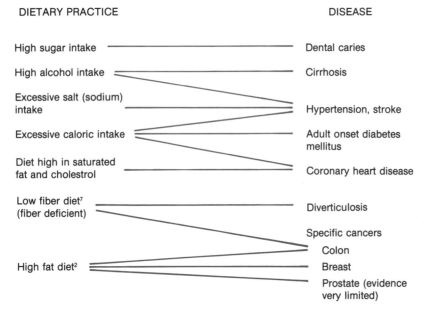

FIGURE 5.4. Dietary practices which have been positively correlated with diseases of overabundance.

DIET AND DISEASES OF OVERABUNDANCE

CIRRHOSIS

A relationship between chronic alcoholism and cirrhosis of the liver has been demonstrated by both retrospective and prospective epidemiological studies. Heavy alcohol use over a period of time tends to result in fatty deposits in the liver and damage to liver cells. In controlled studies, primates fed high levels of alcohol have developed cirrhosis.[8] Not every heavy user of alcohol develops cirrhosis but the risk is high (about 10 to 20 percent).[9] The consequences of cirrhosis are grave, often terminating in untimely death. Efforts should be made to promote moderation in the use of alcohol (or abstinence) to prevent this serious illness.

HYPERTENSION

It is estimated that 20 percent of the adult American population has high blood pressure, with a much higher rate in black Americans and in older age groups.[10]

Various studies have linked hypertension with high salt (sodium chloride) ingestion,[10–12] obesity,[13] and use of alcohol.[14] Metabolic studies with experimental animals indicate that *genetic susceptibility* is required for excessive salt ingestion to result in high blood pressure. Lack of genetic susceptibility may explain why many individuals who make liberal use of salty foods have no problem with their blood pressure.[10]

Hypertension often goes undetected because it causes no discomfort in the early stages. Nonetheless, it begins to harm the body in subtle but serious ways. Hypertension is the most significant risk factor in the development of stroke. It also increases the risk of coronary heart disease. Once high blood pressure has been initiated, it may or may not be completely reversible by changing diet. However, salt restriction[15] and weight loss [16,17] are likely to help reduce hypertension. Presently there is no way to determine if a person is susceptible to hypertension as a result of excessive salt, calorie, or alcohol intake. A family history of hypertension increases the risk that a person will develop this disorder. Limiting intake of salt and alcohol and controlling body weight are prudent methods of reducing the risk of developing hypertension. Meneely[10] suggests that high potassium intake affords some protection as well, by helping to offset deleterious effects of salt.

MATURITY ONSET DIABETES MELLITUS

Retrospective studies indicate that the incidence of maturity onset diabetes mellitus increases with increases in body weight. Overweight by itself does not cause diabetes; a genetic defect is probably involved. Metabolic studies support the view that physiological differences in obese individuals favor the development of diabetes.

CORONARY HEART DISEASE

The role of diet in the development of coronary heart disease has been the subject of great controversy for many years. The nutritional factors which have been most strongly implicated are the type and amount of fatty substances in the diet. The general term "lipid" is often used when referring to fatty substances. Fatty substances which may be relevant to heart disease are described here.

Cholesterol is a lipid normally manufactured (synthesized) in the body by the liver; therefore a dietary supply is not required. Cholesterol and other chemicals made from it are essential for many body processes, such as the functioning of the brain. The amount of cholesterol present in the blood varies with diet, stress, and other conditions. A high blood cholesterol level is one of the three most important risk factors in coronary heart disease. (The two other major risk factors are hypertension and cigarette smoking.) Eating foods high in cholesterol content tends to increase blood cholesterol level. Cholesterol is found *only* in animal products, associated with the fat they contain.

Saturated fats and oils include hard fats such as butterfat, meat and egg fat, coconut oil, and some shortenings. Human metabolic studies have shown that a diet high in saturates tends to increase the level of cholesterol circulating in the blood.

Polyunsaturated oils are characteristically liquid, even at cold temperatures. They include corn, cottonseed, soybean, safflower, sunflower, and fish oils. Polyunsaturated oils tend to *decrease* the amount of cholesterol circulating in the blood.

Monounsaturated fats and oils are present in all fats and oils, but are especially abundant in peanuts, olives, and the oils made from them. Monounsaturates have little influence on blood cholesterol levels.

Hydrogenated or partially hydrogenated (hardened) fats are more saturated (harder) than the oils from which they were made. Hydrogenation is a chemical process which decreases the level of polyunsaturates in a fat. Shortening is usually a partially hydrogenated vegetable oil.

P/S value or ratio refers to the amount of polyunsaturated fat compared to the amount of saturated fact in the diet. A value of 1 (1:1) means that the diet provides equal amounts of each type of fat. A value of 1:1 is considered to be a prudent ratio. A P/S value of 0.25 (1:4) is more typical of the usual American diet.

Epidemiological and metabolic evidence is "very suggestive" that a high fat, high cholesterol diet containing a high proportion of saturated fat increases the risk of a high blood cholesterol level, which in turn increases the risk of developing atherosclerosis and coronary heart disease in susceptible individuals. The risk of developing heart disease is magnified when high blood cholesterol level is accompanied by cigarette smoking or hypertension. If all three risk factors are present, the risk is high indeed.

CANCER

Cancer is initiated by carcinogens (cancer-causing substances). Carcinogens may be present in a variety of forms in the general environment (e.g., air, water, food, dust). It appears that most, if not all, carcinogens are inactive in the usual form in which they occur in the environment. Upon entering the body they may be converted to a form which is more active in the initiation of cancer. Diet may influence the extent to which these conversions take place and/or the sensitivity of specific organs or tissues to the action of carcinogens. Reasearch to date suggests that diet may have opposing effects—both protective and predisposing. The

likelihood that a person will develop certain types of cancer may partially depend on the balance between these two factors.[18] Different types of cancer appear to be influenced by dietary components in different ways.

Cancer of the breast Cancer of the breast is the leading cause of death among women in the U.S. Epidemiologists have been looking for clues explaining differences in breast cancer incidence among nations and some have found that fat content of the diet is highly correlated.[19] Some suspect that the recent dramatic rise in breast cancer in Japanese is due to a change from a low to a high fat diet.[20]*

Since hormone levels are thought to be involved in some types of tumorigenesis (formation and growth of a tumor), metabolic studies have been conducted to investigate the effects of fat intake on hormone levels, e.g., prolactin level.[21,22]

* While the incidence of breast cancer has increased, the incidence of gastric cancer has markedly decreased. This has been linked with other diet changes.

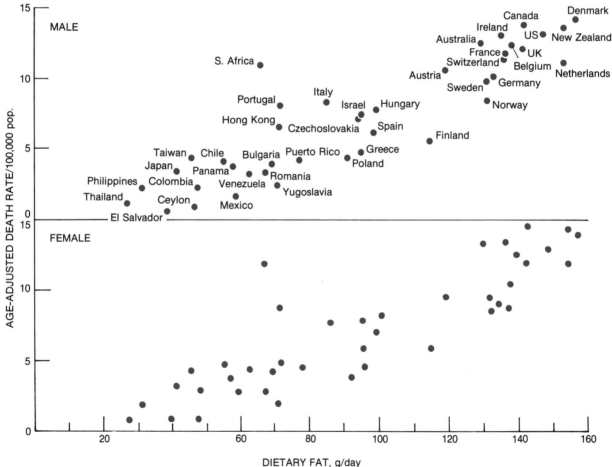

FIGURE 5.5 Positive correlation between per caput consumption of dietary fat and age-adjusted mortality from cancer of the intestine (except rectum). (From Wynder, E. L.: The epidemiology of large bowel cancer. *Cancer Res.* 35:3388, 1975. Used with permission)

The relationship between diet and breast cancer is certainly not clear-cut. For example, there are cultural groups within the U.S., such as American Indians in the Southwest and Mormons residing in Utah, who have low incidence of breast cancer even though their dietary fat intake is not low.

Cancer of the colon Cancer of the colon is second only to lung cancer as a cause of cancer death among American males and is one of the leading causes of death among American women. Incidence of cancer of the colon in populations has been positively correlated with fat content of the diet[23] (Fig. 5.5).

The possibility that fat influences development of colon cancer gains support both from limited metabolic studies[24-26] and from the observation that Japanese immigrants to America who have adopted Western dietary habits have correspondingly experienced increased incidence of colon cancer.[27]

Fat is not the only dietary component that has been correlated with cancer of the colon. Risk appears to increase with *decreasing* fiber intake and with increasing meat intake. Data may be biased by poor reporting of the disease in developing countries.[28] Interpretation of the data is complicated by the fact that there are different types of dietary fiber and that measurement of fiber content of diets tends to be quite inaccurate.[29] Also the difference between a high and low fiber diet usually involves much more than fiber (e.g., high fiber diets are usually low fat diets which are low in meat.)

The hypotheses, as yet unproven, are that fiber protects against colon cancer by one or more of the following means:[29] (1) causing dilution of any carcinogens which may be present, since the water content of the stool tends to be higher on a high fiber diet and fiber can bind bile acids and other substances; (2) decreasing the time for development and/or absorption of carcinogens by decreasing the time the stool remains in the colon; (3) altering the bacterial flora which may be responsible for the production of carcinogens; and (4) reducing formation of potential carcinogens from bile acids.

Well-designed, large-scale prospective studies are needed to prove that changes in diet will reduce incidence of certain types of cancer. Although these are lacking, many consumers may decide that they wish to make prudent diet changes based on information already available. Decreasing fat intake and using more whole grains, fruits, and vegetables are considered to be prudent measures. Health professionals should be aware that using *excessive* fiber (i.e., fiber supplements such as wood pulp or large servings of bran) is not prudent since it might adversely affect nutritional status by decreasing absorption of nutrients.

DIVERTICULOSIS

Diverticulosis of the colon is a condition in which portions of the intestinal wall protrude in pouchlike projections. As with colon cancer, diverticulosis has been negatively correlated with fiber intake. Diverticulosis is reported to be virtually unknown in some parts of the world where fiber intake is high, but it is very common in the U.S., Britain, and other nations where fiber intake is low. Again there are questions about interpretation of the epidemiological data.

Painter and Burkett[30] suggest that increasing the bulk of the stool helps prevent diverticulosis. High bulk increases the diameter of the colon which may decrease pressure within the colon. Theoretically, lowering pressure would reduce the chance that diverticula (pouches) would be forced through any weak regions of the intestinal wall. This remains to be proven. There is conflicting evidence regarding relationships between fiber intake and diverticulosis.

POINTS OF EMPHASIS
Diet and diseases of overabundance

• *High fat intake has been linked with coronary heart disease and with breast and colon cancer—leading causes of death in America.*

• *Because of their high caloric density, high fat diets might indirectly contribute to obesity.*

• *Obesity has been linked with a number of disease conditions.*

• *High intake of salt, sugar, and alcohol and low intake of fiber have also been linked with diseases which are common in America.*

• *Evidence linking diet with disease is largely based on retrospective epidemiological studies. Some metabolic studies support the findings but the evidence is inconclusive.*

• *Results of well-designed, large-scale prospective studies must be available before definite conclusions can be reached about diet in relation to diseases of overabundance.*

• *Until more definitive information is available, many nutrition authorities recommend following a prudent diet.*

DIETARY GOALS FOR THE U.S.

The Senate Select Committee on Nutrition and Human Needs released a report entitled *Dietary Goals for the United States* in February 1977.[31] This report generated considerable public debate.[32,33] It was followed by a second edition of the goals in December 1977.[34] Both reports were based on the Senate hearings previously mentioned, consultation with a variety of experts in health care (primarily physicians and nutritionists), and a review of guidelines published by governmental and professional groups in the U.S. and in eight other technologically developed nations. The second version follows.

U.S. Dietary Goals[35]

1. To avoid overweight, consume only as much energy (calories) as is expended; if overweight, decrease energy intake and increase energy expenditure.
2. Increase the consumption of complex carbohydrates and "naturally occurring" sugars from about 28 percent of energy intake to about 48 percent of energy intake.
3. Reduce the consumption of refined and processed sugars by about 45 percent to account for about 10 percent of total energy intake.
4. Reduce overall fat consumption from approximately 40 percent to about 30 percent of energy intake.
5. Reduce saturated fat consumption to account for about 10 percent of total energy intake; and balance that with poly-unsaturated and mono-unsaturated fats, which should account for about 10 percent of energy intake each.
6. Reduce cholesterol consumption to about 300 mg. a day.
7. Limit the intake of sodium by reducing the intake of salt to about 5 gram a day.

The Goals Suggest the Following Changes in Food Selection and Preparation:

1. Increase consumption of fruits and vegetables and whole grains.
2. Decrease consumption of refined and other processed sugars and foods high in such sugars.
3. Decrease consumption of foods high in total fat, and partially replace saturated fats, whether obtained from animal or vegetable sources, with polyunsaturated fats.
4. Decrease consumption of animal fat, and choose meats, poultry and fish which will reduce saturated fat intake.
5. Except for young children, substitute low-fat and non-fat milk for whole milk, and low-fat dairy products for high fat dairy products.
6. Decrease consumption of butterfat, eggs and other high cholesterol sources. Some consideration should be given to easing the cholesterol goal for premenopausal women, young children and the elderly in order to obtain the nutritional benefits of eggs in the diet.
7. Decrease consumption of salt and foods high in salt content.

Dietary Goals are not meant to be rigid rules but are meant to indicate a healthful direction which people might take when deciding how they want to eat.

One of the effects of following the dietary guidelines might be an increased consumption of some micronutrients because of increased use of unrefined foods. This would help assure adequate intake of essential nutrients, including those for which there are few data regarding amount needed and their bioavailability. Following the guidelines would also result in increased fiber intake. For many Americans meeting the exact percentages set in Dietary Goals for fat and carbohydrate would result in a considerable decrease in intake of animal products from the meat group. Information from studies of vegetarians[36-38] suggests that this need not adversely affect the status of iron nutrition—a concern of many health professionals.

A child or teenager could not follow Basic Four recommendations for milk and meat group intake and meet Dietary Goals at the same time. (Individuals from these age groups would have less carbohydrate and more protein than recommended in Dietary Goals.) Most consumers would find some of the goals very difficult to work with, but the suggestions for food selection and preparation should help them in making prudent choices.

It is important to clarify what is meant by reducing risk. Those consumers who choose to reduce risk by making prudent diet changes may want more practical suggestions than are included with Dietary Goals. Some guidelines follow.

PLANNING A WELL-BALANCED, PRUDENT DIET

Food selection

To help assure nutritive adequacy, Dietary Goals can be used in conjunction with the Basic Four food groups. Recommendations still apply regarding vitamin D, iodine, fluoride, iron, and other nutrients for which adequacy of intake is of concern. Table 5.1 lists prudent food choices for each food group.

Foods which are limited are placed in categories according to the reason for the limitation. This division can help to guide individuals who are more concerned about reducing *particular* risks rather than risks in general. The amounts of foods specified in Table 5.1 will not provide enough calories for weight maintenance for most adults but should otherwise allow for nutritional adequacy. The section "Foods to choose when extra calories are needed for weight maintenance" is important if the balance of the diet is to be maintained. Adhering to these guidelines will not necessarily result in complete conformity with the Dietary Goals but should approach them. It is particularly important to plan for *nutritional adequacy* even if it means that goals will not be exactly met. Table 5.2 shows one possible combination of foods for a prudent diet.

Additional suggestions for decreasing intake of salt, sugar, and fat

1. Use herbs, spices, lemon, and other natural seasonings in place of salt or salted seasonings.
2. Learn simple methods of preparing foods from basic ingredients. Avoid salty commercially prepared foods.
3. Learn to enjoy the natural sweetness and the interesting flavors and textures of fruits in place of desserts loaded with sugar and fat.
4. Try recipes for desserts that are low in sugar and fat. Use spices to enhance sweetness.
5. Try ice water or fruit juice in place of carbonated beverages.

6. Choose cereals which are not obviously sugared, and gradually decrease the amount of sugar you sprinkle on them (if you can't cut sugar out all at once). Try adding chopped dried or fresh fruit to cereal for interest.

7. Experiment with vegetables to find ways to use them more often. Try some of them raw (spinach salad, raw cauliflower, turnip slices, green beans) for a new taste and texture.

8. To make the transition to skim milk easier, add

TABLE 5.1 *Guidelines for choosing foods for a prudent diet*

CHOOSE	LIMIT			
BREAD AND CEREAL GROUP	*HIGH IN SALT*	*HIGH IN FAT*	*HIGH IN SUGAR*	*REDUCED IN FIBER BUT LOW IN SALT, FAT, AND SUGAR*
Use more than four servings daily Use *whole grain* products frequently, such as Whole wheat bread Oatmeal Rye crackers Brown rice Shredded wheat	Corn chips Pretzels Salted crackers Commercially seasoned rice, noodle, and stuffing mixes		Pastries Doughnuts Commercial granola Presweetened breakfast cereals	Refined grains and the products made from them such as: White rice or rice flour Farina Degerminated cornmeal or cornflour Oat flour White wheat flour
FRUIT AND VEGETABLE GROUP	*HIGH IN SALT*	*HIGH IN FAT*	*HIGH IN SUGAR*	*REDUCED IN FIBER*
Use more than four servings daily, including good sources of vitamins A and C Fresh fruits and vegetables, frequently raw Unsweetened frozen and canned fruits Dried fruits Unseasoned frozen vegetables	Potato chips and sticks Commercially-prepared vegetables in sauce Pickled vegetables Regular canned vegetables and vegetable juices	French fries and other fried vegetables	Sweetened canned and frozen fruit and fruit juices	Fruit juices Peeled fruits and vegetables Instant mashed potatoes
MILK GROUP	*HIGH IN SALT*	*HIGH IN FAT**		*HIGH IN SUGAR*
Servings vary with age group. For adults 2 servings Fortified skim (nonfat) milk: fresh, dry or evaporated Lowfat milk (fresh or dry) Lowfat cheeses such as: Cottage cheese Part skim mozarella Sapsago Farmers Plain lowfat yogurt	Processed cheese and cheese foods Salty natural cheeses such as bleu, camembert Most buttermilk	Sweetened condensed milk Ice cream Fountain drinks made with ice cream Malted milk Cream cheese Natural cheddar cheese and most other natural cheeses Sour Cream Whole milk (fresh, evaporated, or dry)		Commercially flavored yogurt Ice milk

Continued on next page

TABLE 5.1 *Guidelines for choosing foods for a prudent diet (Continued)*

MEAT GROUP	HIGH IN SALT	HIGH IN FAT†	HIGH IN CHOLESTEROL

Limit servings of animal products to about 170 gm (6 oz) daily
 	
Fresh or frozen animal products
Most often:
  fish, poultry (no skin), veal, egg whites, egg substitutes, shellfish except shrimp
Less often:
  lean meats—beef, pork, lamb
Plant products
  dried peas, beans, lentils
	Lunch meats
	Sausage
	Corned beef
	Canned meats
	Processed meat main dishes
	Salted nuts
	
	Ham
	Canned fish (i.e. tuna, sardines)
	Chipped beef
	Canned chili or baked beans‡
	Meat analogs (simulated ham, bacon, etc.)
		Duck
		Goose
		Fatty meats
		Unsalted nuts
			Eggs—limit to 3 (yolks) per week
			
			Shrimp
			Organ meats—
			Use occasionally
			Decrease number of egg yolks that week

FOR EXTRA CALORIES, IF NEEDED FOR WEIGHT MAINTENANCE, CHOOSE	HIGH IN CHOLESTEROL	HIGH IN SATURATED FAT	HIGH IN SUGAR
Extra servings from the bread and cereal and fruit and vegetable groups More fat-free milk More legumes, lentils, nuts Polyunsaturated fats in moderation Oils—corn, cottonseed, soybean, safflower, sunflower Margarine Mayonnaise, salad dressing	Animal fats Butter Cream Bacon§ Salt Pork§	Chocolate Coconut Solid shortenings Chocolate Most non-dairy creamers	candy Sweetened coconut Caramels All types of sugar Jam Jelly Honey Syrups Most candies not mentioned above

* All milk products high in fat are also relatively high in cholesterol
† Animal products high in fat are also relatively high in cholesterol
‡ High in sugar
§ High in salt

TABLE 5.2 *Sample menus for a prudent diet that approaches Dietary Goals (ed. 2)*

BREAKFAST	LUNCH	DINNER
½ fresh grapefruit 240 ml oatmeal with raisins 120 ml skim milk Pumpernickel toast or a pumpernickel bagel with margarine* Hot beverage, black *(when desired)* 120 ml skim milk Graham crackers	1½ peanut butter and jelly sandwich on whole grain bread Carrot, celery, and green pepper strips Fresh fruit 240 ml skim milk	85 gm extra-lean ground beef, broiled Large baked potato Steamed spinach with nutmeg Whole wheat rolls Margarine* Tossed salad with oil* and vinegar dressing Fresh fruit

* Total visible fats and oils ± 30 ml (2 Tbsp), depending on caloric requirement.

increasing amounts of it to the whole milk you are used to drinking. Serve very cold. Skim milk used in place of whole milk gives good results in nearly all recipes.

9. Decrease use of fat in cooking and at the table. Skim all the fat off of meat drippings before making gravy. Experiment with fat-free sauces.

10. Cook lean meat and poultry in such a way that excess fat will be lost, as broiling, roasting, or simmering. These are also good methods for cooking fish.

11. Try casseroles as a way of reducing portion size of meat.

12. If desired, try one of the commercial egg substitutes for scrambled eggs, omelets, and other cooking purposes. Try cooking with egg whites in place of whole eggs and feed the yolks to a dog or cat (they handle cholesterol differently than people do).

STUDY QUESTIONS

1. What is a major limitation of using food consumption data to determine how people eat?

2. Why are results of prospective epidemiological studies more valid for drawing conclusions than are results of retrospective studies?

3. What does the following statement mean? "Incidence of stomach cancer has been found to be negatively correlated with ingestion of large amounts of smoked meat and fish."

4. Identify possible advantages and potential drawbacks of making prudent diet changes.

5. What characteristics of foods influence whether they are encouraged or discouraged for a person who is trying to follow a prudent diet?

References

1. *Nutrition and Health.* U.S. Senate Select Committee on Nutrition and Human Needs. Washington DC: U.S. Govt. Printing Office, December 1975.

2. *Diet Related to Killer Diseases.* U.S. Senate Select Committee on Nutrition and Human Needs. Washington DC: U.S. Govt. Printing Office, July 27, 28, 1976.

3. *Diet and Killer Diseases with Press Reaction and Additional Information.* U.S. Senate Select Committee on Nutrition and Human Needs. Washington DC: U.S. Govt. Printing Office, January 1977.

4. *Diet Related to Killer Diseases, II—Part 1. Cardiovascular Disease.* Washington DC: U.S. Govt. Printing Office, February 1, 2, 1977.

*5. *Diet Related to Killer Diseases, II—Part 2. Obesity.* U.S. Senate Select Committee on Nutrition and Human Needs. Washington DC: U.S. Govt. Printing Office, February, 1, 2, 1977.

*6. Brewster, L., and Jacobsen, M. F.: *The Changing American Diet.* Washington DC: Center for Science in the Public Interest, 1978.

7. Burkitt, D. P., and Trowell, H. C.: *Refined Carbohydrate Foods and Disease.* New York: Academic Press, 1975.

8. Lieber, C. S., DeCarli, L. M., and Ribin, E.: Sequential production of fatty liver, hepatitis, and cirrhosis in subhuman primates fed ethanol with adequate diets. *Proc. Natl. Acad. Sci. USA* 72:437, 1975.

9. LaMont, J. T., and Isselbacher, K. J.: Cirrhosis. In G. W. Thorn, et al. (eds.): *Harrison's Principles of Internal Medicine,* New York: McGraw-Hill Book Co., 1977. p. 301.

*10. Meneely, G. R., and Battarbee, H. D.: Sodium and potassium. *Nutr. Rev.* 34:225, 1976.

11. Prior, I. A. M.: The price of civilization. *Nutr. Today* 6(6):2, 1971.

12. Dahl, L. K.: Salt and hypertension. *Am. J. Clin. Nutr.* 25:231, 1972.

13. Bray, G.: The risks and disadvantages of obesity. In L. H. Smith (ed.): *Major Problems in Internal Medicine.* Vol. 9: *The Obese Patient.* Philadelphia: W. B. Saunders Co., 1976.

14. Klalsky, A. L., et al.: Alcohol consumption and blood pressure. *N. Engl. J. Med.* 296:1194, 1977.

*15. Morgan, T., et al.: Hypertension treated by salt restriction. *Lancet* 1:227, 1978.

*16. Reisin, E., et al.: Effect of weight loss without salt restriction on the reduction of blood pressure in overweight hypertensive patients. *N. Engl. J. Med.* 298:1, 1978.

*17. Ramsay, L. E., et al.: Weight reduction in a blood pressure clinic. *Brit. Med. J.* 2:244–245, 1978.

18. Alcantara, E. N., and Speckmann, E. W.: Diet, nutrition and cancer. *Am. J. Clin. Nutr.* 29:1035, 1976.

19. Hankin, J. H., and Rawlings, V.: Diet and breast cancer: a review. *Am. J. Clin. Nutr.* 31:2005, 1978.

20. Wynder, E. L. (statement of) in Senate Select Committee on Nutrition and Human Needs: *Diet Related to Killer Diseases.* Washington DC: U.S. Govt. Printing Office, July 27, 28, 1976, p. 198.

21. Hill, P., et al.: Diet and endocrine related cancer. *Cancer.* 39(4 Suppl):1820, 1977.

22. Chan, P. C., and Cohen, L. A.: Dietary fat and growth promotion of rat mammary tumors. *Cancer Res.* 35:3384, 1975.

23. Reddy, B. S., Mastromarino, A., and Wynder, E.: Diet and metabolism: Large-bowel cancer. *Cancer* 39:1815, 1977.

24. Reddy, B. S., Weisburger, J. I., and Wynder, E. L.: Effect of high risk and low risk diets for colon carcinogenesis of fecal microflora and steroids in man. *J. Nutr.* 105:878, 1975.

25. Reddy, B. S., et al.: Effect of quality and quantity of dietary fat and dimethylhydrazine in colon carcinogenesis in rats (39181). *Proc. Soc. Exp. Biol. Med.* 151:237, 1976.

26. Reddy, B. S., and Wynder, E. L.: Metabolic epidemiology of colon cancer: fecal bile acids and neutral sterols in colon cancer patients and patients with adenomatous polyps. *Cancer* 39:2533, 1977.

27. Wynder, E. L., et al.: Environmental factors of cancer of the colon and rectum. II. Japanese epidemiological data. *Cancer* 23:1210, 1969.

28. Hegsted, D. M.: Food and Fibre: Evidence from experimental animals. *Nutr. Rev.* 35:45, 1977.

29. Huang, C. T. L., Gopalakrishna, G. S., and Nichols, B. L.: Fiber, intestinal sterols, and colon cancer. *Am. J. Clin. Nutr.* 31:516, 1978.

30. Painter, N. S., and Burkitt, D. P.: Diverticular disease of the colon: a deficiency disease of Western civilization. *Brit. Med. J.* 2:450, 1971.

31. *Dietary Goals for the United States.* U.S. Senate Select Committee on Nutrition and Human Needs. Washington DC: U.S. Printing Office, Feb. 1977.

32. Commentary. Dietary Goals: A statement by The American Dietetic Association. *J. Am. Diet. Assoc.* 71:227, 1977.

33. *Dietary Goals for the United States—Supplemental Views.* U.S. Senate Select Committee on Nutrition and Human Needs. Washington DC: U.S. Govt. Printing Office, November 1977.

*34. *Dietary Goals for the United States, 2.* U.S.

Senate Select Committee on Nutrition and Human Needs. Washington DC: U.S. Govt. Printing Office, December 1977.

35. *Dietary Goals for the United States,* ed. 2. U.S. Senate Select Committee on Nutrition and Human Needs. Washington DC: U.S. Govt. Printing Office, December 1977, p. 4.

36. Hardinge, M. G., and Stare, F. J.: Nutritional studies of vegetarians. 1. Nutritional, physical, and laboratory studies. *J. Clin. Nutr.* 2:73, 1954.

37. Ellis, F. R., and Mumford, P.: The nutritional status of vegans and vegetarians, *Symp. Proc.* 26:205, 1967.

38. Harland, B. F., and Peterson, M.: Nutritional status of lacto-ovo-vegetarian Trappist monks. *J. Am. Diet. Assoc.* 72:259, 1978.

* Recommended reading

6

Promoting sound eating habits in different sociocultural situations

Sound nutritional practices abound in different sociocultural groups. Health care providers need to look at the eating practices of others with an open mind. Those who take the time to investigate foodways and food behaviors of the people they serve often find that resulting knowledge and appreciation of the ways of others serve as keys to providing better health care.

The term *foodways* generally refers to ways in which a distinct group selects, prepares, consumes, and otherwise reacts to and uses portions of the available food supply. The term *food behavior* denotes the same kinds of activities, as carried out by an individual. Foodways influence food behaviors. The term *food pattern* usually refers to the characteristic daily diet of a group. To become acquainted with a culture it is more helpful to become familiar with food-related behavior (foodways) rather than to learn just the customary daily fare (food pattern).

Foodways and food behavior tend to be stable and are, therefore, often called *food habits*. The disadvantage of the use of the term "habit" is that it implies static rather than dynamic behavior. Foodways, food behavior, food habits—all are influenced by environmental, sociocultural, physiological, and psychological factors, as illustrated in Figure 6.1.

Groups and individuals can and do change their food habits under a variety of circumstances. This is readily seen by observing changes in a person's food preferences as he matures. It also becomes apparent when food items available today are compared to those available a generation ago.

America is unusually rich in its diversity of foodways and food behaviors. Diversity is due to a number of factors, including geographical location, culture, religious group affiliation, socioeconomic status, and the type of family unit.

Geographical regions of the U.S. have developed distinctive foodways which are quite obvious to visitors. In Texas, for example, chili con carne is a favorite of many families. This meat dish contains hot chili pepper, reflecting the influence of Mexican food ways. Vermonters might be unable to eat a "fiery" dish of chili. Texans, in turn, might react negatively to a Vermonter's custom of eating sugar on snow (boiled-down maple syrup poured over real snow) with pickles.

Culture has numerous effects on foodways and food behaviors. In the traditional sense, culture is a design for living within a society that is transmitted from generation to generation. Through the influence of culture an individual learns how people "should" behave in various situations.

Particular foods and eating behaviors are an integral part of the mosaic of culture. Culture influences what is considered to be acceptable food; the members of a group for whom specific foods are judged most suitable; appropriate methods of food handling, preparation, and storage; table manners; roles food plays in the lives of individuals and their families; purposes for which specific foods are used; attitudes toward eating; attitudes toward obesity and other aspects of body size; and attitudes about relationships of food and health. Cultural practices such as traditional food behaviors promote a sense of stability, security, and belongingness. These feelings provide motivation for maintaining traditional ways.

It can be important to clarify terms when speaking with a person of a different cultural background. A British mother who says she is going home to prepare tea for her children is referring to making an evening meal. "Danish" may mean pastry to one person and ham to another. "Beans" may mean green beans or a specific type of cooked dried beans. Table 6.1 describes assorted ethnic foods.

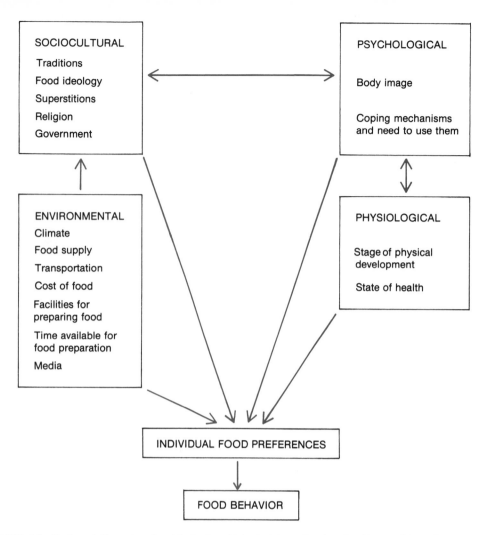

FIGURE 6.1. Factors influencing food behavior. (Adapted from Sanjur, D.: *Puerto Rican Food Habits: A Sociocultural Approach.* Ithaca NY: Cornell University, 1970)

TABLE 6.1 *Brief descriptions of an assortment of ethnic and regional foods*

GRAIN GROUP

Anadama: Cornmeal-molasses yeast bread (New England)

Bagels: Bread dough shaped like a donut, cooked in water, then baked. Chewy. (Jewish American)

Bulgur: Granular wheat product with nutlike flavor, served like rice. (Middle Eastern)

Brioche: Type of egg-rich French roll, often served at breakfast

Challah: Braided eggbread

Chapatis: Unleavened bread used by Indians

Croissants: Flaky crescent-shaped rolls (French)

Crumpets: Muffinlike product cooked on griddle. Often served toasted (British)

Grits: Coarsely ground hominy (Corn product) (Southern USA)

Johnny cake: corn bread (New England)

Kasha: Coarsely ground grain toasted before cooking in liquid

Latkes: Pancakes

Limpa: Rye bread (Swedish)

Mush: Cooked cereal (often cornmeal)

Pasta: Macaroni, spaghetti, noodles in variety of forms (Italian)

Polenta: Cornmeal (Italian)

Scones: Round, flat, unleavened, sweetened bread product (British)

Sopapillas: Fried bread (rich dough) (Mexican)

Tortillas: Thin rounds of leathery dough made from lime-treated corn or from wheat flour, often fried until crisp (Mexican)

FRUIT AND VEGETABLE GROUP

Bok choy: Green leafy, stalk-like vegetable (Oriental)

Chayote: Green or white squashlike vegetable eaten raw, cooked, or pickled (Mexican)

Dandelion greens: Young leaves from wild dandelion plants, eaten raw or cooked

Greens in "pot liquor" ("likor"): Green leafy vegetables such as kale or turnip, mustard or collard greens, cooked with salt pork, served with cooking liquid (Southern USA)

Jalapenos: Hot peppers

Kelp: Seaweed

Papaya: Large, yellow, melonlike tropical fruit

Prickly pear: Fruit of a cactus

Viandas: Starchy tropical vegetables such as sweet potato, cassava, plantain (banana-like in appearance) (Puerto-Rican)

MEAT GROUP

Adobo: Meat, soy sauce (Filipino)
Chitterlings: Pork intestine, tripe (Soul food)
Chorizo: Sausage (Mexican)
Escargots: Snails (French)
Falafel: Mashed chick peas mixed with other ingredients and fried (Israeli)

Feijoada: Blackbeans, meat (Brazilian)
Finnin haddie: Smoked haddock
Frijoles refritas: Refried pinto or calico beans (Mexican)
Gefilte fish: Ground or flaked fish seasoned and shaped into balls (Jewish American)
Hog maw: Stomach of pig (Southern USA)
Jerky: Dried meat strips

Kibee: Fresh raw lamb, ground, seasoned. Eaten uncooked (Middle Eastern)
Kielbasi: Polish sausage
Miso: Soybean paste
Pepperoni: Italian hot sausage
Sauerbrauten: Pot roast marinated in acidic sauce (German)
Sashimi: Raw fish (Japanese)
Teriaki: Broiled beef marinated in sweet soy sauce (Hawaiian)

MIXED DISHES

Couscous: Semolina, meat stew (North African)
Goulash: Stew usually seasoned with paprika (Hungarian)
Gumbo: Okra and meat stew, thickened with filé (pulverized sassafras leaves) (Louisiana Creole)

Hoppin John: Blackeyed peas and rice (Southern US)
Jambalaya: Rice, ham, and seafood (Louisiana Creole)
Moussaka: Eggplant casserole (Greek)

Scrapple: Pork and cornmeal (Pennsylvania Dutch)
Tacos: Fried tortillas filled with meat or beans, vegetables, hot sauce (Mexican)
Wonton: Stuffed dough, fried or cooked in broth (Chinese)

OTHERS

Baklavah: A layered pastry rich in honey (Greek)
Butterhorns: Sweet pastry
Cracklins: Crispy pieces left after pork fat is rendered (Southern)
Fat back: Fat from belly of pig

Kuchen: Cake
Lard: Pork fat rendered to be used like shortening
Salt pork: Salted pork fat, sometimes with bit of meat
Sofrito: Specially seasoned tomato sauce used by Puerto Ricans

Spumoni: Fruit ice cream (Italian)
Strickle sheets: Coffee cake (Pennsylvania Dutch)
Strudel: Paper thin pastry with fruit filling or cheese (German)
Tzimmes: Carrot-prune dessert (Jewish American)

CULTURAL GROUPS IN THE U.S.

Large cultural groups can usually be subdivided into distinctive subcultures. Reference is often made to Chinese Americans, native Americans, Spanish-speaking Americans, and so on. These groupings are unwieldly and tend to overlook important differences within cultures, subcultures, and individuals. Subdivisions listed in Table 6.2 help to distinguish some of the subcultures of a sampling of major cultural groups residing in the U.S. No attempt has been made to identify subcultures of either black or white Americans who are long time residents of the U.S. Americans of any cultural group may have a diverse or a very limited diet depending on such factors as place of residence during childhood, presence of other cultural groups in their immediate neighborhood, desire to maintain an ethnic identity, and other influences discussed later in the chapter.

When viewing traditional cultural food practices, it may seem at first glance that nutrient intake is substandard. Closer examination often reveals that practices peculiar to the culture contribute important amounts of the nutrients in question. A few examples are illustrated in Table 6.3.

Small cultural groups abound in the U.S. In travelling through America one can find clusters of Portuguese, French Canadians, Scandinavians, Germans, Latvians, Vietnamese, Haitians, and many other nationalities. Some of these groups have been in the U.S. for many generations and still maintain their cultural identity, including their foodways.

Religious group affiliation contributes to diversity of food behaviors within a cultural group. Devout Jews of any nationality have some foodways which differ from those of their countrymen. The same holds true for Seventh-Day Adventists, Muslims, and people of many other faiths.

Socioeconomic status should be noted when looking at the practices of any cultural group in America because it influences many food behaviors. The distinctive "soul food" which is a part of the life of many American blacks is food originally accessible to them when they were slaves. Some of it might have been characterized as leftovers, for example the chitterlings, hog maw, and salt pork. Blacks showed ingenuity in transforming humble foods into tasty dishes which are just beginning to be appreciated by white Americans.

Occupation, income, and social class also contribute to the way a person or family eats. A drop in income may prevent the purchase of highly desired ethnic foods and result in a change in food habits. Sometimes members of an ethnic group sever their ties and discard their former foodways when they move up the socioeconomic ladder.

The family unit may either perpetuate or modify cultural practices. For example, the Amish, who value their way of life and have tended to marry within their

TABLE 6.2 *Subdivisions of major cultural groups in the United States*

CHINESE AMERICANS (By region of origin, because of differences in foodways, other customs, and dialect):
  Mainland China
    Northern region (Mandarin)
    Inland region (Szechwan)
    Central coastal region (Shanghai)
    Southern region (Cantonese)
  Taiwan (most residents from Taiwan are not actually Chinese Americans because they are here on a temporary basis, as for educational purposes, rather than citizens)
JAPANESE-AMERICANS
  Isei—Originally this term was applied to first generation Japanese in America. It may be used to refer to those who have retained their cultural identity by continuing the customs and lifestyle of their ancestors
  Nisei—This term refers to second (and later) generation Japanese in America. It implies that the individuals have become acculturated (Westernized).
NATIVE AMERICANS (AMERICAN INDIANS)
  By cultural groups, e.g., navajo shepherds, pueblo farmers, eskimos, and others[1]
  By tribe:
    Approximately 250 to 300 major tribes remain, varying in size from about 100 to 160,000 enrolled members.[2]
    Tribes which comprise a cultural group share certain practices relating to eating, health, and other activities of daily living, but retain many distinctive characteristics
SPANISH-SPEAKING AMERICANS (HISPANIC AMERICANS)
  Mexican Americans
    Settled immigrants (primarily in the Southwest)
    Migrant workers (both legal and illegal residents)
  Spanish Americans
    Descendants of early Spanish settlers (primarily in the Southwest and Colorado)
  Puerto Ricans
    Permanent residents
    Temporary residents who come to the continental U.S. for employment
  Cubans
  People from any of the other Spanish-speaking countries in Central and South America and the Carribean

own group, have made few changes in foodways over a period of many generations. Intermarriage, on the other hand, often results in a modification or sometimes adoption of new traditions. Disruption of the family unit, employment of women, and lack of contact with the extended family tend to weaken cultural traditions and lead to more diversity within a cultural group.

Although America is sometimes characterized by the diversity of its foodways, some foodways have become common for nearly all Americans. Advertising has no doubt been a major force behind the movement toward homogeneity, especially with regard to widespread use of soft drinks and snack foods. Mobility of Americans has also tended to increase homogeneity. Nevertheless, those who move or travel to a different part of the country often find it hard to adjust to differences in the food supply and foodways of the region.

TABLE 6.3 *Examples of cultural practices that promote adequate nutrient intake*

CULTURE	NUTRITIOUS FOODS THAT ARE RARELY EATEN	CULTURAL CORRECTIONS
Chinese	Milk	Cooking bones in acid solution to make soup provides an excellent source of calcium
		Soybean products such as tofu and many Chinese greens are good sources of calcium.
Mexican	Milk	*Corn* tortillas are prepared with lime-soaked corn and therefore contribute significant amounts of calcium to the diet*
Italian	Milk	Calcium rich cheeses are popular
Southern Black	Milk	Buttermilk may be used occasionally
		Calcium rich greens are popular vegetables
Puerto Rican	Bread	Viandas such as plantains are similar to bread in nutritive value
		Rice is popular and is a good substitute if whole grain or enriched

* Lime is a calcium salt

BECOMING ACQUAINTED WITH FOODWAYS AND FOOD BEHAVIOR OF OTHER SOCIOCULTURAL GROUPS

Health care providers need to be prepared to meet the unexpected. When people come in contact with members of a different sociocultural group, they have a tendency to be *ethnocentric*. That is, people are apt to feel that their own beliefs, values, and life ways are better than those of others.[3] People with strong cultural ties may be reluctant to share information about their customs with outsiders; they are inclined to look after their own members.

Sometimes ethnocentricity is aggravated by *cultural shock*—being stunned by seeing or otherwise experiencing the unfamiliar. For example, some Americans might be repelled by seeing an individual eat grubs, squid, horsemeat, or similar wholesome, nutritious items. Americans tend to consider insects to be filth rather than food. What would be your response if a pregnant Chinese-American woman asked you to make arrangements to save her placenta so that she could eat it after her baby was delivered? How do people from other cultural groups react when they observe a middle class white American mother coaxing or forcing her child to finish his meal, regardless of the child's appetite?

Cultural shock often interferes with a person's willingness and ability to deal with cultural differences. While noting differences and similarities among cultures, it is important to avoid being judgmental and quick to find fault. This helps promote communication and development of trust between individuals of different backgrounds and thus facilitates the delivery of sound nutritional care.

The following premises are given as a basis for recognizing and promoting sound nutrition in different sociocultural situations:

1. Groups having a stable history of many generations have foodways and traditions compatible with survival of the group in a particular setting. However the foodways are not always compatible with survival of weaker members of the groups or with achievement of optimal health.
2. Many groups have traditional food habits which are nutritionally superior to those of so-called "ordinary" Americans. "Different" does not imply "inferior."
3. Each food, food behavior, or tradition can be placed in one of three categories, as illustrated in Table 6.4.
4. Since deeply ingrained foodways and traditional foods may help meet an individual's need for security, love, and belongingness, disrupting a tradition may also disrupt psychological health or family stability. When improvement of diet is necessary, guidelines can be built on the solid foundation of the traditional diet using foods which are familiar to and well liked by the cultural group.

The next section of this chapter raises pertinent questions about the foodways of others and provides examples of why the questions may be useful when investigating foodways and behaviors of another cultural group.

HOW IS "GOOD HEALTH" DEFINED AND WHAT VALUE IS PLACED ON IT?

Some cultures view good health as merely ability to function, freedom from pain, or "feeling OK." Those cultures might consider mild symptoms of malnutrition to be normal if those symptoms were prevalent in the community. Other groups, such as the Seventh-Day Adventists, strongly emphasize the value of achieving optimal health. Depending on the culture, either plumpness or thinness may be viewed as an indication of health.

A culture might consider good health to be a gift from God or the result of a proper balance or harmony with nature. Illness might be viewed as a sign of God's displeasure or the result of a hex or of supernatural intervention. Cultures which hold one of these beliefs may fail to relate an adequate diet to good health. De-

TABLE 6.4 *Categories of food behaviors and food traditions*

CATEGORY	DESCRIPTION	EXAMPLES
Beneficial	Promotes health	Eating traditional cultural foods that are rich sources of vitamins, minerals, and/or protein, such as turnip greens with pot liquor, tofu, and tortillas
Neutral	Has no observable or documented effect on health	Using foods infrequently, at times of celebration, such as holiday eggnog, hamantaschen (Jewish pastry), and mince pie
Harmful or potentially harmful	Following the tradition may endanger the health of the individual or of other family members	Substituting bottlefeeding for breastfeeding when an adequate supply of sanitary formula cannot be assured

ficiency states might be blamed on factors beyond the person's control rather than on failure to consume enough essential nutrients.

ARE CERTAIN FOODS OR FOOD COMBINATIONS CONSIDERED TO BE "BAD" OR HARMFUL IN SOME WAY?

It is not unusual for a cultural group to believe that a particular food or combination of foods or ingredients is poisonous or disease producing. Even seemingly unreasonable beliefs can exert a powerful influence upon a person's actions or state of mind. For example, those who consider black pills or liquids to be dangerous would avoid taking prescribed iron tablets if they were black.

If a culture's view of a food is sufficiently negative, the food is considered *taboo* (forbidden), at least under specified circumstances. A food might be taboo only for pregnant women because of a belief that the food causes birthmarks or congenital anomalies in the fetus.

Members of natural food cults may view sugar and food additives as poisons. Many of these people are very well educated and are quite able to back their beliefs with scientifically oriented, although not necessarily accurate, explanations.

IS THERE AN INTANGIBLE ASPECT OF FOOD WHICH THE CULTURE CONSIDERS WHEN COMBINING FOODS OR USING FOODS FOR SPECIFIC PURPOSES?

Some cultural groups hold to either a "yin-yang" theory or a "hot-cold" (caliente-fresco) theory which applies to many aspects of life, including food. The yin-yang belief is prevalent among Chinese Americans, members of macrobiotic cults, and certain other cultural groups having their roots in Eastern religion or philosophy. Hot-cold beliefs pervade many of the Hispanic-American cultures.

According to either theory, health depends upon the proper *balance* between opposing energy forces (yin vs. yang or hot vs. cold). The idea can be illustrated by a discussion of yin and yang. Yin (also called lyang) represents "female," a negative force, emptiness, cold, darkness. Although many of these descriptors make yin sound detrimental, a certain amount of yin is considered necessary. Yin is said to help conserve or restore body energy. Yang (also called bou) represents "male," a positive force, fullness, warmth, light. Despite the desirable connotations of these descriptors, too much yang is believed to be harmful in that it can cause disease. The right amount of yang is believed to help protect the body from outside influence.

It might be easier to grasp this abstract idea by considering night and day and likening them to yin and yang respectively. Although night is dark and perhaps even threatening, it is an excellent time for rest and revitalization of the body. Either too much or too little night could have adverse physical and psychological effects.

The yin-ness or yang-ness of a food depends primarily on the effects that a food is thought to have on the body. Color, texture, flavor, temperature, or other observable characteristics are not necessarily used as the primary basis for classifying food. Season of the year, method of preparation, and some other factors may influence the spot a food occupies on the yin-yang continuum, but does not change it from yin to yang or vice versa. An outsider finds it difficult to distinguish yin foods from yang foods without a thorough orientation to the theory.

In Hispanic-American cultures, the calidad (hotness or coldness) of a food is determined by observing the effects of that food on an illness identified by the cultural group as hot or cold. Occasionally a food may be designated as either hot or cold, depending on how it is prepared. Mexican Americans are shifting toward believing that the calidad of foods is determined by temperature rather than by other characteristics.[4]

In either culture, knowledge of these special attributes of food is transmitted within families by tradition and practice. The family or a folk healer uses yang (hot) foods, herbs, and medicines to treat diseases caused by yin (cold) excesses. (The excesses are not necessarily related to food.) They use the opposite treatment for yang (hot) diseases.

People who believe in the importance of maintaining a balance of opposing elements may pay much more attention to nutritional information if it is put into the framework of their beliefs. For example, if they are not vegetarians and if they believe that anemia is a yin condition, they may readily accept the suggestion of consuming more meat, a yang food, to counteract the anemia.[5]

Currier,[6] Gladney,[7] and Ling[8] present information regarding this type of food grouping. However, when dealing with individuals it is essential to determine *their* particular beliefs.

DOES THE CULTURAL GROUP MAKE USE OF HERBAL SOUPS, TONICS, OR TEAS, OR OF SPECIAL HEALTH FOODS? IS ANYTHING KNOWN OF THE EFFECTS OF THESE?

Practically every culture has a tradition of use of special foods, herbs, and teas for health promotion or for curative purposes. Some Americans still use blackstrap molasses (an iron-rich residue of molasses) as a tonic, but this tradition has been largely replaced by use of highly advertised iron supplements. A Mexican American might brew mulberry leaves into a tea to be used for treating high blood pressure or use garlic to treat diarrhea or bronchitis.[7]

Numerous cultural groups emphasize the value of chicken soup for people who are ill.

A large number of herbs are traditionally used by Chinese Americans for their yin or yang effect or for specific medicinal purposes. One study of 100 Chinese-American babies (2 to 25 months old) found that nearly half of the mothers had taken one or more Chinese herbs while pregnant and that about a fourth of the babies had been fed some Chinese herbs.[8]

Moderate use of traditional herbs or health foods is unlikely to be harmful unless the practice interferes with intake of an adequate diet or with institution of other measures necessary for satisfactory health.

Scientific investigation of the use of herbs, teas, tonics, and "health" foods has been recommended. Many of the herbs, teas, and tonics used by American Indians have already been found to contain substances with impressive pharmacological activity. Investigation could document or refute the efficacy and safety of widely used substances and could indicate whether any would be useful in preventing or reversing specific nutritional deficiencies. Since the popular press is publishing many articles on the health-promoting and curative properties of these products and since health food stores are promoting them, more people are apt to try them even if folk medicine is not a part of their culture.

FOR WHAT REASONS, IF ANY, DOES THE CULTURE PRACTICE FASTING? WHAT TYPE OF FASTING IS PRACTICED AND FOR HOW LONG A PERIOD?

Fasting is most commonly associated with religious observances, but it is practiced by some cultural groups for the purpose of "cleansing the body of poisons." When a person speaks of fasting, it is important to clarify what is meant and whether pregnant and lactating women, children, and individuals who are ill are expected to adhere to the practice. Table 6.5 gives several examples of types of fasting.

DO DIETARY LAWS GOVERN FOOD BEHAVIOR OF MEMBERS OF A RELIGIOUS GROUP?

Some religious groups provide guidelines for food behavior in the form of dietary laws. The Jewish Kashruth and the Muslim dietary laws are very specific and detailed. Some other religions have few if any laws which might be considered to relate to food behavior. A summary of religious dietary laws and traditions is provided in Table 6.5. A few of the religions are discussed briefly here.

Jewish Kashruth Dietary Laws The Jewish Kashruth Dietary Laws, known by the popular term "kosher," provide regulations regarding the selection and preparation of foods that are "fit" for consumption by Jews. Jews who observe these laws do so for *spiritual* reasons rather than out of concern for their physical health.

Orthodox Jews closely observe the dietary laws. Because dietary and other religious regulations are very restrictive, Orthodox Jews generally are unwilling to partake of any food or refreshment except in a home or restaurant which keeps a kosher kitchen.

Conservative Jews may follow the dietary laws at home, but take a more liberal attitude on social occasions. *Reform* Jews are liberalists who observe few, if any, of the dietary laws.

The Kashruth dietary laws (1) distinguish between kosher food and unclean (trayf) food and (2) delineate proper and improper food combinations (Table 6.5). It is more common for Jews to avoid pork products and shellfish than to observe other dietary laws. Meat may be purchased in a kosher meat market to be sure that it meets dietary regulations. The prohibition against improper combinations is so strong that Orthodox Jews use separate utensils, pots, dishes, and sinks or dishpans for meat or poultry and for dairy products. Cooking kosher food in foil and eating it from paper plates with disposable utensils is one way of adapting in a nonkosher kitchen.

That dairy products *can* be combined with fish and/or eggs allows considerable leeway in meal planning. For example, a breakfast that includes juice, an egg, cereal, and milk is perfectly acceptable, as is a lunch of creamed tuna on toast with tossed salad.

Any kosher food described as *pareve* is free of dairy products, meat, and poultry. Pareve foods can be eaten with any other kosher food.

During the Jewish holiday season of Passover, additional food laws apply. Not even a crumb of leavened bread or of ordinary flour is to be in the house. Matzoth and matzoth meal are used instead. If possible, dishes and utensils are reserved for use only during Passover.

Muslim dietary laws The dietary regulations followed by devout Muslims bear some resemblance to the Kashruth. For example, pork and all pork products are unlawful for Muslims as well as for Jews. Laws pertain mainly to meat, pork products, and alcoholic beverages. The term "Hala'l," applied to food, means that the food is lawful for Muslims to eat.

Laws regarding the slaughtering of meat are interpreted differently by different groups of Muslims. Ideally, meat acceptable for consumption is slaughtered in the name of God in a prescribed manner. If any name other than Allah or God is mentioned at the time of slaughter or if the animal is slaughtered by an atheist, that meat is prohibited. In America there is little way of knowing what happened at the time of slaughter except in the case of kosher meat (since kosher meat is prepared under rabbinical supervision). Therefore Muslims might choose to eat kosher meat, abstain from meat entirely (frequently substituting seafood since regulations do not apply to fish), or do their own slaughtering. More liberal Muslims might eat meat slaughtered by either Christians or Jews, but

TABLE 6.5 *Types of prohibited foods and fasting laws*

RELIGION	PROHIBITED FOODS COMMONLY AVAILABLE IN USA	PROHIBITED BEVERAGES	COMMENTS
Jewish	All products obtained from pigs (pork, bacon, ham, lard, animal shortening, ordinary gelatin, and products containing it such as marshmallows and other confections) All fish without scales or fins (as shellfish, eels) Improperly slaughtered meat Foods containing blood Waste products Meat and poultry in combination with dairy products	Any containing milk, cream, or other dairy product with a meat-containing meal or for 6 hr following meat-containing meal	Fast completely for 24 hr on Yom Kippur (Day of Atonement)
Muslim	All products obtained from pigs (see above) Meat that has been slaughtered by someone other than a Muslim, Jew, or Christian (Exceptions can be made if health or life is at stake)	Alcoholic beverages and other intoxicants (Exceptions can be made for medical reasons) Stimulant beverages discouraged	Fast completely from dawn to dusk during month of Ramaden (9th month of Islamic lunar calendar). Other specific fast days are encouraged. Eating is a matter of worship of God
Roman Catholic	None	None	Abstain from eating meat and from eating between meals on Ash Wednesday and Good Friday Some Catholics voluntarily abstain from meat on Fridays.
Orthodox (Eastern, Greek, Russian)	None	None	Fasting can take many forms and is a matter of conscience. Variations include: 1. No animal products at all for 40 days prior to Easter and Christmas 2. Fasting on Wednesday and Friday only 3. Abstention only from meat and poultry
Seventh-Day Adventist	Pork products and shellfish, blood All flesh foods (avoidance is not a tenet of faith) Dairy products and eggs may also be considered harmful, although less so than are other animal products Use of highly spiced foods and of condiments is discouraged	Alcoholic beverages Stimulant beverages Meat broth	Eating between meals is discouraged, 5–6 hr interval between meals is recommended. A light evening meal is encouraged Cereal-based hot beverages such as Postum® are often used in place of coffee or tea
Church of Jesus Christ of the Latter-Day Saints (Mormon)	None	Alcoholic beverages Stimulant beverages	Water and milk are predominent forms of fluid used
Other Christian denominations	Most have no prohibitions. A few prohibit blood	Some prohibit or strongly discourage use of alcoholic beverages Some discourage use of coffee	Some fast by abstaining from meat on Friday

make it a point to mention the name of Allah themselves immediately before eating the meat.

The Muslim prohibition against alcohol even extends to flavoring extracts such as vanilla and almond extract. Not only food but also drugs and cosmetics must be free of alcohol and pork derivatives.

Dietary regulations of religious cults During the late 1960s and the 1970s religious and spiritual cults proliferated in America. It has been estimated that millions of young adults became involved in cults during that time.[9] Most of the cults reflect an influence of Eastern religions or philosophies.

Many of the cults have carefully defined dietary regulations which are part of a system allegedly promoting and maintaining both spiritual and physical health. (In actuality, some cults follow dangerous dietary practices.) These regulations usually require some type of vegetarianism. Balancing of yin and yang is a common finding, receiving most emphasis in groups recommending a macrobiotic eating pattern. Exclusive use of "natural, organically grown foods" is practiced by some groups.

Altered food habits provide members with tangible evidence of a new way of life.[10] Cooking (if practiced) and eating often take on special significance and religious overtones. Some cults choose certain food patterns to produce a "natural high"[11] either as an alternative to drugs (synthetic high) or in conjunction with drugs.

ARE FEASTS OR CELEBRATIONS WHICH FEATURE FOOD AN INTEGRAL PART OF THE CULTURAL TRADITION?

Cultural groups generally have feasts, celebrations, or parties in conjunction with religious holidays, the new year, a day set aside for giving thanks, birthdays, weddings, and "milestones." A traditional barbecue or pot latch is such an important event for members of some tribes of native Americans that they are willing to travel long distances to attend one.

Choice of foods and frequency and elaborateness of celebrations varies widely among cultural groups. A birthday cake aglow with candles and a Thanksgiving turkey are among the most ingrained traditions in American foodways.

Unfortunately, overeating is strongly and positively reinforced by many cultural traditions. A person who tries to exercise moderation in eating at a feast or celebration might be considered to be rude. If an extended family is large or a cultural group is tightly knit, celebrations may be so frequent (graduation, showers, christening, Bar Mitzvah, anniversaries—in addition to previously named celebrations), that overnutrition might become a problem.

On the other hand these same celebrations may enhance the nutrition of those who live alone or have limited ability or interest in feeding themselves well. The conviviality and the wide variety of foods at a party can do much to stimulate a lagging appetite. Leftovers sent home with older relatives may help tide them over until the next party.

WHAT KIND OF FAMILY UNIT IS PART OF THE CULTURAL HERITAGE AND WHAT ARE THE ROLES OF FAMILY MEMBERS?

The extended family remains a strong force in many cultural groups. For example, among Hispanic Americans decisions of the extended family may prevail over those of an individual family member; Godparents may be consulted about family problems, including matters of health.

"Family" encompasses more people for a native American than for an American of English origin. Depending on the kinship system of the tribe to which he belongs, an Indian child might have several sets of grandparents, brothers, sisters, and other relatives, all of whom maintain close ties to the child. Gypsies, a cultural group of nomads, are also noted for having unusually close family lies. No matter what the cultural group, working within the family structure is a key to promoting better nutrition for an individual family member.

Disruption of any family unit or separation from the family may be exceedingly traumatic when there is a strong cultural tradition of close family ties. Separation may adversely affect appetite and eating habits of individuals from many cultures. When separation from the family is unavoidable (as in the case of a Puerto Rican who left family behind on the island), promotion of good nutrition may be impeded by a client's emotional distress.

HOW MUCH PERMISSIVENESS IS ALLOWED WITH REGARD TO CHILDREN'S EATING HABITS?

Native-American tribes may allow small children to eat whenever they are hungry.[12] One study of migrant Mexican-American families reported that children were allowed to eat whatever available food they desired.[13] In contrast, cultural groups such as Orthodox Jews and Seventh-Day Adventists teach their children to observe specific dietary laws and traditions.

ARE THERE ASPECTS OF THE CULTURAL HERITAGE THAT INFLUENCE PATTERNS OF INTERACTION WHICH CAN, IN TURN, INFLUENCE FOOD BEHAVIORS?

Even if help were sorely needed, a Swedish individual might refuse assistance until pressured to accept. A Czech might insist upon making decisions for himself.[14] A Mexican American might become fearful if someone admired his child without also touching the child. (This is called casting an evil eye and is blamed as a cause of illness called *mal de ojo*.) The good intentions of the admirer could interfere with further communication and might cause a mother to refrain from further use of health services. Communication with native Americans might be fostered by knowing that Indians from many tribes are uneasy about direct eye contact and consider it disrespectful.[12] Conversely, a Filipino American develops a sense of trust only if health workers maintain direct eye contact.[15]

WHAT IS THE SIGNIFICANCE OF TIME AND HOW DOES IT INFLUENCE THE PATTERN OF EATING?

Apache Indians may attach little importance to time. Consequently, they often eat at irregular hours, according to convenience and/or hunger.[16] Gypsies may be completely unwilling to arise before late morning.[17]

Definitions of meals are apt to differ depending on the pattern of eating. Breakfast and coffee break may be viewed very differently but often include the same foods.

HOW DO FOODS, FOOD BEHAVIORS, AND STATUS RELATE?

The status of foods is most likely to be high if the foods are expensive, relatively unavailable, endorsed by highly respected individuals, or are part of an age-old tradition. High prestige foods are not necessarily higher in nutritive value than foods for which they are substituted. In fact the opposite may be true.

When the upper class in America appreciates an ethnic food, the label "gourmet food" is sometimes applied to it. In this way some economical foods increase in status. High status associated with natural foods is evidenced by widespread use of the word "natural" on food labels and in advertisements.

DO THE EATING HABITS OF A CULTURAL GROUP REFLECT THE GROUP'S SOCIOECONOMIC STATUS OR THE AVAILABILITY OF FOOD RATHER THAN ACTUAL FOOD PREFERENCES?

Questionable food habits associated with particular cultural groups may be more a result of inadequate income than of disregard for sound nutrition or lack of enjoyment of more nutritious foods. Income affects not only the amount of money available to spend for food but also cooking and eating facilities, time available for cooking, access to a reasonably priced store, ability to take advantage of bargain prices, and many other factors which influence food choices and eating patterns.

Immigrants often find that foods which were dietary staples in their homeland are either unavailable or exhorbitantly expensive in America. Foods chosen as substitutes may not be comparable to traditional foods in nutritive value. If use of traditional foods is impossible, individuals will not necessarily be receptive to suggestions for substitutes similar in nutritive value. The powerful influence of media and of promotional devices in grocery stores has resulted in widespread adoption of American traditions such as overuse of soft drinks, candy, chips, and other sugary, salty, or high fat convenience foods. The poorest food habits of cultural groups in America are those learned from white Americans.

In many cases the quality of the diet has deteriorated. For example, low-income Sioux Indian women in 1970 reportedly ate meals such as these:[18] breakfast—dry cereal with milk and coffee; lunch—bologna sandwich, potato chips, and a carbonated beverage (or perhaps just fried potatoes); dinner—chopped meat and fried potatoes. The limited variety reflects the circumstances in which these impoverished native Americans find themselves, not a cultural tradition. Another observer at the same reservation reported that some Sioux children, when given money, headed eagerly for fresh fruits in the trading post rather than for candy.[19]

The U.S. government provides commodity foods (Appendix 2E) to native Americans living on reservations in an attempt to improve their nutrient intake. Although commodities consist of nutritious foods, there are problems connected with their use which are only gradually overcome by food demonstrations and other special promotional measures. For example, some American Indians have used donated dry egg powder as shampoo instead of cooking with it. This is not surprising since to most people dry egg is an unfamiliar and unattractive food.

The nutritive value of commodity foods or trading post foods is not necessarily comparable to that of traditional Indian foods. For example, corn grown and prepared by Hopi Indians using age-old methods has been found to be exceptionally rich in minerals.[20] By adding ashes from green plants when preparing the corn, they produce a grain product which is richer in calcium, magnesium, iron, zinc, manganese, and other minerals than are the commodity grains provided by the government. (Unfortunately the trend is now to use the more convenient but less nutritious method of adding baking soda instead of plant ash when preparing the corn.)

It has been suggested that the poorest members of some native American tribes may be better off nutritionally than their more affluent neighbors if they resort to gathering nutrient-rich wild plants and animal products (eggs, insects, wild game).

Some of the wild plants used by native Americans have been found to make surprisingly high nutritional contributions to the diet. A single prickly pear fruit (60 gm.) reportedly provides about 500 mg. calcium (as much calcium as in about 420 cc. [1¾ c.] of milk).

IS THERE A STRONG CULTURAL ATTITUDE OR TRADITION WITH REGARD TO THE STORAGE OF FOOD?

The Church of Jesus Christ of the Latter-Day Saints (Mormon) strongly urges its members to always have stores of food on hand in case of emergency. Although not an absolute requirement, a majority of Mormons try to adhere to this practice. The church provides classes and other educational material to promote safe and effective food storage. Since stores of food are useful only if they are reasonably fresh, the storage of so much food influences the eating behaviors of Mormons.

Some cultures have no tradition of storing food. If a well-liked food were brought into the home of a Sioux Indian, for example, the food might be eaten immediately even if a meal had just been consumed.[18]

Some cultures place high priority on fresh food; therefore they shop daily. In some cases an emphasis on prompt consumption of food brought into the home is related to lack of refrigeration rather than to a strong cultural tradition. A family which is unaccustomed to storing food may find it difficult to economize when shopping or to adapt to lack of transportation or mobility.

DO SOME OF THE FOOD HABITS OF THE CULTURAL GROUP CONFLICT WITH SPECIFIC THERAPEUTIC DIET MODIFICATIONS?

Certain cultural food habits may be contraindicated for medical reasons. Prohibiting specific foods may have unintentional adverse effects on overall nutrient intake or may influence a person's willingness to cooperate as described below.

Frequent use of stimulant beverages Many cultures take coffee or tea several times daily. Stimulant beverages may be the major vehicle for milk intake (as in café con leche or tea with milk). Prohibiting use of stimulant beverages might, therefore, result in undesirably low intake of some of the nutrients found in milk. Coffee contains niacin and may be a significant source of this nutrient for some cultural groups. Tea may be a child's only source of fluoride.

Use of wine, beer, or other alcoholic beverages Wine in particular may be a vital part of religious celebrations (as the Seder meal at the beginning of Passover). Many cultural groups routinely take wine with their meals and feel the meal is incomplete without it.

Use of highly salted foods Examples of salty foods used by various cultural groups are listed in Table 6.6. Many of these foods are also high in other essential nutrients which might otherwise be difficult to obtain

TABLE 6.6 *Examples of cultural foods and seasonings that are very high in sodium*

ORIENTAL
Dried and salted fish
Fermented bean curd
Fish cakes
Miso and miso soup
Oyster, black bean, fish, and seafood sauces
Instant noodles
Ra-yu
Soy sauce
Shrimp paste
Salted and pickled vegetables (pickled kelp, tsukudani, kam-chi, miso-quke, umeboshi (salted plums)
Salty preserved eggs-atsuyaki, dalemaki
Tamari
Teriyaki sauce
EUROPE AND BRITISH ISLES
Corned beef
Salty cheeses: feta, blue, Roquefort, Camembert
Sauerkraut
Sauces (Worcestershire, Italian)
Sausage (kielbasi, pepperoni, knockwurst)
GREECE AND THE MIDDLE EAST
Feta cheese
Olives
Pickled vegetables
MEXICAN
Chorizo
Ready-prepared Mexican sauces
SOUL FOOD
Salt pork
Pickled pig's feet or knuckles

from the culture's traditional foods. Some of the foods are exceedingly high in salt because it has been used as a preservative. This is an important consideration when refrigeration is unavailable.

Extensive use of saturated fats Individuals of Scandinavian origin commonly use butterfat (a rich source of vitamin A). Lard, salt pork, and rendered animal fat are the principal fats used by some cultural groups. The flavor provided by these fats promotes consumption of vegetables and other nutritious foods to which the fat is added.

STUDY QUESTIONS

1. When working with a person from a cultural group different from your own, why is it advisable to ask him about his food preferences and food behaviors rather than to rely on information about that culture which is available in books and articles? (Identify several reasons.)

2. A Hispanic American mentions that he has a "hot" disease. What information will help you to give him nutritional advice that he will be willing to follow?

3. A black American states that he never drinks milk because it doesn't agree with him. What foods fre-

quently liked by blacks would be good alternatives from a nutritional standpoint?

4. A native American does not look you in the eye and evades your questions about his usual meal schedule. Is this good reason to suspect that he has poor food habits? Explain.

5. An Orthodox Jew turns down your invitation to have dinner with you at your home. Why would he still refuse if you told him you were going to serve roast lamb? (Give several reasons.)

6. What are some of the common forms of fasting?

References

1. Gonzales, N. L.: Changing dietary patterns of North American Indians. In W. Moore, M. M. Silverberg, and M. S. Read (eds.): *Nutrition, Growth and Development of North American Children.* DHEW Publ. (NIH). Washington DC: U.S. Govt. Printing Office, 1972.

2. Wallace, L. T.: Patient is an American Indian. *Supervisor Nurs.* 8(5):32, 1977.

*3. Leininger, M.: Cultural diversities of health and nursing care. *Nurs. Clin. North Am.* 12(1):5, 1977.

4. Clark, M.: *Health in the Mexican-American Culture,* ed. 2. Berkeley CA: University of California Press, 1970.

5. Wang, M., and Dwyer, J. T.: Reaching Chinese-American children with nutrition education. *J. Nutr. Ed.* 7:145, 1975.

6. Currier, R. L.: The hot-cold syndrome and symbolic balance in Mexican and Spanish-American folk medicine. *Ethnology* 5:251, 1966.

*7. Gladney, V. M.: Food Practices of the Mexican-American in Los Angeles County. County of Los Angeles Department of Health Services. Preventive Health Services. Rev. 1976.

*8. Ling, S., King, J., and Leung, V.: Diet, growth, and cultural food habits in Chinese-American infants. *Am. J. Chin. Med.* 3:125, 1975.

9. Gordon, J. S.: The kids and the cults. *Children Today* 6(4):24, 1977.

10. Erhard, D.: The new vegetarians, Part Two: The Zen Macrobiotic movement and other cults based on vegetarianism. *Nutr. Today* 9(1):20, 1974.

11. Dwyer, J. T., et al.: The new vegetarians: The natural high?" *J. Am. Diet. Assoc.* 65:529, 1974.

*12. Primeaux, M.: Caring for the American Indian patient. *Am. J. Nurs.* 77:91, 1977.

13. Larson, L. B.: Nutritional status of children of Mexican-American migrant families. *J. Am. Diet. Assoc.* 64:29, 1974.

14. Macgregor, F. C.: Uncooperative patients: some cultural interpretations. *Am. J. Nurs.* 67:88, 1967.

15. McKenzie, J. L., and Chrisman, N. J.: Healing herbs, gods, and magic. *Nurs. Outlook* 25:326, 1977.

16. Crockett, D. C.: Medicine among the American Indians. *HSMHA Health Reports* 36:399, 1971.

17. Anderson, G., and Tighe, B.: Gypsy culture and health care. *Am. J. Nurs.* 73: 282, 1973.

18. Bass, M. A., and Wakefield, L. M.: Nutrient intake and food patterns of Indians on Standing Rock Reservation. *J. Am. Diet. Assoc.* 64:36, 1974.

19. Wax, M. L.: Social structure and child-rearing practices of North American Indians. In W. Moore, M. M. Silverberg, and M. S. Read (eds.): *Nutrition, Growth and Development of North American Children.* DHEW Publ. (NIH). Washington DC: U.S. Govt. Printing Office, 1972.

20. Calloway, D. H., Graugue, R. D., and Costa, F. M.: The superior mineral content of some Indian foods in comparison to federally donated counterpart commodities. *Ecol. Food Nutrition* 3:203, 1974.

* Recommended reading

7

Promoting sound eating habits in pregnancy and lactation

Life occurs in cycles, from birth to death, from generation to generation. The course of life throughout infancy and childhood leaves its mark upon the emerging adult. Likewise each childbearing couple has an impact upon the infants and children of succeeding generations. What the childbearing woman eats before and during her pregnancy influences the growth and development of the children she bears. What a person eats as an infant and child affects him, subsequently, as an adult.

Health professionals recognize that different approaches are needed for assisting individuals to meet their particular nutrient needs at each of the stages of the life cycle. This requires knowledge of the influence of various developmental stages on nutrient needs and of realistic methods of meeting those needs.

This chapter and the two that follow provide specific suggestions for promoting sound nutrition for people at various stages of the life cycle.

NUTRITION DURING PREGNANCY

Recommendations for optimal nutritional practices during pregnancy have changed considerably within the last two decades. The new recommendations are based primarily on information compiled by the Committee on Maternal Nutrition of the Food and Nutrition Board. The Committee on Maternal Nutrition was commissioned by the federal government to make a comprehensive study of all the available research literature regarding nutrition and the course and outcome of pregnancy. "Course and out-

come of pregnancy" refers to the presence or absence of complications such as the following:
1. Death of mother or infant (maternal or infant mortality)
2. Miscarriage: interrupted pregnancy prior to the seventh month
3. Preterm (premature) birth: birth of a baby prior to 38-weeks' gestational age
4. Low birth weight (LBW), also called small-for-date (SFD) or small-for-gestational-age (SGA): weight of baby at birth is less than expected for calculated age (can be 28- to 44-weeks' gestation)
5. Congenital anomalies: birth defects
6. Stillborn: dead at birth
7. Toxemia of pregnancy: a potentially life-threatening maternal condition which may occur during pregnancy

Preconceptual nutritional status

In 1970 the Committee on Maternal Nutrition issued a report of their findings.[1] They emphasized that preconceptual nutritional status appears to have an important bearing on the course and outcome of pregnancy. A woman who has a history of good nutritional status and who is well-nourished at the time of conception has an increased chance of delivering a healthy term baby of normal birth weight (2.5 to 4.6 kg. or 5.5 to 10 lb.). Food eaten during pregnancy does count, but entering pregnancy in good nutritional status offers certain advantages. In particular, good preconceptual nutritional status is associated with nutrient reserves and with reasonably sound eating behaviors.

NUTRIENT RESERVES

Nutrient reserves provide a safety margin for a woman who has just become pregnant. Thus if something should happen to interfere with food intake soon after the inception of pregnancy, a well-nourished female will have some reserves to enable her to temporarily provide for the nutrient needs of the fetus.

Large stores of some nutrients can be accumulated if the diet provides extra amounts of them. Other nutrients are not usually considered to be stored in significant amounts, even if the diet has provided an excess. Nonetheless, a well-nourished body has at least a small surplus of all nutrients. Table 7.1 lists nutrients according to storage categories. (These apply to any person, not just to pregnant women.) A woman who has met the RDA for nutrients in the righthand column of Table 7.1 can be expected to have ample stores of them. The fetus can benefit from this nutrient supply without adversely affecting the mother. Unfortunately, it is not unusual for a pregnant woman's stores of some nutrients to be low or absent, especially stores of iron.

Some pregnant women have an inadequate food intake early in pregnancy as a result of nausea and vomiting. Nutrient reserves may then provide a major source of nourishment for the fetus. Adequate nutrition of the fetus is particularly crucial when tissues and organs are being differentiated during the first trimester* of pregnancy. This is the time when adequate nutrition is thought to help protect against certain birth defects.

FOOD HABITS

A woman who is accustomed to eating a varied diet based on a reliable food guide or the RDA will be consuming all of the nutrients needed by the fetus. She should find it easy to adapt her diet to meet the higher RDAs of pregnancy. Waiting until becoming pregnant before adopting good food habits may endanger the fetus, partly because an expectant mother is often well into her first trimester before the pregnancy is confirmed.

* A trimester is a three-month span of time. Thus, the first trimester of pregnancy covers the first three calendar months after conception.

TABLE 7.1 *Potential for storage of nutrients*

STORAGE VERY LIMITED	LARGE RESERVES CAN BE BUILT UP
Protein (amino acids)	Fat, including linoleic
Carbohydrate	acid (the essential fatty
Vitamin C	acid, a component of fat)
B complex vitamins	Vitamins A, D, E
(except B_{12})	Calcium and phosphorus
Vitamin K	Vitamin B_{12}
Most minerals	Iron

Because preconceptual nutritional status may affect the course and outcome of pregnancy, special attention should be directed toward helping girls develop sound eating practices. Any adolescent or adult female contemplating pregnancy in either the near or distant future should be encouraged to learn and apply principles of good nutrition.

Recommendations for dietary management during pregnancy

Once a woman becomes pregnant, she is likely to be receptive to learning about how to meet her increased nutritional needs. The recommendations given in the present chapter are designed for healthy pregnant women. They are based on the report of the Committee on Maternal Nutrition,[1] a handbook prepared by the Committee on Nutrition of the American College of Obstetricians and Gynecologists[2] and on Recommended Dietary Allowances for pregnant women. Every effort should be made to assist pregnant females to meet the recommendations established for this period of life. Special considerations are discussed in Chapter 34.

WEIGHT GAIN

The Committee on Maternal Nutrition has taken a strong stand, based on considerable evidence, that a weight gain of about 11 kg. (24 lb.), with a range of 9 to 11.4 kg. (20 to 25 lb.) is desirable. This amount of weight gain benefits both the mother and the fetus. In particular, the birth weight of the baby is more apt to be in the desirable range. An adequate caloric intake promotes optimal utilization of protein for growth of the fetus.*

The *pattern* of weight gain is more important than the total amount of weight gained. A desirable rate of weight gain is about 0.7 to 1.5 kg. (1.5 to 3 lb.) during the first trimester of pregnancy and 0.36 kg. (0.8 lb.) per week during the remainder of pregnancy. A sharp increase in weight after the twentieth week of pregnancy may be a result of fluid retention. Excessive fluid retention may be a signal that pre-eclampsia, a condition requiring prompt medical attention, is developing.

The recommended pattern of weight gain is illustrated in Figure 7.1. This pattern is recommended even if a woman is overweight or obese at the beginning of pregnancy. If more than the recommended weight is gained over any time span during pregnancy, there should be no attempt to make up for this by restricting weight gain in the remaining weeks. Controlled gain of 0.36 kg. (0.8 lb.) weekly is still the goal. The RDA specifies an increase of 300

* More recently the American College of Obstetrics and Gynecology has recommended that a woman gain 10 to 12.3 kg (22 to 27 lb.) throughout the course of pregnancy.

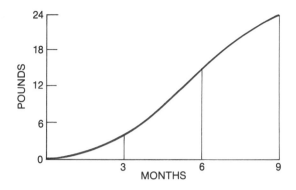

What contributes to this weight?

Baby:	7½ lb (about 3 1/3 kg)
Placenta (afterbirth):	1½ lb (about 2/3 kg)
Uterus:	2 lb (about 1 kg)
Increased blood and fluids:	8½ lb (about 4 kg)
Body changes for breast feeding:	4½ lb (about 2 kg)
TOTAL:	24 lb

FIGURE 7.1. Desirable weight gain during pregnancy. (From Corruccini, C. G.: *Your Weight and Weight Gain.* California Department of Health, 714 P St., Sacramento, CA 95814. 4/77)

kcal. daily above normal caloric requirement to meet the energy demands of pregnancy. This increased caloric intake should result in the recommended weight gain.

Prior to 1970 the belief was widespread that limiting weight gain would help prevent toxemia, one of the feared complications of pregnancy. Despite the fact that this belief was based on very limited evidence, it was customary for health professionals to urge pregnant women to avoid gaining more than about 8.2 kg (18 lb.). Frequently this warning was so forcefully made that women would severely limit food intake, especially toward the end of pregnancy. It would not be unusual for new mothers to boast if they had been able to limit weight gain to 5.5 to 6.8 kg. (12 to 15 lb.). Physicians often placed overweight pregnant women on reducing diets. Because this was common so recently, it is wise to ascertain if a pregnant woman thinks that a gain of 11 kg. (24 lb.) is undesirable, and to clarify any misconceptions she may have.

In planning for nutritional adequacy, the emphasis should be placed on obtaining nutrients from *food,* most of which has undergone minimal processing. All too often individuals think that vitamin-mineral supplements or one or two highly fortified foods can provide for all of their nutritional needs. This is definitely not true. During pregnancy prescribed nutritional supplements serve a useful purpose as *supplements.* They are to be used *in conjunction with,*

not instead of, a nourishing diet. The guidelines for well-balanced diets which have been given in preceding chapters can form the basis for an adequate diet during pregnancy since the same nutrients are needed by everyone.

FOOD GUIDES

There are different points of view regarding recommended meal plans for meeting nutritional needs during pregnancy. The most widely publicized guidelines are those based on the Basic Four Food Groups and those developed by the National Foundation, March of Dimes. The National Foundation is an organization dedicated to the prevention of birth defects. Detailed information about a food plan which coincides with that promoted by the National Foundation has been published in an excellent booklet by the California Department of Health.[3] The two guides are briefly described in Table 7.2. A comparison of the two plans reveals several similarities and differences, some of which are discussed below.

The March of Dimes plan includes six specific food groups. Leafy green vegetables are distinguished from other vegetables and fruits because of their high folic acid content. If two large servings of these vegetables are eaten daily along with the other recommended foods, intake of folic acid will be more apt to meet the greatly increased need for this vitamin during pregnancy. If the Basic Four plan is followed using the minimum amounts specified, average daily intake of folic acid will probably be low or marginal on the average compared to Recommended Dietary Allowances. (This does not necessarily mean that a woman will actually be deficient in the vitamin.)

More high protein foods are recommended in the March of Dimes plan than in the Basic Four plan. This is done to increase intake of vitamin B_6, iron, and zinc, all of which are vital to the developing fetus. Without high intake of high protein foods it is unlikely that the RDA will be met. Use of high protein foods also increases intake of chromium, which may otherwise be marginal during pregnancy.[4] Emphasis on high protein foods increases the cost of a diet. Extensive counseling regarding selection and preparation of relatively low cost, high protein foods might be necessary to enable a woman to incorporate the equivalent of 240 to 360 gm. (8 to 12 oz.) of high protein foods into her diet. Mothers with low incomes may be able to meet this goal if their food dollar is stretched by means of food stamps and/or participation in the Special Supplemental Food Program for Women, Infants and Children (WIC) (Appendix 2B). Alternate sources of zinc, iron, and vitamin B_6 might be suggested for individuals who find it impractical or unpleasant to consume four servings of high protein food. They might be encouraged to increase the number of servings of whole grains, especially yeast-leavened whole grain bread, and to use other foods such as wheat germ, liver, or other organ meats, and perhaps brewers yeast

TABLE 7.2 *Widely distributed guides for meal planning during pregnancy*

TYPES OF FOOD	USDA AND NATIONAL DAIRY COUNCIL	NATIONAL FOUNDATION MARCH OF DIMES, AND CALIFORNIA DEPARTMENT OF HEALTH
Milk and milk products	3 or more c milk or the equivalent daily. If under 17 yr, have an extra 2 c	3 c daily during the first trimester 4 c daily during the 2nd and 3rd trimesters Soybean milk and tofu are included in the choices for this group
Protein foods (animal and vegetable)	3 or more 2-oz servings, a total of 6 oz or equivalent protein	1st trimester: three 2- to 3-oz. servings daily 2nd and 3rd trimesters: 4 servings daily. The total amount from this group is high to achieve the RDA for vitamin B_6, iron, and zinc. The RDA for protein will be greatly exceeded
Grain products	4 or more servings (whole grain, fortified or enriched daily)	3 to 4 servings daily. Use of whole grain products is urged
Fruits and vegetables	4 servings daily, including citrus or source of vitamin C daily, and dark-green and orange vegetables often (at least 3 to 4 times per week)	Vitamin C rich fruits and vegetables: 1 serving daily Leafy green vegetables (vegetables high in folacin): 2 servings daily (1 serving = 1 cup raw or ¾ c cooked. Asparagus, broccoli, cabbage and scallions are among the vegetables in this group Other fruits and vegetables: 1 serving daily
Additional foods to meet caloric requirements	No specific recommendation. Include nutrient-rich foods before adding "others"	Use of some fats and oils is assumed. Emphasis is on increased servings from the food groups and nutritious food combinations

Sources: *Family Fare.* Consumer and Food Economics Research Division, Agricultural Research Service, USDA. Washington DC: Superintendent of Documents. Rev. Nov. 1971.
Partners in Growth. Chicago: National Dairy Council. 1974.
Be Good to Your Baby Before It Is Born. White Plains, NY: The National Foundation-March of Dimes, 1977.
Nutrition During Pregnancy and Lactation. Sacramento CA: California Department of Health, Maternal and Child Health Unit, 1975.

(if it doesn't cause the woman too much gastrointestinal discomfort).

In the Basic Four plan the number of servings is always followed by the words "or more." For example, the recommended number of servings from the grain group is four *or more.* This contrasts with the March of Dimes plan, which merely specifies 4 servings from this group. It seems advantageous to include the phrase "or more" to avoid the implication that calories are to be restricted.

Any plan should stress the importance of avoiding long intervals between meals. Breakfast should be eaten to provide the fetus with the glucose he needs for fuel.

Any plan should also mention the increased need for water during pregnancy, amounting to a total of about 1.5 to 2 L. (6 to 8 c) daily. The need for water can be met by increased intake of a variety of fluids. Alcoholic beverages of any type are not recommended; there is convincing evidence that alcohol increases the risk of birth defects.[5,6] Beverages containing saccharin should perhaps be avoided because of questions relating to saccharin's cancer-causing potential.[7] The relationship between caffeine and outcome of pregnancy has not been determined but is under investigation.[8]

Some cultural groups strongly encourage pregnant women to avoid specific foods or even large groups of foods. For example, Chinese Americans and Mexican Americans who subscribe to yin-yang (cold-hot) beliefs about food may view pregnancy as a yang (hot) condition. Because of this belief Chinese American women may primarily eat yang (hot) foods during pregnancy,[9]

while Mexican Americans may limit intake of "hot" foods.[10]

No matter what diet plan is used during pregnancy, it is advisable to emphasize (1) a variety of foods from each food group, (2) foods which have undergone relatively little processing, (3) safe food preparation methods which retain nutrients, and (4) extra servings from the food groups as needed to achieve desirable weight gain. Sugar and fat may be used in moderation as long as their use does not compromise adequate nutrient intake.

SUPPLEMENTATION

Vitamin-mineral supplements may be prescribed to augment a nutritious diet during pregnancy. Table 7.3 summarizes commonly accepted recommendations for nutritional supplements. The Committee on Maternal Nutrition emphasizes that supplements are not to be substituted for correction of poor food habits and that routine vitamin-mineral supplements are of uncertain value.

Iron The Committee on Maternal Nutrition recommends the use of iron supplements during the second and third trimesters of pregnancy. Extra iron is needed for a variety of reasons in the prenatal period. Iron is required for the fetus, who at term has a hemoglobin level of about 17 mg. per 100 ml. blood. This hemoglobin level is much higher than at any other period of life. The fetus also incorporates iron into muscle tissue and enzymes. During the last trimester of pregnancy the fetus builds up iron stores. These help to see him through his first few months after birth, a time when iron intake tends to be low. The mother requires additional iron for formation of the placenta and to increase her supply of red blood cells. Since only part of ingested iron is absorbed, recommended intake must be much larger than actual need. If multiple births are expected or the mother is found to be deficient in iron, the amount of iron supplementation may be increased above amounts specified in Table 7.3.

Many pregnant women find that iron supplements tend to cause constipation, a condition which can be particularly uncomfortable during pregnancy. Health professionals need to anticipate this problem and give advice about what to do should constipation occur.

Folic Acid Folic acid is a vitamin which is crucial during pregnancy because it is needed for rapid cell division. Supplemental folic acid is particularly important in the case of multiple pregnancy or if there are signs of folic acid deficiency.

Iodine The trace element iodine is needed in increased amounts during periods of heightened metabolic activity such as pregnancy. A pregnant woman who lives in a goitrous region should use iodized salt or some other reliable source of iodine. Although salt intake used to be routinely restricted during pregnancy, this practice has been questioned by the Committee on Maternal Nutrition. In fact the committee feels that sodium (salt) restriction during pregnancy is potentially dangerous.

When supplements are prescribed it is essential to make sure that the woman understands (1) the purpose of the supplements and (2) the fact that supplements alone do not ensure adequate nutrient intake.

TABLE 7.3 *Recommended nutrient supplements for the pregnant woman*

SUPPLEMENT	QUANTITY
Iron	30 to 60 mg daily during the 2nd and 3rd trimesters
Folic acid	200 to 800 μg daily (This equals 0.2 to 0.8 mg)
Vitamin D	400 IU if no fortified milk or fortified soy milk is drunk. Partial supplementation when intake of either type of milk is less than 4 cups daily
Calcium	1200 mg daily if no milk or calcium-rich milk substitutes are consumed. Partial supplementation when some calcium-rich foods are eaten
Vitamin B$_{12}$	4 μg daily for vegans. Partial supplementation for vegetarians consuming goat or soy milk
Iodine	Via iodized salt (Sea-salt is not iodized)

Note: These recommendations are to *supplement* a well-balanced diet. They are not meant to be a substitute for good eating habits.

DEALING WITH DISCOMFORTS OF PREGNANCY RELATED TO DIET

A few changes in dietary habits may make pregnancy more enjoyable by minimizing certain discomforts.

Morning sickness Morning sickness is the term used for a nauseous feeling which often occurs during the first trimester of pregnancy. Actually it may develop at any time of the day and may be accompanied by vomiting. Unlike most familiar types of nausea, the nausea of pregnancy is usually relieved by keeping a small amount of food in the stomach.

If a pregnant woman is bothered in the morning, it may be helpful for her to keep melba toast, plain crackers, or other dry starchy food at the bedside. (Yes, crackers in bed!) She should plan to awaken and eat two or three crackers about 15 to 30 minutes before it is time for her to get up in the morning. (This may save time in the long run.) During the day she may benefit from small, frequent meals which are low

POINTS OF EMPHASIS
Diet during pregnancy

• *Make nutritious food selections with the help of a reliable food guide for pregnancy. Be sure you include several good food sources of folic acid.*

• *Avoid skipping meals, especially breakfast.*

• *Eat enough food to gain weight at a rate of 0.7 to 1.5 kg. (1.5 to 3 lb.) the first trimester and 0.36 kg. (0.8 lb.) weekly during the second and third trimester even if you are overweight.*

• *Do not try to reduce your weight or avoid normal weight gain during pregnancy.*

• *Use moderate amounts of iodized salt in cooking and at the table.*

• *Drink generous amounts of fluid.*

• *If your weight increases suddenly, call your physician. Do not try to handle it yourself by cutting back on food or salt intake.*

• *Do not smoke, or at least try to cut down on smoking, even if it causes you to gain weight a little faster than normal.*

• *Avoid alcoholic beverages and drugs except those prescribed by a physician who knows you are pregnant.*

• *Adjust your food habits as necessary to minimize discomfort associated with eating, but do not let this interfere with recommended nutrient and caloric intake. Do not use medications to combat symptoms without the approval of your doctor or nurse practitioner.*

• *Take nutrient supplements only as prescribed by the doctor or nurse practitioner.*

in fat content. Usually it is helpful to reduce the amount of fluid taken with meals or to eliminate obvious fluid entirely at mealtime. It then becomes imperative to consume juices, milk, and other beverages between meals in order to meet the need for water.

Since strong odors may precipitate nausea, a pregnant woman may wish to avoid cooking foods having this characteristic. Good ventilation in the kitchen may also be helpful, if practical. Avoidance of caffeine-containing beverages, alcoholic beverages, and cigarettes reduces the mother's discomfort and promotes the health of the fetus.

Heartburn and gas Symptoms of heartburn and gas are most apt to be troublesome during the second and third trimesters of pregnancy. Capacity of the stomach and speed of digestion tend to decrease as the fetus exerts increased pressure within the abdomen. Avoidance of caffeine and high fat foods may help prevent development of these symptoms. Small meals taken frequently are usually tolerated well. Eating any food which commonly caused indigestion prior to pregnancy will no doubt continue to do so. Care should be taken to maintain adequate nutrient and caloric intake. Medications should never be used to relieve symptoms unless advised by a qualified health professional.

Constipation and hemorrhoids A diet high in fiber and fluids helps promote normal, easily passed bowel movements. This, in turn, reduces the chance of constipation and hemorrhoids (enlarged veins in the anus, sometimes called "piles"). Using whole grain bread, cereal, and crackers; bran; and raw fruits and raw vegetables is recommended. Prunes, dried fruit, and prune juice may be particularly helpful in avoiding constipation.

LACTATION

Deciding whether to breast feed or bottle feed

During pregnancy serious thought should be given to whether to breast feed or bottle feed.

Until the early 1900s a majority of American mothers breast fed their infants, using bottle feeding only as a last resort. Since then many technological developments such as refrigeration, food processing, improved sanitation, and nipple design have made bottle feeding safer and more practical than it had been previously. With these developments and other changes in society, bottle feeding became the new tradition. Today only about 20 to 25 percent of American babies are breast fed at all[11] and the percentage drops drastically by 6 months of age. There does, however, appear to be a trend toward a return to breast feeding, especially among well-educated women.

New information concerning breast feeding has stimulated a resurgence of respect for this age-old feeding practice. Groups such as the American Academy of Pediatrics, the American Public Health Association, and the World Health Organization recommend breast feeding as the best method of nourishing infants.

Health professionals, whether in the public or the private sector, need to assume responsibility for educating the public about breast feeding versus bottle feeding in a positive, yet objective manner. If this is not done, bottle feeding may be chosen with little thought given to the alternative. Emphasis needs to be placed on which method is best from a nutritional and physiological standpoint for the mother and infant, without overlooking psychological aspects.

Breast feeding is not and has not been well advertised. Many women are unaware of potential advantages of lactation to themselves and to their infants. Many assume they will be happier if they bottle feed. Some women who have tried to breast feed have not received the support they need from health professionals, family, and friends. These mothers may, in turn, discourage others from trying. Perhaps current social and environmental obstacles to breast feeding can be reduced if the value of breast feeding is more widely recognized.

Health care providers should not tell mothers to breast feed their babies or foster a sense of guilt in those who choose to bottle feed. Instead, it would be desirable to create a climate in which breast feeding could be viewed as a desirable way to feed a baby.

Breast milk and formula are similar in their overall nutrient composition; otherwise formula could not support normal growth as it usually does. Nevertheless, the two types of milk differ in innumerable ways, some of which have not yet been clearly identified.

Breast milk has served mankind well for thousands upon thousands of years. There is no evidence yet to indicate that food processors have improved upon or even equalled natural milk for babies. They design their formulas to simulate breast milk. As efforts are made to improve formulas, adjustments in some nutrients might cause imbalances in others, with the possibility of harmful effects on the baby.[12,13]

NUTRITIONAL CONSIDERATIONS

Human milk contains the proper proportions and amounts of all nutrients needed for the growth and health of the infant. The RDA for infants is based on the nutrient composition of breast milk.

The mixture of nutrients in human milk is considered to be ideal for rapid growth of the brain.[14] Human milk is high in the sugar lactose. Lactose is a source of a simpler sugar called galactose which the body uses to synthesize nervous tissue. Formulas vary in lactose content; some are comparable to breast milk. The ratio of cysteine to methionine (two amino acids) in breast milk is thought by some researchers to be more favorable for development of the nervous system than is the ratio of these amino acids in formula.[14]

The biological value of the protein in breast milk is superior to that of protein in formula. This difference is offset by the higher protein content of formula. Protein in breast milk is more readily digested by an infant than is protein in formula.

Breast milk contains a considerable amount of nitrogen in compounds other than protein. There are indications that this nonprotein nitrogen (NPN) may improve the utilization of milk proteins.[15] Overall, the protein and amino acid composition of infant formula differs markedly from that of breast milk.

The fat in breast milk is readily digested by infants and is high in linoleic acid, a component of fat which is essential for growth and health. Formulas vary in digestibility of fat and in their content of linoleic acid.

Breast milk contains much less sodium, potassium, calcium, and phosphorus than do many formulas. The amount is certainly ample to meet the full-term infant's needs but does not put an unnecessary load on the baby's immature kidneys. (The kidneys must excrete more of these minerals if intake is excessive.) The ratio of calcium to phosphorus in human milk is approximately 2.4 to 1. In cow's milk the ratio is about 1.3 to 1. This imbalance may lead to electrolyte disturbances in very young infants, unless cow's milk is diluted or the ratio of these minerals is altered in the preparation of formula.

The availability and balance of trace elements in breast milk is more likely to be optimal in breast milk than in formula.[16] Much remains to be learned about bioavailability of and requirement for trace elements. As recently as 1976 it was found that the level of zinc in two commercial infant formulas was inadequate for optimal nutritional status of healthy term infants, particularly males.[17] (This has since been corrected.) Investigations are continuing to determine if formulas have any other nutrient deficiencies or imbalances that require change. The adequacy of vitamin E content of some formulas has recently been questioned, even though amounts used in commercial formulas equal or exceed Recommended Dietary Allowances.[18]

Breast milk varies in composition during a feeding, from feeding to feeding, from day to day, and over longer periods of time. The difference between colostrum, the fluid secreted during the first few days following delivery, and mature milk is so marked that the two milks even look very different. Colostrum is thicker than mature milk and yellow instead of bluish white. Colostrum is particularly rich in protein (including protective immunoglobulins), zinc, and vitamin A. There is no formula comparable to colostrum.

Some authorities speculate that the increase in fat content of breast milk that occurs during a feeding helps breast fed infants develop an appetite control mechanism and that this in turn helps prevent development of obesity.[19] Formula is constant in composition throughout the feeding and from day to day.

It has been suggested that chronobiological changes (variations in composition of milk over time and from mother to mother) may reflect differences in nutritional requirements of their infants.[20] If this is so, it could not be matched by formula feeding.

The nutritive value of breast milk is likely to be satisfactory unless the mother's diet is grossly inadequate;[21] however, the supply of milk produced may be reduced by a poor diet. When a mother's diet is inadequate, breast milk is more apt to be low in water soluble vitamins and certain trace minerals than in the energy nutrients. Changes in composition of breast milk caused by a somewhat inadequate maternal diet are not apt to be life-threatening to an infant, but improper composition of formula resulting from incorrect formula preparation could have disastrous results.

ANTI-INFECTIVE CONSIDERATIONS

For years the observation has been made that breast fed babies are less susceptible to infection than are bottle fed babies. This was thought to be largely caused by the formula's being easily contaminated in unsanitary environments. However, a number of researchers have thought that the milk itself might be protective. Consequently, breast milk has been examined to determine if it contains substances which afford protection against microorganisms and other harmful substances. The research has been fruitful and has revealed several substances present in fresh breast milk. The presence of these substances is strongly suggestive that breast milk has important anti-infective properties. These substances are the following:

1. The antibody *secretory immunoglobulin A* (SIgA) is thought to bind large molecules of foreign proteins, including viruses, bacteria, and toxic substances. This apparently helps prevent them from being absorbed and harming the infant.
2. Other antibodies, *immunoglobulins G, M, and E* (IgG, IgM, and IgE), in breast milk are structurally similar to corresponding immunoglobulins that are present in blood.[22]
3. *Lactoferrin* is an iron-binding protein which ties up iron in such a way that bacterial growth is retarded. (Some pathogenic bacteria require iron for growth.)
4. *Lysozyme* is an enzyme which may act to destroy bacteria directly by lysing (splitting) their cell membranes. Lysozyme has also been found to act indirectly by increasing the effectiveness of antibodies.
5. *Leukocytes* may be at least partly responsible for providing protection from necrotizing enterocolitis, a life-threatening condition most common among low birth weight infants. Leukocytes have been shown to afford protection in newborn rats.[23]
6. *Macrophages* are living cells which are motile and phagocytic; this means that they can "creep up on" and engulf other organisms. Macrophages also liberate SIgA and *interferon*, a substance which fights viruses.

7. *Bifidus factor* is a specific growth-promoting factor for the bacteria *Lactobacillus bifidus*. This bacterium is thought to interfere with colonization of the intestinal tract by pathogenic bacteria.[24]
8. *Complement, lactoperoxidase,* and *antistaphylococcal* factor are three other defense factors which may contribute to the decreased incidence of infection among breast fed infants.
9. Ingestion of breast milk results in formation of a somewhat acidic stool (the residue of waste products in the large intestine), whereas formula feeding is usually associated with less acid stools. *Increased acidity* of the stool appears to protect against the multiplication of disease-causing bacteria in the colon.

All of the preceding factors appear to give breast fed infants a margin of safety which bottle-fed babies do not have. Ogra and Ogra[25] suggest that breast milk during the first week of life may be crucial in providing the infant with a variety of antibodies at a time when the mucous membranes are too immature to offer full protection.

ANTI-ALLERGENIC CONSIDERATIONS

Babies do not develop allergy to breast milk. Secretory IgA in breast milk binds potential allergens and prevents their absorption. Exclusive breast feeding during the first few weeks after birth may decrease the risk of developing atopic eczema (allergic skin rash) in the first year of life.[25]

On the other hand, formula feeding exposes an infant to a large dose of potential allergens and provides no SIgA to prevent their absorption. Early introduction of potential allergens appears to increase the risk of development of an allergic reaction, particularly if there is a family history of allergy.

PHYSIOLOGICAL EFFECTS ON THE MOTHER

Breast feeding is not a reliable means of family planning. However, when a mother is unwilling to use other methods of contraception, breast feeding may have a child spacing effect *while it is used as the sole means of feeding the infant.* Frequent nursing results in increased blood serum levels of a pituitary hormone, prolactin, which suppresses ovulation.[26]

Nursing a baby stimulates production of the hormone oxytocin; this promotes involution of the mother's uterus back to its normal size. Contractions of the uterus are easily felt by the mother during the first few days postpartum while she nurses the baby.

SOCIOECONOMIC EFFECTS

Cost To determine the cost of breast feeding one should estimate the cost of the additional food used to meet the increased nutrient and caloric requirements of lactation. Cost depends largely on the selected foods. It has been estimated that if low cost foods are selected (such as fortified nonfat dry milk, peanut butter sandwich, orange juice, and spinach) breast feeding costs about the same as feeding an evaporated milk formula and much less than feeding some commercial formulas.[27] Savings on bottles and other equipment might also be considered.

Convenience Advantages of one type of feeding over another from the standpoint of convenience are a matter of opinion. Breast milk requires no shopping or preparation. A mother needs to take precautions to prevent contamination of formula, but contamination is a minor concern when breast feeding. Mothers who feel comfortable nursing in public find it convenient to feed the baby under nearly any circumstance, while those who are more modest may find that breast feeding is incompatible with traveling or other activities outside of the home. It can be difficult, but is not necessarily impossible, for working mothers to continue breast feeding young infants. For about the first month, breast fed infants usually need to be fed more often than formula fed infants of comparable age.

The stool of a breast fed baby has a less offensive odor than that of a bottle fed baby; however, its more liquid consistency may result in extra cleanup and laundry. A breast fed baby is unlikely to be troubled by constipation, whereas this is a fairly common occurrence in some formula fed babies.

PSYCHOLOGICAL ASPECTS

A mother needs to choose the feeding method which seems most suited to her and with which she can be successful. A mother's decision to breast or bottle feed may be influenced not only by many of the previously discussed factors but also by her conception of what would benefit the baby emotionally, her own self-concept and sense of identity, and the feelings of her husband or of significant others. A support group can be vital to a successful experience with breast feeding.[28]

Strong feelings of closeness and attachment develop between a mother and infant during the feeding process. It has been suggested that the bonding between mother and infant which develops during breast feeding may have a positive influence on an infant's psychological development.[29] Certainly, parents who bottle feed can also develop a close physical and emotional relationship with their infant by touching, fondling, and rocking and by singing and talking to the infant.

A mother who feels secure in her ability to breast feed communicates those feelings to her infant; she lets milk down more easily than a mother who is unable to relax prior to feeding. The mother who considers the act of nursing to be objectionable may communicate feelings of anxiety and stress to her infant; feeding, thus, may be an unpleasant experience for the infant.

If a mother is undecided as to how to feed her infant she might be encouraged to try breast feeding, especially if she has people who can provide her with emotional support. Studies have indicated that mothers who have started breast feeding immediately after delivery have continued the practice longer than those who have started breast feeding 24 to 48 hours after delivery.[29] It is easier to initiate breast feeding soon after birth.

Relactation

Sometimes it is possible for a woman to gradually establish a milk supply and to breast feed a baby even though she did not initiate breast feeding after birth. This process is called *relactation*. The same term is also used to describe the process of increasing a dwindling supply of milk. Relactation is more common in developing nations than in America. This process is by no means simple; it requires a highly motivated woman, a hungry baby, and a strong support group for the mother.[30] *The Complete Book of Breast Feeding*[36] briefly describes ways of assisting a mother with relactation.

Indications for formula feeding

Formula feeding may be indicated because of specific illnesses of the mother (such as tuberculosis), specific illnesses of the infant (including certain genetic defects), toxic substances in the milk (as from use of certain pharmaceutical agents or addictive drugs), inability of the infant to nurse, or absence of the mother. In all but the first case, if the condition is *temporary* a mother might choose to maintain her milk supply by manual expression or use of a breast pump at regular intervals. Breast milk can be collected in a sterile container and be fed to the infant immediately or stored in the refrigerator for 24 hours if desired (Fig. 7.2).

Advance preparation

It is advantageous for a mother to read about breast feeding prior to delivery of the baby. Many mothers will benefit from informative books such as *The Complete Book of Breast Feeding*[31] or *The Womanly Art of Breast Feeding*.[32] Others will find brief publications adequate for meeting their needs.

After a woman decides to breast feed, she may want to contact the LaLeche League in her area. LaLeche League International is a world-wide organization which promotes breast feeding. Local groups hold informal educational and supportive meetings for expectant mothers and for mothers who are nursing their babies. A small fee is charged unless a person is unable to pay. Experienced LaLeche members offer help with problems by telephone and, if necessary, by home visits. Some large communities have an organization such as a nursing mothers' council which offers services similar to those provided by LaLeche.

Nutrition during lactation

A woman who decides to breast feed should be provided with information about the nutritive needs of lactation and how to meet them. Apparently this information is often overlooked by health care workers.[33]

A nutritious diet which meets the Recommended Dietary Allowances for the lactating woman is of benefit to both the mother and infant. Such a diet provides a sufficient quantity of nutrients to prevent maternal reserves from being depleted. It promotes an adequate supply of high quality milk for the baby. It should be noted that a nutritious diet does not guarantee a successful nursing experience. Success is also influenced by such factors as adequate suckling stimulus and a relaxed attitude toward nursing. The health care team needs to help inexperienced mothers learn techniques of breast feeding. Mothers need to know that frequent nursing stimulates the production of milk and that

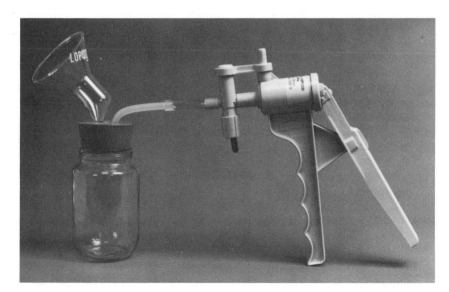

FIGURE 7.2. A hand operated breast pump which may be used to maintain milk supply when baby must be away from mother, or may be used in other situations. The collection jar is on the left with the cuplike breast shield attached. To the right is the pump body. Vacuum is created by squeezing its handles together. (Courtesy of Lopuco, Ltd., 1615 Old Annapolis Rd., Woodbine MD 21797)

early introduction of supplemental formula or of solid foods may decrease milk production. Excellent suggestions for assisting nursing mothers can be found in references listed at the end of Part One.

Nutrient demands of lactation are considerably higher than those of nonlactating mothers, but similar to those of pregnancy. Lactation increases caloric demands even more than pregnancy does. A lactating woman can enjoy large helpings of food without the usual worry about "getting fat." A lactating woman needs to meet her usual nutrient requirements and take in additional nutrients to cover those lost in breast milk and those required for making the milk. Drinking extra milk does not supply all of the extra nutrients needed during lactation. The need for calcium, phosphorus, protein, and riboflavin would probably be met in this manner. However, milk does not provide enough micronutrients such as folic acid, vitamin B_6, vitamin C, zinc, magnesium, and iron to meet increased demands of lactation. Although the loss of iron in milk is small, it increases the iron requirement of lactating women significantly. Human milk, unlike processed cows' milk, is a good source of vitamin C. Therefore the dietary supply of this vitamin should be high enough to cover this increased loss. Vitamin D has only recently been discovered to be present in substantial amounts in breast milk.[34] Researchers are investigating whether lactating women should increase intake of vitamin D above the 400 IU daily currently recommended.

Food guides

Food guides which have been developed for lactating women are identical to those for pregnancy (Table 7.3) with the addition of one more cup of milk daily. Thus the Basic Four plans recommend 1 L. (4 c.) of milk daily (1.5 L. for adolescents under 17 years of age) or the equivalent. The California Department of Health recommends 1.2 L. (5 c.) of milk or the equivalent daily. Because the recommended intake of folic acid remains high during lactation (two times normal), use of generous servings of green leafy vegetables should be strongly urged.

Weight changes, nutrition, and milk supply

The caloric requirement of a lactating woman is affected by the amount of milk she produces. Once the milk supply is well-established, milk production usually averages about 600 to 700 ml. daily.[10] It is usually lower if the baby is given solid food.[12,20] This amount of milk represents about 400 to 460 kcal. not including the energy required to make the milk. The lactating woman, therefore, needs to consume a substantial amount of extra calories (usually in excess of 500 kcal. daily) to maintain an adequate milk supply and/or avoid excessive weight loss. The Recommended Dietary Allowances, which suggest adding 500 kcal. to the diet of the lactating woman, assumes that some fat

loss will take place. Thin individuals should definitely consume more than 500 extra calories to cover the caloric requirement of lactation.

Appetite is probably the most reliable guide to total food intake during lactation. Attempts to curtail food intake to achieve rapid weight loss are likely to interfere with milk production. Strict dieting, if needed, is best delayed until after the baby is weaned. Gradual weight loss is normal during the first weeks after delivery because the blood volume and uterus return to normal size. Many nursing mothers find that they lose some body fat gradually even while maintaining a high food intake.

A nursing mother should consume extra fluid to make up for that lost in the milk. Establishing a pattern of taking extra fluid before or during nursing the baby may be helpful.

Effects of ingested substances on human milk and the baby

There are no commonly used foods that are definitely contraindicated during lactation. A possible exception is freshwater game fish from certain areas, which may contain hazardous amounts of the insecticide PCB. Fish purchased in the market should be safe. Some foods, such as onions or garlic, may change the flavor of breast milk. If the infant seems to object to the taste of the milk, the mother may decide to avoid those foods temporarily. Occasionally a specific food will have a laxative effect on the infant. Usually, however, disorders in the infant are not related to the mother's milk and the advice of a health professional should be sought. If no physiological reasons for probems are found, a mother may be advised to observe for symptoms after she has eaten a specific food, and repeat the trial at intervals. Eliminating wholesome foods during lactation is seldom desirable or necessary.

A lactating woman should probably avoid taking oral contraceptives for at least 6 weeks following delivery. If taken sooner, there is likely to be a decrease in the quality and quantity of breast milk produced and successful nursing may be impossible to establish.[26]

A number of drugs should be avoided during lacta-

POINTS OF EMPHASIS
Nutrition during lactation

• *Follow a reliable food guide for lactating women.*
• *Make sure that intake of vitamin D from food or supplements is 400 IU daily.*
• *Do not restrict calories, but make calories count.*
• *Continue to supplement diet with 30 to 60 mg. elemental iron daily for 2 to 3 months, or longer on physician's recommendation.*
• *Drink about 3 L. (3 qt.) fluid daily. If urine is concentrated, increase fluid intake more.*

tion because they are secreted in the milk and may adversely affect the baby. Suggested sources of this information are included at the end of Part One. It may be advisable to avoid use of saccharin during lactation.[7]

STUDY QUESTIONS

1. A woman whose intake of essential nutrients is habitually low says she will improve her diet as soon as she becomes pregnant. Name several reasons why she should be encouraged to improve her eating behavior before she conceives.

2. An obese woman comes for her first prenatal checkup when she is 3-months pregnant. She says that she has been very careful about her diet and has gained no weight since she became pregnant. What amount of weight gain should be recommended for her? Why should she be encouraged to gain weight even though she is obese? How would you discuss this with her?

3. List several reasons why it is desirable for a pregnant woman to take supplemental iron rather than to depend only on the iron in the food supply.

4. Why should a pregnant woman be urged to eat a well-balanced diet during pregnancy even though prenatal vitamin supplements plus iron are prescribed?

5. Plan a well-balanced diet which you would be willing to eat if you were pregnant. How would you change it if you were lactating?

6. Discuss reasons why lactating women may need extra support and assistance even though breast feeding is a natural process. What can health professionals do to help make breast feeding a more appealing option?

7. Identify how different types of nutrient deficiencies are apt to affect the quality or quantity of breast milk.

8. Why is it impossible for a formula to duplicate colostrum?

References

1. *Maternal Nutrition and the Course of Pregnancy.* National Research Council, Food and Nutrition Board, Committee on Maternal Nutrition. Washington DC: National Academy of Sciences, 1970.

2. *Nutrition in Maternal Health Care.* Committee on Nutrition, American College of Obstetricians and Gynecologists. Chicago: American College of Obsettricians and Gynecologists, 1974.

*3. *Nutrition During Pregnancy and Lactation.* Sacramento CA: Maternal and Child Health Unit, California Department of Health, 1975.

4. Mahalko, J. R., and Bennion, M.: The effect of parity and time between pregnancies on maternal hair chromium concentration. *Am. J. Clin. Nutr.* 29:1069, 1976.

5. Ouellette, E. M., et al.: Adverse effect on offspring of maternal alcohol abuse during pregnancy. *N. Engl. J. Med.* 297:528, 1977.

*6. Erb, L.: The fetal alcohol syndrome (FAS). *Clin. Pediatr.* 17:644, 1978.

7. *Cancer Testing and Saccharin.* Washington DC: Office of Technology Assessment. U.S. Govt. Printing Office, October 1977.

8. Hopkins, H.: The GRAS list revisited. *FDA Consumer.* 12(4):13, 1978.

9. Ling, S., King, J., and Leung, V.: Diet, growth, and cultural food habits in Chinese-American infants. *Am. J. Chin. Med.* 3:125, 1975.

10. Abril, I. F.: Mexican-American folk beliefs: How they affect health care. *MCN* 2:168, 1977.

11. Fomon, S. J.: What are infants fed in the United States? *Pediatrics* 56:350, 1975.

12. Jelliffe, E. F. P.: Infant feeding practices: Associated iatrogenic and commerciogenic diseases. *Pediatr. Clin. North Am.* 24(1):49, 1977.

13. Jelliffe, D., and Jelliffe, P.: Alleged inadequacies of human milk. *Clin. Pediatr.* 16:1140, 1977.

14. Jelliffe, D., and Jelliffe, E. F.: Nutrition and human milk. *Postgrad. Med.* 60:153, 1976.

15. Lonnerdal, B., Forsum, E., and Hambraeus, L.: A longitudinal study of the protein, nitrogen and lactose contents of human milk from Swedish well-nourished mothers. *Am. J. Clin. Nutr.* 29:1127, 1976.

16. Hambidge, K. M.: The role of zinc and other trace metals in pediatric nutrition and health. *Pediatr. Clin. North Am.* 24(1):95, 1977.

17. Walravens, P. A., and Hambidge, K. M.: Growth of infants fed a zinc supplemented formula. *Am. J. Clin. Nutr.* 29:1114, 1976.

18. Asfour, R., et al.: Folacin requirements of children. III. Normal infants. *Am. J. Clin. Nutr.* 30:1098, 1977.

19. Hall B.: Changing composition of human milk and early development of an appetite control. *Lancet* I:779, 1975.

*20. Alfin-Slater, R. B., and Jelliffe, D. B.: Nutritional requirements with special reference to infancy. *Pediatr. Clin. North Am.* 24(1):3, 1977.

21. Lonnerdal, B., et al.: Breast milk composition in Ethiopian and Swedish mothers. II. Lactose, nitrogen, and protein contents." *Am. J. Clin. Nutr.* 29:1134, 1976.

22. Hambraeus, L.: Proprietary milk versus human breast milk in infant feeding. *Pediatr. Clin. North Am.* 24(1):17, 1977.

23. Review. The role of milk leukocytes in protection from necrotizing enterocolitis." *Nutr. Rev.* 36:190, 1978.

24. Goldman, A. S., and Smith, C. W.: Host resistance factors in breast milk. *J. Pediatr.* 82:1082, 1973.

25. Ogra, S. S., and Ogra, P. L.: Immunologic aspects of human colostrum and milk. *J. Pediatr.* 92:547, 1978.

26. Jackson, R. L.: Long term consequences of suboptimal nutritional practices in early life." *Pediatr. Clin. North Am.* 24(1):63, 1977.

27. Lamm, E., Delaney, J., and Dwyer, J. T.: Economy in the feeding of infants.*Pediatr. Clin. North Am.* 24(1):71, 1977.

28. Nielsen, I. L.: Breast feeding for knowledge, confidence, and support." *Issues in Comprehensive Pediatric Nursing* II (1):35–42, January/February 1977.

29. Klaus, M., and Kennell, J.: *Maternal-Infant Bonding.* St. Louis: C. V. Mosby Co., 1976.

30. Brown, R. E.: Relactation with reference to application in developing countries. *Clin. Pediatr.* 17:333, 1978.

31. Olds, S. W., and Eiger, M. S.: *The Complete Book of Breast Feeding.* New York: Workman Publishing Co., 1976.

32. *The Womanly Art of Breastfeeding,* ed. 2. Franklin Park IL: LaLeche League International, 1963.

33. Sims, L. S.: Dietary status of lactating women. I. Nutrient intake from food and from supplements. *J. Am. Diet. Assoc.* 73:139, 1978.

34. Lakdawala, D. R., and Widdowson, E. M.: Vitamin D in human milk *Lancet* I:167, 1977.

8

Promoting sound eating habits during infancy

Food and nutrition play a very important role in the life of an infant. The infant needs adequate amounts of nutritious food to support his rapid growth. The atmosphere and manner in which an infant is introduced to food strongly influence the food habits he begins to develop. The development of sound eating habits should begin in infancy.

Growth during the first 18 years of life is remarkable. A healthy child's weight increases approximately 20 times and his height increases more than 3 times. Likewise, marked social, psychological, and intellectual changes occur as a child moves from infancy to adulthood.

Balanced and varied meals provide a child with the energy and nutrients needed to make this amount of physical growth possible. If these varied meals are presented in pleasant surroundings, eating also provides a child with learning experiences that support normal development.

Nutrition during infancy and the establishment of sound eating and feeding practices during the first year of life are discussed in this chapter. A general discussion of growth and development is included with some of the factors promoting or retarding growth and development.

GROWTH AND DEVELOPMENT

Types of tissue growth

Growth denotes an increase in size. Growth of tissue involves hyperplasia and/or hypertrophy. *Hyperplasia* is an increase in the total *number* of cells composing a particular tissue. *Hypertrophy* is an increase in the

size of a cell within a tissue. During the initial growth of a tissue there is a period of rapid hyperplasia when the number of cells is increasing. Gradually, as these cells begin to hypertrophy or increase in size, hyperplasia slows down. During the last stage of tissue development hypertrophy is dominant.

The period of hyperplasia is said to be critical to tissue development. It is primarily at this time that the number of cells forming a tissue is determined. During hyperplasia the demand for nutrients to support tissue development is great. Developing tissues are extremely vulnerable to lack of nutrients and to other environmental stressors. If there is a lack of nutrients or energy, the total number of cells may be undesirably small. If there is ample material for growth, a greater number of cells may be formed. The genetic plan limits the number of cells which may be formed in all tissues except adipose tissue.

Much attention has been directed recently toward growth of brain tissue and adipose tissue during the critical hyperplasia period. It is suspected that malnutrition during fetal development and the first two years of life may lead to retarded brain growth and impaired intellectual development.[1] Excessive calories, on the other hand, are thought to result in a permanent increase in the number of fat cells. This greater number of fat cells may be a factor contributing to obesity later in life.[2]

Patterns of growth and development

Although each child grows and develops in a unique manner, there is a predictable pattern of events. Different parts of the body grow at different times and at different rates. Each tissue has a specific period of rapid growth marked by rapid cell differentiation and change in form. Nutrient requirements change somewhat as the focus of growth changes. For instance, periods of rapid bone growth increase the calcium requirement, while muscular growth increases the iron requirement.

The overall growth rate changes at different periods of childhood. It is most rapid in infancy and adolescence. At those times nutritional and energy requirements for growth are especially high. At any age, about an extra 5 to 8 kcal. are needed for each gram of body tissue gained.[3] When growth slows, the demand for energy diminishes.

The caloric requirement for infants gradually increases as their overall body size increases. However, the number of calories required *per unit* of body size becomes smaller, primarily because growth proceeds at a slower rate.

Factors influencing growth

Physiological, environmental, and behavioral factors influence whether or not a child grows to his maximum potential.

PHYSIOLOGICAL FACTORS

The genetic makeup a child receives from his parents contributes to the determination of his adult size and body build. The endocrine system regulates the rate of growth and development by several means: (1) Growth hormone from the pituitary gland participates in the regulation of metabolism and skeletal growth. (2) Thyroid hormone helps maintain a normal rate of energy metabolism. If thyroid hormone is lacking, there is a marked slowing of linear growth and maturation. (3) Insulin and certain other hormones affect growth in a variety of ways.

ENVIRONMENTAL AND BEHAVIORAL FACTORS

Whether or not a child is provided with an adequate supply of nutrients and energy for growth is greatly influenced by his environment. The foods commonly used in a particular locale may be low in one or more nutrients. In developing nations where the food supply is limited, some children develop a protein-deficiency disease called *kwashiorkor*. The principal food in their diet may be yams or another low-protein plant food. Children with kwashiorkor are significantly stunted in their growth and development. In the U.S. an infant may not be given enough nutritious food because parents lack purchasing power or the ability to budget.

Sometimes an adequate food supply is available but the mother fails to provide her child with a balanced diet. This may be the result of her lack of knowledge as to what or how to feed her infant, or it may be due to a problem in the maternal-child relationship.

Catch-up growth Any period of undernutrition or illness may result in a lack of growth or decreased growth rate. In most instances, correcting the cause results in a dramatic acceleration of growth. This type of rapid growth is referred to as *catch-up growth*. It continues until the child has caught up to the level of growth expected for his chronological age and genetic makeup. After this the infant or child resumes a more normal rate of growth. The amount of catch-up growth occurring in infants whose weight is low for gestational age tends to be less than that for preterm infants.

Limitations of Growth Measurements

Growth is frequently measured by both parents and professionals to determine how an infant or child is progressing. A child's progress is often seen as an index of success or failure in providing care. While growth certainly is an important assessment criterion it is not the only measure of success. The infant's level of physical activity, his appetite, and his interest in activities other than eating affect his rate of growth. Measurement of growth may precipitate a problem if a breast fed infant is compared to a bottle fed infant. A breast fed baby is usually smaller than the bottle fed one. The overanxious mother who is breast feeding sometimes interprets this to mean that her milk supply is inadequate. After all, she has no good way to estimate how much milk the baby is consuming, and Americans tend to take the attitude that "bigger is better." In most instances, the breast fed infant receives adequate nutrition and grows at an acceptable though somewhat slower rate.

POINTS OF EMPHASIS
Factors influencing growth

• *Physiological factors such as genetic makeup and hormonal regulation influence an individual's adult size.*

• *Environmental factors such as geographical location, financial resources, a mother's knowledge of nutrition, and a family's emotional climate affect a child's growth.*

• *Undernutrition and illness may slow growth.*

• *Catch-up growth may follow a period of undernutrition or illness.*

• *A variety of parameters should be used to determine how growth and development is progressing.*

Behavioral characteristics

Development is dependent upon the processes of maturation and learning. Maturation consists of physical changes in body tissues which are necessary for new kinds of behavior to occur. An infant cannot learn to hold his own cup to feed himself until the nerve tissue to his arm and hand has developed so he can move his hand purposefully to his mouth. When sufficient eye-hand coordination develops, the infant reaches for the cup. Initially the infant is clumsy in his actions. With practice he soon is able to hold the cup and feed himself adeptly.

Food and eating behaviors assist the child's development in a variety of ways. The introduction of new foods provides the infant with opportunities to try out and adjust to new experiences. He learns about new tastes, textures, colors, sounds, and odors as new foods are introduced. Mealtime offers the older infant varied ways to develop motor skills as he learns to feed himself. When an infant first begins to hold his own bottle or cup, he practices and masters gross motor movements. Later, when the infant develops the pincer grasp, he practices and learns fine motor movements while picking up small bits of food such as cooked green beans. When the older infant purposely drops some food item or an eating utensil from his high chair he is learning to "let go." The mother who does not recognize this may get caught in a frustrating game of drop-and-retrieve.

The home is the healthy infant's primary environment. Within the family atmosphere the infant begins to develop a pattern of behavior and attitudes toward food. Initially an infant depends on his parents for food. The parents determine what he will eat and influence the amount consumed. As an infant grows he exerts more control over his food intake. He accepts and rejects various foods. How and what a child learns to eat lay a foundation of attitudes toward food and eating upon which adult eating behavior may be based.

Eating is one of the infant's first ways of interacting with other people, particularly his mother. The infant who is snugly held and cuddled during feedings feels warm and secure. From the tone of his mother's voice and her expression of smiles, the infant feels love. A warm comfortable feeling follows the filling of his tummy with milk or other foods. The infant comes to associate food with happy experiences. Food thus associated is usually well accepted. Because of these early associations, food may come to represent love and security to an individual later in life. On the other hand, if the family atmosphere is tense and unhappy, mealtime may be strained. As a result an infant may come to dislike specific foods or become uninterested in food altogether.

Feeding an infant helps him to acquire a sense of trust that the world and the people in it will meet most of his physical and psychological needs. For example, if an infant is usually fed when he signals that he is hungry, he learns that approaching people and making his state of discomfort known leads to gratification of his needs. Each infant is an active participant in the process of trust development. Each one shows a unique variety of behaviors toward his mother.

Some infants are irritable, responding to a stress such as hunger pain by vigorous crying. Others are more passive and cry only when the discomfort has become quite intense. Some infants quiet quickly when fed; others continue to fuss. The kinds of feelings a mother develops toward her infant are related to the responses the infant makes. It is important for a mother to be "tuned in" to her infant, particularly during the feeding experience, to promote positive experiens for both of them.

Some normal healthy infants develop *feeding problems* which relate to one or more of the following: (1) the manner in which they are fed, (2) what they are fed and how much and (3) the current emotional climate of the family. Figure 8.1 lists signs and symptoms of some common infant feeding problems and suggests some corrective measures.

Malnutrition and development

Malnutrition has been a frequent intruder in developing nations throughout history. Only recently, malnutrition has been acknowledged to be a problem of some communities of the U.S., particularly where living conditions are substandard. Here or elsewhere, factors such as the amount and kind of food available, adequacy of housing and sanitation, and the rate of infection influence the kind of malnutrition and degree to which it occurs.

The age of onset and type of malnutrition in Third World countries is changing. More young infants are suffering from a mixed type of protein-energy malnutrition which is due to an overall decrease in nutrient and calorie intake. This change may be related to an alarming trend in developing countries to wean infants from the breast at an early age and switch to bottle feeding. Because of the high cost of infant formula relative to income in these nations, mothers may dilute the formula excessively. This overdiluted formula does not supply the infant with adequate calories or nutrients. Moreover, the formula is likely to harbor many disease-causing organisms as a result of lack of refrigeration and inadequate supply of clean water for its preparation. If gastroenteritis results from ingestion of unsanitary formula, malnutrition is likely to be intensified.

Vitamin A deficiency is frequently seen in children suffering from protein-energy malnutrition. Vitamin A deficiency is an important cause of childhood mortality and of xerophthalmia. Xerophthalmia is a preventable disease causing irreversible blindness in its victims.

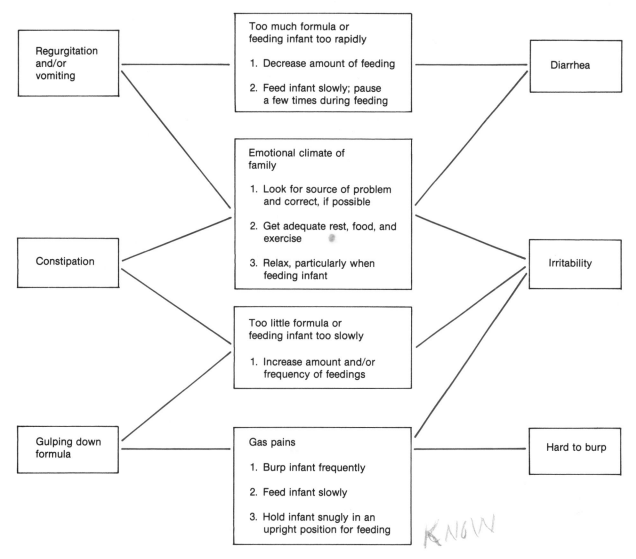

FIGURE 8.1. Common infant feeding problems and corrective measures.

Severe prolonged malnutrition can have devastating effects on growth and development. This is particularly the case during critical periods of hyperplastic tissue development, when some of the damage may be irreversible. If malnutrition does not occur until later (during periods of tissue hypertrophy), subsequent dietary improvement may result in catch-up growth with no noticeable side effects.

Malnutrition and brain development Severe malnutrition during the first 2 to 3 years of life has been positively correlated with a decrease in head circumference and a decrease in the size of the brain.[4] The specific relationship between brain size and intellectual development has not been determined. Most malnutrition occurs in settings where the socioeconomic and educational levels are low, appropriate environmental stimuli for the infant are lacking, sanitary conditions are poor, and recurrent infections are prevalent. Since these factors all influence intellectual development, it is difficult to pinpoint specific effects of malnutrition.

CONCERNS ABOUT INFANT FEEDING PRACTICES

Some infant feeding practices commonly seen in the U.S. may have adverse effects on health during infancy or in later years of life. Most of these feeding practices involve some type of overnutrition.

HIGH RENAL SOLUTE LOAD

The *renal solute load* is the amount of waste products which the kidneys must process. Excretion of solutes causes loss of water since the kidneys can excrete wastes only in solution. The infant's immature kidneys have limited ability to concentrate urine and thus cannot prevent excessive water loss. Any feeding which produces a high renal solute load because it is high in protein and/or minerals may severely reduce an infant's body fluid reserves, predisposing the infant to dehydration. A very dangerous feeding practice is giving formula which requires prefeeding dilution (as opposed to ready-to-feed formula) without diluting it properly. Concentrated formula can quickly cause life-threatening dehydration because it causes a high renal solute load without providing adequate fluids.

SODIUM INTAKE

There is considerable disagreement regarding the long term effects of high sodium intake during infancy. No prospective studies have been conducted to determine the relationship between sodium intake during infancy and the development of hypertension during the adult years. An intake of 6 to 8 mEq. (138 to 184 mg.) of sodium is considered adequate, but a baby who drinks about 800 ml. of home prepared formula daily gets more than twice that much sodium. Solid foods have the potential of adding much more sodium if the parents add salt to it or feed the baby foods already high in sodium. One survey verified that the salt intake of infants under 8 months of age decreased after manufacturers lowered the salt content of some commercial baby foods. However, studies indicate the salt intake of older infants remains high.[5]

Preference for a high salt intake is a *learned behavior*. Infants enjoy unsalted foods. Considering that salt may contribute to the development of hypertension in persons at risk, it seems reasonable to limit sodium intake early in life. The salt will not be missed and a healthier eating pattern might be established.

EXCESSIVE CALORIE INTAKE

Providing the infant with an excessive amount of food, even if it is appropriate in quality, can have harmful effects. The consequences of *over*feeding may extend into adulthood. The resulting unnecessary weight gain may contribute to obesity later in life. There is evidence that the total number of fat cells increases when an individual is overfed in infancy. The implications for health have not been clearly established. Some obese infants have developed into obese children and adults while others have lost their excess baby fat.[6] Although obesity in infancy has not been directly linked to physical disease, adult obesity has been. Feeding habits leading to adult obesity should certainly be avoided.

Early dietary influences could be crucial in the development of infantile obesity. While there is evidence suggestive of a strong genetic component, parents have control over the amount and type of food infants and young children eat. An excessive caloric intake is always necessary for the development of obesity. Early addition of solid foods to the infant's diet may add unnecessary calories. For example, if an infant is overfed by about 100 kcal. per

day, the infant could conceivably be 4.6 kg. (10 lb.) overweight at the end of a year.

Parents who overfeed tend to respond to a broad range of infant cues and signals as if they indicated hunger. Often when an infant begins crying a mother attempts to pacify him by offering food rather than first trying to determine the source of discomfort and then providing an appropriate remedy. Parents need to distinguish the infant's expressions of hunger from thirst or other needs. In hot, dry weather, for example, it is sensible to offer an infant water if he cries between feedings. Parents also need to assist the infant to recognize nutritional needs, but not other needs, as hunger.

Parents do not always realize when an infant is satiated. They may encourage him to finish the last drop of milk in the bottle. They may be concerned about avoiding waste, they may be trying to give the infant pleasure, or they may be trying to make the infant sleep a long time so that he will not require so much attention. When parents are not certain how much to feed, they usually feel it is better to err on the side of excess. Chubbiness and rapid growth of infants are admired ideals by Americans of many cultures. Since some deposition of fat is normal and desirable, parents need help in distinguishing between appropriate weight gain and obesity.

There are a number of ways to reduce the chance that an infant will become obese.

1. Breast feed for at least 3 months.[7]
2. Stop feeding when the baby stops sucking or pushes the nipple out of his mouth and shows no further interest in feeding.
3. Delay introducing solid food until the infant is 4 to 6 months old.
4. Use plain vegetables, meats, and fruits rather than mixed dinners and sweet desserts which have a high calorie content.
5. Provide the baby with lots of non-nutritive stimulation, such as cuddling. The infant needs an opportunity to suck for about 20 minutes at each feeding. He may cry because he wants more sucking and cuddling rather than more food.

POINTS OF EMPHASIS
Concerns about infant feeding practices

• *Feeding an infant a highly concentrated formula or undiluted cow's milk results in a high renal solute load. If adequate fluids are not provided, dehydration will develop.*

• *Excessive sodium intake may contribute to the development of hypertension in susceptible persons. Preference for salty foods is a learned behavior.*

• *Overfeeding in infancy may be a crucial factor in both the development of infantile obesity and obesity later in life. Infantile obesity is preventable.*

6. Allow infants free movement of their whole bodies and extremities.
7. Avoid comparing baby's intakes and feeding milestones with those of another baby, even if from the same family.
8. Consult a doctor or nurse practitioner regarding the baby's rate of growth to make certain it is adequate without being excessive.

DEVELOPING SOUND EATING HABITS IN INFANCY

Under most circumstances, both breast and bottle feeding are considered to be acceptable methods of providing an infant with a complete and adequate diet for about the first 6 months of life. Many health professionals view breast feeding as the preferred method of providing the young infant with energy and nutrients. There are some differences in the composition of breast milk, cow's milk, and selected proprietary (commercially prepared) formulas as shown in Table 8.1.

Breast feeding

If the mother's diet is high in nutritive value her milk will contain adequate amounts of nutrients for the infant with the exception of fluoride. The breast fed infant needs a fluoride supplement when he is 3 to 6 months old.[8] A water-soluble form of vitamin D has recently been discovered in breast milk, giving credence to LaLeche League's recommendation that vitamin D supplements are probably not needed by breast fed infants.[9]

Although the iron content of breast milk is low, there is evidence to indicate that the amount of iron present may be sufficient to meet the infant's needs for the first year of life. A recent study of four infants who had been fed breast milk exclusively for 8 to 18 months revealed that all had normal hemoglobin and serum iron levels. The iron in breast milk is apparently more available to the infant than that in cow's milk.[10]

Normally, considerable iron is transferred from the mother to the fetus during the last 3 months of pregnancy. Some of the iron needed by the fetus is not needed immediately after birth and is, consequently, stored in the liver. The term infant uses up most of these iron stores by 4 to 6 months of age.[10] The American Academy of Pediatrics Committee on Nutrition recommends that iron supplements from one or more sources (iron fortified cereal, iron fortified formula, or medicinal iron) be added to all infants' diets no later than 4 months of age in term infants.[11] Premature infants and those infants whose mothers were anemic during pregnancy require iron supplements by 2 months of age since they have not been born with adequate stores. Building up iron stores during infancy can help prevent iron deficiency during the preschool years, when it may be more difficult to provide for adequate intake.

Most breast fed infants get the correct amount of milk naturally. As the infant empties the breast, milk is produced for the next feeding. Thus, normally, a supply of milk adequate to meet the infant's demand is produced. It is not likely that the infant will be

TABLE 8.1 *Approximate composition per liter of breast milk, cow's milk, and selected proprietary formulas*

| | | | PROPRIETARY FORMULAS | | |
EXAMPLES OF PRODUCTS	HUMAN BREAST MILK*	COW'S MILK (UNMODIFIED)†	CONVENTIONAL MILK-BASED FORMULA‡§	"HUMANIZED" MILK-BASED FORMULA‖	SOY-BASED FORMULA¶
Energy (kcal)	750**	660	700	700	700
Protein (gm)	11**	35	15	15	18–25
Fat (gm)	45	37	37	36	30–36
Minerals††					
Calcium (mg)	340	1170	536	445	700–950
Phosphorus (mg)	140	920	454	300	500–690
Sodium (mEq)	7	22	11	6	9–24
Vitamins					
A (IU)	1898	1025	1650	2650	2100–2500
Thiamine (µg)	160	440	510	710	400–700
Riboflavin (µg)	360	1750	620	1060	600–1060
Niacin (mg)	1.5	0.9	9	9	5.0–8.4
Ascorbic acid (mg)	43	11	52	58	50–55
Vitamin E (IU)	2	0.4	12	9	9–11

Adapted from Hambraeus, L.: Proprietary milk versus human breast milk. *Ped. Clin. North Amer.* 24(1):1736, 1977.

  * The composition of human milk may vary greatly
  † Homogenized milk
  ‡ Milk-based formulas are similar and interchangeable
  § Enfamil, Similac
  ‖ SMA–SMA has a relatively low renal solute load
  ¶ Isomil, Neo-Mull-Soy, ProSobee, Nursoy—the soy-based formulas listed do not contain milk protein or lactose
  ** Values from Fomon, S.: *Infant Nutrition.* Philadelphia: W. B. Saunders Co., 1974.
  †† Levels of trace minerals would be difficult to interpret because of differences in bioavailability

overfed since he influences the amount of milk produced.

Although some individuals feel that breast fed infants should not receive supplemental bottle feedings, there are no scientific contraindications to giving occasional supplemental feedings once the mother's milk supply is well established.

Bottle-feeding

TYPES OF FORMULAS

There are a variety of artificial infant formulas available commercially which somewhat resemble human milk in composition. If an infant is bottle fed, these proprietary formulas provide the best alternative to breastfeeding except in terms of cost. A mother may be introduced to a particular proprietary formula in a hospital following her infant's birth. Many of the companies making proprietary formulas give mothers complementary packages of formula when they are discharged. "Discharge packs" may contain nursettes, a can of ready-to-feed formula, a can of concentrated formula, and a brochure about infant feeding and formula preparation. The discharge pack provides formula for the trip home and for the first few home feedings. The pack may also give a mother the opportunity to try various forms of one brand of formula. Health professionals should review commercially prepared brochures to see that they are appropriate for a mother to use.

Before a mother and infant are discharged, a health care provider should consult with the infant's pediatrician or nurse practitioner to determine the kind and amount of formula recommended for the infant. This information can then be carefully reviewed with the mother.

Iron-fortified proprietary formulas provide nutrients (except fluoride) in amounts believed to be appropriate for infants. Table 8.1 compares the composition of some commercial formulas. Commercial formulas come in a variety of forms: powdered, condensed, liquid, ready-to-feed liquid, and formula prepackaged in bottles. Cost and amount of preparation vary among the different types. The powdered form is relatively inexpensive but involves the most preparation. The prepackaged form is the most convenient but also the most expensive. Using proprietary formulas instead of making formula "from scratch" saves time and reduces the chance of mixing errors. There is less risk of contamination with ready-to-feed formulas than there is with other types.

Health professionals should encourage mothers to check the tops of formula cans for a "use by" date. Formula which is out of date should not be used. Many brands of concentrated formula have a statement in bold lettering on the top of the can about diluting the formula before feeding. Mothers should be encouraged to carefully read and follow the directions for preparation on cans of formula unless they have received special instructions from their doctor.

Home-prepared formula If a mother decides to prepare her own formula she must be given careful instructions for its preparation. Evaporated whole milk is preferred over fresh homogenized milk. Evaporated milk is sterile and inexpensive and its heat-treated protein is more easily digested than is the protein in fresh whole milk. Fresh whole milk is not recommended because it may irritate the intestinal tract of infants under 1 year of age, causing a small but significant loss of blood.[12] Goat's milk may be used for preparing formula. If it is, the infant should be given supplemental vitamin B_6 (pyridoxine).

Use of some types of milk is unacceptable except in emergency situations. Sweetened condensed milk is much too high in sugar to be used. Skim milk, either fresh or powdered, does not provide linoleic acid (a component of fat needed for normal growth and health). Skim milk is low in calories. Taking extra skim milk to make up for it low calorie content would result in an excessive intake of protein and minerals, increasing the renal solute load. If an infant does not make up the calorie deficit caused by using skim milk, his rate of growth may decrease or halt and he may fail to gain a desirable amount of body fat.

The composition of cow's milk needs to be modified to be suitable for the young infant. Milk for infant formula requires dilution to decrease the concentration of protein and minerals and thus the renal solute load. Evaporated milk requires much more dilution than does fresh whole milk. Since dilution lowers the caloric value of milk, carbohydrate is added to compensate. Either corn syrup or Dextrimaltose, a commercially prepared carbohydrate, may be used. Table sugar, while it too may be used, is very sweet tasting and does not dissolve as readily. Infants on home-prepared formulas need a reliable source of vitamin C and iron.

Fluoride supplements are recommended for all infants beginning at about 6 months of age unless the water used in formula preparation provides the recommended amount. Vitamin D should be given if the milk used is not fortified.

Methods of formula preparation There are three main methods of formula preparation: (1) the terminal method of sterilization, (2) the aseptic technique, and (3) the clean technique. Sterile disposable plastic liners are available and can be used in combination with either the clean or aseptic technique. Some liners are not appropriate for the terminal method of sterilization as they may melt or burst during the boiling process; other liners state clearly "may be boiled" on the package.

In the *terminal method*, clean bottles are filled with formula and then placed in boiling water for about 25 minutes. This method of preparation requires some planning ahead since the formula must cool about 2 hours before it can be used. More rapid cooling might result in cracked bottles. The terminal method minimizes the danger of contaminating the bottles during preparation.

With the *aseptic method*, the bottles, nipples, and all equipment used in formula preparation are sterilized by being boiled in water for a specified length of time. If tap water is used in preparation of the formula, it is boiled for 5 minutes. Equipment or bottles not used immediately can be stored covered in the pan they were boiled in, after the water has been drained off. There is much room for error with this method of preparation. If the mother does not fully understand the concept of sterile technique she may inadvertently contaminate the bottles or formula. For example, a mother might touch the inside of the nipple when putting it on a bottle.

In the *clean technique*, the formula is prepared using clean bottles and equipment. A safe source of formula and tap water must be available. The mother needs to know what *clean* preparation and handling means. For example, if she drops the nipple on the freshly washed floor, the nipple is dirty even though it still looks clean. For maximum safety, infant formula should be sterilized using either the terminal or aseptic method of preparation. Good sanitation may make the clean technique acceptable in some situations.

The mother's willingness and ability to follow the specific procedure should be considered when determining the method of preparation most appropriate for her to follow. The general cleanliness of the home environment gives an indication of the value the family places on cleanliness, as well as some indication of the mother's understanding of the term "clean." Some mothers may think that rinsing the baby's bottle in dirty dishwater makes it clean.

TYPES OF NIPPLES

There are two main types of nipples manufactured—the traditional nipple and the nipple designed to resemble a mother's nipple. Infants suck differently with the traditional nipple as opposed to the breast. There is no evidence that one is preferable to the other. Since the method of sucking may vary, one type or the other should be used consistently. The infant who is breast feeding may more easily accept supplementary bottle feedings if the breast-shaped nipple is used. The type of opening and the stiffness of nipples also vary. These affect the rate of flow of formula and how vigorously the infant must suck. The opening should not be so large and the nipple should not be so soft that the infant receives too much formula at once and chokes.

AMOUNT AND FREQUENCY OF
BOTTLE FEEDING

The approximate amount of formula to feed an infant can easily be calculated by a health professional and divided among approximately six daily feedings. Formula needs should be calculated on an individual basis. Most infants receiving appropriate amounts of formula gain 0.3 kg. (7 to 8 oz.) of weight per week although a wide range of normal weight gain can be expected.

A newborn who weighs 3 to 4 kg. (6 to 9 lb.) has such a small stomach that he can initially hold only about 30 ml. (⅛ c.) of milk. Stomach capacity quickly increases; however, during the first month of life, frequent small feedings are necessary, perhaps as often as every 2 to 3 hours. As the capacity of the infant's stomach increases the infant will not need to be fed as frequently. If started on a demand schedule, infants will usually establish their own pattern of eating within a few weeks. Gentle nudging toward a schedule rather than rigid control is desirable. When the infant's body has grown enough so he can go 6 to 7 hours without eating, he may begin sleeping through the night. This usually occurs after the infant is about 2-months old.

Infants should be offered unsweetened water (sterile for the very young infant) at least twice a day. In warm weather or if an infant has an elevated temperature, extra water should be offered.

Solid foods

Parents often need advice from health professionals regarding when and how to introduce solid foods (foods other than breast milk or formula). In the U.S. the introduction of solids tends to be based more on current trends than on the nutritional and developmental needs of the infant. There have been many changes in infant feeding practices in the last 20 years. During that time the variety and kinds of special commercial food products for infants greatly increased. Parents often need advice regarding when and how to introduce solids.

The mother's readiness and desire to introduce solid foods is influenced in many ways. Well-meaning relatives, friends, and neighbors may exert considerable pressure on a mother to follow their advice about introducing solid foods. Some people feel that solids should be introduced when the infant weighs 4 kg. (9 lb.). Others urge giving solids when the infant is consuming nearly a liter (1 qt.) of milk daily. Often feeding solids is begun as a method to get the infant to sleep through the night. (Studies have not shown that giving solids makes any significant difference in an infant's sleeping pattern.[13]) A mother who thinks her infant is gaining weight too slowly may decide to give solids to speed up the process. Another mother may be concerned about introducing solids because of either positive or negative experiences with previous siblings. Different cultural groups have characteristic patterns of adding solid foods to their baby's diet.[14] Finally, eating solids is seen by some as a significant accomplishment by the infant.

When early introduction of solid foods was first

recommended by health professionals, one of the reasons stressed was the desirability of introducing the infant to a variety of foods to increase his acceptance of them before he actually needed them. There is no good evidence that this is a valid reason. The infant's sense of taste is not well-developed until he is three- to four-months old. An infant who starts on solids early may reject some of them when his sense of taste is better developed.

Nutritionally it is not necessary to introduce solid foods before 4 to 6 months of age, especially if the infant is receiving supplemental iron from formula or is being breast fed. Introduction of solids at 4 months of age for formula fed infants may help compensate for any unrecognized inadequacies of formula.

Throughout the first year of life, breast milk or infant formula is preferable as the main source of nutrients. Solids should be used primarily to provide nutritional and caloric supplements when necessary and to provide learning experiences.

Semisolids and strained foods can be introduced when the infant is 4- to 6-months old and is sucking voluntarily. If solids are given much earlier the infant's tongue reflexively rolls forward (protrusion reflex) pushing much of the food out of the infant's mouth. When the protrusion tongue reflex has faded, it is easier for the infant to keep food in his mouth and swallow it.

Solids requiring some chewing can be offered when the jaw musculature is sufficiently developed for the infant to bite and chew. Infants begin making chewing movements before teeth actually erupt. Chewing in fact facilitates the eruption of the teeth. Usually the central incisors come in first, so the infant initially chews his food rabbit style. A mother may misinterpret this to mean that the infant is spitting out the food.

How readily the infant accepts new experiences and adapts to change should affect how soon and how quickly new foods are introduced. A mother need not be concerned if her infant initially refuses solids. She can wait awhile and try introducing them later.

Guidelines for introducing new foods

The introduction of new foods ought to be based on nutritional needs and on cues indicating the infant's readiness for them. There are no rigidly set rules. The suggestions given here foster safety and may help make mealtime a pleasant experience for both mother and baby.

1. Initially dilute solid food to make it fairly liquid, about the consistency of a thin cream soup.
2. Warm new food to the temperature of the breast milk or formula.
3. Hold the infant as if to bottle feed. This increases the infant's sense of security and the upright position facilitates swallowing.
4. If the infant is very hungry offer him some milk first to take the edge off his appetite.
5. Offer new foods when the infant is moderately hungry, before offering the breast or bottle.
6. Try introducing new experiences at a time when they are apt to be well-tolerated, such as in the morning when the infant is well-rested.
7. Try reintroducing food which the infant initially rejects, after waiting a few days. If the food is continually rejected, respect the infant's preference and move along to other foods.
8. Give only one new food at a time. Offer that new food several times and observe how the infant reacts to make sure that it is tolerated. Discontinue feeding of a new food if the infant vomits, develops diarrhea or constipation, or continually draws his knees up to his chest and cries following the addition of it.
9. Increase the amount of the new food just a little with each feeding, starting off with a half tsp. and increasing to about 1 tbsp. at the end of a week.
10. Introduce foods with the attitude, "I'm sure this tastes good." Most infants are hungry and will try new foods easily.
11. Place food well back on the tongue, using a small blunt-ended spoon.
12. If a new food is not well-accepted, try mixing a small amount with a well-liked food. Meats are generally not as well-liked as fruits and vegetables. Initially, meats might be given with a well-liked vegetable. Gradually the amount of vegetable is decreased and the amount of meat is increased.

HOME PREPARATION OF BABY FOOD

For home-prepared meats, vegetables, and fruits, high quality fresh or plain unsalted frozen food is cooked in a minimal amount of water, taking care to conserve the nutritive value. Canned meats and vegetables should be avoided due to their high salt content. Some authorities recommend avoiding home-prepared carrots, beets, and spinach for the infant under 6 months of age. The nitrate content of these vegetables, when prepared at home, may be high enough to be toxic to the very young infant. Commercially prepared products have lower nitrate levels and are safe for use. Canned fruit is acceptable to use if it is packed in its own juice or water without added sugar.

To achieve suitable consistency, food is pureed in a blender, food grinder, or food mill. These pieces of equipment are a potential breeding ground for dangerous bacteria if not kept scrupulously clean. Fat, skin, connective tissue, and seeds should be removed from food before it is pureed. Some of the cooking liquid may be added to thin the food to an appropriate consistency. Sugar, salt, monosodium gluta-mate, and other seasonings should not be added to food served to babies. Infants will eat foods without salt or sugar. Once food is prepared it should be fed or refrigerated. Extra food may be frozen in ice cube trays or dropped by spoonfuls on a cookie sheet. Once the food is frozen it should be stored in tightly sealed plastic bags. Cleanliness in preparation and storage is essential.

COMMERCIALLY-PREPARED BABY FOODS

If commercial foods are used, the labels should be read carefully to determine those which provide the desired nutrients without excess calories. Many products are now prepared without added sugar. In general, using single foods rather than commercial mixtures (such as high-meat dinners) is recom-mended. Single foods provide more nutritive value for the money and allow the infant to be exposed to distinctive flavors.

Before a jar of baby food is opened, it is important to check the expiration date and the seal. If the jar is properly sealed there will be a depressed area in the lid. Jar lids and rims need to be washed with clean water to remove any dirt or debris; otherwise the dirt may be sucked into the jar by the vacuum created when the seal is broken.

Unless the whole container of food is to be used, the portion to be served should be put in a dish for two reasons. (1) Enzymes in the baby's saliva may be transferred via the spoon to the food being eaten. There they will begin to break down the starch in the food. This is not desirable if an unused portion is to be stored. (2) Bacteria, while harmless in small concentrations in the mouth, may become patho-genic if transferred to warm food where they can multiply. Open jars of baby food may be covered and stored in the refrigerator for a maximum of 2 to 3 days.

THE SEQUENCE IN WHICH NEW FOOD IS INTRODUCED

There are a variety of acceptable sequences for the introduction of solids. Solids should be selected to provide adequate nutrients and appropriate amounts of calories. The sequence suggested in Table 8.2 is based on observation of infants' preferences as well as on meeting nutrient needs. The order certainly can be changed. Suitable foods are described here.

Cereals and grains Rice cereal is usually the first cereal introduced because it is considered to be the least allergenic of the cereals. Introduction of single cereals such as barley or oatmeal should precede introduction of mixed varieties. If the infant does not

tolerate a particular type of cereal, it can easily be identified.

There is a great deal of variation in the amount of protein and iron provided by cereals. Precooked dry infant cereals are recommended for their high iron content. Whole grain or enriched cereals used by the family are suitable only if fully cooked without added salt and then strained. Labels provide in-formation for making a nutritious selection; iron content should be noted in particular.

Mixing cereal with formula in the bottle is not recommended because it deprives the infant of learn-ing experiences provided by other methods of eating. The nipple has to have such a large hole for this method of feeding that the danger of choking is great. If the baby is not ready for spoon feeding, there is no nutritional reason to introduce solid foods.

Vegetables Many strained cooked vegetables are good sources of vitamin A and other micronutrients. It may be helpful to introduce mild-flavored vege-tables (e.g., carrots, green beans, peas) before the more strongly-flavored ones.

Meats and other high protein foods Strained meats are an excellent source of protein, minerals, and vitamins. It may be easiest to introduce strained chicken first because its bland flavor is often well-accepted by infants. Once the infant is used to the consistency of meat he may accept strained liver if it is offered in small amounts at the beginning of the meal. Strained cooked egg yolk is often added during the middle of the first year. Introduction of egg white or whole egg is usually delayed until the end of the first year because egg white frequently causes allergic reactions. Egg yolk may be cooked, mashed, and mixed with a small amount of water or food. Eggs should not be given raw, as they may contain salmonellae, bacteria that can cause an in-testinal infection. Commercial soups, mixed dinners, and high protein dinners for babies are not eco-nomical sources of protein and contain a significant proportion of empty calories.

Fruits Mashed ripe bananas or strained cooked fruit such as applesauce, peaches, and pears are usually well accepted by infants. This is probably because the infant enjoys the natural sweetness of these foods. A number of commercial strained fruits for babies are available without added sugar. Strained orange juice is occasionally introduced early (if there is no family history of allergy) as it is a good source of vitamin C. Some physicians suggest that mothers postpone introduction of orange juice because it carries some risk of causing allergic reactions. Most commercial *baby* juices such as apple and grape are fortified with vitamin C. They may be used as re-liable sources of this vitamin. Strained fresh or un-sweetened canned juices used by the family may be

TABLE 8.2 *Introducing new foods into an infant's diet*

WHEN TO INTRODUCE	APPROXIMATE TOTAL DAILY INTAKE OF SOLIDS*	DESCRIPTION OF FOODS AND HINTS ABOUT GIVING THEM
4–5 mo (6–7 mo if infant is breastfed)	Dry cereal: Start with ½ tsp (dry measurement), gradually increase to 2–3 Tbsp Vegetables: Start with 1 tsp, gradually increase to 2 Tbsp Fruit: Start with 1 tsp, gradually increase to 2 Tbsp Divide food among 4 feedings per day (if possible)	Cereal: Offer iron-enriched baby cereal or plain Cream of Rice first. Begin with single grains (rice, barley, corn). Mix cereal with an equal amount of breast milk, formula, or water Vegetables: Try a mild-tasting vegetable first (carrots, squash, peas, green beans). Stronger-flavored vegetables (spinach, sweet potatoes) may be tried after the infant accepts some mild-tasting ones Fruits: Mashed ripe banana and unsweetened, cooked, bland fruits (apples, peaches, pears) are usually well-liked. Apple juice and grape juice (unsweetened) may be introduced. Initially, dilute juice with an equal amount of water Introduce one new food at a time and offer it several times before trying another new food Give a new food once a day for a day or two; Increase to twice a day as the infant begins to enjoy the food. Watch for signs of intolerance Include some foods that are good sources of Vitamin C (other than orange juice)
5–6 mo (6–7 mo if infant is breastfed)	Dry cereal: Gradually increase up to 4 Tbsp Fruits and vegetables: gradually increase up to 3 Tbsp of each Meat: Start with 1 tsp and gradually increase to 2 Tbsp Divide food among 4 feedings per day (if possible)	Meat: Offer pureed or milled poultry (chicken or turkey) followed by lean meat (veal, beef); lamb has a stronger flavor and may not be as well-liked initially. Liver is a good source of iron; it may be accepted at the beginning of a meal with a familiar vegetable Continue introducing new cereals, fruits, and vegetables as the infant indicates he is ready to accept them, but always one at a time
6–8 mo (7–9 mo if infant is breastfed)	Dry cereal: Up to ½ c Fruits and vegetables: Up to ¼ to ½ c of each Meats: Up to 3 Tbsp Divide food among 4 feedings per day (if possible)	Soft table foods may be introduced; e.g., mashed potatoes and squash and small pieces of soft, peeled fruits Toasted whole grain or enriched bread may be added when the infant begins chewing If introduction of solids is delayed until now, it is not necessary to use strained fruits and vegetables Continue using *iron-fortified* baby cereals
8–12 mo	Dry cereal: Up to ½ c Bread: About 1 slice Fruits and vegetables: Up to ½ c of each Meat: Up to ¼ c Divide food among 4 feedings per day (if possible)	Table foods may be added gradually. Cut table foods into small pieces. Start with ones that do not require too much chewing (cooked, cut green beans and carrots, noodles, ground meats, tuna fish, soft cheese, plain yogurt). If fish is offered, check closely to be sure there are no bones in the serving Mashed, cooked egg yolk and orange juice may be added at about 9 mo of age Sometimes offer peanut butter or thoroughly cooked dried peas and beans in place of meat

* Some infants do not need or want these amounts of food; some may need a little more food.

given, but some of them, such as unfortified apple and prune juice, are poor sources of vitamin C. Fruit drinks should be avoided.

Dairy products Small amounts of plain yogurt, cottage cheese, and mild processed cheese may gradually be added to the older infant's diet after he has begun chewing. The amount of formula or milk offered can be decreased somewhat and other fluids, such as fruit juice and water offered more often.

American mothers tend to switch to whole milk much earlier than is now recommended by pediatricians, probably because it is easier and more convenient. This is especially common among Puerto Rican mothers.[14] There is increasing concern about the relationship between whole milk and iron deficiency anemia in infants. Therefore pediatricians recommend continuing the use of proprietary formula (preferably iron-fortified) or suitably modified evaporated milk until the end of the first year. Diluted evaporated milk may be the most *realistic* choice for low income families unless they are able to participate in a WIC (Supplementary Food for Women, Infants and Children) program.

Amount of food to serve an infant

The number of servings of the Basic Four food groups is the same for an older infant as for an adult, except that more servings of milk are recommended for the infant. The size of the servings will be smaller (Table 8.2). With the addition of solids to an infant's diet a gradual shift can be made to a pattern of three meals a day with between-meal feedings appropriate to the infant's needs, appetite, and activity level.

Promoting self-feeding

Gradually, as an infant's central nervous system matures, he can consciously direct the movement of his hands and mouth and can begin to learn to feed himself. At about 6 months of age the infant can reach for and grasp an object. Everything goes into the infant's mouth. This is one of the infant's main ways of exploring his environment.

At this time an infant can be encouraged to begin to hold his own cup or bottle. Offering food he can easily pick up in his hand such as dry toast, or a similar product such as rusk or zwieback, encourages self-feeding. It is best to avoid underripe fruits and vegetables. Foods which should be avoided because they are dangerous include stringy foods (such as celery) and nuts, berries, and raisins (which may cause choking).

By 9 to 10 months an infant usually tries to use a spoon to feed himself. The infant should be offered opportunities to learn to use it properly. Sitting in a high chair which provides good support to the back and feet makes self-feeding easier.

Weaning

The weaning process is a major modification in the infant's manner of interacting with his environment. When he gives up the breast or the bottle he foregoes pleasurable sensations he derived from this method of eating. At the same time he gains a measure of independence. The actual switch from the bottle or breast to the cup should be gradually made after the infant demonstrates the ability to swallow voluntarily, approximate his lips to the rim of a cup, and grasp objects and bring them to his mouth.

There is some controversy as to what is the best time to discontinue breast feeding.[15,16] The mother should not be pressured to follow strict guidelines. Breast milk from a well-nourished mother is an excellent form of milk to offer throughout the first year of life. Some mothers may begin to wean the infant to a bottle or a cup when the infant starts to make chewing movements and his first teeth appear. Since the infant can be taught not to bite the breast, breast feeding can be comfortably continued if the mother desires to do so.

Whether the breast fed infant is weaned to a bottle or a cup depends on his developmental age when breast feeding is discontinued. Weaning from the breast should take place very gradually if possible, since abrupt discontinuance results in discomfort for the mother due to breast engorgement. Gradual weaning from the breast results in a gradual decrease in the milk supply which facilitates the weaning process.

Encouraging completion of the weaning process from the bottle by the end of the first year of life can be desirable in America for two reasons. Prolonged bottle-feeding has been implicated as a factor in the development of both iron deficiency anemia and bottle-mouth syndrome (a disease characterized by rapidly progressing tooth decay). If the baby is under stress such as illness, separation from his family, or the birth of a sibling, he may continue to need the security of the bottle or breast for a while longer.

In developing nations prolonged breast feeding is often advantageous to the infant since it is a safe source of high quality protein and other essential nutrients.

When an infant of strict vegetarian parents is weaned from the breast he should be weaned to fortified soy milk containing vitamin B_{12}. The label of the soy milk preparation should be check to determine the amount of vitamin B_{12} it contains. According to the RDA, an infant under 1 year of age needs 1.5 μg. daily and an infant over 1 year needs 2.0 μg. daily. Vitamin supplements or a vitamin B_{12} fortified yeast supplement may be acceptable alternatives. If there is objection to commercial soy milk it can be prepared at home using a special procedure to destroy toxic substances present in raw soybeans.[17] Other adequate vegetarian formulas can be devised, but care must be taken since there seems to be a tendency to overdilute them.

Establishment of sound eating practices at the beginning of infancy will be of assistance in completing the weaning process. For example, the use of rocking or singing as a method of settling an infant for sleep is preferable to offering the breast or bottle if nutritional needs have been met. The transition occasioned by weaning should occur in a relaxed, unhurried manner. The following suggestions may be implemented over the second half of the first year.
1. Begin using a cup at mealtime.
2. Follow the meal with breast or bottle feeding.

3. Gradually increase the amout of fluid given from the cup and decrease the amount from breast or bottle.

4. Discontinue morning breast or bottle feeding, then afternoon feeding, and finally discontinue the evening feeding when the infant is taking most of his fluids from a cup at mealtime.

5. Provide pleasurable distraction for the infant at the times when the bottle or breast had been offered.

6. Provide for periods of continued close physical contact with the infant.

POINTS OF EMPHASIS

Promoting normal growth and development by developing sound eating habits

- *Offer single foods so that the infant may learn to appreciate them.*
- *Introduce a variety of different food shapes and textures.*
- *Make mealtime a pleasant learning experience for the infant.*
- *Allow the infant an opportunity to learn to feed himself.*
- *Enjoy the infant's babyhood; let the feeding and eating process unfold naturally.*

STUDY QUESTIONS

1. Identify three health problems which may develop in an infant as a result of overnutrition. Suggest several ways to prevent each problem.

2. Describe some of the ways an infant's experiences with food help to shape his development.

3. A group of expectant mothers asks you to conduct a discussion of both breast and formula-feeding. List points you would discuss under each topic.

4. Following each of his first three feedings a newborn infant regurgitates about half of his meal. His mother is upset and states that she feels like a failure. What suggestions might a nurse make to help correct the situation?

5. The mother of a 6-week-old infant asks if she can begin giving her infant solid food to help him sleep through the night. List several reasons why it might be desirable to discourage her from introducing solids this early, and describe how you would respond to the mother.

References

1. Dobbing, J.: Undernutrition and the developing brain. *Am. J. Dis. Child* 120:41, 1970.
2. Dwyer, J. T., and Mayer, J.: Overfeeding and obesity in infants and children. *World Rev. Nutr. Diet.* (No. 18) 123, 1973,
*3. Pipes, P.: *Nutrition in Infancy and Childhood.* St. Louis: C. V. Mosby Co. 1977.
4. Dobbing, J., and Sands, J.: Quantitative growth and development of the human brain. *Arch. Dis. Child.* 48:757, 1973.
5. Salt intake and eating patterns of infants and children in relation to blood pressure. American Academy of Pediatrics Committee on Nutrition. *Pediatrics* 53:115, 1974.
6. Poskih, E. M. E., and Cole, T. J.: Do fat babies stay fat? *Br. Med. J.* 1:7, 1977.
7. Taitz, L.: Obesity in pediatric practice: Infantile obesity. *Ped. Clin. North Amer.* 24(1):107, 1977.
*8. Foman, S. J.: DHEW. *Nutritional Disorders of Children: Prevention Screening and Follow-up.* Washington DC: U.S. Govt. Printing Office, 1976.
9. Lakdawala, D. R., and Widdowson, E. M.: Vitamin D in Human Milk. *Lancet* (I):167, 1977.
10. McMillan, S. A., et al.: Iron sufficiency in breast-fed infants and the availability of iron from human milk. *Pediatrics* 58:686, 1976.
11. Iron supplements for infants, Committee on Nutrition, American Academy of Pediatrics. *Pediatrics* 58:765, 1976.
12. Eastham, E. J., and Walker, W. A.: Effect of cow's milk on the gastrointestinal tract: A persistent dilemma for the pediatrician. *Pediatrics* 60:477, 1977.
13. Pipes, P.: When should semisolid food be fed to infants. *J. Nutr. Ed.* 9:57, 1977.
14. Bowering, J., et al.: Infant feeding practices in East Harlem. *J. Am. Diet. Assoc.* 72:148, 1978.
*15. Heimann, L.: Weaning to prevent nutritional anemia. *Ped. Nurs.* 3(3):8, 1977.
*16. Jelliffe, D., and Jelliffe, P.: Alleged inadequacies of human milk. *Clin. Ped.* 16:1140, 1977.
*17. Robertson, L. Flinders, C., and Godfrey, B.: *Laurel's Kitchen.* Petaluma CA: Nilgiri Press, 1977, pp. 134–136.

* Recommended reading.

9

Promoting sound eating habits during childhood and adulthood

The family, as the basic social unit, influences the development of eating behaviors not during infancy only, but throughout the life cycle. Families are the primary vehicles through which children learn culturally acceptable food behaviors. Each family unit establishes and passes on to its members food preferences and eating behaviors that are unique. Families can successfully promote good nutrition among their members in many ways, including (1) providing a variety of wholesome food which promotes optimal nutritional and health status, and (2) establishing enjoyable and satisfying eating habits which meet psychosocial as well as physical needs.

Emphasis in this chapter is placed on developing and following sound eating habits from early childhood through old age. Nutritional needs as well as patterns of food behavior are considered in relation to growth, development, and aging. Common nutritional problems related to basic food habits are discussed.

THE TODDLER STAGE

Toddlerhood is the transition period between infancy and childhood, extending from about 1 to 3 years of age. It is an opportune time for parents to introduce their child to good food habits. Parents who are in tune with their child's progress can easily assist him to develop food habits which will foster optimal nutritional status and promote health. While the growth and development of each child is unique, growth and development progress in an orderly manner. Knowledge of this process can serve as a guide for fostering good eating habits.

Growth and development

During the second year of life the rate of growth slows. A toddler gains about 2.5 to 5 kg. (5 to 10 lb.) and 7.5 cm. (3 in.) per year.[1] Correspondingly the toddler requires less food and he is not as hungry as he was during infancy. A toddler's psychomotor skills (mind-directed muscle actions) improve. He progresses from eating with his fingers and hands to using utensils to eat. His movements are initially clumsy and awkward but slowly become more coordinated; he has a tendency to turn the spoon over enroute from a dish to his mouth. Both time and practice are necessary to improve his skills. When he is tired or hurried he may temporarily revert to eating with his fingers and his sloppiness may increase.

The process of teething continues during the toddler years until sometime between the second and third year. With the eruption of the molars (the large grinding teeth found toward the back of the mouth) a toddler is able to chew food more easily. Foods which require *more* chewing such as chunks of chicken or crunchy vegetables can be added to his diet in increasing amounts.

BEHAVIORAL CHARACTERISTICS

A toddler strives for autonomy, that is he tries to gain a sense of self-control. His desire for autonomy is reflected in his demands to feed himself and to decide whether or not he will eat and what he will eat. As the toddler's language skills increase he more specifically asks for food or refuses it. "Want" and "No" are frequently used words. When offered some foods the toddler may say "No" because he does not want or like them. He may also say "No" meaning "I want to decide for myself, I don't want you to tell me what to eat." "No," used in the latter manner, is an example of negativism. Negativism is part of the process by which the toddler gains control over the world around him. Offering the toddler a choice between two nutritious foods such as tomato juice or orange slices gives the toddler some control yet assures appropriate food selection. His mother's listening to his food requests and meeting those which are reasonable gives the toddler a sense of being in control and indicates respect for him as a person.

The toddler is growing less self-centered, directing more of his attention to the world around him. His curiosity prods him to explore and learn about his environment. His mouth and hands continue to be important ways of gaining information. He is a messy eater because he is learning. He "mushes" his hands in his food to see how it feels. Then he puts the food in his mouth, tasting it and feeling the texture. He may spit the food out to see what it feels like to spit or because the texture or taste is strange. The toddler's whole body often gets involved in eating. He may have peanut butter in his hair or oatmeal between his toes and a lot of food on the floor. Some advance preparation makes it easier to clean up after a toddler eats. Old newspapers or a plastic cloth on the floor around the toddler catch the spills. A large jacket-type bib helps keep the toddler's clothes clean.

In his quest for knowledge, a toddler may practice potentially dangerous food behaviors if not adequately supervised. He may stuff a pea or small piece of carrot in his nose or ear. His increased mobility allows him greater accessibility to food and other items. He can open a cupboard and get himself a box of cereal or he can wander into the living room and help himself to a glass of beer and some peanuts, if left unattended. Items other than food may go into the toddler's mouth as he does not always differentiate between what is edible and what is not. When young children persist in eating nonedible substances, the practice is called *pica*. The cause of pica is unknown, but it seems to be more common in children from lower socioeconomic groups who live in emotionally impoverished environments. Studies have shown that some children with pica are deficient in iron.[2,3]

Young children require close supervision to prevent them from ingesting harmful substances. Often the environment can be arranged so that a young child cannot reach nonfood items.

The toddler's attention span is short. He is easily distracted from eating and finds it hard to sit still for the length of time necessary to eat a whole meal with the rest of the family. It is helpful to a small child to establish a mealtime routine and to consistently follow it. Calling a child to the table, eating food only at the table, and keeping distractions to a minimum (no toys at the table, TV turned off) help him focus his attention on eating. Still, he needs to have some freedom to get up during a meal, move around and then return to eat a few more bites.

The toddler's behavior is uneven. One minute he wants to feed himself, the next minute he wants assistance. The person who recognizes a toddler's ambivalence can provide him with some extra assistance when he wants and needs it. A toddler continues to need security as he moves away from his previous close attachment to his mother or primary caretaker. One of the ways he finds security in the world around him is by carrying out certain activities in a ritualistic manner. Rituals often relate to eating. The toddler may have a special cup or bowl and be unwilling to eat without it. Security is particularly important when the toddler is in an unfamiliar environment. A toddler may feel more comfortable and eat better when away from home if his caretaker brings along his own dishes and utensils.

THE PRESCHOOLER STAGE

The preschool years are the period of time before a child begins his formal education (approximately 3 to 5 years of age). During these years children continue to develop new food behaviors.

Growth and development

Growth continues at a slow, although not always uniform, rate. The preschooler gains about 1.8 kg. (3 to 5 lb.) and grows about 6.3 cm (2½ in.) taller each year.[1] His bones and muscles grow larger and stronger. The rather chubby body appearance of the toddler gives way to a lean appearance in most children. This is due to the proportionately greater increase in height relative to weight. Parents often become concerned when their children "thin out" that they are not receiving adequate nutrition. Being aware of normal body changes which occur during the preschool years helps alleviate this concern.

Muscle control continues to develop, especially fine motor movements. Dexterity in handling eating utensils increases. By age 4 or 5 a child can begin to use a blunt-edged knife to cut up some of his own food.

A preschooler seems to have boundless amounts of energy. He is active, often restless. His caloric needs increase in proportion to his increased energy expenditure. Offering the child frequent small nutritious snacks not only supplies needed calories but also can add essential nutrients to his intake. The following list suggests nutritious snacks for children (young and old) which are relatively noncariogenic (do not promote tooth decay).

Raw vegetables: such as carrots,* cucumbers, celery,* green beans, green pepper, mushrooms, turnips, broccoli, cauliflower, tomatoes
Fresh fruits: such as apples, oranges, pears, peaches, grapes,* cherries,* melons
Unsalted whole grain crackers
Whole grain bread: cut to finger-sized sticks; plain, toasted, or with peanut butter
Small sandwiches
Natural cheese: cut in cubes
Cooked meat: cut in small chunks or sliced thinly
*Nuts**
*Sunflower seeds**
Cookies: made with lightly sweetened whole grains
*Plain popped corn**
Yogurt: plain or with fresh fruit added

BEHAVIORAL CHARACTERISTICS

A preschooler strives for initiative; he wants to learn to do things competently. He wants to learn to pour his own milk; he may ask to help with meal preparation. He needs to be provided with opportunities to practice and succeed in carrying out simple tasks.

A preschooler is inquisitive about the world around him. "Why" is a word which frequents his vocabulary. He is eager to learn about everything—not just what it is, but *why* it is and how it works. He develops concepts from labels attached to events and things. Labels appropriately attached to foods help him form the idea that foods which are good to eat are those which are nutritious. Young children begin to associate certain foods with social occasions. They know that a birthday means there will be cake and ice cream; going to Grandma's house for dinner means whole wheat rolls, fresh out of the oven. The preschool years are an opportune time to begin teaching a child simple concepts about food.

The preschooler, like the toddler, imitates adult behavior. In his play he acts out real life situations, such as grocery shopping. If he observes good food habits he is likely to imitate them and integrate them into his own behavior patterns. Unfortunately, he is also likely to adopt poor food habits if these are what he sees. Parents who observe their children playing can learn much about their own behavior and about how their children perceive them. It is not unusual to see a small child admonishing his teddy bear for not eating his vegetables or sending a doll to bed without supper for misbehaving. Parents can consider whether or not these are the messages and ideas they want to give their children about food.

Relationships with siblings become increasingly important as a small child grows. A preschooler may

---

POINTS OF EMPHASIS
Guidelines for helping children learn about food

- *Relate food to body functions.*
- *Take children grocery shopping, spending time at the fresh produce, meat, and dairy departments.*
- *Name foods and explain in simple terms where they come from.*
- *Take children on trips to see, for example, that milk comes from cows, that eggs come from chickens, and vegetables grow in a garden.*
- *Let a child grow a few vegetables outdoors or in a window box.*
- *Read children stories that tell about wholesome food and eating.*
- *Emphasize safety in handling and eating food, namely washing hands before eating, not sharing food which has been tasted, not eating directly out of storage containers, returning perishable food to the refrigerator.*

---

emulate an older brother or sister. If he sees his siblings eating a variety of wholesome foods he is likely to do the same. A preschooler needs praise for his own accomplishments rather than to have his behavior compared to the achievements of his older siblings.

A preschooler's thought processes are concrete and absolute. He tends to see only one way to do things. It is difficult for him to understand why he cannot eat in front of the television if his parents do. He is more agreeable to accepting and following rules when parents abide by them too.

A preschooler's limited experience makes it difficult for him to evaluate information he receives about food. Television bombards the preschooler with food messages. Catchy rhymes, colorful ads, animated cartoon characters, and other children have a significant impact on a young child. In the grocery store a preschooler may raise a great fuss about wanting a particular food item he saw advertised on television. Acknowledging hearing the child's requests and then asking him to choose from a nutritious assortment of foods may help solve this problem. Bypassing the cereals until just before entering the checkout line avoids disruption of the entire shopping trip. Leaving a young child home with a sitter or a friend while a parent shops is an alternative solution.

A preschooler has increased contacts with children and adults outside his immediate family. These individuals begin to influence his eating behavior. If the child next door is eating a candy bar, the preschooler wants the same. He has a difficult time understanding and accepting that some foods are not the most appropriate ones for him to eat. Rather than emphasizing that what the other child is eating is bad or wrong,

---

* Children under 2 years may choke on nuts, seeds, popcorn, celery strings, or carrot sticks. It is best to avoid offering these foods until the preschool years.

parents can try to find suitable alternatives for their child. Inviting the child's playmate over for a nutritious snack may help.

Many preschool children are enrolled in nursery or day care programs. If food is served, both the manner in which it is presented and the kinds of food offered are significant. A preschool program may broaden a child's acceptance of foods and reinforce positive food habits. If children eat in groups they learn that mealtime is an opportunity for socializing and sharing with others. When selecting a nursery school or day care center, concerned parents inquire about the school's philosophy and attitude toward food as well as the foods provided for meals and snacks. Observing children at snack and mealtime gives a good indication of the manner in which food is presented to children and the amount of emphasis placed on developing sound food habits. Sample meal and snack plans may reveal whether or not a child will be offered a nutritious variety of foods.

Inappropriate use of foods   Food is sometimes used to reward, punish, or bribe a child, or it is sometimes used as a substitute for meaningful relationships. Sugary foods, candies, cakes, and cookies used as rewards relay messages like "I love you," and "you've been good." A child may have an increased sense of self-esteem when he eats "reward" foods. "Reward" foods quickly become highly desirable foods to a child. Trying to bribe a child with food also conveys the message that some foods are more desirable than others. This is particularly the case if, for instance, a child is told he can have a dish of ice cream after he eats all his vegetables. Eating, on the other hand, becomes an unpleasant experience when food is used as a punishment. Requiring a child to sit at the dinner table until the last spoonful of food is consumed is inappropriate.

When under stress, a child may revert to earlier forms of behavior including eating behavior. For instance, when a new baby joins the family the young child may suddenly ask for a bottle or to nurse from his mother's breast.

Areas of concern about the young child's eating behavior

Parents express concern over their young child's *decreased* food intake. Most often a young child eats less because he does not need as much food. A young child's appetite varies with his rate of growth and with his activity level. A child may eat ravenously one day and very little the next. If a child is healthy and demonstrates characteristics of good nutritional status, he is probably getting enough to eat.

There are other reasons why a young child may have a decreased food intake, namely, the child (1) is overtired, (2) is unhappy at mealtime, (3) is seeking attention, (4) is physically ill or has decayed, painful teeth,

or (5) is emotionally disturbed. Most of these problems can be easily remedied; if the child is physically or emotionally ill, medical attention may be needed.

The young child learns very quickly that he can capitalize on his parents' concerns about his food intake. He tries modifying his eating habits to manipulate his parents. If a child wants to stay up late to watch TV he may refuse to eat unless parents agree to his request. Most young children will not starve themselves. Removing food after a reasonable period of time and ignoring undesirable behavior go a long way toward solving this problem. Sometimes a young child doesn't eat simply to get extra attention. If this is the case, focusing more attention on the child at mealtimes and at other times during the day may be helpful. Emotional problems related to eating may develop if parents' expectations are too rigid or unrealistic for their child. Coaxing and forcing a child to eat may further decrease his appetite.

Many young children occasionally go on *food jags.* They want to eat the same few foods morning, noon, and night. Parents may wonder if their child will become malnourished when this occurs. Usually food jags are temporary; a child resumes eating a more varied diet within a few days. During the time of the food jag parents can continue to offer a variety of foods without making an issue about what their child eats.

Eating too much of one food over a prolonged period of time may lead to inadequate nutrition. Many parents do not recognize that 500 to 750 ml. (2 to 3 c.) of milk is plenty for a young child and they may encourage him to take more. Excessive milk intake dulls the child's appetite for a variety of foods. Offering water and juices, particularly when the child is thirsty, helps decrease milk intake.

Iron deficiency is a nutritional problem frequently occurring in early childhood. It often develops in young children who drink too much milk. If severe, a child may develop a blood disorder called iron deficiency anemia. Children with iron deficiency anemia look pale, have little energy, and are often irritable. Children are likely to develop iron deficiency if (1) they have not built up adequate iron stores during infancy or (2) they do not eat iron-rich foods such as iron-fortified cereals (preferably unsweetened), foods from the meat group (including legumes), and dark green leafy vegetables. Too much milk crowds these foods out of the diet.

Promoting good food habits

Parents who are concerned about their children's nutritional status establish guidelines to assist their children in developing desirable food habits. The food which is available to young children is largely determined by parents' food preferences.

Mothers and sometimes fathers act as "gatekeepers" selecting and preparing the food offered to their children. A simple way to limit the intake of foods which are not nutritious is to keep them out of the home. To increase a child's intake of nutritious foods, parents might follow guidelines such as those below.

Atmosphere at mealtime A warm, relaxed, friendly atmosphere at mealtime contributes to making eating a happy experience. Young children benefit from eating some of their meals with other family members. Eating is facilitated by a comfortable chair within easy reach of the table and appropriately-sized utensils and dishes. In time, children learn manners through imitation. A child who is continually scolded and corrected is likely to feel unsuccessful in eating. Establishing reasonable rules, reinforcing desired behavior, and ignoring undesirable behavior promotes good eating habits.

Serving size and food selection Observing a child eat provides information about what he likes and how much he eats. Combining this information with a reliable food guide can serve as a basis for determining how to feed a child. Young children have an acute sense of taste and smell and are very sensitive to texture. Eggs fried "sunny side up" and baked custard have a "slimy" texture which children may reject. Young children usually prefer simple, mild-flavored foods such as ground meat, chicken, fruits, whole grain breads, and cereals. Serving less than a child wants is a better way to end up with a "clean plate" than is forcing a child to finish unwanted food. Allowing a child to decide when he has had enough to eat helps him develop appetite control.

Gradually introducing new foods and providing ample variety in the young child's diet helps assure adequate nutrition. Young children are more likely to accept new foods when they are offered at the beginning of a meal. New foods may be rejected because the taste is strange. Offering small amounts at intervals encourages their acceptance.

Some suggestions to encourage children to eat vegetables include the following: (1) Eat vegetables yourself and show that you enjoy them. (2) Offer an assortment of vegetables. (3) Let children help in selection and preparation. Encourage tasting at this time. (4) Introduce new vegetables along with familiar well-liked ones. (5) Serve small amounts of vegetables at the beginning of a meal when a child is hungriest. (6) Offer vegetables for snacks. (7) Cook vegetables so they are tender crisp and retain their bright colors. (8) Offer vegetables in a variety of forms: raw, cooked, juice, and mixed in a casserole or stew. (Raw ones may be preferred.) (9) Cut vegetables into different shapes to make them more interesting.

Self-feeding It is easier for a child to feed himself if foods are cut into bite-sized pieces which can be readily lifted to his mouth on a spoon or fork. Complementary flavors and textures make eating more enjoyable. A moist food such as applesauce might be offered with a dry food such as ground meat. A crunchy vegetable such as raw green beans complements a soft vegetable such as mashed potato. Children may be intrigued by the noise produced when food is chewed. Children often prefer foods which are at room temperature and will delay eating if foods are too hot or too cold. Finger foods are easily handled by children. They like fresh oranges and apples cut into wedges, small carrot sticks, small chunks of cheese and small sandwiches. Nutritious finger foods can be prepared in advance and make excellent snacks.

THE SCHOOL YEARS

The school years (the age range of 6 to 10 years) are often considered to be an uneventful period of growth and development. Changes are not dramatic; however, during these years children continue to grow and develop. Each year brings unique changes as children mature.

Growth and development

Growth proceeds at a slow pace, marked by small spurts and plateaus. Children gain about 3.2 kg. (7 lb.) and grow about 6.3 cm. (2½ in.) annually.[1] Height and weight vary greatly among children because of genetic makeup and environmental influences.

During the school years baby teeth are shed and replaced by permanent ones. For the short period of time when the front teeth are missing, biting may be difficult. Cutting food into small pieces and serving food which is easy to bite such as bananas and orange slices makes eating easier for the child. Promotion of dental health during the school years pays long term dividends.

BEHAVIORAL CHARACTERISTICS

The school-aged child develops a sense of industry by participating in real-life situations. A sense of pride and accomplishment comes from activities such as gardening, cooking, setting the table, helping with dishwashing, and going to the grocery store for milk.

During the school years a child spends an increasing amount of time away from home. He begins to make his own food selections. School friends and adults other than his parents have increasing influence on his food habits. A child's friends are important to him; he enjoys having friends come over for dinner. Children like to share their experiences with parents and others who will listen. Parents are thus provided with an opportunity to inquire about what their child eats when away from home. They can discuss food choices with him and show approval of his nutritious selections.

While school-age children do like an increasingly larger variety of foods, some likes and dislikes from early childhood persist. A child may strongly reject foods parents try to push on him. Often the school-aged child gets involved in activities and he forgets or is reluctant to stop and eat. Stress related to school work, competitive activities, and illness also influence his appetite.

Areas of concern about eating behavior

Skipping breakfast If a child rushes to get to school, breakfast is hurried or missed altogether. If eaten, breakfast may consist of highly sweetened convenience foods. Some children do not have much of an appetite first thing in the morning or they may not like the foods served them. Without breakfast they often become cranky, inattentive, and less able to perform well in school.[4]

Providing different foods may make breakfast more appealing to a child. Foods which are nutritious and appetizing for lunch and dinner are no less nutritious or less appropriate for breakfast. A milkshake, hamburger, peanut butter sandwich, or cheese on toast may prompt a child to eat breakfast.

POINTS OF EMPHASIS
Suggestions for breakfast

• *Plan breakfast in advance with family members.*
• *Rise early enough to allow an adequate amount of time to eat.*
• *Keep nonperishable breakfast foods together in a handy location.*
• *Allow for some food choices.*
• *Keep easy-to-prepare, nourishing foods on hand for occasions when time is short.*
• *Encourage family members to share responsibility for preparing breakfast.*
• *Eat together when possible.*

Weight problems Excessive caloric intake and insufficient exercise are two primary reasons for obesity in childhood. Children who eat much food high in sugar and/or fat may quickly exceed their calorie requirements. Little energy is expended in sedentary activities such as watching TV. Children who eat a lot of sugar-rich foods may not feel satiated; because of this they may eat more frequently. Some children turn to food "to protect" themselves from various psychosocial stresses such as going to school and being separated from home and family.

Collecting some information about a child and his family is useful in establishing a program to help a child *control* his weight. Information which may be useful includes (1) family's and child's attitude toward food and nutrition, (2) family's and child's eating and activity patterns, and (3) whether or not the child wants to be at a normal weight. A desire to control weight makes it easier to modify eating habits and to increase activity level. Often appealing to a child's

vanity may help motivate him to change his behavior. Except in extreme cases emphasis is placed on weight control rather than weight reduction. Limiting weight gain while a child is growing corrects moderate degrees of overweight.

Promoting good food habits

Appropriate food practices begun in early childhood need continued emphasis and reinforcement during the school years. At this time children begin to form *values about food*. With help they can learn to evaluate information about food and nutrition. This is an appropriate time to introduce the idea that TV and other media do not always tell people what is best to do. Parents may want to investigate the nutrition messages conveyed at school and take action if indicated.

Children who have an allowance or who earn spending money have an opportunity to decide whether to spend the money on food and what kinds of food to spend it on. With reliable information, guidance from knowledgeable adults, and at least some palatable, nutritious food choices, children can learn to make sound decisions for themselves.

CHILDHOOD TO ADULTHOOD

The boundaries between the stages of life from the school years through adulthood are blurred. It is difficult to clearly identify the beginning and end of each period for several reasons: (1) The biological changes marking the beginning and end of adolescence do not occur at precisely the same time for everyone. (2) There are marked differences from adolescent to adolescent in the rate and amount of physical change occurring. (3) The effects of aging differ among individuals. (4) Psychological and social development from the onset of adolescence through adulthood is influenced by an ever-increasing number of variables, including physical change, school and peer group activities, family attitudes, cognitive development, occupation, marital choice, use of leisure time, economic factors, and cultural influences.

Specific nutrient needs and eating habits vary among individuals in the same stage of the life cycle as well as among persons who are in different periods of life. Care needs to be taken in making and applying generalizations for any two individuals of the same age.

ADOLESCENCE

Adolescence is a transition stage in the life cycle, linking childhood to adulthood. Adolescents are often labeled as "difficult to manage" and as having "poor food habits." For many adolescents these labels have not been earned and are not deserved. Unfortunately, the amount of reliable scientific data about adolescents' growth, development, and nutritional needs is limited. Studies have shown that teenagers do have some sound nutrition knowledge.[5] Data from the Health and Nutrition Examination Survey on mean dietary intake suggest that adolescents' intake of most nutrients is adequate.[6] Some common areas of concern are discussed later in the chapter.

It is helpful to distinguish between early adolescence and late adolescence when discussing teenagers' nutritional needs and eating habits. Definitions of these adolescent periods and other related terms as they are used in this text are presented in Table 9.1.

Growth and development

Several specific biological changes occur during adolescence, namely (1) the growth rate increases during early adolescence, (2) height and weight increase, (3) body composition (the proportions of various tissues in the body) changes, and (4) sexual maturity is

TABLE 9.1 *Terms commonly used in reference to adolescence*

TERM	DESCRIPTION
Pubescence	The period of time when a young person's reproductive organs begin to mature and secondary sexual characteristics start to develop. This term may be equated with *early adolescence.*
Prepubescence	The two years preceding pubescence. It is marked by a rapid increase in growth.
Early adolescence	The period of prepubescence and pubescence.
Puberty	The point in time when a person reaches reproductive maturity. The onset of menstruation in girls and presence of spermatozoa in boys are often used as reference points for the beginning of puberty. However, reproductive capability is probably not well established for about two years in girls and several years in boys.
Late adolescence	The period beginning at puberty.
Secondary sexual characteristics	Characteristics identifying the sex of a person but not directly related to reproduction.
Menarche	The time when the first menstrual cycle occurs.
Peak height velocity	The single year during which the increase in height is greatest.
Lean body mass	The bulk of metabolically active tissue in the body (mainly muscle).
Adipose tissue	Fatty tissue which serves to insulate the body and provide storage.

achieved. There are significant variations between the sexes in the process of growth and development. On the average, girls begin the adolescent growth spurt between the ages of 10 and 12 years. The male growth spurt generally begins 1½ to 2 years later, between 12 and 14 years of age. The velocity of growth, the rate at which growth proceeds, is greater in males than in females. During adolescence (10 to 18 years of age) the average American male almost doubles his weight, gaining about 30 kg. (67 lb.). He grows about 34 cm. (13½ in.). During the same time period adolescent females gain about 22 kg. (49 lb.) and grow about 24 cm. (9 in.).[1] Most adequately nourished girls develop a layer of adipose tissue which remains throughout life. Most boys have a substantial increase in lean body mass which gives them a lean, muscular appearance.

It has been suggested that the rate of a child's growth may correlate with sexual maturation. For example, in most girls menarche occurs after the peak height velocity. However, studies indicate that there may not be a direct correlation between the growth pattern and the appearance of secondary sexual characteristics. The order of the appearance of secondary sexual characteristics varies among youngsters.[7]

There are several important nutritional implications related to the adolescent growth process, namely:
1. More food is needed to support growth at this time of life.
2. Girls need to increase their food intake at an earlier age than boys.
3. Boys need more food than girls (when they begin the growth spurt) since boys gain substantially more lean body mass.
4. Compared to females, males continue to need more food to maintain their large lean body mass.
5. Nutrient needs may correlate with an adolescent's stage of sexual maturation, probably being greatest *before* menarche in females and when secondary sexual characteristics appear in males. With the onset of menses girls need to increase their intake of iron.

The young adolescent is much like the older school-aged child in his behavior. At the time when his nutrient and caloric needs begin to increase he is likely to agree to suggestions made by his parents and other significant adults about his eating habits. Parents can provide balanced meals and a variety of nutritious snacks to help the adolescent maintain adequate nutritional status. Caloric requirements for most healthy adolescents are high. (RDA for boys 11 to 14 years is 2800 kcal. and for girls 11 to 14 years 2400 kcal.) When food is abundant boys have an advantage over girls. Their higher caloric requirement makes meeting nutrient needs easier. Adolescents who eat nutritionally sound meals may meet their needs for specific nutrients and still need extra calories. This may prompt frequent snacking. Many adolescents can eat some high calorie foods such as soft drinks, cookies, and donuts without gaining excess weight. However, eating this type of food may not be a wise practice for maintaining good health throughout the life span.

BEHAVIORAL CHARACTERISTICS

During later adolescence many changes occur in a youth's behavior because he is struggling to become an adult. The nature of these changes influences the adolescent's eating habits and, in turn, his nutritional status. One of the adolescent's major tasks is to achieve a sense of identity, that is, to know who he is as a person, what he values, and the direction he wants to take in adulthood. To accomplish this task the adolescent must separate himself from his parents and family and try out different roles or ways of behaving.

The separation process may be reflected in an adolescent's food habits. He may reject parental suggestions and skip breakfast or refuse to eat certain foods as a means of asserting himself. The values and opinions of the peer group exert a great influence on the adolescent's food selections. A teen may choose to buy chips and soda for lunch at school because that is what his friends do. Parents can help the adolescent maintain adequate nutritional status and yet allow him the freedom to be independent. Keeping a supply of nutritious snacks on hand or putting a sandwich in a teen's book bag for a morning snack may do more to promote adequate nutrition than making an issue of what a teen is eating.

Eating habits and nutritional status influence the adolescent's developing sense of identity. If an adolescent eats well and gets enough exercise and rest, he may have positive feelings about his body and its capabilities. On the other hand, if inadequate food intake leads to lack of energy and poor body performance, the result may be a sense of low self-esteem.

Unfortunately the adolescent may not relate nutrition to body function. Many adolescents are far removed from illness and death and do not have a clear appreciation for human vulnerability. They do not see that their daily activities, including what they eat, may have an impact on their health now or in the future. Many of them are more likely to see food as gratifying a current need, like hunger.

Physical changes cause an adolescent to focus attention on his body as he tries to incorporate his new appearance into his developing sense of identity. Many adolescents go through stages when they are preoccupied with their appearance and body function. They may see nutrition as helpful or harmful to their developing body image. A boy may show concern about his body in relation to athletic ability. He may want to eat more to increase his weight and muscle mass to play football. He may think, incorrectly, that eating large portions of meat is the only way to do this. Conversely, he may want to diet to lose weight to make the wrestling team.

TABLE 9.2 *Teenager's meals and snacks for a day compared to the Basic Four*

1 English muffin 1 cup of tea with 　milk and sugar	ham sandwich 1 cup of milk 1 med. banana	hamburger patty (90 gm) 　(3 oz) buttered noodles 1 slice of bread and butter sm. dish of ice cream
Snack donut	*Snack* sm. bag of potato chips glass noncarbonated soft 　drink	*Snack* can carbonated soft drink

SUMMARY OF FOODS EATEN *BASIC FOUR*	*SUGGESTIONS TO IMPROVE THE* *NUTRITIONAL QUALITY**
Vegetables and Fruits 　0 servings of excellent source of 　vitamin A 　0 servings of excellent source of 　vitamin C 　1 serving of other vegetable or fruit	Have pumpkin pie for dessert or raw 　carrot with lunch Add a glass of orange juice for 　breakfast or orange for an after- 　noon snack Have a potato or french fries in place 　of noodles for dinner
Whole grain or enriched breads and cereals 　6 servings	
Milk Group 　Equivalent to 300 ml (1¼ c.)	Add cheese to sandwich at lunch and 　have a glass of milk with donut in 　morning or instead of soft drink
Meat group 　Equivalent to 150 gm (5 oz)	

* This teen's diet is far from prudent. However, the fewer the number of changes made, the greater the chance that they will be adopted by the teen.

The deposition of fat which normally occurs in an adolescent girl may cause her to become concerned that she is getting fat. She may eliminate from her diet foods she regards as fattening. High carbohydrate foods such as potatoes and bread have a particularly bad, but undeserved, reputation for being fattening. If she decides to eliminate potatoes and bread, milk and/or meat to lose weight, she eliminates valuable sources of nutrients. Limiting caloric intake at this time may interfere with linear growth. Growing adolescents are highly sensitive to caloric restriction.

With his often busy schedule an adolescent may rush off to school without eating breakfast. In the evening, rather than waiting for dinner, he may grab a snack so he can spend the evening with friends or get to baseball practice on time. Consequently, he eats fewer meals at home where parents can provide him with nutritious foods. When away from home an adolescent often eats meals that are readily available, inexpensive, and acceptable to his peer group. This may mean snacks in the form of "fast foods." Fast foods and ready-to-eat foods obtained from vending machines or from the corner grocery store are frequently referred to as "junk" food. To most people "junk" food means food that is very salty, sugary, or has a high fat content (e.g., chips, candy bars). However, other foods sometimes classified as "junk" such as pizza, hamburgers, and french fries do supply needed nutrients. In fact, some studies have shown that adolescents obtain many of the nutrients they need from the "fast" food they consume.[8,9]

Eating "junk" food *in moderation* does not pose a serious threat to the nutritional status of an adolescent whose basic food habits are nutritionally sound. However, when carried to extremes or when practiced by the adolescent who does not and/or has not had good food habits, these practices may compromise growth and maintenance of body functions. Looking at the adolescent's intake of specific nutrients as well as comparing his food intake to the Basic Four gives an indication of the diet's adequacy. Nutrients to be checked include iron, vitamin A, vitamin C, riboflavin, thiamine, and calcium. Surveys have indicated that these nutrients are likely to be in short supply in the diet of teens.[9] Both boys and girls need an increased amount of *iron* during adolescence. A girl's need for iron increases with the onset of menstruation; a boy needs more iron because of the increase in lean body mass. Table 9.2 shows a teen's diet compared to the Basic Four and suggests ways to improve its nutritional quality.

Parents can encourage open discussion of nutrition and food habits and come up with constructive suggestions rather than criticism. Ways to promote sound eating habits include setting a good example, keeping nourishing ready-to-eat foods on hand, involving a teen in meal planning, and making nutrition information available (such as "Your Food—Chance or Choice").[10] The adolescent needs the opportunity to apply nutrition knowledge himself. He is more likely to respond positively when allowed to make his own decisions than when told what to do.

Areas of concern about eating behavior

Obesity The onset of obesity during adolescence is less common than onset during the school years. Many obese adolescents have been obese since childhood. Overweight teens are usually not very active physically. In fact, it has been suggested that low energy expenditure rather than excessive calorie intake may be responsible for adolescent obesity.[11,12] Obesity during adolescence may contribute to a number of psychological problems. It may interfere with the development of a positive body image and result in the adolescent's having a low sense of self-esteem. Overweight teens are sometimes very sensitive about their appearance. Consequently they may withdraw from various school and social activities. The adolescent's obesity may be the focus (not the cause) of family conflict characterized by continual harassment of their teen about losing weight. The task of trying to lose weight is not easy; failure does little to promote the adolescent's sense of accomplishment.

The adolescent needs assistance in setting realistic goals to control or lose weight. Reaching goals has important psychological benefits to the teen. It is important to be certain the adolescent has adequate calories and nutrients to support growth. Physical exercise and emotional support are important aspects of an adolescent weight control program.

Cigarettes, alcohol, and drugs Smoking, ingesting alcohol, and abusing drugs are habits that often begin during the teenage years. In many cases their effects on nutritional status are much less dramatic than their effects on overall health.

Cigarette smoking impairs the senses of taste and smell. It also appears to increase the amount of vitamin C required to maintain a given serum level of the vitamin.[13] When dietary intake of vitamin C is comparable, serum levels of vitamin C are about 25 percent less in smokers (up to 20 cigarettes daily) than nonsmokers. The effect is even more marked in people who smoke 20 to 40 cigarettes daily; their serum vitamin C averages 40 percent less than that of nonsmokers. Cigarette smoking appears to decrease absorption of vitamin C. Metabolism, storage, and excretion are not significantly affected. It has been suggested that adjustments be made in vitamin C "requirements" to compensate for reduced bioavailability of the vitamin in smokers.[13]

Excessive intake of alcohol is a problem that has been increasing in teens. Chronic abuse is related to some serious nutritional disorders, such as vitamin deficiency states. Moderate use of alcohol may be of concern because of the "empty calories" it provides.

Drug abuse may take any one of a number of forms, from use of illegal drugs to overdosing on vitamin pills to misuse of drugs to control appetite. Indiscriminate use of drugs can cause some nutritional problems. Changes in food habits often accompany drug abuse. Habitual drug users require special medical attention.

Acne vulgaris Acne vulgaris is a common skin disorder occurring during adolescence. Most adolescents are concerned about controlling and preventing acne since they feel extremely self-conscious when their face has "broken out." Eliminating foods such as chocolate, nuts, fried and fatty foods, and soft drinks has long been suggested as a method of treatment. However, there is no documentation that diet plays a major role in this disorder. Nutrient supplements, either topical or systemic, should not be used for treatment of acne, except under close supervision of a competent dermatologist.

Dehydration Large water losses may accompany vigorous physical activity. Athletes who train hard or compete on a hot day are at great risk of becoming dehydrated.[14] Adolescent athletes need to increase their water consumption. Satisfaction of thirst is not always a reliable indicator that water needs have been met.

POINTS OF EMPHASIS
Guidelines for developing sound eating habits during adolescence

*   *Encourage adolescents to:*
1. *Enjoy food*
2. *Try new foods*
3. *Eat some food in the morning*
4. *Join the family for meals*
5. *Select nutritious snacks*
6. *Occasionally invite friends for dinner (if the food budget allows)*
*   *Aim for at least one mealtime a day as an enjoyable time for sharing family experiences.*
*   *Within reason, find out about a teen's schedule in advance so that mealtimes won't conflict with activities which are important to him.*
*   *Provide basic facts about food and nutrition from which adolescents can make informed decisions about their food intake.*
*   *Present nutrition information in a competent manner; state values clearly without imposing them.*
*   *Give specific examples of how to put sound nutrition knowledge to work.*
*   *Stress immediate tangible effects of a good diet such as improved vitality and increased physical endurance.*
*   *Consistently reinforce an adolescent's selection of nutritious foods and ignore poor food choices.*
*   *Stock the refrigerator with healthful snack foods.*
*   *Encourage the adolescent to assume responsibilities related to meal planning, grocery shopping, cooking, and gardening.*

Scheduled drinking of water, juices, or other non-diuretic beverages may be necessary to assure adequate fluid intake. It is a good idea to keep a record of weight when in training. Loss of 0.5 to 1 kg. per day signals a potential problem of dehydration.

EARLY ADULTHOOD

For practical purposes early adulthood will be considered as the period of time from 18 to 30 years of age and middle adulthood from 30 to 65 years of age. During early adulthood physical growth and development cease. Correspondingly, the amounts of specific nutrients needed by adults decrease to a maintenance level. As age increases the metabolic rate slowly decreases, accompanied by a gradual decrease in the number of calories needed to meet the body's basal energy needs. On the other hand, psychosocial development continues but it does not follow a predictable pattern. The adult may adopt any one of a number of lifestyles, each of which has unique influences on food habits and nutrient needs. Major events such as beginning a career, marrying, and having a family occur at different ages for different people.

Diet and psychosocial considerations

Moving away from home requires many adjustments. The process is easier if the person has learned and practiced some basic food preparation and menu planning skills at home. Using some nutritious convenience foods initially may be helpful for the person who is an inexperienced cook or who has a busy schedule.

Away from home an individual is often confronted with food preferences different from his own. This is especially likely to occur when a person marries, shares an apartment with friends, or eats in a cafeteria or boarding house. New foods are less apt to cause problems if a person has previously adopted an adventuresome attitude toward eating. Single adults and working couples without children may choose to dine out rather than to prepare their own meals. They may be able to select nourishing meals if they eat at a restaurant which offers a varied menu including fresh fruits and vegetables. Since many restaurants feature large portions and use salt, fat, and sugar liberally when preparing foods, eating prudently may be difficult. When eating out some people have only two meals daily so that they can maintain weight without losing money. There is no evidence that this pattern is harmful to healthy individuals. Other individuals bring their uneaten food home from a restaurant in a "doggy bag." The leftovers are then used for the next day's lunch or dinner. If this is done, it is important to use safe methods of food storage.

Nutrition and the growing family

Pregnancy and the addition of children to a family often focus adults' attention on diet and nutrition. Women may be concerned about their own diet during pregnancy. Following pregnancy they may have questions about what foods they should eat and how to lose weight. Parents frequently express concern about feeding their children nutritiously and about teaching them good food habits. This is a good time to encourage parents to consider whether they want their current food habits to be imitated by their children.

Anticipatory guidance may help a mother avoid developing the habit of snacking frequently when she is home most of the day with children. Parents may want to avoid "cleaning" their children's or each others plates at the end of a meal, since this can be a source of unneeded calories. It is also an unsanitary food practice which children may imitate.

Birth control and nutrition   Two methods of birth control, use of an intrauterine device (IUD) or of oral contraceptive agents (OCA), may affect a woman's nutritional status. The use of an intrauterine device, a small object inserted into the uterus to prevent pregnancy, has been noted to increase menstrual blood loss. This greater blood loss increases the need for iron. Women who use an IUD can increase their intake of foods high in iron to counter the loss. If menstrual flow is extremely heavy, it may be advisable to monitor for iron deficiency anemia or to consider another means of birth control.

Oral contraceptive agents, commonly called birth control pills (often "the Pill"), prevent pregnancy by inhibiting ovulation. They exert a variety of nutritional and metabolic effects on the body. OCAs have not been reported to cause *overt* nutrient deficiencies except in a few women who were already malnourished for reasons other than being on the Pill. Studies suggest OCAs may alter a woman's requirements for a variety of vitamins and minerals.[15] Blood (serum) levels of vitamin B_2 (riboflavin), B_6 (pyridoxine), vitamin C, folic acid, and vitamin B_{12} are probably decreased in women who use OCAs. Levels of vitamin A may be elevated. Iron requirements may be reduced owing to reduction in menstrual blood loss. There is not enough evidence to recommend that women on OCAs take nutritional supplements such as multivitamin preparations prophylactically.[16] However, to ensure adequate nutrition while using an OCA, women at risk should receive (1) counseling regarding intake of foods which are good sources of the nutrients which may be affected, (2) monitoring for nutritional deficiencies, and (3) corrective measures if specific deficiencies are identified. Women who become pregnant within 6 months of taking OCAs should also have their nutritional status closely monitored since malnutrition may affect an unborn child.

MIDDLE ADULTHOOD

As an individual approaches middle adulthood, visible signs of aging begin to appear. However, as an individual reaches 40 or 50 he finds that "middle age" is not as old as it once seemed. People in this age group may adopt regular forms of exercise such as tennis and jogging if they have not already done so. Exercising helps maintain lean body mass which in turn keeps the metabolic rate stable. Without regular exercise weight may gradually increase if caloric intake is not decreased. At this stage of life, concern about maintaining health often precipitates a new surge of interest in prudent eating, giving up smoking, and weight control.

Studies confirm the common concern that cessation of smoking often leads to weight gain. The gain is usually in the range of 10 to 15 percent above ideal body weight. Although this amount of weight gain is annoying, it does not contribute significantly to the risk of heart disease[17] and should not be viewed as a deterrent to giving up cigarettes. Weight gain is probably the result of changes in eating habits which occur after an individual stops smoking. An individual who is alerted to these possible changes can take steps to control his food habits and to avoid gaining weight. The American Heart Association's pamphlet "Guidelines for a Weight Control Component in a Smoking Cessation Program" gives suggestions that may be particularly helpful to a former smoker.

Eating prudently and maintaining a high level of exercise help minimize problems of heartburn, constipation, and lack of vitality which are common complaints during the middle years. Individuals who have practiced and continue to practice measures to promote dental health may avoid tooth loss and chewing difficulties.

Some individuals erroneously attribute gums which bleed easily to a deficiency of vitamin C. They may take large doses of vitamin C in an effort to correct this problem. However, bleeding gums are more likely to be due to poor oral hygiene and periodontal disease.

Requirements for nutrients remain stable throughout the adult years, except for iron. A woman's need for iron is higher than a man's because of menstruation. This need for iron decreases when a woman reaches menopause.

OLDER ADULTHOOD

Older adults are usually described as being individuals 60 to 65 years of age and older. The nutritional status of older persons (senior citizens), is influenced by the process of aging. Aging begins at the moment of conception; however, decreased renewal of cells and tissues does not become obvious for many years.

Although the precise role nutrition plays in the aging process has not been determined, certainly nutrition influences the development and course of many chronic and degenerative diseases which often accompany old age. One motivation for eating prudently throughout life is increasing the chance of being able to enjoy "old age" in a state of good health. There is no guarantee that disease will not strike but, even if it does, sensible eating helps a person feel as well as possible under the circumstances. Old age can be a time for new opportunities if an individual has looked after the health of his body.

Physical characteristics

The types of normal degenerative changes occurring over the years affect numerous body tissues and physiological processes. For example, taste buds become less effective in detecting taste, gastric secretions decrease, the kidneys' ability to concentrate urine diminishes, and motor function and physical strength decrease. Many older persons who have consistently practiced sound eating habits adapt gradually to normal changes and maintain adequate food intake. For other individuals these same degenerative changes may interfere with processes necessary to nourish the body. These changes can also make eating less pleasurable than it was earlier in life. Fortunately, most of the problems caused by minor degenerative changes are easily remedied.

A decrease in the acuity of taste and smell causes some people to complain that "food doesn't taste the way it used to." Most older people appreciate suggestions to promote an interest in eating. For instance, small servings of familiar foods that look good and smell good stimulate the appetite. An occasional "treat" (perhaps an expensive cut of meat which is easy to chew or a favorite fresh fruit) can renew interest in eating.

A decrease in gastric secretions makes an older person more vulnerable to symptoms of indigestion. Eating small frequent meals, chewing food thoroughly, and decreasing intake of poorly tolerated foods help prevent indigestion. He needs to be sure to include ample amounts of foods which are good sources of iron, calcium, and vitamin B_{12}. Absorption of these nutrients may be limited because of decreased gastric secretions.

Sufficient fluid intake, e.g., water, is needed to promote adequate kidney function since the kidneys are less able to change the concentration of the urine. Avoiding *excessive* intake of foods which increase the renal solute load is also desirable.

Many older adults remain physically active even though motor function and strength decrease with age. It's not unusual to see an older person riding a bike, swimming, or even skiing. An older person who exercises regularly can eat more without gaining weight than can an individual who is inactive. The more calories an individual can prudently consume, the more easily he can meet his nutrient needs.

For some persons, years of inadequate nutrition and chronic debilitating illness have interfered with eating and resulted in depletion of nutrient stores. It is particularly important for these individuals to have assistance in obtaining an adequate diet.

Many older people focus attention on their bowel habits. Eating a diet which contains some bulk-forming foods such as fruits, vegetables, and whole grains and drinking several glasses of water in addition to other liquids each day helps prevent constipation.

Loss of teeth, periodontal disease, or ill-fitting dentures, though not direct results of aging, occur in individuals who previously did not take steps to maintain their oral health. Some individuals without teeth may be able to "gum" food and eat reasonably normally. Other persons who have problems with chewing seem to avoid eating meat in particular. Quite a few have described the practice of simmering meat a long time "to get all the good out of it." They consume the broth and discard the meat (and thus the protein and other nutrients). They may turn to a diet of tea, toast, cream soups, and other foods which are easy to chew. These individuals may benefit from suggestions of easy-to-chew foods which add more variety and nutrients to their diets.

Psychosocial and economic factors

The number of individuals 65 years of age and older is growing rapidly. Many of them are active, live independently, and enjoy good health. The ability of an older person to care for himself, if he is motivated to do so, should not be underestimated. Many are fiercely independent and take pride in "doing for themselves." Nonetheless, studies indicate that segments of the older population eat poorly and suffer from some degree of malnutrition.[18] Those who have the most trouble are those without friends, family, and adequate income. In order to combat nutrition problems of the elderly it is necessary to develop constructive solutions to economic and social problems. Individuals might be encouraged to eat some of their meals at a senior citizens center. A warm, friendly atmosphere often stimulates a new interest in life and, in turn, increases a person's self-esteem (see Appendix 2C).

Lack of nutrition knowledge in combination with long-held food practices and beliefs are often thought to be the cause of poor food selections by older persons. Old people are characterized as being opinionated and resistant to change. Actually older people are knowledgeable; they have a lifetime of experiences behind them. When some attention is paid to them and some genuine interest in their well-being is clearly expressed, most of them willingly listen to suggestions. With a little support and motivation an individual can make changes in his lifestyle and eating habits. Encouragement to use nutritious convenience foods, such as instant potatoes, might make it possible for some elderly people to continue preparing their own meals.

Studies have indicated that older individuals who regularly consume alcoholic beverages may reduce their intake of food.[19] The more alcohol consumed, the lower the intake of food. Alcohol does not provide any nutrients. For many elderly who need to limit their caloric intake, alcohol is a poor choice. For others, a glass of wine or beer before or with dinner may stimulate the appetite and increase the enjoyment of the meal.

The fixed low income of many older people may limit (1) the kind and quality of food purchased, (2) the cooking and storage facilities available to him, (3) transportation to and from the grocery store, and (4) outlook on life. Poor food choices and poor budgeting of the food dollar have been identified as factors contributing to undernutrition. Senior citizens should be encouraged to use community services such as free bus service to local supermarkets.

Physical disabilities that interfere with meal preparation can be overcome. Many people adapt to progressive disabilities such as loss of eyesight. On the other hand, drastic changes in lifestyle, such as the death of a spouse, may cause changes in food behavior that become difficult to overcome.

Loneliness, for example, is often associated with poor appetite and apathy toward food. Those who find themselves living alone or without the support and companionship of friends and family may develop a sense of low self-esteem. An individual with low self-esteem may think it is not worth going to the bother of cooking a meal just for himself. A person like this might jump at the opportunity of preparing or helping prepare a group meal, as for a family gathering or church supper.

Older people often take a variety of medications—some prescribed and some over-the-counter. Many of these interfere with absorption and/or utilization of nutrients. These persons should be knowledgeable about ways to modify their diets if this is indicated.

POINTS OF EMPHASIS
Guidelines for promoting healthful eating in later years

• *Develop a regular pattern of food intake. (Often small frequent meals are preferred by the elderly.)*

• *Eat with a friend, relatives, or at a senior citizen center if possible.*

• *Identify and use family and community resources to obtain a variety of nutritious foods.*

• *Try new food, new seasonings, and new ways of preparing foods.*

• *Avoid totally relying on convenience foods and canned goods.*

• *Keep physically active.*

• *Keep some easy-to-prepare foods on hand for times when energy level is low.*

STUDY QUESTIONS

1. Why should health care workers emphasize establishing sound eating habits for the entire family when a child is found to have a nutritional problem?
2. Describe how several factors may affect a healthy child's appetite.
3. What points should a health care worker discuss with a mother (or caretaker) who states, "I don't worry about my toddler's food intake as long as he drinks plenty of milk."
4. What are the major differences in the nutritive needs of male and female adolescents? Explain.
5. Discuss some of the factors that influence children's food preferences.
6. What physical factors may contribute to nutritional problems in elderly persons?
7. Identify how each of the following problems may interfere with a person's nutritional status. Suggest several ways of overcoming each problem:
   a. limited income
   b. lack of transportation to grocery store
   c. inadequate cooking and storage facilities
   d. social isolation

References

*1. Marlow, D.: *Textbook of Pediatric Nursing,* ed. 5. Philadelphia: W. B. Saunders Co., 1977.

2. Guteluis, M. F., et al.: Nutritional studies of children with pica: Controlled study evaluation nutritional status; 2. Treatment of pica with iron given intramuscularly. *Pediatrics* 29:1012, 1962.

3. Lankowsky, P.: Investigation into aetiology and treatment of pica. *Arch. Dis. Child.* 34:140, 1959.

4. Tuttle, W. W., et al.: Effect on school boys of omitting breakfast. *J. Am. Diet. Assoc.* 30:674, 1954.

*5. Kaufman, N. A., Poznanski, R., and Guggenheim, K.: Eating habits and opinions of teenagers on nutrition and obesity. *J. Am. Diet. Assoc.* 66:264, 1975.

6. DHEW. National Center for Health Statistics, HANES Dietary Intake Findings, 1971–1974.

7. Marshall, W. A., and Tanner, J. M.: Variations in the pattern of pubertal changes in boys. *Arch. Dis. Child.* 45:13, 1970.

*8. Finberg, L.: Fast foods for adolescents: Nutritional disaster or triumph of technology? *Am. J. Dis. Child.* 130:362, 1976.

*9. Appledorf, H., and Kelly, L. S.: Proximate and mineral content of fast foods. Pizzas, Mexican-American style foods and submarine sandwiches. *J. Am. Diet. Assoc.* 74:35, 1979.

*10. ———: Your food—Chance or choice. Chicago: National Dairy Council,1971.

11. Hammar, S. L., et al.: An interdisciplinary study of adolescent obesity. *J. Pediatr.* 80:373, 1972.

12. Huenemann, R. L.: Food habits of obese and non-obese adolescents. *Postgrad. Med.* 51:99, 1972.

13. Pelletier, O.: Vitamin C and cigarette smokers. *Ann. N.Y. Acad. Sci.* 258:156, 1975.

14. Water deprivation and performance of athletes. Committee on Nutritional Misinformation. Food and Nutrition Board NAS-NRC. *Nutr. Rev.* 32:314, 1974.

15. Roe, D.: *Drug-Induced Nutritional Deficiencies.* Westport CT: Avi Publishing Co., 1976.

* Recommended reading

16. Wynn, V.: Vitamins and oral contraceptive use. *Lancet* 1:561, 1975.

17. Rode, A., Ross, R., and Shephard, R. J.: Smoking withdrawal programme. Personality and cardio-respiratory fitness. *Arch. Environ. Health.* 24:27, 1972.

*18. Winick, M.: Nutrition and aging. *Contemporary Nutr.* 2(6), June 1977.

19. Barboriak, J., et al.: Alcohol and nutrient intake of elderly men. *J. Am. Diet. Assoc.* 72:493, 1978.

* Recommended reading

10
The changing nutritional scene

TECHNOLOGICAL CHANGES AND THE FOOD SUPPLY

Today, as a result of applications of science and technology, our food supply has many new characteristics. There are new varieties of edible plants, large-scale methods of agriculture and animal husbandry, rapid means of transporting food over long distances, and large-scale processing and storage methods for the preservation and preparation of food. Increasingly, the food Americans eat is grown and prepared away from home, with the result that agribusiness and the food processing industry exert much control over the food supply.

Effects of these changes are both positive and negative. Seasonal foods are available throughout the year. Perishable items last longer. Food is likely to be cleaner, more uniform, and easier to prepare. Whether or not the palatability of food has improved appears to be a matter of opinion.

Nutritional quality definitely depends on what happens to a food between farm and table. Many developments have helped to increase the availability of nutritious foods, such as food sources of vitamin C in the winter. On the other hand, developments such as the widespread use of highly refined and unfamiliar ingredients have caused nutrition-conscious individuals to wonder if new foods really are as nutritious as the manufacturers would have the public believe.

TRANSPORTATION OF THE FOOD SUPPLY

The decline of small farming operations has increased the distance between the farm and the supermarket. High speed means of transportation have made it possible to obtain fresh meat and produce in any season—sometimes from the other side of the world. Usually the nutritive value of produce declines in proportion to the length of time between harvesting and use. Nutritive value, therefore, depends on whether modern transportation actually reduces the time taken for food to reach the market.

Characteristics of some of the food with which Americans are supplied have been purposely altered to make the food travel better. Fruits and tomatoes being sent to distant markets may be picked before they are ripe. The effect of early picking on palatability is often detrimental; the effect on nutritive value is variable. New varieties of plants have been developed to enable produce such as tomatoes and strawberries to better withstand the rigors of shipping. While these changes increase the variety of foods available, quality is often sacrificed.

The rising cost of transportation has placed increased pressure on the food industry to process food to reduce its bulk prior to shipping it long distances. Great space saving may be achieved by preparing concentrated juices from fresh fruit. With rising fuel costs, the pressure to reduce transportation costs will no doubt increase, and fresh meat and produce may become less available.

FOOD PROCESSING

The term "food processing" encompasses all of the ways in which agricultural and livestock products are treated to preserve them and/or to prepare them for consumption as food. Preservation methods include canning, chilling or freezing, drying, fermenting (such as pickles and sauerkraut), and adding chemical preservatives (as in curing of meat, highly salting, and more recent innovations). Food processing has been going on for thousands of years, e.g., cheese making. Historically much of the processing has been carried out in the home. However, in technologically developed nations a very large proportion of food processing is now carried out by industry.

Generally food processors have not ranked nutritive value as a major quality factor in their products.[1] Instead they have emphasized safety, overall acceptability, and convenience—all features of immediate concern to the consumer. Attention should also be directed toward the nutritional quality of food. Although some processing methods produce improvements in nutritional quality, more often some nutrient loss occurs. In some cases reduction of nutritive value is absolutely necessary to assure safety. For example, canned foods must undergo rigorous heat treatment to destroy all microorganisms even though this also destroys some vitamins. The degree and type of processing affect the extent of nutritive loss.

An increasing percentage of food available on the market is now highly processed. This is partially in response to consumers' wishes, but in many cases the food industry has created a market for its new products and packaging methods.

Advantages of processing

Food processing serves a number of functions vital for an adequate food supply. Food preservation prevents food from deteriorating quickly and becoming inedible. Preservation, including packaging, also reduces losses caused by insects and rodents. Thus, processing for preservation, although it causes some loss of nutrients, is *absolutely essential* if we are to have an adequate supply of nutrients throughout the year in all parts of the nation.

Some types of processing improve the safety of foods. The washing of fruits and vegetables and the pasteurization of milk are important examples. In some cases processing improves the nutritional value of foods by destroying or decreasing content of antinutritional factors. Heating soybeans in the presence of moisture has this effect.

Processing can result in a change in appearance or taste of food that is pleasing to some consumers. Homogenization of milk fits in this category. Thus some types of processing might encourage consumers to select nutritious food.

Processing to minimize the amount of food preparation necessary in the home offers obvious advantages for mothers in the labor force, for handicapped persons who might otherwise have difficulty maintaining their independence, and for anyone else needing to save time or effort.

Processing also provides food uses for byproducts resulting from the preparation of other foods. Whey, a watery but nutritious fluid remaining after the manufacture of cheese, is now being incorporated into a variety of processed foods.

Disadvantages of processing

The uproar by consumer activists regarding processed foods often revolves around those which are highly refined or undergo many processes causing loss of nutrients. Some wholesome foods undergo so many changes during processing that the end product bears little nutritional resemblance to the original. A classic illustration is provided by potatoes which are peeled, cooked, mashed, dehydrated, rehydrated with additional ingredients, shaped, and fried. This produces fabricated potato chips, a popular snack food with low nutrient density, high caloric density (resulting from added fat), and high sodium content.

ADDED SALT, SUGAR, AND FAT

Much criticism is directed toward the addition of salt, sugar, fat, and a host of other substances to a broad spectrum of foods. Salt is, with certain exceptions, added for taste and *not for preservation* of food. The amounts added are sometimes far in excess of what would be used at home. Young and old consumers alike often become accustomed to the salty taste of commercially seasoned food and may think that home-prepared food tastes flat unless it is highly salted. As long as salt is copiously used in the preparation of many convenience foods, it will be difficult for Americans to reduce salt intake to 5 gm. daily as recommended in "Dietary Goals."

The sugar content of many processed foods is unnecessarily high. Some ready-to-eat breakfast cereals are more than 50 percent sugar by weight. Processed fruits and certain vegetables frequently contain much added sugar. Manufacturers may add sugar for reasons other than its sweetening effect. For example, it is easier to make muffins tender when extra sugar is used. A product can be high in nutritive sweeteners even if the word "sugar" does not appear on the label. Some of the names that indicate added sugar include dextrose, maltodextrins, corn syrup, corn syrup solids, corn sweeteners, refiner's syrup, honey, and molasses.

Fat is being used extensively in many new processed foods. The fat used is likely to be saturated to prolong the shelf life of the product. Crispy snack foods such as specialty crackers and chips usually have a high fat content. Vegetables can be purchased prebuttered; meat, fish, and potatoes come prefried; and even some breakfast cereals now contain added fat.

Many health professionals are concerned that American children are learning to equate saltiness, sweetness, and the texture provided by fat with good taste.

SUBSTITUTION OF INGREDIENTS IN FAMILIAR FOODS

Some of the controversy regarding processed food concerns the alteration of ingredients in familiar products, such as the substitution of sodium caseinate for nonfat dry milk solids in ice cream or the use of caramel coloring to make a bread appear to be "whole grain." Small changes in nutritional value can be additive. Ignoring a series of small decreases in nutrient content in many staple foods could possibly lead to significant nutritional deficits in the long run.

TYPES OF FOOD PRODUCTS

Processing holds the key to an adequate, safe, palatable, and nutritious food supply but it also has the possibility of delivering inferior products. For a better understanding of this it is helpful to consider different types of food products.

Conventional Foods Conventional foods are usually single entity foods that have been traditional in the diet for decades. Eggs, apples, milk, corn on the cob, spinach, soybeans, and potatoes are but a few examples. Simple prepared foods such as cheese and unrefined basic ingredients such as whole wheat flour are usually considered to be conventional foods or "familiar foods."

Convenience Foods If a food is partially or completely prepared before the product is offered for sale, it becomes a convenience food. The purpose of these products is to save time and/or work in food preparation.

Convenience foods are not necessarily low in nutritional value. If made primarily from basic, nutritious ingredients, some convenience foods are equal in nutritive value to comparable products prepared at home or are higher than the latter. In the winter canned tomatoes may be higher in vitamin content than are immature fresh tomatoes. (Tomatoes are usually at or close to their peak in nutritive value when canned, and relatively little vitamin destruction occurs during canning and proper storage.)

Not all convenience foods made from basic ingredients compare favorably with home-prepared foods. Reheated frozen TV dinners tend to be very low in folic acid. A range of 5.8 to 29.3 μg. folic acid per dinner (RDA = 400 μg, for adults) was reported for unfortified products with additional loss after the required heating.[2] Many varieties of dinners have also been found to be very low in thiamine, vitamin B_6, and/or vitamin E. Nevertheless, these dinners may be more nourishing than meals consisting primarily of snack foods.

Fabricated or "engineered" foods Fabricated foods are either imitations of conventional foods or new food forms. Ingredients such as soy protein isolate, modified food starch, corn sweeteners, and sodium caseinate are combined to achieve a particular result which would not be possible with ordinary food ingredients. Nondairy creamer, nondairy imitation cream cheese, imitation pecans, and breakfast bars are but a few of the many fabricated foods on the market. A list of the ingredients of one fabricated food, orange flavor instant breakfast drink, follows:

Sugar, citric acid (for tartness), calcium phosphates (regulate tartness and prevent caking), modified starches (provide body), potassium citrate (regulates tartness), cellulose gum (vegetable gum—provides body), natural orange flavor, vitamin C, hydrogenated coconut oil, artificial flavor, artificial color, vitamin A palmitate, BHA (a preservative).

Some fabricated foods are called food analogs, such as meat analogs which are made from extruded soy protein or other forms of textured vegetable protein. Changing soybeans into a meatlike food involves extensive "engineering."

If a food is made to resemble a familiar or conventional food, the FDA requires that it be called "imitation" unless it is "nutritionally equal to the original" in all respects except fat content and caloric value.[3] If the fabricated food contains at least as much of each of the vitamins, minerals, and protein as does the food it resembles, it need not be called imitation but instead may be given a new name which is descriptive to the consumer. Thus a simulated applesauce might be called "Imitation Applesauce" or perhaps "Apple Flavored Saucey Delight," depending on its nutritional value. Neither product would have to contain any real apple.

This FDA regulation governing the naming of fabricated foods implies that scientists know more about the nutritive qualities of these foods than is actually the case. Engineered foods which by chemical analysis appear to be the nutritional equal of conventional foods are sometimes found to be inferior when compared in animal feeding studies.[4,5,7]

Formulated foods The term "formulated foods" usually applies to foods designed to meet special needs. Infant formulas provide a classic example. Many products used in hospitals for total or supplemental feedings are formulated foods, as are some liquid diet products. Formulated foods have also been defined as mixtures of two or more ingredients, other than seasonings, processed or blended together. By this definition innumerable convenience foods and all fabricated foods are formulated foods.

Dietetic foods Most large supermarkets have a section for "dietetic" foods. These are convenience foods processed in a manner which is supposed to make them suitable for use by individuals on certain types of modified diets. The foods may have been prepared without added sodium and/or sugar. They may have been specially processed to be low in cholesterol and saturated fat. Some products are unusually low in calories. The term "dietetic food" provides no specific information about the type of diet for which the food is appropriate, if any. Individuals on modified diets need advice from health professionals as to the suitability of these foods because it may be difficult to interpret the labels correctly.

FOODS AVAILABLE AWAY FROM HOME

Other changes in foods eaten by Americans result from the practice of eating meals away from home. This option has become increasingly popular because of the convenience of fast food restaurants and vending machines. The impact of the fast food industry has been so great that supermarkets are perceiving it as a threat. They are responding by getting into the fast food business themselves. Some food manufacturers have tried to meet the fast food challenge by promoting their products as quick, easy, and economical substitutes for fast food. One survey of customers at fast food restaurants revealed that a majority of them purchased fast food infrequently. Only 11 percent bought fast food items six or more times weekly, and a large number of purchases were for snacks (such as cola, coffee) rather than meals.[6]

FAST FOOD CHAINS

More is known about the nutritional value of foods offered by fast food chains than by local coffee shops and restaurants. The food offered by the chains is made from commercially standardized ingredients using specified methods of preparation. Turnover of food is usually so rapid that cooked foods are not kept warm long enough to cause serious nutrient loss. The nutritive value of many products offered by fast food chains has been determined. Nutrient analyses of some representative samples is given in Appendix 3C.

A number of reports of the nutritional value of fast food meals have indicated that they are higher in nutritive value than many people expect. The meat used in the hamburgers, for example, is usually lean, and suitable for use in a prudent diet. In most food chains it is possible to select meals providing at least one fourth of the RDA for several of the micronutrients. However, vitamin A, vitamin E, folic acid, vitamin C, and several trace elements are likely to be in short supply. Many chains offer nothing that is a significant source of vitamin A except milk and sometimes cheese and tomato juice. Shakes are not a source of vitamin A if they are not made with ice cream. The most commonly available source of vitamin C in fast food chains is french fries. Cole slaw, tomato and/or orange juice are available at some establishments. Much of the vitamin C in pizza may be lost (chemically destroyed) during handling and cooking.

Actual meals selected often provide low intakes of several nutrients, with the intake of vitamin A and calcium being especially low. The presence of good calcium sources on the menu (milk, shakes) does not necessarily result in their being ordered.

Major nutritional drawbacks of eating at fast food restaurants include:
1. Lack of variety.
2. High caloric density of some of the foods offered.

A meal of a hamburger, french fries, and shake provides about 2 percent of the 1974 RDA for vitamin E, 4 percent of vitamin A, 11 percent of folic acid, 34 percent of calcium, 45 percent of protein, but 37 percent of the RDA for calories for an average adolescent female. Careful food selection throughout the remainder of the day would be necessary to achieve recommended intake of the vitamins named above.

3. High sugar content of most beverages. The most nutritious beverages offered generally cost more than the carbonated ones when equal volumes are compared.
4. High proportion of saturated fat. Fat used in frying is usually saturated (depending on the food chain). Milk, if available, is usually whole.
5. High sodium content of many foods. The amount of sodium provided by some fast food meals is almost as high as the amount recommended in Dietary Goals for an entire day's intake. Some fast food chains will "hold" the added salt upon request, but this usually means that the order will take longer to fill.
6. Preponderance of refined foods and lack of food sources of fiber.

FOOD IN VENDING MACHINES

The nutritional quality of food in vending machines depends primarily on the choices offered. Unfortunately most machines feature soft drinks and candy. Where turnover is large, perishables such as milk, fruit, and sandwiches can also be stocked in vending machines. This is seldom done unless consumers request that such items be made available.

NEED FOR LABELING

Nutritional labeling was initiated on a wide scale in 1973 to inform consumers about the nutritional value of processed food. Many consumers still complain that labels fail to provide all of the information they want, and some have difficulty interpreting the information which is included. In the fall of 1978 the Food and Drug Administration, Federal Trade Commission, and United States Department of Agriculture held public hearings to gather information and opinions on food labeling. Their aim was to develop a strategy for providing consumers with useful nutrition-oriented information on the labels of food products. Topics covered included ingredient labeling, nutritional labeling and other dietary information, open date labeling, imitation and substitute foods, food fortification, the total food label, and safe and suitable ingredients. At the time of writing, changes in regulations had not been completed. The following information, therefore, is subject to change. Health professionals are urged to contact the Food and Drug Administration (Appendix 1) for updated information.

TABLE 10.1 *Mandatory general information on food labels*

A. REQUIRED INFORMATION ON ALL FOOD LABELS

> 1 Seasoned Rye Crackers
>
> 2 Net weight 1 lb (454 gm)
>
> 3 Super Cracker Co.
> Crackertown, CA

1. Name of product
2. Net contents or net weight. It is customary for the weight to be expressed in the metric as well as in the avoirdupois (household) system. Under the Metric Conversion Act of 1975, manufacturers are voluntarily converting to the metric system in a gradual, easily understood manner. If the product is packed in liquid, the weight of both is included. Manufacturers are, at their option, providing information on the solids content, i.e., the weight of the food before the addition of liquid. FDA is developing a regulation which will require declaration of the drained weight.
3. Name and address of the manufacturer, packer, or distributor.

B. ADDITIONAL REQUIRED INFORMATION ON FOODS FOR WHICH THERE IS NO STANDARD OF IDENTITY

Ingredient present in greatest amount by weight	INGREDIENTS: Sugar, Nonfat Dry Milk, Dextrose, Cocoa, Salt, Soya Lecithin (an emulsifier), Vanillin	Food additives which must be listed by name

MANDATORY GENERAL INFORMATION ON FOOD LABELS

Although the FDA has been regulating the labeling of food products in interstate commerce for years, mandatory information included only those items shown in Table 10-1. This information is still mandatory today.

Ingredient labeling is not mandatory for foods for which a *standard of identity* has been established. A standard of identity is something like a required "recipe"—one that must be used if a particular name is given to a product. There are about 300 standardized foods including catsup, tomato sauce and paste, mayonnaise, ice cream, cheddar cheese, canned fruits, vegetables, and jelly. Optional ingredients may be added to a number of the standardized foods; the FDA requires that these be listed on the label. Some manufacturers have taken the initiative of listing all ingredients in standardized foods as a consumer service.

Even though ingredient listing is required on the labels of all nonstandardized foods, this still provides the consumer with limited information about nutrient value (Table 10.1). Ingredients must be listed in descending order by weight, but in most cases there is no way to tell if the first ingredient comprises 90 or 50 or some other percent of the total weight.

Because of FDA regulations, the name of some mixed foods indicates the minimum proportion of meat which must be present. The trouble is that the consumer needs to have access to the "code" to be able to use this information. A few examples are included in Table 10.2.

TABLE 10.2 *A sample of federal standards for products made with meat*

TYPE OF FOOD		PERCENT OF MEAT IN THE FOOD
Baby food	High meat dinner	30
	High poultry dinner	18¾ (meat, skin, fat and giblets)
	Meat and broth	68
	Poultry and broth	43
	Vegetables and meat	8
General convenience foods	Beef with gravy	50
	Gravy with beef	35
	Turkey with gravy	35
	Gravy with turkey	15

Source: Standards for meat and poultry—a consumer reference list. Animal and Plant Health Inspection Service. U.S. Department of Agriculture. Washington DC, Rev. 1973.

NUTRITIONAL LABELING

In conjunction with mandatory general food labeling, nutritional labeling is supposed to arm the consumer with facts needed to compare the nutritive value of similar products, determine good sources of specific nutrients, evaluate the nutritive value of new products, determine good food buys, and plan more nutritionally balanced meals. It is unrealistic to expect that these objectives will be met on a wide scale unless consumers are taught how to make effective use of nutritional labeling. It is hoped that nutritional labeling will upgrade the nutritional quality of the food supply since the food industry has increased responsibility to determine what nutrients are actually contained in the food they are selling and to reveal the facts plainly.

Unfortunately, nutritional labeling is in many instances not mandatory but, rather, a voluntary service provided by manufacturers if they so choose. Nutritional labeling is mandatory only if: (1) The food has been enriched or fortified with one or more nutrients. (When nutrients are added for reasons other than nutrition, such as sodium chloride for flavor or ascorbic acid to prevent discoloration of fruit, nutritional labeling is not required.) (2) A nutritional claim has been made for the product, on the label or in advertising, such as "low fat" or "a good source of iron." Dietetic foods make nutritional claims and, thus, must be nutritionally labeled.

Description of nutritional labeling

The FDA expended considerable time and effort in developing a method of presenting nutrition information clearly, concisely, and simply. Compromises were necessary because so many different nutrients are

TABLE 10.3 *A sample nutritional label*

NUTRITION INFORMATION PER SERVING

Serving Size: ⅔ cup (1 oz)
Servings per Container: 18
Shredded Wheat

	1 oz.	With ½ cup whole milk
Calories	110	190
Protein	3g	7g
Carbohydrate	23g	29g
Fat	1g	5g
Sodium	**	60mg

**Not more than 10 mg/100 gm
Not more than 10 mg/1 ounce serving

Placed here because it is the weight of sodium which is important to consumers who wish or need to restrict intake. There is no U.S. RDA for sodium

PERCENTAGE OF U.S. RECOMMENDED DAILY ALLOWANCES (U.S. RDA)

	1 oz.	With ½ cup whole milk
Protein	4	10
Vitamin A	*	2
Vitamin C	*	*
Thiamine	4	6
Riboflavin	*	10
Niacin	8	8
Calcium	*	15
Iron	6	6
Phosphorus	10	20
Magnesium	8	10
Zinc	4	6
Copper	6	6

Indicator or leader nutrients

These could have been omitted or other nutrients could have been listed at the manufacturer's option

* Contains less than 2 percent of the U.S. RDA of these nutrients

INGREDIENTS: Shredded wheat is 100 percent natural whole wheat. BHT, a preservative, is added to the packaging to retain the natural whole wheat flavor.

Shredded wheat contains 2.0 percent non-nutritive Crude Fiber (0.57 gm. per 1 oz. serving).

Key: Optional information

involved and the recommended intake of each varies with sex, stage in the developmental cycle, and other factors. The nutrition information panel shown in Table 10.3 follows the regulations set by the FDA in 1973.

United States Recommended Daily Allowances (U.S. RDA) as a reference standard

The standard used for declaring nutrient content on food labels is the U.S. Recommended Daily Allowances (U.S. RDA). The content of each nutrient listed on a label is expressed as a percentage of the U.S. RDA.

The similarity of this name to Recommended Dietary Allowances (RDA) can be a source of confusion. Values used for the U.S. RDA may differ considerably from an individual's RDA, as illustrated in Table 10.4.

Unlike the Recommended Dietary Allowances, the U.S. RDA values are standard for nearly all individuals above 4 years of age. (Special U.S. RDAs have been developed for children under 4 years and for pregnant and lactating women.)

A major problem in interpreting food labels can result from exclusive use of the U.S. RDA. If consumers try to achieve 100 percent of the U.S. RDA for all family members, for all listed nutrients, they are likely to find that this is difficult unless they select mainly highly fortified foods or take vitamin-mineral supplements. This may reduce their intake of less known but equally essential nutrients. Consumers need to know that the U.S. RDA is not a satisfactory guide for planning for adequate nutrient intake since it is very high for some nutrients, about right for some, and omits other nutrients entirely.

Although the U.S. RDA does not accurately reflect the nutrient requirements of any one individual, it does provide a satisfactory means of comparing products and finding foods which are good sources of a particular nutrient.

Degree of accuracy required in nutritional labeling

Consumers should recognize that the nutritional values displayed on labels represent average figures which have been rounded off. Rounding off reduces the likelihood that the consumer will make meaningless comparisons. For example a ½ cup serving of orange juice providing 76 percent of the U.S. RDA for vitamin C is not significantly different from a different brand of juice providing 79 percent of the same nutrient. The labels for both will read 80 percent because of the rounding off procedure. In general, the stated nutritional value should not differ from the actual nutritional value by more than 20 percent, but fortified or fabricated foods *must* contain at least the amounts of nutrients declared on the label.

REQUIRED INFORMATION AND FORMAT

Serving size and number of servings Serving size is determined by the manufacturer, but can be challenged by the FDA if it seems unduly large. The size selected is supposed to be suitable for consumption as part of a meal for an adult male who engages in light activity. The nutritive value and number of portions per container will be expressed only for that serving size. Manufacturers frequently designate larger portion sizes than are customarily eaten by many people. A 1 cup serving of vegetables would be much too large for most children and for many adults. One-half cup of raisins would, likewise, be more than the usual serving.

Nutrient content If any nutrient is to be declared, all of the nutrients shown in black type in Table 10.3 must also be listed, even if the food is an insignificant source of some of those nutrients. The first eight nutrients listed under "Percentage of U.S. RDA" are called *leader* or *indicator* nutrients. The assumption is made that if the intake of these nutrients is adequate, intake of other micronutrients should also be adequate. This assumption is not necessarily valid.

Nutrients in conventional food combinations which are more predictive of adequate content of other nutrients are vitamins A and B_6, folacin, pantothenic acid, calcium, magnesium, and iron.[7]

OPTIONAL NUTRITIONAL INFORMATION

If the manufacturer desires, he may also reveal nutritional information about the nutrients shown in red type in Table 10.3. Optional information is commonly given for highly fortified convenience or fabricated foods and for a few of the more conventional foods that are good sources of particular micronutrients. Fiber content, if indicated, is always given in terms of *crude* fiber. The crude fiber content underestimates

TABLE 10.4 *Comparison of the U.S. RDA with the RDA for two age groups (selected nutrients)*

	VITAMIN A	VITAMIN C	THIAMINE	CALCIUM	IRON	VITAMIN B_{12}
U.S. RDA	5000	60	1.5	800	18	6.0
RDA for 9-yr-old child	35000	45	1.2	800	10	3.0
RDA for a woman 23–50-yr old	4000	60	1.0	800	18	3.0

the total amount of naturally occurring fiber in most products.

Another option for the manufacturer is display of the content of cholesterol. Polyunsaturated and saturated fat content may be identified only if the fat content of the product exceeds 2 gm per serving. The format for this type of information is shown in Table 10.5. The sum of the polyunsaturated plus the saturated fat is less than the total fat content since the product also contains monounsaturated fat. This means of presentation reveals the P/S ratio of the product. In Table 10.5 the P/S ratio is 5/3. When information about cholesterol and/or polyunsaturated and saturated fat is included as part of nutritional labeling, the statement shown in red type must appear on the label.

Sugar content At the time of writing, the only type of product that includes specific information about the amount of added sugar is ready-to-eat breakfast cereal. Some cereal companies specify the amount of sucrose and other sugars in gm. per serving (serving size given in grams). If desired, the consumer can use this information to calculate the percent of sugar contained in the product. The method is shown below for a presweetened cereal that contains 13 gm. sugar per 28 gm. serving:

$$\frac{13 \text{ gm sugar}}{28 \text{ gm serving}} = \text{What } \% \left(\frac{X}{100}\right)? = \frac{13}{28} \times 100 = 46\% \text{ sugar}$$

Guidelines for use of labeling in investigating the nutritional value of foods

The suggestions given here are designed to assist consumers in using nutritional labeling in appropriate ways.

1. Use nutritional labeling primarily as a supplement to a reliable meal planning guide. The nutritional information available on labels is not sufficiently complete to provide an adequate basis for determining if nutritional needs are being met.
2. If you feel too rushed to use nutritional labeling in the supermarket, check labels at your leisure at home. Look at advertisements in newspapers and magazines as well. The next time you shop, avoid foods you have found to be nutritionally inferior.
3. Compare the serving size indicated with the portion you intend to use and adjust the nutritional information as appropriate. For example, if the designated portion is 1 cup and you intend to use ½ cup, cut the nutritional values in half.
4. Check labels to learn which foods are good sources of specific nutrients, for example fruits and vegetables which are good sources of vitamin C.
5. Determine differences of similar products that are nutritionally labeled, making sure the portion sizes are the same. In particular, check for nutrients that appear to be less abundant in your family's diet.
6. Determine if processing has conserved the nutritive value of a food. Does a canned stew or frozen dinner provide the nutrients you would expect from a freshly prepared meal? Does the main dish provide more of the nutrients you need than would other quick and easy foods?
7. Find out if processing has caused a significant change (either increase or decrease) in caloric value. For example, find out if a new style of vegetable is laden with extra calories. If you are trying to control your weight, use nutritional labeling to identify low calorie foods high in nutrients.
8. Compare a fabricated food which is attractive to you because of its convenience, cost, texture, or taste with a food for which you might substitute it. Look at ingredient listing as well as nutrient content.
   a. Assume that foods made from refined ingredients will contain few nutrients other than those declared on the label.
   b. Recognize that a high number of grams of carbohydrate is compatible with a prudent diet unless the carbohydrate is provided primarily by some type of sugar or refined starches or flours.
   Try not to be unduly pressured by hard-sell advertising if the product is high in sugar, salt, and/or fat.
9. Recognize that nutritional labeling may be misleading. Do not jump to the conclusion that it is better to buy a fortified product than an unfortified, lightly processed, conventional food because it con-

TABLE 10.5 *Part of nutrition information panel revealing information on fat and cholesterol content*

Fat	16 gm
% of calories from fat*	73%
Polyunsaturated*	5 gm
Saturated*	3 gm
Cholesterol* (10 mg/100 gm)	0 gm

* Information on fat and cholesterol content is provided for individuals who, on the advice of a physician, are modifying their total dietary intake of fat and/or cholesterol.

POINTS OF EMPHASIS
Nutritional labeling

• *Nutritional labeling is voluntary for many products. Its absence does not necessarily indicate nutritional inferiority.*

• *Nutritional labeling facilitates identification of good sources of specific nutrients and of the caloric value of foods.*

• *The amount of information given on nutritionally labeled foods is insufficient to use as the sole basis of selecting foods for good health.*

TABLE 10.6 *Comparison of toaster pastries with whole wheat toast and butter*

TOASTER PASTRIES NUTRITION INFORMATION PER SERVING		WHOLE WHEAT TOAST SPREAD WITH 1 TSP. BUTTER OR MARGARINE	
		(BREAD)	(BUTTER)
Serving size 1 pastry		1 slice*	1 tsp*
Serving per container	4		
Calories	190	70	35
Protein	2 gm	3 gm	0
Carbohydrate	35 gm	13 gm	0
Fat	5 gm	1 gm	5
Percentage of U.S. Recommended Daily Allowances (U.S. RDA)			
Protein	2	4	0
Vitamin A	10	0	2
Vitamin C	10	0	0
Thiamine	10	4	0
Riboflavin	10	0	0
Niacin	10	4	0
Calcium	0	0	0
Iron	10	4	0
Vitamin B$_6$	10		

INGREDIENTS: Enriched wheat flour, rye flour, sugar, partially hydrogenated soybean oil, corn sweeteners, corn flour, apples, tapioca starch, whey, corn starch, salt, citric acid, leavening, niacinamide, vitamin A, spices, benzoate of soda, vitamin B$_6$, vitamin B$_2$, vitamin B$_1$, and artificial flavor.

INGREDIENTS: Whole wheat flour, stone ground whole wheat flour, water, unsulfured molasses, cottonseed oil, corn syrup, fresh yeast, nonfat dry milk, salt, wheat gluten, dough conditioner, calcium propionate.

INGREDIENTS: Not listed

* A smaller serving size than is usually indicated on the label

tains more of the listed nutrients. It is inexpensive and easy for the manufacturer to add 25 percent or more of the U.S. RDA of vitamins and minerals to a product. If you already have an adequate intake of these nutrients, extra amounts will provide no additional benefit. Moreover, if you choose four foods, each of which provides 25 percent of the U.S. RDA for protein and listed vitamins and minerals, those foods will not necessarily promote optimal health. They will no doubt still be low in unlisted vitamins and minerals.

Nutritional information about two quickly prepared breakfast items is given in Table 10.6. It is not immediately apparent how to interpret the information given in the table. At first glance the toaster pastries appear to be far superior to the buttered toast. However, the difference in calories should not be overlooked. Two slices of toast with one pat of butter could be eaten without reaching the number of calories in the pastry. The broader spectrum of nutrients in the whole wheat toast (Mg, Zn, K, pantothenic acid, folic acid, and others) is not apparent from the information given. Since all of the basic ingredients in the toaster pastries are highly refined, except the rye flour, one can assume that the pastries lack significant amounts of other essential nutrients. It is impossible to determine the proportion of each ingredient used in the pastries. The weight of one of the flours might greatly

exceed the weight of sugar or be nearly the same. The combined weight of sugar and corn sweeteners might exceed the weight of one of the flours. Thus it is even hard to predict how sweet the product will taste. At least it is encouraging to find that the weight of the apples exceeds the weight of the salt. The vegetable shortening used in the pastries probably has a P/S ratio similar to that of the butter used on the toast, but there is no way to tell for sure from this label.

STUDY QUESTIONS

1. What are major nutritional drawbacks of consuming a majority of your daily food intake at a fast food restaurant?
2. If a product is labeled as follows, how much can you tell about its sugar content?
   Ingredients: white flour, oat flour, corn flour, white sugar, corn sugar, brown sugar, honey, coconut oil, salt. . .
3. Should all family members try to select foods supplying 100 percent of the U.S. RDA for nutrients? Explain.
4. How do the leader nutrients used for nutritional labeling compare with those identified by Pennington as being most predictive of overall nutritive adequacy of the diet?

References

1. Review. Nutritional quality and food product development. *Nutr. Rev.* 31:226,1973.

2. Hoppner, K., Lampi, B., and Perrin, D. E.: Folacin activity of frozen convenience foods. *J. Am. Diet. Assoc.* 63:536, 1973.

*3. Morrison, M.: A consumer's guide to food labels. *FDA Consumer.* 11(5):4, 1977.

4. Weininger, J., and Briggs, G.: Nutrition Update. *J. Nutr. Ed.* 6:139, 1974.

5. Instant breakfasts. Nutritious junk food. *Consumer Reports* 42:324, 1977.

6. Greecher, C. P., and Shannon, B.: Impact of fast food meals on nutrient intake of two groups. *J. Am. Diet Assoc.* 70:368, 1977.

7. Pennington, J. A.: *Dietary Nutrient Guide.* Westport CT: Avi Publishing Co., 1976.

* Recommended reading.

11
Menu planning and the purchase of food

Providing varied, appealing, nutritious, economical meals requires creativity, knowledge, and skill in food management. A variety of guidelines and resource materials can aid experienced and inexperienced individuals in successfully managing food.

Food management, as it is used in this text, refers to knowledge and skills necessary to (1) plan meals, (2) purchase food and store it safely, and (3) prepare and serve meals. This chapter discusses information related to planning meals and purchasing food. Chapter 12 discusses safe food storage and preparation. The individual who is responsible for food management is referred to as the food manager* (a term interchangeable with homemaker). Information in this chapter can not only guide the food manager but also should be considered by health professionals who are assisting clients to improve their diets.

MEAL PLANNING

The first step in food management is meal planning. The main goals of meal planning are to (1) serve food that is appealing and appetizing to those eating it, (2) provide a variety of wholesome foods that meet the nutritional needs of individual family members, and (3) keep within the available food budget. Among the factors influencing how meals are planned for a specific family are meal patterns and the family's resources.

Meal patterns

A meal pattern is a description of (1) the number of meals eaten by an individual or family within a specified time period (e.g., daily, weekly), (2) approximate

* The food manager may be male or female; the pronoun "he" is used when referring to the food manager.

times when meals are eaten, and (3) components of individual meals. The lifestyle and composition of a family, special needs of individual family members, and cultural factors influence the kind of meal pattern a family adopts.

Lifestyle The traditional pattern of three meals a day does not fit the lifestyle of many contemporary Americans. Therefore it is important to recognize that any number of meal patterns can meet the nutritional needs of healthy people. The pattern should be chosen with the needs and preferences of family members in mind. Varied work schedules and school hours may make a uniform meal pattern impossible. In this case, ways to make it easy for family members to "fend for themselves" and still meet their nutritional needs in an enjoyable fashion should be incorporated into the meal plan. Developing a satisfactory meal pattern may depend upon making arrangements for family members to share domestic chores. The food manager's work is easier when responsibility for food shopping, preparation, and cleanup is divided among family members.

Some families choose to follow one meal pattern during the week and another one on the weekend. If families manage to eat only a few meals together during the week, weekend meals may take on special meaning. Not only can food be eaten more leisurely then, but also there is more time for meal planning and preparation. Weekend cooking has become a hobby for many individuals, as have growing and preserving one's own food.

A survey of how American consumers spend their food dollars showed that the share of the food dollar going to frozen plate dinners, entrees, and soups each increased about 20 to 25 percent from 1965 to 1975, while the purchase of ready-to-eat cereals increased

TABLE 11.1 *Skeleton menu*

MORNING OR A.M. MEAL
  juice
  cereal or toast
  milk
  •
  grain product or fruit
  beverage

AFTERNOON OR LIGHT MEAL
  sandwich   soup
  vegetable   or   salad
  beverage   beverage
  •   •
  fruit   grain product

EVENING OR HEAVY MEAL
  protein main dish
  grain and/or potato
  vegetable
  beverage
  •
  milk
  grain product

approximately 40 to 45 percent. These items, however, accounted for less than $1.00 out of every $100.00 spent for food. Overall, the survey found that families spent money for food in 1975 in much the same manner as they did in 1965. This was the case whether foods were categorized by the Basic Four food groups or by the degree of processing. Fresh and unprocessed foods accounted for 46 percent of the food dollars spent in both 1965 and 1975.[1]

Family composition   The number of family members, their age distribution, and their special nutritional needs influence family food patterns. The amounts and kinds of food served to various family members and the frequency of eating differ according to body size, activity level, and growth and development. A growing teenager may eat a large serving of potatoes, while an elderly person or a small child may only need half as much.

Cultural factors   A food manager will usually incorporate the family's cultural food preferences into the meal pattern. In mixed marriages or a group setting, he may need to make compromises in order to provide food that individuals from differing cultural backgrounds will eat. Health professionals who give guidance in meal planning may be more successful if they consider the impact of culture on family food habits.

Determining a family's meal pattern   To determine the family's meal pattern, the food manager identifies the number of meals and kinds of food eaten by various family members each day. He should be cognizant of the kinds and amount of food family members eat away from home and as snacks. These foods contribute nutrients and calories.

Using the preceding information, the food manager can develop a skeleton menu such as the one shown in

Table 11.1. This skeleton menu is an adequate meal pattern in that it provides for (1) a somewhat regular daily intake of food, (2) some food in the morning, and (3) a variety of foods from the four food groups each day.

Family resources

Before actually planning meals and snacks a well-organized food manager considers family resources including (1) knowledge and skills of family members who will be participating in meal preparation and cleanup, (2) time available for food related activities, (3) energy level of food preparers and their willingness to spend time on food preparation, (4) available equipment and storage facilities, (5) food on hand that should be used, and (6) amount of money that can be allocated for food.

The food manager might also consider the kinds of learning experiences he wants to provide for children in the family (e.g., popping corn, baking bread, preparing fresh vegetables). Since a clean table, attractively set in comfortable surroundings, enhances the appearance of food and helps set the mood for mealtime, the food manager might want to plan at least some meals so there will be time to accomplish these things.

KNOWLEDGE AND SKILL OF THE FOOD MANAGER

The knowledge and attitudes of the food manager and his food management skills have an impact on the kinds of meal he prepares and ultimately on the nutritional status of the family. Nutrition knowledge is not necessarily synonymous with the ability to prepare good-tasting meals.[2] However, studies have identified a positive relationship between a food manager's level of formal education and the information he has about food purchases and nutrient needs of the family. In general, higher levels of education are related to higher levels of nutritional knowledge.[3]

A person's nutrition knowledge is modified by attitudes toward food and nutrition.[4] Family attitudes and food beliefs influence the food manager's choice of foods and methods of preparation. Husbands, for example, may indirectly influence the composition of meals by making their food preferences known to wives. It is well documented that children influence food selection.[5-8]

Family dietary concerns tend to shift as a family progresses through the life cycle. One study of families identified that (1) young families with young children were most concerned about economizing on the food budget, (2) middle-aged families composed of working couples and school-aged children were concerned with food budgeting and with using time for food management economically, (3) older couples without children were concerned about decreasing calories and about amounts of cholesterol and saturated fats in their diets, and (4) elderly couples were concerned about decreasing calories, cholesterol, and saturated fats, and they were very concerned about economizing on their food budgets.[9] Health professionals who are providing guidance in meal planning should determine if their clients share any of these concerns and want assistance in dealing with them.

When food managers have little knowledge or experience in preparing food it is sensible for them initially to plan simple meals, making judicious use of convenience foods. For example, meal preparation can be made easier by using some lightly processed foods that are packaged with directions for preparation (e.g., frozen vegetables), some fully prepared foods (e.g., rolls) and only one or two foods that involve the learning of new preparation skills. Since fresh meat, fruits, and vegetables rarely come with directions for preparation, these foods may pose a challenge to a beginning cook. Actually, many fresh foods are easy to prepare.

Even if a person knows how to prepare many different foods he may have difficulty coordinating meal preparation so that everything is ready at the right time. If this is the situation and no "helpers" are available, a wise food manager will limit the number of different food items to be prepared.

Following a few time guidelines such as those given here may streamline meal preparation when time is limited. Time guidelines can be helpful for an inexperienced cook such as a new widower, a disabled or debilitated person, or an individual who is not interested in spending much time on food preparation.

1. Plan meals and do shopping for at least a week at a time.
2. Plan meals around foods that are easy to prepare, e.g.:
   a. one pot meals
   b. main dishes which can be cooked quickly or eaten cold
   c. pan-broiled meats such as hamburger and chops
3. Serve fruits and vegetables raw some of the time.
4. Avoid use of complicated recipes. When possible use cooking appliances that decrease preparation time, e.g., pressure cooker.
5. Include the use of leftovers in the menu plan.
6. Plan for some make-ahead and freeze dishes, if possible.
7. Minimize cleanup chores by:
   a. limiting the number of pots used for cooking
   b. serving food from kitchen on dinnerplates
   c. soaking dishes and pans immediately after use
8. Delegate some food management tasks to other family members.

EQUIPMENT FOR FOOD PREPARATION AND STORAGE

Food storage and preparation require resources such as a food cooking unit and a refrigerator. Cooking appliances, the number of utensils, and space in the kitchen determine the kinds of meals which can be conveniently prepared. The size of the refrigerator, whether or not there is a freezer, and the amount of other safe storage space influence the kind and quantity of food a family is able to purchase at one time. Some families have difficulty controlling vermin such as cockroaches and mice. Unless they have a good supply of storage containers that can be tightly sealed it may be necessary for them to limit the amount of food stored in order to keep it from being contaminated.

FOOD ON HAND

When planning meals the food manager should check to see what food is on hand. He should plan menus to use up perishable food items before they spoil and to rotate nonperishable items in stock within a reasonable period of time.

FAMILY FOOD BUDGET

The recent sharp increase in the cost of foods has caused many families to plan economical meals, shop more carefully for food, and do without certain luxury items. Using food money wisely is particularly important for families with limited incomes. Limited purchasing power limits food selection. This, in turn, may lower the nutritional quality of the diet.

It is difficult to say specifically how much a family needs to budget for food. Many variables influence family food expenditures, including:

1. Family size and composition. Large families tend to spend less money per family member for food than small families.[10] Families with several growing children may have greater food expenditures than a group of elderly individuals.
2. Family income. When a family's income is low, the proportion of the income spent for food is likely to be high. Conversely, as income rises the portion spent for food usually decreases.[11] Federal food programs and the Food Stamp Program stretch the food budget of certain families (Appendix 2).
3. Differences in food costs. The prices of foods vary with the season of the year and the area from which they come. Foods cost less when they are in season. Foods in northern states tend to cost more than foods in southern states. Food purchased near the source of its production is generally less expensive than food transported from one place to another.
4. Importance of food in relation to other family needs. Families who are interested in maintaining health may place added emphasis on trying to adequately meet nutritional needs.
5. The ability of the food manager to use cost-saving factors. The food manager who knows amounts of foods needed to meet nutrient needs and how to make suitable substitutes can decrease food expenditures. A food manager who is creative, resourceful, and skillful can minimize food costs.
6. Place of purchase. Some families have access to foods that are inexpensive if, for instance, they be-

long to a food co-op or live near a farm stand. Growing and preserving foods at home is another way of obtaining food for the family. It takes time and may or may not save money. Home food production often increases the variety of foods served to a family.

7. Types of food purchased. Frequent use of convenience foods increases food cost.
8. Entertaining. Having guests for meals increases food costs.
9. Meals purchased away from home. Meals purchased away from home may cost up to 30 to 50 percent more than meals prepared at home.[10]
10. Use of fuel. Some food managers try to control expense and reduce the waste of natural resources by careful use of fuel when cooking. Some suggestions to minimize fuel expenditure when cooking are listed here:
    a. Cook one pot meals.
    b. Cook oven meals instead of using both the oven and the surface heating units.
    c. Plan to do baking when the oven is being used to cook a meal.
    d. Use a pressure cooker, small electrical appliances, or a microwave oven when possible.
    e. Cook several meals or foods at once and store properly for later use.
    f. Keep lids on pans.
    g. When boiling, use just enough heat to maintain a *slow* boil.

Economy-minded food managers examine family characteristics to determine acceptable ways to cut food costs. Health professionals can give food managers assistance with this task.

Components of meals

Many combinations of food make appetizing, satisfying meals and snacks and provide adequate amounts and kinds of nutrients. The food manager chooses foods which fit in the family's skeleton menu. He aims to (1) meet Basic Four guidelines, (2) provide variety during the day and from day to day (more or less according to family preference), (3) choose nutritious foods that family members enjoy, and (4) combine foods in appetizing ways. Menus should include all food prepared at home whether or not it is eaten there.

BASIC FOUR GUIDELINES

The Basic Four food groups serve well as a foundation for planning meals. The food manager can identify the family's usual eating times and distribute foods from the Basic Four groups among the various meals. Unless a person is on a reducing diet, extra foods from the four food groups or from the "other" group will need to be added in order to meet energy needs. Meals are more likely to meet nutrient needs if they are planned for a period of several days or a week. When a pattern of three daily meals is followed, inclusion of *at least three* of the Basic Four food groups in each meal simplifies meeting the guidelines for the day. This becomes less important when nutritious snacks are selected to supplement meals.

VARIETY

Some variety from meal to meal and day to day can add to the enjoyment of meals and can increase the likelihood of meeting nutrient needs. Serving foods from each of the Basic Four food groups gives balance to a meal. Creativity and a willingness to try new foods and recipes adds variety to meals. Some families may have to limit the variety of foods they eat for economic reasons. Many other people are set in their ways; they enjoy eating many of the same foods every day. Moderation helps avoid overuse of any potentially harmful foods.

A number of different foods can easily be served at a meal when several people are eating. With some advance planning and a little creativity, a variety of foods can also be served when only one or two people are eating.

AMOUNT OF FOOD PREPARED

The amount of food prepared at one time depends on the needs of family members and on whether leftovers are desired or are likely to be discarded. Families differ widely in their attitudes toward leftovers. If a family dislikes them, unusually careful planning may be needed in order to avoid waste. Extra food encourages overeating if it is placed on the table. It may be more economical to cook a little less rather than a little extra. If someone is still a little hungry at the end of a meal a slice of bread might be added or a nutritious snack might be eaten later. An alternative to skimping is to prepare an extra amount of a food which can easily be used as a snack if some is left over. Leftover cooked meat or raw celery and carrots can easily be used for the next day's lunch. Leftover cooked vegetables can be appetizing if added to soup or marinated overnight and served in a salad.

In some instances, cooking larger quantities than are needed at a given meal provides leftovers for other meals. Leftover sauce or stew may taste better the second day. Cooking a whole chicken and using the leftover meat for sandwiches or for a combination chicken dish provides variety and saves time and work.

PALATABILITY

No matter how nutritious food is, if it is not palatable to the eater it is likely to end up in the garbage. Palatable food suits the palate; it is acceptable and appealing. A few ways in which the palatability of food can be enhanced are briefly described here.

Flavor The natural flavors of many foods, when prepared in a simple manner, are delightful and enjoyable. Flavor contrasts such as fish and lemon stimulate the appetite. Spice and herbs, lightly used, enhance natural flavors in foods. Condiments and relishes used sparingly brighten bland-tasting foods such as rice or pasta. Serving only one strong-flavored food per meal avoids overwhelming the taste buds.

Texture Soft foods and crisp foods complement each other as do moist foods and dry foods. When opposite textures are included, a meal is likely to be more interesting. For example, raw vegetables contrast with a creamed entree (main dish).

Temperature Most individuals prefer hot foods hot and cold foods cold. Young children are an exception. They dislike extremes of temperature. Timing is a crucial factor in serving foods at the right temperature.

Color The color and appearance of food is quite important to the palatability of a meal. Coordination of colors increases a meal's attractiveness. A meal consisting of roasted chicken which is golden brown, snowy-white mashed potatoes, and tender crisp green broccoli provides a variety of colors and stimulates the appetite. Drab foods can be brightened up with a vegetable or fruit garnish. Many herbs and spices add color to food. Paprika, for instance, gives fish a touch of warm red-orange color, as well as adding a pleasant flavor.

Form A variety of shapes and forms can make a meal more attractive. Using different portion sizes, for example, serving some foods whole or in large pieces and other foods in small pieces, adds interest.

Serving sizes Food may be placed on individual plates in the kitchen or served at the table. It is important to consider the amount of food served. Too much of one food may dull a person's appetite for other foods. At the end of a meal a person functions best if he has a feeling of satiety but not of having overeaten.

Meals which are nutritious, appealing, and appetizing to a family are the result of appropriate food combinations. Nutrients which complement each other should be eaten together when possible. For example, iron is absorbed better in the presence of vitamin C. Serving an orange in the same meal with oatmeal increases iron absorption. Providing all the essential amino acids at each meal favors optimal protein utilization. This can be accomplished by providing even a small amount of complete protein such as milk, eggs or meat at each meal. This can also be accomplished by serving plant proteins which complement each other at the same time, for example, grain with legumes.

Food plans

Food managers can use food plans as an aid in planning meals that are nutritious and good to eat. Health care workers who are familiar with food plans can use them when counseling clients. The U.S. Department of Agriculture (USDA) publishes four food plans: the thrifty plan, the low-cost plan, the moderate plan, and the liberal plan. Each plan is designed to provide enough appropriate food to meet the Recommended Dietary Allowances for most family members within a specified income range. The plans reflect typical U.S. food consumption patterns. Presently the plans are not designed for prudent eating. The plans, however, do restrict the use of eggs to four per week. The two low-cost plans provide some control over cholesterol and fat by limiting the amount of meat used and by suggesting that low grade (low fat), inexpensive meats and low fat milk be used. A family can determine which plan to use based on its income and number of family members.

Each of the plans includes recommendations for the amounts of food to buy on a weekly basis for 15 food groups and for 14 age-sex categories. Allowances are made for food waste in preparation, loss of nutrients in cooking, and plate waste. When compared to the moderate and liberal plans, the thrifty and low-cost plans include use of (1) less expensive foods from each of the food groups; (2) smaller amounts of meat, poultry, fish, fruits, and vegetables; (3) more servings of dried beans and other legumes, bread, cereal, and peanut butter; and (4) more home-prepared food rather than ready-to-cook and ready-to-eat food. Comparing food purchases and the amount of money spent to an appropriate USDA food plan may give a family an indication of whether it is spending its food dollars sensibly and economically.

POINTS OF EMPHASIS
Meal planning

- *Plan meals in advance.*
- *Plan meals based on family's lifestyle and food preferences, nutritional needs of individual family members, and family resources.*
- *Use a skeleton menu to simplify meal planning.*
- *Plan meals which provide for a somewhat regular intake of food, distribute food intake throughout the day, and provide a variety of foods from the Basic Four food groups.*

The USDA also publishes several guides to good nutrition. "Family Food Budgeting" gives directions for using each of the four food plans. "Food for the Family—A Cost Saving Plan" includes (1) guides for planning and preparing well-balanced meals at low cost and (2) tips for economical food shopping. Families who use the thrifty food plan, particularly families receiving food stamps, might benefit from using the sample menu plans, food lists, and recipes in "Food for Thrifty Families." Information about obtaining these and other useful government publications is given in Appendix 1.

FOOD PURCHASING

Grocery shopping can be a challenging and rewarding experience. With careful planning and shopping, food managers can make wise food purchases and still provide interesting, tasty foods for the family.

Shopping lists

Individuals who write and adhere to shopping lists are more likely to make economical food purchases than those who do not. Lists can be made from weekly menu plans. Keeping an ongoing grocery list is a habit which helps eliminate the need for extra trips to the store. Staples such as flour, cereal, margarine, coffee, and spices can be added to the list as needed.

The food manager may want to modify his menu plan to take advantage of food specials advertised in the local newspaper. He may also want to read the paper for USDAs report on foods which are in plentiful supply. These foods are not necessarily the most economical sources of nutrients, but since they are in season they are more reasonably priced than at other times of the year. It is important to remember that food is a bargain only if the family will eat it. Discount coupons can save money, but only if they are used for food which is needed and liked by the family.

Before going to the store, the food manager should check the grocery list against foods on hand to avoid buying unneeded items. Shopping time can be saved by arranging the list in the order in which foods are arranged in the store.

Where and when shopping is done influences the amount of money spent and the quality of food obtained. Food managers can compare stores with regard to the types of food available, quality, and prices. A food manager's choice of where to shop may be influenced by the kind of transportation available to and from the grocery store and whether or not there is a parking lot adjacent to the store.

Shopping wisely for nutritious palatable foods

There is no magic formula for making nutritious and economical food purchases. However, food purchase decisions should be based on (1) the wholesomeness and safety of products, (2) the nutritional value of products, (3) the sensory characteristics of products, and (4) price.

CONDITION OF FOOD AT TIME OF PURCHASE

Although several government agencies provide services which regulate the wholesomeness and safety of food it is important to look closely for clues about the condition of food when it is purchased, namely, (1) check the condition of packages and containers, and avoid buying crushed or unsealed packages and dented cans; (2) look for a date on the product package to help you determine if the food is still at its peak quality and is safe; (3) evaluate quality and cleanliness of fresh fruits, vegetables, and meats; and (4) determine whether or not the store has handled foods properly (Are eggs refrigerated? Are bulk foods covered? Is meat slicer kept cold and clean? Do thermometers in refrigerators and freezers register less than 5°C. (40°F.) and −12° C. (10° F.) respectively?).

LABELS

Shoppers should read labels carefully to determine which foods best meet their needs, especially if they are inexperienced shoppers or are interested in trying a new form of food. Nutrition labeling; ingredients; net weight, measure, or count; number of servings; dating; product guarantee; and price might all enter into the decision about what foods to buy. This information should also be checked occasionally with reference to regularly purchased items since products change from time to time.

DATING

Products can be dated in five different ways, considered under Open Dating and Code Dating.

Open dating The four types listed here can be directly used by the consumer and are, therefore, called *open dating*. Some states require open dating of certain food products.

Pack date indicates the age of the product since it represents the date of processing or packing. It is helpful in selecting the most recent products on the grocer's shelves and in making sure that the older products in the cupboard are used first. Pack date gives no information regarding the length of time the product maintains its original quality if properly stored. *Pull* or *sell date* is the last date on which the product should be sold, but it allows for some storage in the home refrigerator. Dairy products, cold cuts, and refrigerated fresh dough products usually have a pull date. *Freshness date* is very similar to a pull date, but usually applies to bakery products. After the freshness date has arrived, these products may be sold for a limited time at reduced cost. *Expiration date* indicates the last date on which the product should be used. Expiration dates appear on products such as yeast and infant formula. After the expiration date the quality of the product has usually deteriorated.

Code dating Although code dating is mandatory, it is of little use to the consumer unless he knows the code. Manufacturers will send literature describing the method of interpreting the code to consumers upon request. (This code identifies exactly when and where the product was packed, information which is required by the FDA to facilitate recall, if necessary.)

FOOD GRADING

Being informed about food grading and product names may help consumers identify quality of food products. Food grading is a process used to classify a food product according to selected criteria. Many individuals erroneously think foods with higher grades are more nutritious. A higher grade does *not* mean higher nutritive value.

Presently, criteria used to grade food are based mainly on sensory characteristics such as taste, flavor, color, and external appearance. Some food grading may help a consumer determine which food he prefers. Other gradings are not particularly useful and may be a source of confusion to a consumer. Maple syrup, for example, may be graded Fancy, Grade A, and Grade B. Fancy is a pale maple syrup with a light delicate flavor; Grade A is darker in color and has more maple flavor; Grade B is even stronger in flavor. If a person wants *maple flavor*, Grade A or B would be preferable to Grade Fancy. Each specific food category poses special problems in grading. Consequently, there are several grading systems.

A consumer who is familiar with the way a few kinds of foods are graded may be better able to make selections that meet his needs. The foods most often graded include meats, poultry, eggs, and butter. Some cheese, instant nonfat dry milk, jams, jellies, and canned, frozen, and fresh fruits and vegetables are also labeled by grades. Tables 11.2 and 11.3 include detailed information on specific food grades and how to use them.

Food grading is conducted by the USDA only if the food processor or packer requests it and pays the required fee. The Food Safety and Quality Service provides grading services for food. In some instances, grading service is provided in cooperation with state departments of agriculture.

The use of food grading has declined over the years, particularly of fruits and vegetables. Many manufacturers have their own quality control programs both to comply with government regulations and to assure their customers of high quality products.

TABLE 11.2 *Comparing costs of grains, fruits and vegetables*

	SPECIAL FACTORS TO CONSIDER WHEN COMPARING COST	RELATIVE COST		
		USUALLY MORE ECONOMICAL		USUALLY MORE EXPENSIVE
Grains	Compare cost of bakery products and cereal by weight rather than by volume	day-old bread	vs	fresh bread
		bread	vs	rolls, buns
	Compare servings per pound when comparing cost of to-be-cooked and ready-to-eat cereals	white enriched products	vs	whole grain
	Whole grain and enriched products have more nutrients than unenriched products	to-be-cooked cereal	vs	ready-to-eat cereal
	Bran cereals provide extra fiber	unsweetened cereal	vs	presweetened cereal
	Wheat germ adds extra nutrients to a grain dish	plain rice and pasta	vs	seasoned rice and pasta
		regular rice	vs	parboiled and instant rice
Fruits and Vegetables (Fresh)	Consider freshness and quality; it may affect nutritive value	fresh produce in season and in abundant supply	vs	fresh produce out of season and in limited quantities
	Avoid produce with large bruises, cuts, or spots of decay			
	Buy only amount that can be used before spoiling	locally grown produce	vs	produce transported a long distance
	Consider amount of waste (i.e., inedible peel, outer leaves, core, pit, tough stalks, green areas on potatoes)			
	Oversized vegetables may be tough			
Fruits and Vegetables (Canned and Frozen)	Graded A, B, C; all grades approximately equal in wholesomeness and nutritive value	cut up or sliced	vs	whole
		diced or short cut	vs	fancy cut
	Canned produce contains some cooking fluid which accounts for a percent of weight	mixed sizes	vs	all same size
		fruits in light syrup	vs	fruits in heavy syrup
	Frozen produce has little or no waste	frozen orange juice	vs	whole oranges
		plain vegetables	vs	mixed vegetables or vegetables in sauces

TABLE 11.3 *Comparing costs of protein foods and dairy products*

	RELATIVE COST	NUTRITION INFORMATION	PALATABILITY
Meats (beef, veal, lamb, and pork)	Among the most expensive types of food Cost for edible portion (EP) rises if meat contains high percent of bone, fat, gristle Generally 450 gm (1 lb) uncooked meat yields 3–4 servings (3 oz each); if percent of inedible portion is high, yield is less; cooked meat with no waste may yield more Ground meat may be made from a variety of cuts Ground beef (hamburger) usually has most fat, costs less than ground beef with less fat	High grades—well marbled with fat Low grades—lower in fat Tough cuts equal in nutritive value to tender ones (EP) *Different* types of meats (e.g., veal, pork) are similar in nutritive value; pork is highest in thiamine Organ meats higher in vitamins and minerals; lower in fats but higher in cholesterol Some meat products (bologna, hot dogs) high in fat; low in protein and micronutrients	Graded—prime, choice, good, standard Cut affects tenderness more than grade does Meat usually most palatable when cooked in manner suggested for it Tough cuts can be more flavorful than tender cuts in dishes such as stew, pot roast Tough cuts can be cooked in several appetizing ways to make them tender
Poultry	Whole birds usually cost less than parts Well-fleshed large birds have larger EP than small birds	Less iron than meats but still a good source	May be graded—Grade A Young poultry more tender than mature poultry (fowl, hen, stewing chicken) Mature poultry suitable for stewing, soups, salads, casseroles
Fish	Cost of fish varies with season and region Fresh fish usually more expensive than frozen Fillet and steaks yield greatest EP, dressed fish yields less EP, whole fish has lowest EP Some shellfish more expensive than other fish Canned fish has high EP Canned flaked or grated less expensive than solid or chunk	Most fish is low in fat Regular canned fish usually has much higher sodium content than fresh or frozen Federal inspection of fish and fishery products is voluntary Less iron than meats but still a good source	Fresh fish usually has more desirable flavor Frozen fish may have rancid taste, texture variable Some fish bony
Eggs	Inexpensive form of protein and minerals Sizes—peewee, small, medium, large, extra large, and jumbo Difference in sizes about 10% by weight. Buy larger size eggs when their price is less than 10% higher than next smaller size (e.g., buy large eggs at 97¢ per dozen when medium eggs cost 89¢ per dozen—89¢ + 9¢ [10% of 89] = 98¢)	White and brown shelled eggs are equally nutritious Difference in color of yolk not significant in terms of nutritive value Size and grade have no relation to nutritive value An egg substitute is equivalent to an egg in some, but not all, nutrients	Graded AA, A, B Grade A eggs are firm, good for all uses, especially if appearance is important Grade B eggs have a thin white which spreads; the flavor is not as delicate as grade A; they are satisfactory for general cooking
Dairy Products	Nonfat dry milk least expensive, fortified skim milk next, whole milk most expensive Yogurt, cottage cheese, and ice cream or ice milk more expensive than milk Aged or sharp natural cheese more expensive than mild natural cheese Imported cheese more costly than domestic Pasteurized processed cheese usually costs less than natural cheese	Fortified nonfat dry milk has most of protein, vitamins, and minerals of whole milk, only water and fat have been removed Milk has approximately twice as much calcium as ice cream *Imitation* milk products are not comparable to milk in nutritive value Most processed cheeses have a higher sodium content than natural cheeses	To make instant dry milk tastier (1) mix a few hours before using, (2) serve ice cold, (3) mix equal parts of reconstituted dry milk with whole milk Canned and dry milk can be used satisfactorily in cooking and baking Cottage cheese spoils more quickly than other varieties of cheese

RELATIVE COST	NUTRITION INFORMATION	PALATABILITY
Individually wrapped sliced and grated more expensive than wedges Mild cheddar, swiss, and cottage cheese relatively inexpensive Compare cost of a pound of cheese to a pound of meat; it may serve as a meat substitute occasionally	Cheese does not provide iron which meat does	

BRAND NAMES AND PRIVATE LABELS

A *brand* is a name which differentiates the goods of one seller from those of another. The term brand name (or national brand) usually refers to a product produced by a particular food processing company and for sale in many different retail stores. Many name brand products are heavily promoted by advertising; they are usually more expensive than other labels. Many individuals think that name brands are better because they cost more.

Many large chain stores have products distributed under their own names. These are called *private or house labels* and are found only in stores belonging to the chain. Private store brands account for a sizable portion of food products sold. They are usually less expensive than name brand products of similar quality. Consumers can compare different brands and select the ones they prefer. They have some assurance that the quality of these products will remain the same.

Recently a third form of product labeling has appeared in large chain supermarkets—*generic labeling.* Generic products, also known as no-frills or no-name products, consist of every-day food products packaged in plain wrappers. These foods are less expensive than either brand name or private label foods. Some food companies state that the lower cost is due to the products' simplified labeling and packaging. They also state that generic foods may be a lower grade or lower quality product than name brand or house labeled products. This may or may not be the case; it does not mean that generic products are nutritionally inferior. In a limited study the Consumers Union found that generic products saved the consumer 30 percent over similar name-brand products and 19 percent over similar house brand products.[12]

Making economical food purchases

Knowledge of the economical range of choices within a food group helps the food buyer make wise food choices. Nutritional value and palatability should also be considered when making food choices. Tables 11.2 and 11.3 compare the costs of various foods within each food group. Comments on nutritional value and palatability are noted when appropriate.

COST OF PROTEIN

Many Americans like to include large amounts of meat in their diets. This may not be economical or necessary for meeting nutrient needs. In addition, eating large amounts of meat is incompatible with a prudent diet. Since meat and other protein-rich foods tend to be expensive, the food manager may wish to decrease the amount used and to select them carefully in order to economize.

The price per unit measure (grams, pounds) does not always reflect the true cost of protein because the amount of protein provided by meats and meat alternatives varies greatly. One way to identify good buys among various protein foods is to compare the costs of amounts of them that provide equal amounts of protein. The USDA periodically publishes a list of the cost of 20 gm. of protein* from meats and meat alternatives. This list shows, for example, that hot dogs are relatively much more expensive than hamburger. It takes 3½ hot dogs but only 115 gm. (4 oz.) of hamburger to provide 20 gm. of protein.

> **POINTS OF EMPHASIS**
> *Ways to reduce protein costs*
>
> • *Use small servings of meat, poultry, and fish.*
> • *Use lower grades and less tender cuts of meat.*
> • *Use legumes, peanut butter, and eggs for some meals.*

CONVENIENCE FOODS

Some convenience foods save time and cost no more to buy than the combined cost of their ingredients. Most baked products made from dry mixes cost about the

* 20 gm protein equals one third of the RDA for an adult male.

same as products made at home from basic ingredients. Other convenience foods are expensive. Usually, foods with added ingredients (such as seasoned rice or vegetables in sauce) are more costly than their plain counterparts. Answers to the following questions can be helpful when evaluating convenience foods: Are they liked by the family? Do they contribute to the nutritive value of the day's meals in a manner similar to a homemade product? Do they *really* save time? Is the cost reasonable when compared to other foods? Are they packaged in amounts that can be used easily?

COMPARING COST OF VARIOUS FOOD ITEMS

Unit pricing   Unit pricing makes it easier for the consumer to compare prices between packages of the same product which are of different weight. Unit pricing shows price per gram or ounce, liter or quart, or other unit of measure. This allows the consumer to determine which brand and size gives the greater weight or amount for money. Many stores display the cost per unit on the shelf near a particular food item.

POINTS OF EMPHASIS

Making wise food purchases

* *Plan menu for at least several days to a week at a time.*
* *Make shopping list and stick to it.*
* *Use a budget for food items and stay within it.*
* *Consistently check ads to find bargains.*
* *Compare labels on products to get good nutritional value.*
* *Use unit pricing to determine price comparability.*
* *Use dating to be certain fresh products are being obtained.*
* *Understand grades and cuts of meats and use them in selecting meats.*
* *Resist buying overpriced foods when you can buy them for less elsewhere.*
* *Return spoiled or damaged products and products which do not live up to their guarantee, if they have been handled properly after purchase.*

Cost per serving   For some foods the number of servings per unit measure varies depending on the form of the food. For instance, fresh peas in the pod yield 2 servings per pound, canned peas yield 3 to 4 servings per 16 oz. can, and a 9 to 10 oz. frozen package yields 3

servings. On the other hand, fresh green beans yield 5 to 6 servings per pound and 3 to 4 servings per 16 oz. can or 9 to 10 oz. frozen package. Cost comparisons should be done several times per year to determine which food is least expensive.

STUDY QUESTIONS

1. Give several suggestions for meal planning to make meal preparation easier.
2. Before a person purchases food in bulk for the family, what things should he consider?
3. What nutritional advantage may low grades of beef have over prime beef? How does grade influence nutritional value of other kinds of foods? Explain.
4. Describe how to estimate whether the amount spent for food for the family is reasonable for the family's income.
5. Plan menus for three days for a family of four (man 52-years old, woman 49-years old, boy 16-years old, girl 10-years old). Both adults work and the children are in school. Family income is limited (low to middle income).

References

1. Cromwell, C., and Kerr, R.: How food dollars were divided 1965 and 1975. *Fam. Econ. Rev.* Summer: 12, 1977.
2. Schwartz, N. E.: Nutrition knowledge attitudes and practices of high school graduates. *J. Am. Diet. Assoc.* 66:28, 1975.
3. Wang, L. V.: Food information of homemakers and 4-H youths, facts and fallacies reported in a Maryland survey. *J. Am. Diet. Assoc.* 58:215, 1971.
*4. Sims, L.: Dietary status of lactating women. II. Relation of nutritional knowledge and attitudes to nutrient intake. *J. Am. Diet. Assoc.* 73:147, 1978.
5. Crawford, P., Hamkin, J., and Huenemann, R.: Environmental factors associated with preschool obesity. *J. Am. Diet. Assoc.* 72:589, 1978.
*6. Clandy-Hepburn, K., et al.: Children's behavior responses to T.V. advertisements. *J. Nutr. Ed.* 6:93, 1974.
*7. Gussow, J.: Counternutritional messages of T.V. ads aimed at children. *J. Nutr. Ed.* 4:48, 1972.
*8. Lewis, C. E., and Lewis, M. A.: The impact of television commercials on health-related beliefs and behaviors of children. *Pediatrics* 53:431, 1974.
*9. Cross, B., et al.: Effects of family life cycle stage on concerns about food selection. *J. Am. Diet. Assoc.* 67:131, 1975.
*10. Peterkin, B.: Family food budgeting . . . for meals and good nutrition. USDA Agricultural Research Service. Home and Garden Bull. No. 94. Washington DC: U.S. Govt. Printing Office, 1976.
11. ——— Food takes more of needy budgets. *Community Nutrition Institute Week.* May 1, 1975.
12. ——— Big savings in small packages. *Consumer Reports* 43:315, 1978.

* Recommended reading

12

Food preparation and the safe handling of food

Anyone who chooses to eat a well-balanced diet wants it to taste good, provide the nutrients needed for good health, and have no undesirable consequences. No matter how carefully selected the meal, the food will satisfactorily nourish a healthy individual only if (1) it is eaten, (2) it has been handled in such a way that major losses of nutrients are avoided, and (3) it is not a source of foodborne illness. Those responsible for buying food and handling it after purchase have great impact on these three areas. For the most part practices which contribute to either nutrient retention or safety also contribute to palatability of the food.

RETAINING NUTRIENTS IN FOODS

It makes good sense to try to store and prepare foods in such a way that they retain most of their nutritive value. The methods are easy to learn and put in practice, they result in food which tastes good, and they help assure that nutrient intake is adequate for maintaining optimal health.

Loss of nutrients

Knowing how nutrients can be lost provides some clues as to what needs to be done to prevent their loss. Nutrients are lost by either being *discarded* or *chemically changed*. Nutrients differ in their susceptibility to loss, depending on their chemical characteristics and their location within a food.

DISCARDING OF NUTRIENTS

Trimming losses Nutrients are commonly lost by throwing away part of a food. This can be desirable, as in the trimming of fat from meat. Trimming is also essential for removal of decayed or otherwise inedible parts. Often parts of food are discarded for reasons of palatability, even if the part is edible.

Some types of trimming of fruits and vegetables can significantly reduce the micronutrient content of food for two reasons: (1) micronutrients tend to be more concentrated in a thin layer right under the skin than they are in the inner part of many fruits and vegetables and (2) the dark outer leaves of vegetables such as lettuce, broccoli, and celery are higher in micronutrients than are other parts of the vegetable.

Trimming cannot be considered to reduce an individual's nutrient intake if it results in greater acceptance and, therefore, greater consumption of the food by family members.

Solution losses Water-soluble nutrients (vitamin C, the B complex vitamins, and a wide range of minerals) readily diffuse out of food into cooking or soaking water. This occurs during preparation processes such as soaking, boiling, simmering, and pressure cooking. Boiled vegetables might lose nutrients in this way. Nutrients in the cooking liquid will not be lost if the liquid is incorporated into other foods, such as soup. Salting raw vegetables to draw out the water also draws out water-soluble nutrients. Water-soluble nutrients will not diffuse into oil. Therefore stir-fried vegetables (vegetables cooked in a small amount of oil in a covered pan) retain nutrients well.

Much of the water-soluble nutrient content of

canned fruits and vegetables is found in the surrounding liquid. Meat drippings and broth contain water-soluble micronutrients. In general, solution losses of protein are insignificant.

The amount of nutrient which diffuses into solution can be limited by:

1. Keeping the surface area of the food small. This is easily achieved by leaving the food whole or in large pieces.
2. Decreasing the amount of water to which the food is exposed. Steaming can greatly reduce solution losses while minimizing danger of scorching.
3. Decreasing the length of time the food is exposed to the water. Vegetables that are cooked just until tender retain more nutrients, color, and flavor than vegetables that are overcooked. Pressure cooking shortens cooking time.
4. Avoiding changing the water in which the food is cooked.
5. Avoiding soaking raw, cut-up vegetables or fruits in water for a period of time before cooking.

Loss of fat-soluble vitamins in cooking oil is not generally a problem when cooking vegetables. Either the amount of oil used is small and is consumed with the vegetable (stir frying) or the vegetable is not an important source of fat-soluble vitamins (french fried potatoes).

CHEMICAL STABILITY OF NUTRIENTS

A variety of factors affects the stability of nutrients. These include enzymes, heat, exposure to air, trace metals, light, and pH. Fortunately only a few nutrients are easily inactivated by ordinary cooking practices. Good food preparation practices can limit destruction of nutrients.

Enzymes Enzymes are protein substances which catalyze (speed up) chemical reactions. Enzymes present in uncooked foods can increase the rate at which certain vitamins are chemically changed (inactivated). This is particularly true at *warm* temperatures. Enzyme activity is likely to increase in fresh fruits and vegetables when cell walls are destroyed. Enzyme activity can be curbed and vitamin loss reduced by handling fresh produce gently and by using a sharp rather than a dull knife for cutting.

Some types of enzymes can increase the nutritive value of foods. Enzyme activity which occurs when bread dough is allowed to ferment (rise) increases the bioavailability of zinc, iron, and calcium from whole grain products.

Heat Heat accelerates chemical reactions and causes considerable vitamin destruction if other conditions are favorable. Part of the carotene in vegetables is inactivated during cooking.[1] Vitamin C, thiamine, and folacin are also easily destroyed by heat. The shorter the cooking time the less the destruction of vitamins will be.

Heat can also have positive effects with regard to nutrient retention and availability. Quick heating of raw vegetables by putting them in rapidly boiling water results in less chemical loss of vitamins than does slow heating. Cooking eggs destroys a factor called avidin which is normally present in raw egg white. Cooking prevents avidin from binding biotin (a B complex vitamin) and, thus, increases bioavailability of the vitamin. Heat destroys other antinutritional factors as well, such as certain substances present in raw soybeans.

Cooking softens cellulose. This reduces the bulk of many vegetables, makes them easier to chew, and encourages consumption of a larger portion than would be eaten raw. This is especially true of leafy vegetables such as spinach.

Mild heating of protein increases its digestibility. Overheating protein reduces its nutritive value. The effect is most marked if certain sugars are also present. Highly toasted cereals such as many ready-to-eat breakfast cereals usually have lower protein efficiency ratios than the untoasted grain prepared as a cooked cereal.

Temperature also affects vitamin retention during storage of food. The warmer the storage temperature, the greater the vitamin destruction which will occur in a given period of time. Refrigeration helps to reduce chemical destruction of nutrients.

Exposure to air A number of vitamins, upon exposure to air, are inactivated by the chemical process of oxidation. Among these are vitamins A, C, and E and folacin. Unsaturated fats gradually become rancid and lose both their food value and palatability when exposed to oxygen. Since linoleic acid (the essential fatty acid) is polyunsaturated, it is destroyed by oxidation.

Oxidation is reduced by measures limiting exposure of food to air. Grating, mashing, or whipping fruits and vegetables and storing foods in oversized containers are practices which invite oxidative destruction of vitamins.

Trace metals Trace metals such as iron and copper can catalyze the chemical oxidation of nutrients such as vitamin C and unsaturated fats. If the storage container is made of one of these metals, the nutritive value of the food will decrease more rapidly than usual. Use of glass and plastic containers avoids this problem.

Light With time, ultraviolet (UV) light catalyzes chemical changes resulting in destruction of riboflavin. Both artificial and ultraviolet light catalyze oxidative destruction of unsaturated fats.

Acidity of the food or cooking solution The amount of hydrogen ion present in a food or cooking solution affects enzyme activity and the ease with which chemical changes occur. Vitamin C and thiamine are two vitamins which are rapidly destroyed in alkaline solution (high pH). Vitamin C is quite stable in acidic orange juice. However, it is quickly destroyed in vegetables such as broccoli if they are cooked in water which is made alkaline by the addition of baking soda. Thiamine is rapidly destroyed in bakery products if an excessive amount of baking soda is used in their preparation.

Significance of measures to conserve nutrients

Using food preparation methods maximizing nutrient retention is of most importance when the diet contains few good sources of nutrients. Occasional use of methods which cause considerable nutrient loss is not a cause for alarm. However, if few nutritious foods are eaten, conserving the nutritive value of food gains importance.

Fortunately, methods which help retain the nutritive value of foods are methods which result in tasty, attractive food—food which entices the eater to enjoy a nutritious meal. The following suggested methods reduce loss of flavor and color, as well as loss of nutrients. They are also economical. Many of them save time.

POINTS OF EMPHASIS
Conserving nutritive value

- *Many foods lose vitamins during storage, especially at warm temperatures.*
- *Nutrients are lost by unnecessary trimming, dissolving in soaking or in cooking water, and overcooking.*
- *Nutrient losses caused by popular food preparation methods should be weighed against benefits of those practices.*

DURING STORAGE

The following suggestions minimize nutrient loss during storage:
1. Avoid bruising soft fresh produce such as berries and peaches.
2. Store perishable items at the recommended temperature, usually in the refrigerator or freezer (Fig. 12.1).
3. Store foods, except fresh meats, in containers which allow little room for air or wrap in moisture-vapor proof material.
4. Package green vegetables in such a way that they stay crisp. Keep them slightly moist, not wet. (Washed lettuce keeps well if wrapped loosely in a clean towel and enclosed in a plastic bag.)
5. Store less perishable items (such as canned foods, dry cereals, cooking oils) in a cool dry place.
6. If foods are not stored in opaque or colored glass containers, store away from the light.

7. Plan for fast turnover of food on the shelf or in the refrigerator to avoid long storage times. Use leftovers as soon as possible.

DURING PREPARATION

Measures to conserve the nutritive value of food during preparation include:
1. Prepare fresh produce as close to time of use as is practical.
2. Use very sharp knife for cutting fresh produce.
3. Avoid soaking cut-up fruits and vegetables, especially if they are your major source of any water-soluble nutrients.
4. When appropriate, scrub vegetables instead of paring them and leave them whole instead of cutting them up.
5. If paring is desired, pare as thinly as possible. If practical (as for beets and potatoes), peel after cooking.
6. Use clean fresh vegetable parings for making stock for soup.
7. Use the liquid from canned fruit as an ingredient in homemade fruit punch.
8. Save time, fuel, and nutrients by eating raw fruits and vegetables often.
9. Avoid reheating leftover cooked vegetables by using them in salads.

DURING COOKING

In order to maximize nutrient retention during cooking, use the following measures:
1. Cook for the shortest time possible, just until tender.
2. If cooking any type of vegetable in water, make sure it is boiling rapidly before vegetable is added.
3. Cook vegetables in the smallest amount of water practical for the type of pan, but take care not to scorch them. A small volume of water is especially helpful to reduce nutrient loss when cooking vegetables that are cut in small pieces. Cover the pan tightly to minimize the amount of water needed.
4. Steam, microwave, or pressure cook clean, whole, unpeeled vegetables.
5. Stir fry vegetables the Chinese way.
6. Plan the meal so that vegetables can be served as soon as they are cooked.
7. Heat canned vegetables in the liquid in which they are packed.
8. Use cooking liquid from vegetables and drippings from meat for gravy, sauces, soup stock, or for cooking grains such as rice. Small amounts of cooking liquid can be saved and stored in the freezer.
9. Do not add baking soda when cooking vegetables, even though it makes green vegetables stay brightly colored.

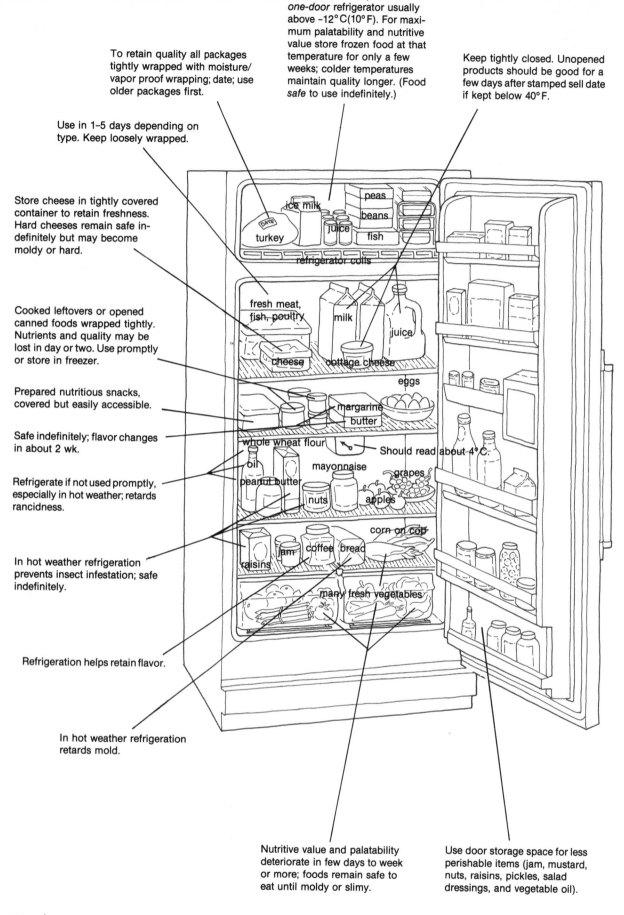

To retain quality all packages tightly wrapped with moisture/vapor proof wrapping; date; use older packages first.

Frozen food compartment of *one-door* refrigerator usually above -12°C(10°F). For maximum palatability and nutritive value store frozen food at that temperature for only a few weeks; colder temperatures maintain quality longer. (Food *safe* to use indefinitely.)

Keep tightly closed. Unopened products should be good for a few days after stamped sell date if kept below 40°F.

Use in 1–5 days depending on type. Keep loosely wrapped.

Store cheese in tightly covered container to retain freshness. Hard cheeses remain safe indefinitely but may become moldy or hard.

Cooked leftovers or opened canned foods wrapped tightly. Nutrients and quality may be lost in day or two. Use promptly or store in freezer.

Prepared nutritious snacks, covered but easily accessible.

Safe indefinitely; flavor changes in about 2 wk.

Refrigerate if not used promptly, especially in hot weather; retards rancidity.

In hot weather refrigeration prevents insect infestation; safe indefinitely.

Refrigeration helps retain flavor.

In hot weather refrigeration retards mold.

Should read about 4°C.

peas

beans

fish

ice milk

DATE

turkey

juice

refrigerator coils

fresh meat, fish, poultry

milk

juice

cheese

cottage cheese

eggs

margarine

butter

whole wheat flour

oil

peanut butter

mayonnaise

nuts

grapes

apples

corn on cob

jam

coffee

bread

raisins

many fresh vegetables

Nutritive value and palatability deteriorate in few days to week or more; foods remain safe to eat until moldy or slimy.

Use door storage space for less perishable items (jam, mustard, nuts, raisins, pickles, salad dressings, and vegetable oil).

10. Avoid browning grains (such as granola or rice) to a dark color if the food makes up a large fraction of the diet.

SAFE FOOD HANDLING

Under all circumstances, safety measures should take priority in food preparation. Occasionally safety requires that delicious food be discarded completely. Sometimes safety measures result in considerable loss of nutrients. However, the benefits of safety measures far outweigh possible losses. Nutrients are of little use if they are accompanied by substances which cause illness. Food has high potential for being a source of infection or of toxic substances.

The severity of foodborne illness varies widely, depending on the type of organism or toxin, the amount consumed, and the susceptibility of the individual who ingests a potentially dangerous food. Infants, the elderly, and sick individuals are particularly likely to be seriously affected by any form of foodborne illness.

The Center for Disease Control (CDC) publishes reports each year on foodborne and waterborne illness in the U.S.[2] These reports substantiate the need for safe food handling even though they document only a small fraction of the total number. (Many cases are not brought to a physician's attention or are passed off as "a touch of the flu.") Estimates of the incidence of foodborne illness range from 2 million to 10 million cases annually.

One study indicated that many people are in need of practical information about food safety because they commonly practice at least one high risk food handling measure.[3] Health professionals are in a good position to identify families at high risk of foodborne illness and to assist them to learn and to use safe food handling practices. The latter requires knowledge of the safety of the food supply.

Governmental efforts to promote safety

Foods can be unsafe to eat if they contain excessive levels of potentially dangerous organisms or toxins. Potentially toxic substances are present in foods inherently (as toxins in certain seafoods) or as a result of accidental contamination (e.g., mercury in fish), action by mold or bacteria, or intentional addition of pesticides, antibiotics and certain food additives by food producers and processors.

To protect the consumer from unsafe foods, laws have been written and agencies charged with their enforcement at the federal, state, and local levels. The federal agencies most directly concerned with the safety of the food supply are the Food Safety and Quality Service (FSQS) of the USDA and the Food and Drug Administration (FDA) of the Department of Health, Education, and Welfare (DHEW). The Environmental Protection Agency (EPA) has responsibilities relating to safeguarding of public drinking water.

FOOD SAFETY AND QUALITY SERVICE (FSQS)

The Meat and Poultry Inspection Staff of the FSQS enforces laws to protect consumers from unwholesome meat and poultry. The inspection staff inspects the slaughtering and processing of all livestock and poultry sold in the U.S. Inspection covers points such as the health of the animals, methods of processing, and sanitation of the processing plant. If standards are not met, animals will be condemned and disposed of or meat will be seized and destroyed; plants may be closed.

It is important to note that inspection does *not* assure freedom from microorganisms. Fresh meat and poultry always harbor some potentially dangerous bacteria and pork commonly harbors a parasite that can cause the disease trichinosis. Nevertheless, products that pass inspection are wholesome and safe if properly handled and cooked before they are eaten.

FOOD AND DRUG ADMINISTRATION (FDA)

The Federal Food, Drug, and Cosmetic Act, as amended October 1976, gives the FDA the authority to conduct a variety of activities to promote food safety. The law applies only to food in interstate commerce, that is, food prepared by companies which ship at least some of their products over state lines.

The FDA periodically inspects food establishments and examines food to determine if it is adulterated. Adulterated food has been defined by law* to protect against a wide range of unsafe and deceptive practices and products. A food is considered to be adulterated if it contains dangerous amounts of poisonous substances or filth, if it was processed or stored under unsanitary conditions, or for several other reasons. This definition of adulteration allows the FDA to monitor environmental contaminants, toxic substances produced by microorganisms, bacterial levels, and extraneous matters in foods. Since it is considered impossible for a food to be 100 percent pure, tolerances are established for different types of contaminants. Thus a certain number of bacteria or insect fragments may be allowed in specific foods. Zero tolerance can be set for very hazardous substances.

The FDA has set a low tolerance level for aflatoxin, a potent carcinogenic compound which may contaminate peanuts and peanut butter, nuts, grains, and ani-

---

* Food and Drug Law, as amended 1976.

FIGURE 12.1. Recommended storage of perishable foods. (Adapted from *Consumers All, The Yearbook of Agriculture.* Washington DC: U.S. Govt. Printing Office, 1965, p. 433.)

mal products (if the animals are fed contaminated grain). Aflatoxin is called a mycotoxin because it is formed by the action of certain types of mold. Aflatoxin may be produced while plants are growing; therefore the FDA does not feel that it can be completely eliminated from the food supply. However, the FDA does prohibit interstate distribution of any products found to contain more than 15 ppb (parts per billion) of aflatoxin. Manufacturers aim to achieve lower levels.[4]

The FDA commonly finds violations of sanitary regulations, seizes food contaminated by rat droppings or other filth, and takes appropriate action to prevent recurrence of the problem.* The FDA also checks imported foods to make sure they comply with U.S. laws.

The FDA provides a number of other services to guard the safety of the food supply:

1. Investigation of consumer complaints of contaminated products. Complaints of farmers resulted in FDA action which helped pinpoint the source of accidental contamination of feed with the hazardous chemical PBB.
2. Supervision of the recall of defective products from the market. In the case of the toxic feed mentioned above, FDA quickly recalled and prevented its further distribution.
3. Assisting (if necessary, prodding) industry to comply with the law.
4. Enforcement of safe limits on pesticide residues on food crops. FDA may prohibit use of any pesticide considered to be hazardous to the public health.
5. Regulation of veterinary drugs and medicated livestock and poultry feed. Regulation is intended to:
   a. prevent harmful residues from remaining in edible animal products
   b. prevent bacteria which can infect humans from developing resistance to antibiotics used for humans
6. Inspection of foods contaminated by fires and "disasters" and overseeing removal of unsafe products from the market.
7. Assisting states in setting safety standards for eating establishments.
8. Monitoring the safety and proper use of food additives and food colorings.

The FDA has established guidelines to determine whether a food additive is safe for its proposed use. If a food processor wants to use a new food additive, he must petition the FDA for approval, presenting information regarding (1) practical methods for detecting and measuring the additive in foods and (2) reports of controlled studies of the additive's safety, using at least two animal species.

Since no substance, not even water, is safe to use in unlimited amounts, tolerance levels must be set for food additives. The tolerance level can "not exceed the smallest amount needed, even though a higher tolerance may be safe." Controlled studies financed by industry determine the maximum amount of the food

additive that will not produce any undesirable effect on the test animals used, and normally only 1/100th of that amount may be used. The intent of the FDA is to provide a wide margin of safety. No margin of safety is allowed for potentially carcinogenic food additives; their use in foods is prohibited.

Decisions regarding the safety of food additives are not made lightly, and they may be reversed if new information shows an additive to be a significant health hazard. In fact, in 1977 the FDA initiated a comprehensive review of *all* permitted food additives, to determine if they meet up-to-date, strict guidelines for safety. Included in the reevaluation is the GRAS list of substances used in food, direct food additives (including colorings), and indirect additives. Additional funds have been allocated to the FDA by Congress to make these activities possible. Once completed, the review is to be conducted periodically. This reassessment should do much to assure the safety of processed food but, if previously approved additives are found to be carcinogenic or otherwise harmful, legal procedures will no doubt cause delays in removing them from the market. It is more difficult to remove an additive from the market than to prevent its initial introduction. Hence premarketing clearance is a dominant feature of food and drug law.[5]

ENVIRONMENTAL PROTECTION AGENCY (EPA)

The Safe Drinking Water Act was passed in 1974 to safeguard public drinking water supplies* and to protect public health. The EPA establishes minimum drinking water standards, setting maximum levels for contaminants that may adversely affect health. The states are responsible for enforcement of the regulations, but the EPA may take action if a state is negligent. The EPA has been conducting research in water safety, such as an assessment of suspected carcinogens in drinking water.[6]

STATE AND LOCAL PROTECTION

State and local health departments establish sanitation codes and other food safety regulations for food processing plants, markets, and food service establishments (e.g., restaurants). The strictness of the regulations for food processing may be more or less stringent than are FDA regulations. How strictly regulations are enforced depends on the state or local department of health or sometimes on the state attorney general.

The consumer should realize that foods produced by a small local operation may seldom be monitored for toxicants and bacteriological safety. Although they usually are safe, local products sometimes hold some risk. For example, locally made cider might be made

---

* Seizures and judgments are reported monthly in *FDA Consumer.*

* Every community water supply serving 15 or more connections or 25 or more people.

from unwashed apples, many of which might be moldy and therefore a source of a potential carcinogen called patulin. Some stores sell unpackaged food which is susceptible to contamination. Rather than avoiding locally processed foods or restaurant meals, the consumer might (1) buy from food processors or from establishments which appear to strictly enforce hygiene measures and (2) take action to promote improved sanitation and food preparation practices when they appear to be needed.

All states have strict regulations to assure the safety of dairy products. Dairy products sold in the U.S. are either pasteurized or, less commonly, certified. (Pasteurization is a heat treatment which destroys pathogenic bacteria. Certified milk is raw milk from herds which are carefully inspected to rule out the possibility of contamination by a diseased animal.) State and local health departments set standards for pasteurization, certification, and cleanliness of dairies; conduct inspections; and monitor bacterial counts in dairy products.

Pasteurization is a very important public health measure. Because of it, dairy products that formerly were potentially dangerous are now uniformly wholesome. Pasteurization does not render dairy products free of bacteria. What it does is to virtually eliminate the possibility that they will transmit tuberculosis, brucellosis, or certain other serious infectious diseases to humans.

Causative agents of foodborne illness

The consumer should not expect all food in the market place to be safe to eat "as is." It is not feasible from the standpoint of cost or of manpower to examine all food for the presence of dangerous organisms or toxins. However, foodborne illness is largely preventable if consumers take appropriate precautions.

In order to handle foods safely, it is helpful to be aware of types of pathogenic organisms or toxins that may be present in food as purchased or introduced in the home. Microorganisms that have caused many cases of foodborne illness in the U.S. are described briefly here.

BACTERIA

The most prevalent type of foodborne illness is that associated with bacteria. Some types of bacteria cause disease directly by causing infection within the digestive tract or bloodstream. Other types of bacteria cause illness by forming toxins that produce symptoms.

Bacteria are present in all unsterilized food. The presence of bacteria does not necessarily mean that food is unsafe, but does mean that food must be properly handled to remain safe. If relatively few pathogenic bacteria are present, they are likely to be harmless. Likewise, toxins made by bacteria will not be a problem if toxin-forming bacteria have not had a chance to multiply.

Salmonella has been found to be the cause of foodborne illness associated with a wide range of foods including poultry, eggs, snow cones, ham, lettuce, and candy bars. A person who is infected with salmonellae can transmit the illness to others.

Staphylococcus aureus (staph) is associated with secretions of the nose and throat and with skin infections including acne. Staph organisms are introduced into food by careless food handlers. Ham, potato and meat salads, and other foods whose preparation involves considerable handling are potential sources of the organism. Given the opportunity, these bacteria produce a tasteless, odorless, and colorless toxin that is extremely resistant to destruction by cooking, including boiling. If the toxin is present the food cannot be made safe to eat.

Clostridium perfringens is an anaerobic spore-forming bacterium most commonly associated with fresh or frozen meat such as roast beef and poultry.[7] The active bacteria are destroyed by ordinary cooking, but the spores survive and proliferate rapidly when given the opportunity.

Clostridium botulinum is another spore-forming, anaerobic bacterium. The toxin it produces may be found in any improperly processed nonacidic canned food (meat and most vegetables). Improperly handled smoked fish has also been a source of the toxin. Since commercial food canners adhere to strict regulations to destroy these bacteria, the greatest danger is associated with home-canned foods. In 1977, home-canned peppers served in a restaurant (an illegal practice) caused an outbreak of botulism which resulted in hospitalization of 44 individuals.[8]

The substance made by *C. botulinum* is a neurotoxin, which means that it affects the nervous system. The toxin is so powerful that just a taste of a food containing it may produce severe illness (botulism) or death. The toxin can be destroyed by boiling.

PARASITES

Trichinella spiralis, sometimes simply called trichina, is a tiny, unnoticeable roundworm. This organism may be present in raw pork and pork products such as sausage. Occasionally hamburger is adulterated (illegally) with pork. Grinding hamburger with a meat grinder that had previously been used for pork can have this effect. Bear and walrus meat can also be a source of trichina. *Trichinella spiralis* causes the serious, sometimes fatal, disease called trichinosis.

Toxoplasma gondii, a single-celled protozoan, may be harbored in raw red meat and may also be transmitted to food either by insects (cockroaches, flies) or by food handlers, especially if they have been in contact with cats or "kitty litter."[9] Toxoplasmosis, the disease caused by this organism, is generally mild. However, if a pregnant woman contracts the disease, it may severely damage her unborn child, possibly causing stillbirth or eye or brain damage.

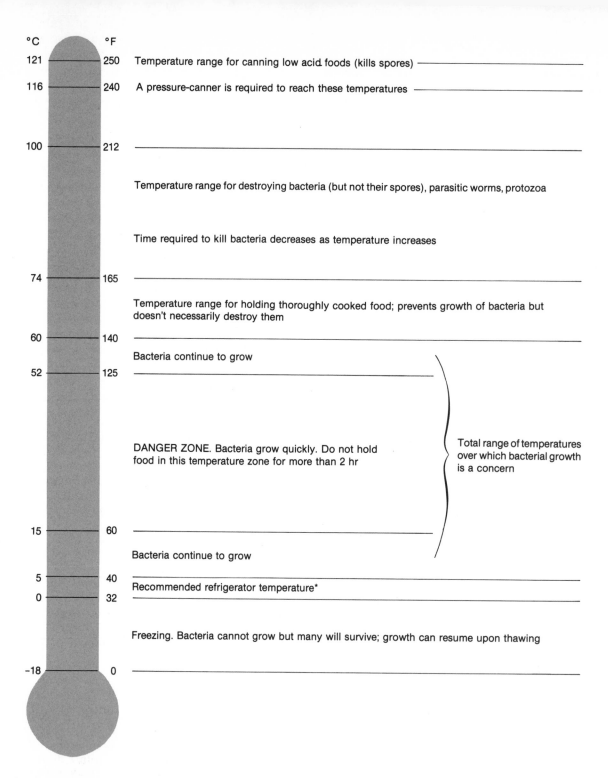

°C   °F

121 — 250   Temperature range for canning low acid foods (kills spores) ───────

116 — 240   A pressure-canner is required to reach these temperatures ──────

100 — 212   ───────────────────────────────

Temperature range for destroying bacteria (but not their spores), parasitic worms, protozoa

Time required to kill bacteria decreases as temperature increases

74 — 165   ───────────────────────────────

Temperature range for holding thoroughly cooked food; prevents growth of bacteria but doesn't necessarily destroy them

60 — 140   ───────────────────────────────

Bacteria continue to grow

52 — 125   ───────────────────────────────

DANGER ZONE. Bacteria grow quickly. Do not hold food in this temperature zone for more than 2 hr

Total range of temperatures over which bacterial growth is a concern

15 — 60   ───────────────────────────────

Bacteria continue to grow

5 — 40   Recommended refrigerator temperature*

0 — 32   ───────────────────────────────

Freezing. Bacteria cannot grow but many will survive; growth can resume upon thawing

-18 — 0   ───────────────────────────────

*Store raw meats for no more than 5 days and poultry, fish, and ground meat for no more than 2 days at refrigerator temperature

FIGURE 12.2. Effects of temperature on organisms that cause foodborne illness. (Adapted from Temperature guide to food safety. *Food and Home Notes,* USDA, No. 25. June 20, 1977)

VIRAL HEPATITIS

Food is a convenient vehicle for the transmission of type A viral hepatitis, formerly called infectious hepatitis. Since type A viral hepatitis appears to be most infectious prior to the onset of symptoms, carelessness in handwashing and food handling on the part of seemingly healthy individuals is often at fault. Children especially might spread the disease to other family members. Outbreaks of hepatitis involving many people have been traced to eating establishments where an infected individual prepared food. Hepatitis can also be transmitted by eating of shellfish obtained from polluted water.

FOOD TOXINS

Most of the toxic substances inherently present in foods pose no hazard under normal conditions of use. For example, a cyanide-containing compound that occurs naturally in lima beans grown in the U.S. does not cause illness because its concentration is so low. A varied diet helps to limit the intake of any one natural toxicant and thus decreases the chance that it will reach a hazardous level. However, an average portion of certain types of seafood occasionally contains enough of a toxin to produce symptoms of illness. For example, a number of cases of foodborne illness in Florida and Hawaii have been traced to ciguatoxin (from grouper fish) and to scrombotoxin (from mahi-mahi fish) respectively.

Ingestion of large amounts (1.5 gm. or more) of monosodium glutamate (MSG), a flavor enhancer, can cause susceptible persons to develop unpleasant symptoms including burning sensations, pressure over the face, and/or a heaviness of the chest.[12] These symptoms are often called the Chinese restaurant syndrome because they are most commonly associated with Chinese food. Some Chinese restaurants will omit MSG from food at the consumer's request.

Safeguarding food after purchase

A majority of cases of foodborne illness can be prevented by keeping food clean, preventing bacteria from multiplying, and adequately cooking fresh and frozen meat, fish, poultry, and eggs.

Since a majority of cases of foodborne illness are caused by bacteria or by bacterial toxins, it is important to know what factors influence bacterial growth. Retarding bacterial growth is an essential step in keeping food safe to eat.

Multiplication is definitely a descriptive term to use for the growth of bacteria. If conditions are favorable, the number of bacteria quickly increases by geometric progression: $1 \rightarrow 2 \rightarrow 4 \rightarrow 8 \rightarrow 16 \rightarrow 32$, etc. Thus, even a few pathogenic bacteria and favorable conditions are present, a harmless food can quickly become a source of foodborne illness.

FAVORABLE CONDITIONS FOR BACTERIAL GROWTH

Bacteria thrive in food that is moist, warm, a good source of protein, and low in acid. Fresh and cooked meats, fish and poultry, eggs, milk, puddings, and casseroles are but a few of the foods that have these char-

acteristics. Although broth is not a good source of protein for humans, bacteria find its protein content quite adequate. If given the opportunity, illness-causing bacteria reproduce rapidly in broth, meat-based soups, and gravy.

Temperature Bacteria thrive in food only if kept at a temperature that can support their growth. They are most active between 15° and 52° C. (60 and 125° F.), the "danger zone"; but temperatures all the way from 7° to 60° C. (45 to 140°F.) are considered potentially dangerous (Fig. 12.2). At proper refrigerator temperatures (preferably less than 5°C.) bacteria multiply slowly enough that short-term storage is safe. Fish needs to be stored at very low temperature, as on ice. Bacteria do not grow at all below 0° C. (32° F.), but many of them survive freezing temperatures.

Food may be safely held for a while if the temperature is above 60° C., although nutritive value and palatability are apt to suffer. Temperatures above 74° C. (165° F.) result in destruction of most bacteria. However, if the bacteria are spore formers, as is true of *C. perfringens* and *C. botulinum*, normal cooking processes *will not destroy them completely*. Even boiling food for several hours will not prevent spore-forming bacteria from multiplying once the food is returned to more favorable conditions for growth.

Moisture Bacterial growth is very slow or absent in foods with a low water content. Uncooked grains and freeze-dried main dishes are examples of foods that do not support bacterial growth. If moisture is added to dried food, bacteria can usually flourish. Cooked rice, for example, can support the growth of disease-causing bacteria.[10] Foods which are *very* high in salt or sugar, even if they appear moist, do not readily support bacterial growth. Salt and sugar draw moisture out of bacteria and, thus, have a drying effect. This is why foods such as highly salted cod and fudge do not allow proliferation of bacteria.

Acidity Acid retards growth of most pathogenic bacteria. For this reason yogurt stays bacteriologically safe for a longer time than does fresh milk. Vegetables pickled in vinegar do not support bacterial growth, whereas most nonacid cooked vegetables do. Most fruit juices and tomatoes, because of their acidity, do not allow multiplication of harmful bacteria. However, improperly handled spaghetti sauce has been linked with foodborne illness.

The lower the pH of a food, the greater the retardation of bacterial growth. Adding a small amount of acid to a food in which bacteria ordinarily thrive retards bacterial growth at least a little. Adding pickle relish to meat-based sandwich spreads has this effect.[11] Acidic ingredients should *not* be depended upon to provide complete protection.

Oxygen Some bacteria thrive only in the absence of oxygen. These bacteria, called anaerobes, multiply best in improperly canned foods and in deep containers filled with food (as at the bottom of a large pot of soup or sauce). Many kinds of bacteria grow well in environments having varying percentages of oxygen. Thus they can grow either near the surface or in interior parts of food.

POINTS OF EMPHASIS
Bacteria and foodborne illness

• *Bacteria are the major cause of foodborne illness.*

• *Bacteria thrive in warm, moist environments.*

• *Foods held at a temperature between 15° and 52°C. (60 and 125°F.) for more than 2 hours may not be safe to eat.*

• *Cooking food which has been improperly stored may not make it safe to eat.*

Common errors to avoid

All family members should be taught to handle food safely. Practices that minimize the likelihood of foodborne disease may occasionally take a few extra minutes of time, but the price of haste can be severe discomfort or perhaps even death. Making a *habit* of safe food handling is excellent preventive "medicine." The following section lists common unsafe practices and identifies practices that should greatly reduce risk of foodborne illness.

COMMON TYPES OF CONTAMINATION

A large number of careless practices cause contamination of clean food with potentially pathogenic microorganisms. The more common ones are summarized here:

1. If hands are not thoroughly cleansed following a bowel movement, harmful bacteria and viruses can easily be transmitted to food (fecal-oral route).
2. Sneezing or coughing into food, or touching food after blowing one's nose, will introduce germs into food. Open sores, boils, and some other types of skin infections can be a source of contamination.
3. Cross contamination of food can easily occur if clean food comes in contact with food which harbors bacteria. This happens inadvertently and indirectly. For example, drippings from raw poultry may contaminate another food with salmonellae by falling on the food or by being transmitted by hands or equipment.
4. Insects such as flies and cockroaches can transmit germs to food.
5. Rodents such as mice can transmit germs via their feet or contaminate food with their droppings.

CLEANLINESS AND AVOIDANCE OF CONTAMINATION

Hygiene measures can prevent many problems, especially if the temperature of food will be in the danger zone for a significant period of time before, during, or after cooking.

1. Thoroughly wash hands with hot soapy water and rinse under running water prior to handling food. Always thoroughly wash hands after handling raw meat, fish, poultry, or eggs.
2. Make sure that cleaning cloths, sponges, and dish and hand towels are clean. Bacteria can multiply rapidly in a damp sponge that contains food particles.
3. Make sure counters, boards, equipment, and dishes are thoroughly clean and rinsed before being used. (Using bleach in the rinse water helps to sanitize cutting boards.)
4. Be especially careful to use hot soapy water to wash all countertops, utensils, cutting boards, and other pieces of equipment which have come in contact with raw meat, fish, poultry, and eggs—as soon as possible after use.
5. Carefully wash fresh produce to remove residual insecticide as well as dirt. Do not use home-grown vegetables which have been treated with insecticide just before being harvested. (Check label on insecticide container to be sure.)
6. If possible, cut foods to be eaten raw (such as salad ingredients) on a clean board reserved for that purpose. If the same board must be used for both meat and other foods, save cleaning time and maximize safety by cutting vegetables and other items *before* cutting meat. Remember that washed cutting boards may have harmful bacteria lodged in the cracks and uneven surfaces.
7. Try using utensils rather than hands to pick up and mix foods.
8. Wash the tops of cans and jars before opening them.
9. When preparing foods, keep hands away from nose, mouth, and hair. Keep hair pulled back away from food. Avoid coughing or sneezing over food even when you are healthy.
10. If possible, do not allow food to be prepared by anyone (yourself included) with an infectious disease or a skin infection. If there is no alternative, use extra precautions to prevent contamination.
11. Cook stuffing separately from poultry.
12. Transfer a portion of food to a dish rather than eat out of the container in which food is to be stored.
13. Minimize pest infestation by keeping windows and doors screened, promptly cleaning up spills, disposing of garbage, and caulking cracks around sinks and pipes.
14. If insecticides must be used, exercise extreme caution in cooking and eating areas to prevent contamination of food.
15. Make sure that pottery does not contain lead if it is to be in contact with food.

PRACTICES WHICH MAY RESULT IN THE MULTIPLICATION OF BACTERIA AND THE PRODUCTION OF TOXINS

Bacteria are given more favorable opportunities to incubate than many people realize. The time-temperature relationship is critical.

Anytime bacteria are in a favorable temperature zone (the danger zone), they can multiply (see Fig. 12.2). This means bacteria can multiply when a food is warming up in an oven or on the stove. The stuffing inside a turkey is a delightful place from the bacteria's point of view, because it stays warm for a long time. Salmonellae (from the turkey itself) can multiply to a dangerously high level and will be destroyed only if the temperature of *all* parts of the stuffing exceeds 165° F. If staph were introduced when mixing the stuffing and if the stuffing were slowly cooked inside the bird, the bacteria would have ample opportunity to multiply and produce toxin. Toxin could be present in the cooked stuffing in high enough concentration to cause illness.

Bacteria can also multiply when a *cooked* food is cooling because the cooking process does not make food free of bacteria. This is particularly true of large roasts, big pots of soup or sauce, and other large volumes of food. Unless special precautions are taken, these foods will stay within the danger zone for several hours after being cooked. People have a tendency to overlook this danger, thinking that cooked food is safe.

Other common practices which may result in dangerous multiplication of bacteria are (1) allowing meat, egg, or tuna sandwiches to stand at room temperature for several hours in a "brown bag" lunch (cheese or peanut butter sandwiches would be safe under the same conditions); (2) allowing groceries to sit in a warm car while other errands are run; and (3) allowing perishable foods to stand at room temperature for a long time during meal preparation. (This can be dangerous even if foods are to be cooked.)

MINIMIZING INCUBATION TIME

A number of steps can be taken to minimize opportunities for bacteria to multiply to dangerous levels.
1. Buy perishable foods last at the supermarket. Get them home and into the refrigerator promptly.
2. Make sure your refrigerator maintains a temperature of *less than* 7° C. (45° F.). Many refrigerators checked in a recent study did not.[3]
3. Avoid allowing perishable foods to stand at room temperature (or at any temperature within the danger zone) during food preparation.
4. Do not allow food that will support growth of pathogenic bacteria to remain in the range of 15 to 60° C. (60 to 140° F.) for more than 2 hours.
5. Store fresh poultry, fish, ground meat and liver for no more than 2 days in the refrigerator. Store uncooked meat no more than 5 days in the refrigerator.

6. Quickly chill foods that require refrigeration. Refrigerate a roast or other perishable cooked food while it is still hot. Just be sure that the hot food is not in contact with a cold food in the refrigerator. If practical, spread hot food into long flat pans to hasten cooling, or place container of food into a larger container of cold water before refrigerating it. (This saves fuel.)
7. If cooked food is to be kept warm before eating, make sure the temperature is maintained above 60° C. (140° F.). Use a cover or a warmer temperature to make sure that the surfaces of the food stay above 60° C.
8. Thaw frozen meat in the refrigerator, in an insulated container, or, if essential for quicker thawing, in cold water.
9. If you insist on stuffing poultry, stuff immediately before roasting. Remove the stuffing before refrigerating leftovers.
10. When taking food on a picnic or when packing a lunch, use insulated containers to keep hot foods hot and cold foods cold. Preheat or precool them for extra safety. Use ice to be sure that meats, salads, and other highly perishable foods stay cold.

ADEQUATE COOKING

Adequate cooking of fresh and frozen meat, fish, poultry, eggs, and main dishes helps to reduce risk of a variety of types of foodborne illness, including some of the less common types. Thorough cooking can (1) temporarily reduce the number of bacteria in a food, (2) destroy parasites such as *T. spiralis*, fish tapeworms, and *Toxoplasma gondii*, and (3) destroy viruses. It should be emphasized, however, that cooking will not necessarily make a mishandled food safe to eat.
1. Cook meat to recommended safe temperature. (Check USDA guidelines or a reliable cookbook. Note that new recommendations suggest cooking beef to 63° C. (145° F.) or above.) Cook ground meat thoroughly for maximum safety. Cook pork and pork products such as uncooked ham and sausage to an internal temperature of *at least* 60° C. (140° F.) to destroy any *Trichinella spiralis* that may be present. Never taste uncooked sausage or ground beef. (Sausage accounts for nearly half of the reported cases of trichinosis.) *Never partially cook* meat one day to reduce cooking time at a later date.
2. Reheat leftover meats (if you want them hot), gravies, casseroles, and meat sauces to an internal temperature of *at least* 74° C. (165° F.) and hold at that temperature or above for several minutes.
3. Boil home-canned low acid foods before tasting them, even if there are no signs of spoilage. Corn, spinach, meats, and poultry will be safe after 20 minutes of boiling. Other vegetables require only 10 minutes of boiling.[12]
4. If home canning, carefully follow reliable instructions such as those available from the USDA. Do not

take any shortcuts. Be wary of instructions found in old cookbooks or with water-bath canners. Sometimes these are unsafe and could lead to botulism.

Deciding if a food is safe

There is no way for consumers to determine definitely if a food is safe to eat. If food is suspected of being bacteriologically unsafe for any reason, it should not be used. It is essential to remember that food will not necessarily be made safe by boiling. Helpful questions to ask in judging bacteriological safety are:
1. Can bacteria multiply easily in the particular food? (Is it moist, nonacidic, and a source of protein?)
2. What are the chances that disease-causing bacteria are in the food? (Was it handled at home or in the store? Does the food commonly contain disease-causing organisms?)
3. What is the total time that the food has been in the danger zone? (Did it sit on the table for 2 hours before and after being refrigerated?) The adage to follow is: WHEN IN DOUBT, THROW IT OUT.
   Some additional information regarding the safety of food may be helpful to consumers. Common areas of concern are briefly discussed here:
1. Defrosted food is probably safe if no part of it has had a chance to remain in the danger zone for more than 2 hours. (This includes time prior to freezing as well as during and after defrosting.)
2. Bubbly fruits and fruit juices are undergoing fermentation. They will have an off-taste, but are not usually harmful.
3. Canned food stored in the original opened can in the refrigerator is apt to undergo flavor and sometimes color changes (due to reactions with the metal) but these are not harmful.
4. The safety of moldy food is questionable. Discard moldy food to be on the safe side. To avoid aflatoxin carefully examine peanuts and other nuts; discard any that are moldy, shriveled, or damaged. (Children will need assistance with this.) If you use store-ground peanut butter, find out if the peanuts are examined and discarded when moldy; otherwise well-known commercial brands may be safer. Cheese purposely made with mold (e.g., bleu, roquefort) is safe to use. Trim the mold off hard or semihard cheeses such as parmesan and cheddar. Discard moldy cottage, cream, or other high moisture cheeses.
5. Even a small taste of a spoiled food might be harmful. *Never* taste a food that is suspected of being bad, especially from a can that is bulging, spurts upon being opened, or has split seams.
6. Eggs that were cracked at the time of purchase may harbor salmonellae. Discard them.
7. Oil that has an "off" (rancid) odor is spoiled. Discard it.
8. Some wild plants are highly poisonous. Do not eat "wild" plants such as mushrooms or miscellaneous weeds unless an expert has trained you to correctly identify edible varieties.
9. High temperature cooking (as pan broiling), smoking meat, and charcoal broiling may cause formation of potentially carcinogenic substances on outer surfaces of the food. If you want to minimize this possible problem, cook hamburgers and steak by baking them in the oven, cooking them in a microwave oven, or cooking them over low heat on top of the range, but expect the taste to be different. (The degree of risk associated with these carcinogens has not been established.)
10. Eat a wide variety of conventional foods to decrease hazards associated with natural food toxicants.[13] Avoid diets that emphasize only one or two foods.

STEPS TO TAKE IF A FOOD IS DETERMINED TO BE UNSAFE

If a food is determined to be unsafe, measures should be taken to protect others. A commercial food that appears to be spoiled (despite proper handling after purchase) may endanger other consumers who do not recognize warning signs. Prompt action might prevent widespread serious consequences. Follow these brief guidelines:
1. Dispose of unsafe home-prepared food in such a way that it will not endanger other people (such as children) or pets.
2. If *upon opening* a commercially canned food you suspect that its contents are unsafe, contact the nearest branch of the FDA or your local health department. Be prepared to relate information about the label, code marks, name and address of store where purchased, and date of purchase. Health authorities may want to examine the contents. Wrap and label the can and its contents and store in such a way that no one will use it by mistake. If meat or poultry is involved, contact USDA rather than FDA.
3. If a commercially prepared food is suspected of having caused foodborne illness, wrap and store any remaining food and the original container as above, and contact the local health department.

STUDY QUESTIONS

1. Pat likes to cook broccoli in a large amount of water because he thinks it tastes better that way. What nutrients would be most apt to be lost by this cooking method? Should he be advised to make any changes in his cooking method? Explain.
2. List two reasons why the recommendation is made to use leftover vegetables as soon as possible.
3. Part of the contents of a can of commercially-processed soup spurt out when the can is opened. What steps should be taken, if any, to assure maximum safety? Why?
4. A large rolled roast is cooked to a temperature of 60° C. (140° F.). It is allowed to stand on the table at room temperature for 2 hours and is then refrigerated. The roast is sliced the next morning for

sandwiches to be taken to school for lunch. Would there be any danger of foodborne infection from the sandwiches? If so, of what type and why? What food handling measures would be safer?

5. Thorough handwashing prior to food handling provides some protection from what types of foodborne illnesses?

References

1. Sweeney, J. P., and Marsh, A. C.: Effect of processing on provitamin A in vegetables. *J. Am. Diet. Assoc.* 59:238, 1971.

2. *Foodborne and Waterborne Disease Outbreaks, Annual Summary 1975*. DHEW. Public Health Service. Center for Disease Control. Publ. No. (CDC) 76-8185. Washington DC: U. S. Govt. Printing Office, 1976.

*3. *Food Safety: Homemakers' Attitudes and Practices*. USDA, Economic Research Service. Agricultural Economic Report No. 360. Washington DC: U. S. Govt. Printing Office, 1977.

4. Rodricks, J. V.: Hazards from nature. Aflatoxins. *FDA Consumer* 12(4):16, 1978.

5. Schmidt, A. M.: Food and drug law: A 200-year perspective. *Nutr. Today* 10(4):29, 1975.

6. *Preliminary Assessment of Suspected Carcinogens in Drinking Water. Report to Congress.* Environmental Protection Agency, Office of Toxic Substances. Washington DC, Dec. 1975.

7. Trakulchang, S. P., and Kraft, A. A.: Survival of C. perfringens in refrigerated and frozen meat and poultry items. *J. Food Sci.* 42:518, 1977.

8. Food poisoning notes. *J. Am. Diet. Assoc.* 71:64, 1977, citing Morbidity and Mortality Weekly Report, April 8 and 22, 1977.

9. Toxoplasmosis. DHEW. Public Health Service. National Institutes of Health. Publ. No. (NIH) 75-308. Washington DC: U. S. Govt. Printing Office, 1975.

10. Terranova, W., and Blake, P. A.: Bacillus cereus food poisoning. *N. Engl. J. Med.* 298:143, 1978.

11. Longree, K., White, J. C., and Lynch, C. W.: Bacterial growth in protein-base sandwich fillings. *J. Am. Diet. Assoc.* 35:131, 1959.

12. Keeping food safe to eat. USDA. Agricultural Research Service, Consumer and Food Economics Institute. Home and Garden Bulletin No. 162. Washington DC: U. S. Govt. Printing Office. Rev. 1975.

*13. Coon, J. M.: Natural food toxicants—A perspective. *Nutr. Rev.* 32:321, 1974.

* Recommended reading

Part 1

Bibliography and additional recommended readings

Assessment of Maternal Nutrition. Task Force on Nutrition, American College of Obstetricians and Gynecologists, The American Dietetic Association, Chicago, 1978.

Bass, M. A., Wakefield, L., and Kolasa, K.: *Community Nutrition and Individual Food Behavior.* Minneapolis: Burgess Publishing Co., 1979.

Bradley, H., and Sundberg, C.: *Keeping Foods Safe.* Garden City NY: Doubleday & Co., 1975.

Clydesdale, F. M.: Nutritional realities—Where does technology fit? *J. Am. Diet. Assoc.* 74:17, 1979.

Dickman, S.: Breast-feeding and infant nutrition. *Family Community Health* 1:19, 1979.

Ethnicity and Health Care. New York: National League for Nursing. Publ. No. 14-1625, 1976.

Fleishman, R.: Eating rituals and realities. *Nurs. Clin. North Am.* 8:91, 1973.

Gussow, J. D.: *The Feeding Web: Issues in Nutritional Ecology.* Palo Alto CA: Bull Publishing Co., 1978.

Katzen, M.: *Moosewood Cookbook.* Berkeley CA: Ten Speed Press, 1978.

Lowenberg, M. E., et al.: *Food and People,* ed. 3. New York: John Wiley & Sons, 1979.

Martin, J.: School nutrition programs in perspective. *J. Am. Diet. Assoc.* 73:389, 1978.

McNutt, K. W., and McNutt, D. R.: *Nutrition and Food Choices.* Chicago: Science Research Associates, 1978.

Moore, W., Silverberg, M. M., and Read, M. S. (eds.): *Nutrition, Growth and Development of North American Children.* DHEW Publ. No. (NIH) 72–26, Washington DC: U. S. Govt. Printing Office, 1972.

Nutrition Labeling: How It Can Work for You. Washington DC: The National Nutrition Consortium, 1975.

Olson, R. E.: Are professionals jumping the gun in the fight against chronic diseases? *J. Am. Diet. Assoc.* 74:543, 1979.

Pipes, P.: When should semisolid food be fed to infants? *J. Nutr. Ed.* 9:57, 1977.

Smith, G. V., Calvert, L. J., and Kanto, W. P.: Breast feeding and infant nutrition. *Am. Fam. Physician* 17:92, 1978. (Includes information about drugs and breast feeding.)

Whitney, E., and Hamilton, M.: *Understanding Nutrition.* St. Paul: West Publishing Co., 1977.

Worthington, B. (ed): Nutrition. *Nurs. Clin. North Amer.* 14(3), 1979.

Worthington, B.: Nutritional considerations during pregnancy and lactation. *Family Community Health* 1:13, 1978.

Your Moneys Worth in Foods. Agricultural Research Service, USDA. Home and Garden Bull. No. 183. Washington DC: U. S. Govt. Printing Office, 1977.

Relationship of Nutrients to Normal Body Function

13
Digestion, absorption, storage, excretion

Food has not entered the internal environment of the body when it is placed in the mouth and swallowed. Instead it has entered a long hollow tube with numerous compartments which is called the gastrointestinal tract or alimentary canal (Figs. 13.1–3). This tube places a barrier between the food and the interior parts of the body. Most ingested substances cannot actually enter the body (be absorbed) without extensive processing. Many useless or potentially dangerous substances cannot gain entrance at all. Instead they are

excreted via the feces or stool. The functioning of the gastrointestinal tract is one of the major determinants of nutritional status.

DIGESTION—THE PHYSICAL AND CHEMICAL ALTERATION OF FOOD

Food is a variable mixture of nutrients, fiber, food additives, and other extraneous materials which must undergo a variety of changes. Most naturally occurring forms of protein, fat, and carbohydrate are large molecules which cannot be absorbed through the intestinal wall. Sometimes the nutrients are trapped by other food components and are not exposed to chemical digestion unless physical processing takes place.

Physical alteration of food

The most important types of physical processing include mechanical breakdown, mixing, and emulsification.

Mechanical breakdown Mechanical breakdown occurs during the act of mastication or chewing of food. The powerful grinding forces exerted by chewing with the molars greatly multiply the surface area of the food. The rate of chemical digestion of food increases with increased surface area of the food. Mastication of fruits and vegetables breaks cell walls, releasing nutrients contained within the cells. Since the cell walls of plant foods are resistant to chemical digestion in humans, chewing increases the availability of nutrients from these foods. Unchewed or poorly chewed

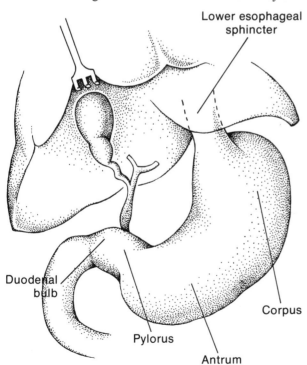

FIGURE 13.1. The alimentary tract showing the three parts of the stomach.

Lower esophageal sphincter

Duodenal bulb

Pylorus

Antrum

Corpus

TABLE 13.1 *The major digestive enzymes*

NAME OF ENZYME	SUBSTRATE	PRODUCTS OF REACTION	SOURCE OF ENZYME	SITE OF ACTION
ACTION OF ENZYMES THAT DIGEST CARBOHYDRATE				
Salivary amylase (ptyalin)	Starch (amylose) as in grains, potatoes, legumes	Dextrins, maltose, glucose	Secretions from parotid and sub-maxillary glands (saliva)	Mouth—if chewing is very thorough Some in fundus of stomach if mixing with acidic gastric juice is delayed
Pancreatic amylase	Starch	Dextrins, maltose, glucose	Secretions from pancreas	Small intestine
	Dextrins	Maltose, glucose		
Disaccharidases	Disaccharides	Monosaccharides	Mucosal cells of small intestine	Brush border of intestinal wall
Maltase	Maltose (in corn syrup, beer)	Glucose		
Sucrase	Sucrose (in table sugar, fruits)	Glucose and fructose		
Lactase	Lactose (in milk)	Glucose and galactose		
ACTION OF ENZYMES THAT DIGEST PROTEIN				
Pepsin (protease)	Protein	Large peptides	Chief cells of gastric mucosa (secreted as the inactive pro-enzyme pepsino-gen*)	Stomach
Trypsin	Protein and polypeptides (Polypeptides are primarily from the partial digestion of protein)	Polypeptides, dipeptides, amino acids	Pancreas (secreted as the inactive pro-enzymes trypsino-gen, chymotrypsin-ogen, and procar-boxypeptidase*)	Lumen of the small intestine
Chymotrypsin				
Carboxypeptidase				
Aminopeptidase	Polypeptides	Smaller peptides, amino acids	Mucosal cells of small intestine	Brush border of small intestine
Dipeptidase	Dipeptides	Amino acids		
ACTION OF ENZYMES THAT DIGEST FAT (TRIGLYCERIDE)				
Pharyngeal lipase†	Triglycerides (in foods containing fat such as meat, butter, nuts, cheese)	Fatty acids, diglycerides, monoglycerides	Mucosa of pharynx	Fundus of stomach
Gastric lipase†	Short-chain triglycerides (dairy fats)	Short-chain fatty acids, diglycerides, monoglycerides	Gastric mucosa	Stomach
Pancreatic lipase	Triglycerides, diglycerides	Diglycerides, monoglycerides, fatty acids (short, long, and medium chain)	Pancreas	Lumen of small intestine

* Activation of proenzymes takes place in the lumen of the intestinal tract
† Not essential for adequate digestion of fat.

fruits, vegetables, and seeds may pass through the entire alimentary canal and be excreted unchanged in the stool.

Mixing Mixing occurs in every part of the gastro-intestinal tract except the pharynx and esophagus. Mastication and the action of the tongue mix food with saliva. This mixing causes chemical digestion to begin (Table 13.1). More importantly, this initial mixing with secretions facilitates passage of swallowed food to the stomach. Mixing activity varies in the three parts of the stomach (see Fig. 13.1).

When a large meal is eaten, food is temporarily stored in the corpus or body of the stomach. Except for some continued digestion of starch by saliva, digestion of the "stored" food is at a temporary standstill. Farther down the stomach there is vigorous activity. Mixing waves, which usually begin at about the midpoint of the stomach, move gastric secretions and the outer layer of stored food toward the antrum (see Fig. 13.1).

In the antrum the food is vigorously churned with the gastric secretions. Chyme is the name given to the mixture of food and secretions passing out of the pylorus into the small intestine (duodenum).

In the small intestine, mixing continues as a result of both segmentation (mixing) contractions and propulsive contractions (peristalsis) which spread out the chyme. *Segmentation contractions* occur at regular intervals when the gut is distended with chyme. As one set of contractions relaxes, a new set begins at intermediate points, resulting in "chopping" and mixing of the chyme with digestive secretions. This process allows all of the chyme to come into contact with the intestinal mucosa, thus promoting maximum absorption of nutrients. The function of peristalsis is usually viewed as one of propulsion, even though it results in some mixing of the chyme.

Slow mixing occurs in the colon and results in gradual exposure of all fecal material to the surface of the large intestine, thus increasing absorption of water.

Emulsification Emulsification is the process during which lipids, including fats and other fat-soluble substances, are broken up and evenly dispersed in an aqueous medium. Emulsification occurs in the small intestine when bile salts are mixed with intestinal contents. Bile salts are emulsifying agents which are synthesized by the liver and released in the bile. They promote the breakdown of fat globules into minute particles by lowering their surface tension. This emulsifying action of bile salts is similar to the action of detergents in removing fat from greasy dishes. Emulsification greatly increases the surface area of lipids, enhancing their chemical digestion and absorption.

POINTS OF EMPHASIS
Physical alteration of food

• *Mechanical breakdown, mixing, and emulsification of food increase the contact between nutrients and digestive secretions, promoting chemical digestion.*
• *Mechanical breakdown and mixing with digestive secretions facilitate movement of food along the alimentary tract.*
• *Mixing movements are different in different parts of the tract, but serve similar purposes.*
• *Mixing movements in the intestines increase contact between nutrients and the intestinal wall, promoting absorption.*

Chemical alteration of food

Chemical digestion breaks down nutrients in food to a form which can be absorbed into the body. The energy nutrients (carbohydrate, fat, and protein) in food are chemically altered during digestion by a process called *hydrolysis*. The vitamins which occur in bound forms also undergo hydrolysis prior to absorption. Hydrolysis involves the splitting of a molecule with the addition of water. The reaction takes place at body temperature only if particular digestive substances called enzymes are present. Very large molecules are hydrolyzed (broken down) to hundreds of much smaller molecules. This dramatic change takes place by stages in the digestion of starch and protein. Some nutritive substances such as sugar and fat require that only one or two units be split off by hydrolysis in order for the end products to be of a size and form suitable for absorption. Some foods contain nutrients such as simple sugars which require no digestion whatsoever. The desired end products of the digestion of energy nutrients are *monosaccharides* (simple sugars) from carbohydrates; *amino acids* and *dipeptides* from protein; and *fatty acids, monoglycerides,* and *glycerol* from fat. These are the only forms in which significant amounts of the energy nutrients can be absorbed. Alcohol (ethanol) is absorbed without undergoing any chemical change.

As indicated in Tables 1.1 (p. 4) and 13.1, there are many different amino acids and several types of disaccharides, monosaccharides, and fatty acids. It is sometimes important to be able to distinguish the different types since they may be handled differently by the body and they may have different physiological effects.

ENZYMES

The major chemical changes involved in the digestion of food are a result of digestive enzyme activity. Enzymes are biological catalysts, that is, they speed up chemical reactions.

Some terminology has been developed to make it easier to discuss and identify enzymes. The substance upon which an enzyme acts is called its *substrate.* In the naming of enzymes, the stem of the word refers to the substrate and the ending "ase" signifies "enzyme." Thus, lactase is the enzyme that digests the sugar lactose.

All enzymes have the following characteristics in common:
• Enzymes are organic compounds, protein in nature, synthesized by cells. They control most of the chemical reactions occurring in living organisms.
• There are many types of enzymes. One kind of enzyme cannot substitute for another.
• A very small amount of enzyme can greatly speed up (catalyze) a specific chemical reaction of a large amount of substrate.
• Increases in temperature increase enzyme activity. Enzymes are relatively unstable compounds, which are destroyed by high temperatures.
• Enzymes function most efficiently within a narrow range of pH which is specific for each enzyme. They may become completely inactive outside of their optimal pH range.
• Most enzymes require one or more minerals in ionic form, such as Cl^- or Mg^{++}, in order to be active.

The digestive enzymes include all of the enzymes in the gastrointestinal tract which chemically break down nutrients into smaller compounds by the process of hydrolysis.

The digestive enzymes may be categorized according to the types of nutrients upon which they act. The names of the major digestive enzymes and pertinent information relating to their activity are summarized in Table 13.1. The food sources and products of digestion of each disaccharide are particularly important to note. Fiber is not included in Table 13.1 since humans lack enzymes capable of hydrolyzing cellulose or other fiber.

In most cases the amount of digestive enzyme secreted is adequate to meet digestive needs. However many people lack the particular enzyme called lactase, which is required for the digestion of the sugar in milk.[1]

Lactose intolerance   Nearly all human infants produce sufficient lactase to hydrolyze usual intakes of lactose to glucose and galactose. However, for a majority of the world's population it is *normal* for lactase activity to progressively decrease. After infancy, as lactase activity decreases, the ability to digest the disaccharide lactose also decreases. Loss of ability to digest lactose may become evident after about 3 to 5 years of age.[2,3] Caskey,[4] however, reports that native Americans tend to retain ability to digest lactose until adolescence.

Differences in lactase activity have been noted for different ethnic and racial groups. The population groups that are most apt to *retain* lactase activity are Caucasion Northern Europeans, their many descendants in other countries (as the U.S. and Canada), and some pastoral tribes in Africa. Most adults (85 to 95 percent) from these ethnic backgrounds retain the ability to digest milk sugar. However, 60 to nearly 100 percent of the adults from other ethnic backgrounds lose much or all of their ability to digest milk sugar.[1,5-7]

If lactose cannot be digested, it passes along the small intestine without being absorbed. This causes changes to take place within the gut which often result in cramps, flatus (gas), distention, and diarrhea. These unpleasant symptoms may occur in many normal healthy blacks, Orientals, native Americans, and other ethnic groups within half an hour to 4 hours of drinking a glass of milk.

Individuals who respond to ingestion of lactose with these symptoms are described as "lactose intolerant." (Lactose malabsorption does not necessarily cause symptoms.[5,8]) Lactose intolerant persons may experience more discomfort from drinking skim milk than whole milk.[9] Some lactose intolerant individuals apparently can tolerate sweetened milk beverages such as chocolate milk,[10] perhaps because the added sucrose causes the milk to be released from the stomach more slowly.

Many lactose intolerant individuals are not bothered by symptoms if the amount of lactose they ingest at one time is small. Some say that they drink milk because they desire its laxative quality. Lactose may be tolerated better if taken with a meal rather than in milk alone.[11] Many lactose intolerant individuals can tolerate up to 6 gm. lactose at a time, the amount of lactose in 120 ml. (½ c.) milk, or even more.[2,6]

Several kinds of milk products are reduced in lactose content. Most cheeses, for example, are very low in lactose and, therefore, do not cause discomfort in lactose intolerant individuals. When milk has been fermented (e.g., *cultured* buttermilk, yogurt, and sour cream), part of the lactose is changed to lactic acid. These cultured dairy products are usually well tolerated by individuals who have low lactase levels.[12]

POINTS OF EMPHASIS
Lactose intolerance

• *Much of the world's adult population is unable to digest lactose.*
• *Failure to digest lactose may, but does not always, result in unpleasant symptoms.*
• *Most healthy lactose intolerant individuals can comfortably use dairy products to help meet nutrient needs by limiting the amount of milk consumed at a time, taking milk with other foods, and/or using dairy products reduced in lactose content.*

ROLE OF SECRETIONS

The digestive enzymes would have little effect on food without the benefit of other components of digestive secretions. The principal nonenzymatic components of secretions aiding chemical digestion are water, electrolytes, and bile salts.

POINTS OF EMPHASIS
Chemical digestion of food

• *Digestive enzymes catalyze the hydrolysis of protein, fat, and carbohydrate to simpler forms which can be absorbed.*
• *Digestive secretions contain ions which promote the activity of digestive enzymes.*
• *The end products of chemical digestion of energy nutrients are monosaccharides, amino acids, fatty acids, and glycerides.*

Water provides a medium for diluting nutrients, thus increasing the effectiveness of enzyme action. The stomach secretes *hydrochloric acid*, which lowers the pH of gastric contents, activates the enzyme pepsin, and helps to dissolve minerals such as iron, calcium, and zinc. The *bicarbonate* ions which are secreted by the pancreas neutralize the acid in the chyme after it enters the duodenum. The resulting increase in pH stops the action of pepsin but is essential for the activity of the digestive enzymes in the small intestine. *Sodium* ions (which are also present in pancreatic secretions) appear to function primarily in absorption rather than in digestion. *Bile salts,* by their emulsifying action, allow pancreatic lipase to hydrolyze triglycerides.

PROPULSION

The rate at which food moves along the digestive tract needs to be controlled so that it is slow enough for digestion and absorption but fast enough to adequately supply the nutrients needed and to promote the individual's comfort. The nature of the intestinal contents and hormonal and nervous controls influence the rate of propulsion.

EFFECT OF OSMOLARITY

The osmolarity* of the intestinal contents affects the amount of dilution and the rate of propulsion. Osmolarity varies with the number of particles dissolved in a given amount of solution. The greater the number of particles per liter, the higher the osmolarity. If the osmolarity of the chyme is higher than that of the blood, water will be drawn from the blood into the lumen of the intestinal tract to mix with the chyme.

The osmotic effect of a given weight of a substance is related to the size of the particles produced when that substance is dissolved. For example, 10 gm. sugar dissolved in 100 ml. water has a much higher osmolarity than does 10 gm. protein. (Sugar molecules are very much smaller than are protein molecules and, therefore, many more particles are present when the sugar dissolves.) Consequently sugar and other nutrients which form small particles in solution can greatly increase the dilution of chyme by osmosis and this, in turn, can increase the rate at which the chyme is propelled through the gut.

GASTRIC EMPTYING

One of the major functions of the stomach is controlling the rate at which chyme enters the duodenum. "Gastric emptying time" refers to the amount of time required for the chyme to pass from the stomach to the duodenum. If gastric emptying *time* is increased the chyme leaves slowly. If the *rate* of gastric emptying is increased the chyme leaves more quickly.

The type and amount of food eaten influences the rate of gastric emptying as follows:
- Excessive stretch, as when the volume of the stomach contents exceeds 1 L., slows gastric emptying.

* Specifically, osmolarity refers to the number of milliosmoles per liter of solution. Osmolality refers to the number of milliosmoles per kilogram of water. Both are measures of the osmotic pressure exerted by the solution. For clinical application the two terms can be considered to be essentially the same.

- Liquids leave the stomach faster than do solid foods.
- Foods with high osmolarity tend to remain in the stomach until diluted by gastric secretions to make a nearly iso-osmolar solution.
- Carbohydrate leaves the stomach more quickly than do other energy nutrients.
- Protein slows gastric emptying rate.
- Fat markedly decreases the rate of gastric emptying, causing a fatty meal to remain in the stomach for a long time.

Because fat slows gastric emptying, a high fat meal may make a person feel uncomfortably full for a long time. This is probably the basis for the commonly heard statement, "Fats are hard to digest." Healthy individuals digest and absorb all but a tiny fraction of the fat they eat, but it does take a while.

PROPULSION IN THE SMALL INTESTINE

Chyme normally moves analward (toward the anus) through the small intestine at a variable rate, usually requiring 3 to 10 hours to pass from the pylorus to the ileocecal valve (Fig. 13.3). Along the way the composition changes greatly as a result of the absorption of nutrients. If for some reason the osmolarity of the chyme is high or an irritating substance is present, the chyme passes more quickly. Either situation causes water to be drawn into the lumen of the intestine. The resulting distention stimulates a *peristaltic rush* which sweeps the chyme into the large bowel.

PROPULSION IN THE COLON

Mass movements, rather than the usual peristaltic movements, propel the feces through the colon. These movements occur only a few times daily. They are most likely to occur in the morning following breakfast, or even after just a glass of a liquid such as juice. Distention in the colon and rectum may stimulate *defecation* (a bowel movement).

Mechanisms for stimulating gastrointestinal activity

The activity of the gastrointestinal tract and its accessory organs is under both hormonal and nervous control. The mechanisms are complex; they can result in either stimulation or inhibition of activity.

HORMONAL REGULATION

Hormonal regulation occurs in response to local stimuli within the gut, such as the presence of fat in the duodenum. Hormones are chemical substances which travel through the bloodstream and stimulate their target glands or organs. A variety of gastrointestinal

TABLE 13.2 *Hormones that influence the functioning of the gastrointestinal tract*

HORMONE	STIMULUS FOR ITS PRODUCTION	TARGET GLANDS OR TISSUES OR ORGANS	EFFECT ON SECRETIONS	EFFECT ON MOTILITY
Gastrin	Myenteric reflexes caused by: Distention of stomach with food	Gastric glands	Increased secretion of gastric juice which is rich in HCl	Increased motility of stomach, decreases time required for gastric emptying
	Secretagogues: Partially digested protein; caffeine; other substance(s) present in regular and decaffeinated coffee; alcohol; extractives			Relaxation of ileocecal sphincter Excitation of colon Constriction of gastroesophageal sphincter
Enterogastrone (?) (has not been isolated and identified)	Fat in duodenum (?)		Decreased secretion of gastric juice	Decreased gastric motility Relaxation of sphincter of Oddi, increased contraction of gallbladder
Cholecystokinin	Fat in duodenum	Gallbladder	Release of bile into duodenum	
		Pancreas	Increased production of enzyme rich pancreatic secretions	
		Stomach	May inhibit gastric secretion somewhat	
Secretin	pH of chyme in duodenum below 4.0–5.0	Stomach	May inhibit gastric secretion somewhat	Inhibits stomach contractions
		Pancreas	Increased production of bicarbonate-rich pancreatic juice	

hormones are produced by the gastrointestinal mucosa as indicated in Table 13.2. Hormonal control serves to regulate secretions as they are needed for digestive or protective functions.

NERVOUS REGULATION

The activity of the alimentary tract can be altered just by the thought of food. If the thoughts are pleasant and an individual is hungry, impulses transmitted via the vagus nerve stimulate gastric secretions. The same effect can result from smelling or tasting a well-liked food. Conversely, secretions and motility are inhibited by unpleasant odors, tastes, textures, or thoughts of food. These reactions to thought, smell, taste, and feel of food are referred to as the "cephalic stage of digestion." The important influence of the cephalic stage of digestion should be considered when trying to promote a good appetite.

Local stimulation of the gastrointestinal mucosa can result in marked increase in secretions via nervous reflexes. Chemically irritating substances can cause copious secretion, such as the increase in salivation caused by sucking a lemon. Tactile stimulation alone may produce increase in secretion and motility. Thus the entrance of food into the stomach or into the small intestine stimulates the activity of that part of the gastrointestinal tract. Increasing the intensity of the

tactile stimulation, as occurs in overdistention of the small intestine, markedly increases propulsion of chyme via activation of the myenteric reflex.

Parasympathetic or sympathetic stimulation can affect the activity of the entire alimentary tract or of more limited parts of it. Parasympathetic innervation is provided mainly to the esophagus and stomach (via the vagus nerves) and to the distal portion of the large intestine. Parasympathetic stimulation causes general increase in motility and secretions in these areas and inhibits sphincter tone. Stimulation of the sympathetic nerves inhibits activity of the gastrointestinal tract and increases sphincter tone, sometimes leading to constipation.

POINTS OF EMPHASIS
Propulsion in the gastrointestinal tract

• *Nervous and hormonal regulations promote propulsion of food at a rate which favors its digestion and absorption.*

• *Changes in rate of propulsion can serve to protect the integrity of the intestinal tract.*

• *Strong emotions and other factors which influence the autonomic nervous system readily change the rate of propulsion.*

ABSORPTION AND TRANSPORT

The design of the small intestine provides an enormous mucosal surface area. This makes possible the absorption of large amounts of nutrients. The capacity for absorption greatly exceeds the usual demand. Not only is the small intestine long (nearly 7 meters) but also its surface is covered with tiny projections called villi which, in turn, have minute projections called microvilli (Fig. 13.2). The microvilli make up the "brush border" mentioned in Table 13.1. The projections increase the surface area of the mucosa hundreds of times.

MECHANISMS

Absorption of most water-soluble nutrients is by active transport through the brush border and, therefore, requires energy. Carriers are apparently essential for the active absorption of amino acids, monosaccharides, calcium, iron, and probably for some of the other minerals. Carriers are substances enabling these nutrients to penetrate the mucosal cell wall. Normal functioning of at least some of the transporting mechanisms requires stimulation by nutrients in the digestive tract.

Some large molecules may gain entrance into the mucosa by being engulfed by cells of the brush border following prolonged contact between nutrient and cell. This means of entering cells is called *pinocytosis.* A few small ions, notably chloride, can freely diffuse out of or into the lumen of the gut. Water passes in and out by the process of osmosis.

Fat-soluble substances, such as fatty acids, monoglycerides, and fat-soluble vitamins, can pass readily

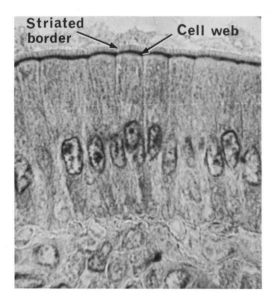

Striated border
Cell web

FIGURE 13.2. Brush border composed of microvilli. (Reprinted from Ham, A. W.: *Histology,* ed. 7. Philadelphia: J. B. Lippincott Co., 1974)

into the intestinal epithelium. Bile salts facilitate this contact by "ferrying" these lipids from the lumen of the gut to the mucosa. The bile salts themselves remain in the lumen and, thus, are able to continue the ferrying action along the length of the duodenum and jejunum.

Alcohol passes so readily through the musoca that some is even absorbed from the stomach.

Extent of absorption of nutrients

Essentially all of the carbohydrate, fat, and protein which has been digested is normally absorbed in healthy individuals. The energy nutrients are, thus, described as having high *bioavailability.* The percent absorption of a few minerals (the monovalent ions: sodium, potassium, chloride, fluoride, and iodide) is likewise high.

Other minerals (divalent and trivalent ions) are less well absorbed. This is especially true for iron. A well-nourished adult absorbs, on the average, only about 10 percent of ingested iron. Less is known about absorption of some of the other trace minerals, but zinc absorption is estimated to be about 20 to 30 percent.[12] Calcium absorption varies, but may be about 40 percent of the amount ingested.

Mechanisms in the small intestine regulate the absorption of divalent mineral ions (Fe^{++}, Ca^{++}, Zn^{++}, and others). This helps protect the body since excessive absorption can result in toxicity, even death.

The percent of iron and calcium absorbed is correlated with need for the particular mineral. Some examples follow:

- When the diet is low in calcium or iron over a period of time, the percent absorption of the mineral tends to increase, helping to safeguard against deficiency.
- Growth periods, including pregnancy, increase the metabolic demand for these minerals and percent absorption tends to increase.
- Blood loss results in improved iron absorption and accounts for higher percent absorption by women than by men.
- When body stores of calcium or iron are large, percent absorption decreases.

However, even in individuals whose need for iron appears to be similar, there is considerable variation in percent iron absorption.[14]

The most significant factor influencing calcium absorption is an adequate supply of active vitamin D.

A number of other factors can influence the absorption of iron, calcium, zinc, and other divalent minerals. Bioavailability depends in part on the chemical form of the minerals in foods or supplements and partly on the presence of other substances.

Heme iron, the form of iron found in flesh foods, is absorbed much more readily than is iron from plant foods. If meat or fish is included in a meal, not only is the heme iron well absorbed, but the heme iron improves the absorption of iron from plant foods. The iron in egg yolk is poorly absorbed.

Although ferric iron (Fe^{+++}) is poorly absorbed, much of the iron in food is in the ferric form. Iron absorption will be improved if Fe^{+++} is reduced to Fe^{++} within the intestinal tract. This reaction is favored by an acidic medium such as that found in the stomach and proximal duodenum. Vitamin C is particularly effective in reducing ferric to ferrous iron, greatly improving the absorption of supplemental inorganic iron and iron from plant foods. Vitamin C also reduces the chance that ferrous iron will be oxidized back to the ferric form within the intestinal tract. Including a good to excellent source of vitamin C with an iron-containing meal or with an iron supplement is an effective means of promoting iron absorption.

Minerals that have formed insoluble compounds with food components are poorly absorbed even if the need for those minerals is great. Table 13.3 identifies examples which are most apt to be of nutritional significance.

Most of the water-soluble vitamins are readily absorbed, but the absorption of two of them—vitamin B_{12} and folic acid—should receive special note. Many forms of folic acid (folates) occur in food, some of which are exceptionally large molecules that require digestion before they can be absorbed. Folates vary in their bioavailability.

Vitamin B_{12} (cyanocabalamin) requires *intrinsic factor* for its absorption. Intrinsic factor, which is normally secreted by the *gastric* mucosa, binds vitamin B_{12} and protects it from being destroyed by digestive enzymes. The bound vitamin B_{12} travels to the ileum where it is *ad*sorbed onto the musoca, and transported into the cells (by pinocytosis). Eventually, free vitamin B_{12} is released into the blood.

The fat-soluble vitamins A, D, and E all require bile salts for effective absorption. The form of vitamin K found in foods (K_1) also requires bile for its absorption. Vitamin K_2, which is formed by bacteria in the intestinal tract, apparently can be absorbed by passive diffusion.[17]

ABSORPTION SITES

The duodenum, jejunum, and ileum differ in their ability to absorb specific nutrients. Figure 13.3 indicates where maximal absorption of nutrients occurs.

Normally, when chyme moves from the small intestine to the colon, it is practically devoid of nutrients with the exception of water and some electrolytes. Active absorption of sodium occurs in the proximal half of the colon, with absorption of water following. Chloride diffuses out of the mucosa but is also actively absorbed in exchange for bicarbonate. Some vitamins, notably vitamin K and biotin, are synthesized by bacteria in the colon, and perhaps in the ileum, and absorbed. Bacterial synthesis in the gut is one of the most important sources of vitamin K for humans.

TABLE 13.3 *Influences of food components on the bioavailability of minerals*

MINERAL	FOOD COMPONENT THAT CAN BIND THE MINERAL	SOURCES OF FOOD COMPONENT	BIOAVAILABILITY
Calcium	Oxalate	Rhubarb, spinach, dandelion greens, swiss chard, beet greens, tea	Calcium naturally present in these foods is bound and cannot be absorbed. The absorption of calcium from other foods is not significantly reduced except perhaps by rhubarb.
Zinc, calcium, iron, other divalent ions	Phytate (a phosporus-containing compound)	Bran, whole grains (whole grain yeast-leavened bread is lower in phytate than the grain from which it is made)	Absorption of zinc, calcium, and iron present in these foods is reduced. This is especially significant when unleavened whole grain bread such as chapati makes up the bulk of the diet, as in certain parts of India and the Middle East.
Calcium, iron, zinc, magnesium, other divalent ions	Fiber	Bran, refined cellulose, and wood fiber added to processed foods	Under investigation. Concern is voiced regarding decreased absorption resulting from *excessive* fiber intake. (Use of fruits, vegetables, and whole grain breads and cereals is not considered to result in excessive fiber intake)
Iron	EDTA*	Food additive in beer, carbonated beverages, salad dressing, mayonnaise, sauces and sandwich spreads	Absorption of iron is significantly reduced[15,16]

* Ethylenediamine tetraacetic acid, an antioxidant

Transport of nutrients to the general circulation

After being absorbed, nutrients follow one of two possible routes for entering the general circulation. Water-soluble nutrients and most short- and medium-chain fatty acids (fatty acids having 12 or fewer carbon atoms) enter the capillary blood of the villi and are carried via the portal vein to the liver (see Fig. 13.2).

The other route of entry into the bloodstream is via the lymphatic system. Long-chain fatty acids (14 or more carbon atoms) and monoglycerides, after being absorbed into the epithelial cells of the brush border, are resynthesized into triglycerides by enzyme action. These triglycerides are coated with a small amount of protein, making water-soluble particles called *chylomicrons*. Chylomicrons pass from the epithelial cell into the lacteal in the center of the villus (see Fig. 13.2). From there chylomicrons are transported into the thoracic duct of the lymphatic system. They enter the general circulation via the great veins of the neck, without having been processed by the liver. Choles-

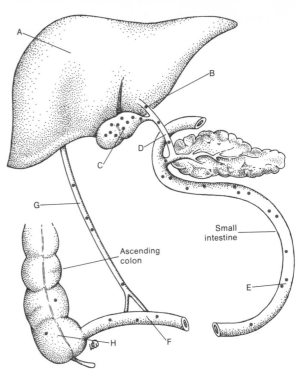

FIGURE 13.4. Enterohepatic circulation of bile salts (size of salts exaggerated). (A) Bile salts synthesized from cholesterol in liver and, (B) secreted by liver into hepatic duct. (C) Bile concentrated in gallbladder. (D) Contraction of gallbladder forces passage of bile into common duct and duodenum. (E) Bile salts emulsify fatty substances and ferry them to intestinal mucosa for absorption; bile salts refused by small intestine. (F) About 95% of bile salts are reabsorbed into portal blood in distal portion of ileum; (G) they enter liver and are recirculated. (H) About 5% are lost in feces.

terol (both from the diet and from the bile) and phospholipids, being fat soluble, are absorbed and transported in the same manner.

RECIRCULATION OF BILE SALTS

Although bile salts* are not nutrients, their absorption from the ileum is essential to the maintenance of an adequate supply of these salts for digestive purposes. Absorption of bile salts is one of the steps in the *enterohepatic circulation.* The enterohepatic circulation (recirculation of bile salts) minimizes the need to synthesize bile salts, maintains a pool of these salts, and prevents most of them from entering the general circulation. The entire process is described in Figure 13.4.

If for some reason the absorption of bile salts is greatly decreased, synthesis of bile salts can increase approximately six- to eightfold.[18] Normally, however, bile salts are recirculated and reused many times a day. Diets high in certain types of fiber, such as pectin, appear to reduce the absorption of bile salts, thereby increasing the rate at which bile salts are synthesized.[19]

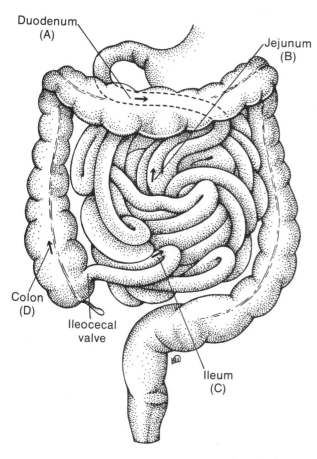

FIGURE 13.3. Absorption sites along the intestinal tract. (A) Minerals (especially divalent cations, e.g., Fe, Ca, Zn, Mg); some digested energy nutrients and vitamins; (B) Major portion of energy nutrients and vitamins; Na, K, chloride; some H_2O. (C) Vitamins B_{12} and K; Na, K, chloride; H_2O; some energy nutrients and vitamins that escaped prior absorption; bile salts. (D) H_2O; Na, K, chloride; vitamin K; biotin(?).

* Sometimes the term bile acid is used instead of bile salt.

EXCRETION

The material remaining in the colon provides little additional nourishment to the body—only water and a few micronutrients. Wastes simply await the act of defecation. However, there is growing evidence that certain characteristics of the feces may influence the health of individuals.

The composition, pH, and amount of feces varies with diet, bacterial action, and state of health. The following types of substances are normally present in stool. All except water are waste products.

POINTS OF EMPHASIS
Excretion

- *The stool contains a variety of unabsorbed substances originating both from without and within the body.*
- *Unabsorbed substances are held in the colon awaiting their elimination during a bowel movement.*
- *In health, the composition, pH, and amount of feces depend on diet and emotional status.*

- *Water.* The amount varies with the type of fiber present and inversely with the length of time the feces has remained in the colon. The amount of water in stool does *not* increase as a result of excessive fluid intake.
- *Microorganisms.* The population of microorganisms, especially bacteria, is large. Nonpathogenic bacteria help to retard the multiplication of pathogens and thus help to maintain health. The food eaten affects the composition of the flora to some extent, but the results are not usually predictable for adults. In infants there is a difference in the proportions of various types of bacteria in the colon depending on whether the baby is fed breast milk or a cow's milk formula. Pathogenic organisms (such as Pseudomonas, Proteus, and various species of Clostridia) are more prevalent in the stools of formula-fed babies.[20]
- *Fiber.* Cellulose, hemicellulose, lignin, pectin, gums, and certain other substances from plants resist the action of digestive juices and, therefore, need to be excreted. Some types of fiber may be partially digested by the colonic bacteria. Fiber holds water and small amounts of some other nutrients and increases the bulk of the stool.
- *Constituents of digestive juices.* Some enzymes (mainly inactive), bile salts and their metabolites, brown-colored derivatives of bilirubin (from bile), cholesterol metabolites, and some ions appear in the feces. Little bicarbonate remains. Some is used to neutralize acids produced by bacteria.
- *Undigested or unabsorbed nutrients*
- *Sloughed-off cells from the mucosa*
- *Products of bacterial action.* Acids and gases are produced when bacteria act on undigested nutrients. Part of the gas produced is absorbed into the portal circulation.
- *Nonfood items.* These may have been ingested inadvertently; chewing gum, fruit pits, hair, and paper are common examples.

When these waste products are excreted during a bowel movement, the gastrointestinal tract has completed an amazingly complex processing of food in a period of about 24 to 36 hours.

SELF-PROTECTION AND RENEWAL

The gastrointestinal tract has a remarkable ability to maintain its integrity in the face of continuing threats. The alimentary canal must be able to withstand potential injury from ingested substances and its own digestive secretions. The gut is regularly exposed to digestive enzymes, microorganisms, and other potentially irritating, abrasive, or toxic materials, such as hydrochloric acid in gastric juice. Protective mechanisms are described briefly here.

Dilution Saliva helps to wash pathogenic bacteria out of the mouth, reducing the chance of tissue destruction and dental caries. The moistening of food greatly reduces the concentration of chemical irritants which may be present and, along with mastication, softens some otherwise abrasive foodstuffs (such as crackers). Extensive dilution occurs in the stomach and small intestine when necessary.

Lubrication Mucus is secreted by cells along the entire length of the alimentary canal. It allows food to slip easily along the gastrointestinal tract because it coats the wall of the gut and can also coat ingested foods. It prevents damage to the epithelium by preventing actual physical contact with food and other particles. The mucus-secreting Brunner's glands in the duodenal bulb (see Fig. 13.1) provide protection against digestion by gastric juice before the acid is neutralized by pancreatic secretions.

Valves and Sphincters Valves and sphincters provide protection by limiting the exposure of sensitive parts of the gastrointestinal tract to irritants. The stomach is the only part of the body which can withstand prolonged contact with hydrochloric acid. The lower esophageal sphincter (LES) and flutter valve closure at the distal end of the esophagus serve to prevent backflow of acidic gastric contents into the esophagus, even when a person is in a recumbent position. The pyloric valve prevents excessive loads of acidic or otherwise irritating chyme from entering the duodenum. It also helps prevent backflow of bile into the stomach. (The stomach is poorly resistant to the detergent-like action of bile.) The pyloric valve may also stay closed in response to toxic substances of external origin, preventing them from damaging the small intestine.

Renewal of the mucosa The integrity of the gastrointestinal tract is maintained by rapid turnover of cells. Mature cells lining the gut continually desquamate (flake off) and are replaced by new cells. Complete renewal of the surface lining of the stomach and intestine requires approximately 3 to 5 days. Small injuries to the gut, therefore, may be repaired very quickly.

Bactericidal and bacteriostatic substances in secretions Bactericidal substances destroy bacteria. Bacteriostatic substances prevent bacteria from multiplying. Saliva contains at least two bactericidal substances (an enzyme and the thiocyanate ion) which help to reduce the bacterial population of the mouth. The hydrochloric acid secreted by the stomach destroys some bacteria and prevents the proliferation of most of those which survive.

Neutralization and buffering Mucopolysaccharides (a special type of protein) in the mucus can neutralize small amounts of either acid or base. Bicarbonate ions, present in greatest amount in pancreatic secretions, neutralize acid, protecting the walls of the small intestine from the action of acid.

Normal bacterial flora The bacteria normally present in the colon help to prevent infection by yeast, fungi, and some potentially pathogenic bacteria.

Anorexia, nausea, and vomiting Anorexia (lack of appetite) and nausea are sometimes evoked by the odor, sight, or taste of spoiled food. These reactions reduce the chance of exposure to certain foodborne diseases. Vomiting and diarrhea may eliminate some toxic substances from the gastrointestinal tract.

Discomfort Discomfort felt as a result of overeating, overdrinking (as of alcoholic beverages or coffee), consuming too little fiber, or otherwise stressing the intestinal tract is usually a result of the gut's attempts to protect its integrity. Although the alimentary canal has a remarkable ability to protect itself, it can do so most efficiently if symptoms of discomfort are heeded and the behavior causing the discomfort is changed.

Adequate nutrition is essential to provide the materials and energy needed for maintaining the integrity of the gastrointestinal tract.

STUDY QUESTIONS

1. List several factors which prolong gastric emptying time. How does a prolonged gastric emptying time help avoid intestinal problems?
2. Taking enzyme tablets does not promote digestion as well as digestive secretions do. After considering the way digestive enzymes function, list several possible reasons why.
3. Explain why inability to digest lactose may result in flatus (gas) and diarrhea.
4. Name two substances which improve the absorption of iron from plant foods.
5. How does the absorption of most types of fat differ from the absorption of amino acids and sugars?
6. Where are bile salts and vitamin B_{12} absorbed?
7. Identify several ways in which gastrointestinal secretions help to protect the integrity of the intestinal tract.

References

1. Kretchmer, N.: Lactose and lactase. *Sci Am.* 227(4):70, 1972.
2. Review. The lactose intolerance test and milk consumption. *Nutr. Rev.* 34:302, 1976.
3. Johnson, J. D., Kretchmer, N., and Simoons, F. J.: Lactose malabsorption: Its biology and history. *Adv. Pediatr.* 21:197, 1974.
4. Caskey, D. A., et al.: Effect of age on lactose malabsorption in Oklahoma Native Americans as determined by breath H_2 analysis. *Am. J. Dig Dis.* 22:113, 1977.
*5. Bayless, T. M., et al.: Lactose and milk intolerance: clinical implications. *N. Engl. J. Med.* 292:1156, 1975.
6. Newcomer, A. D., et al.: Tolerance to lactose among lactase-deficient American Indians. *Gastroenterology* 74:44, 1978.
7. Simoons, F. J.: New light on ethnic differences in adult lactose intolerance. *Am. J. Dig. Dis.* 18:595, 1973.
8. Fernandes, J., et al.: Respiratory excretion as a parameter for lactose malabsorption in children. *Am. J. Clin. Nutr.* 31:597, 1978.
9. Gudmand-Høyer, E., and Simony, K.: Individual sensitivity to lactose in lactose malabsorption. *Am. J. Dig. Dis.* 22:177, 1977.
*10. Welsh, J. D.: Diet therapy in adult lactose malabsorption: present practices. *Am. J. Clin. Nutr.* 31:592, 1978.
11. Bayless, T. M., and Paige, D. M.: Lactose tolerance by lactose-malabsorbing Indians. (Editorial) *Gastroenterology* 74:153, 1978.
12. Gallagher, C. R., Molleson, A. L., and Caldwell, J. H.: Lactose intolerance and fermented dairy products. *J. Am. Diet. Assoc.* 65:418, 1974.
13. Prasad, A. S.: Nutritional aspects of zinc. *Dietetic Currents* 4(5) September/October 1977.
14. Olszon, E., et al.: Food iron absorption in iron deficiency. *Am. J. Clin. Nutr.* 31:106, 1978.
*15. Underwood, E. J.: Trace element imbalances of interest to the dietitian. *J. Am. Diet. Assoc.* 72:177, 1978.
16. Cook, J. D., and Monsen, E. R.: Food iron absorption in man. II. The effect of EDTA on absorption of dietary non-heme iron. *Am. J. Clin. Nutr.* 29:614, 1976.
17. Review. Interaction between Vitamin K-1 and fat absorption. *Nutr. Rev.* 34:314, 1976.
18. Deckelbaum, R. J., et al.: Failure of complete bile diversion and oral bile acid therapy in the treatment of homozygous familial hypercholesterolemia. *N. Engl. J. Med.* 296:465, 1977.
19. Kay, R. M., and Truswell, A. S.: Effect of citrus pectin on blood lipids and fecal steroid excretion in man. *Am. J. Clin. Nutr.* 30:171, 1977.
20. Review. The effect of a breast milk substitute on stool flora. *Nutr. Rev.* 32:136, 1974.

* Recommended reading

14

Nutrients as a source of fuel

Nothing is more important to the body than having a supply of energy. Death would rapidly ensue if either fuel or the oxygen required to burn it became unavailable. Fortunately the body is intricately designed to regulate the fuel supply to the cells even in the face of extremes such as starvation or gluttony. This ability to regulate the internal fuel supply increases freedom of activity. Imagine how different life would be if one had to continually take in very small amounts of fuel just as one must breathe oxygen around the clock! Knowl-

edge of how the body uses fuel is a valuable asset to the health professional when assisting clients with eating problems or metabolic disorders.

BODY COMPOSITION IN TERMS OF FUEL VALUE

It is not necessary to eat continuously because a large fraction of the energy nutrients absorbed following a meal are deposited in body tissue as usable forms of

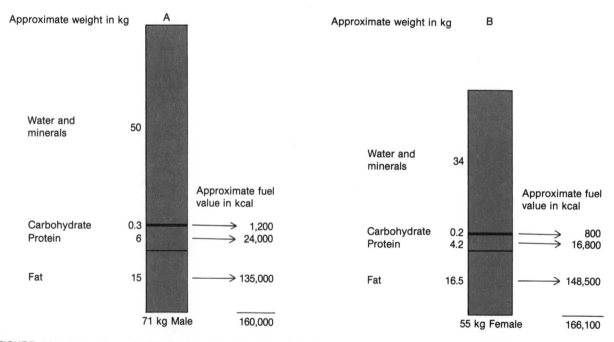

FIGURE 14.1. Approximate fuel value of A, man of normal weight; B, woman of normal weight. Marked variations in fuel value occur among individuals of the same weight because of differences in the proportion of lean body mass and adipose tissue.

fuel. These energy reserves can be mobilized whenever fuel is needed. A look at the composition of the body in terms of its fuel value gives an indication of the extent and relative importance of the energy reserves (Fig. 14.1). Figure 14.1 clearly indicates that carbohydrate reserves are very small. A normal active adult would not be able to meet his energy needs for a day from internal sources of carbohydrate alone. On the other hand, fat stores in an adult of desirable body weight contain enough potential energy to meet fuel needs for weeks or months.

Body protein is also a potential source of energy and is often used as such. However, because of the need for protein to serve other functions, survival depends on limiting the amount of protein used for energy. Body protein used for fuel is not some extra protein tucked away somewhere, but it is an integral part of desirable body tissue such as muscle cells. This tissue is rapidly replaced once the diet provides the necessary amino acids and energy. If body protein is used for fuel without being replaced, however, this is soon accompanied by a noticeable decrease in muscle mass, a feeling of weakness, and other undesirable changes.

Adipose tissue

Adipose tissue is made up of many cells called adipocytes. These cells are in a dynamic state in which *lipogenesis* (fat formation) is balanced against *lipolysis* (fat breakdown). If lipogenesis exceeds lipolysis, the adipocytes increase in size and a person becomes "fatter." Likewise, if lipolysis predominates, the adipocytes shrink and the person becomes thinner.

Lipogenesis Since the body can convert carbohydrate, alcohol, and amino acids into triglycerides, any of these substances can eventually end up as body fat. Figure 14.2 illustrates what happens. Endogenous triglycerides (fat made within the body) are formed in the liver and carried via the blood to the adipocytes. Glucose can also enter adipocytes directly from the blood and then be converted to triglyceride within the adipocytes.

Fat from the diet (exogenous triglyceride), after traveling as chylomicrons, becomes part of adipose tissue. An enzyme in cell walls called lipoprotein lipase breaks down chylomicrons, allowing the fatty acids they contain to enter the cell. Within the cell these fatty acids are combined with glycerol, forming new fat molecules (triglycerides).

Lipolysis Specific enzymes in cell walls of adipocytes can break down fat contained within the cell and release free fatty acids into the bloodstream. Free fatty acids travel attached to a blood protein called albumin. The level of free fatty acids in the blood normally remains low because fatty acids are metabolized by liver and muscle tissue. Turnover is rapid—any one fatty acid molecule remains in the bloodstream an average of only 2 to 3 minutes.

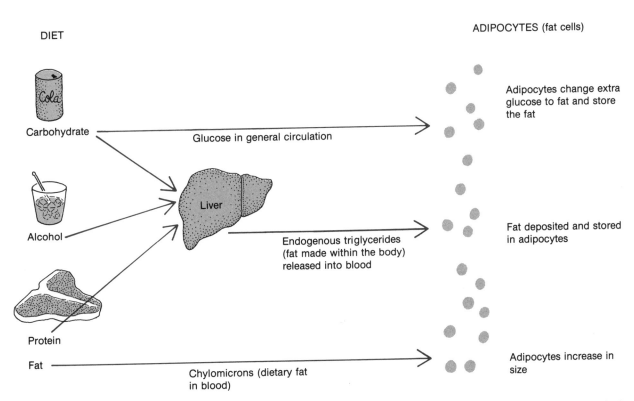

FIGURE 14.2. Lipogenesis (fat formation).

REGULATION OF FUEL LEVELS FOLLOWING A MEAL

Energy nutrients enter the bloodstream primarily in the form of monosaccharides, amino acids, short- or medium-chain fatty acids, and chylomicrons (triglyceride "coated" with protein) (Table 14.1). All except the chylomicrons travel directly to the liver via the portal vein. If alcohol is ingested, it also travels directly to the liver.

The liver acts like a chemical factory and processes the nutrients with which it is supplied. If the body's demand for carbohydrate or specific amino acids is high at that moment, the liver releases the nutrients into the bloodstream. If the supply of carbohydrate or amino acids is much greater than the demand, the liver alters the nutrients chemically. The liver also metabolizes alcohol, but can only do so at a fixed rate which is independent of the supply of alcohol.[1]

Carbohydrate

The amount of carbohydrate absorbed from a meal could quickly overload the system were it not for a number of regulatory processes. After all, just one slice of bread provides much more carbohydrate than is supposed to be in the blood at one time. Regulation of carbohydrate is primarily regulation of glucose. After the monosaccharides fructose and galactose are absorbed from the intestine, they undergo chemical changes in the liver. Sorbitol, a sugar alcohol used in some dietetic foods, may also be chemically changed by the liver. The result of the liver's processing of fructose, galactose, and sorbitol is that the principal carbohydrate entering the general circulation is glucose.

Several processes help to keep the level of glucose in blood from rising too high or remaining at an elevated level. These processes are described here.

REGULATION BY THE LIVER

Glycogenesis (Synthesis of glycogen) Some of the extra glucose is converted to glycogen, a starchlike polysaccharide, and stored in the liver. This occurs only if liver glycogen stores are not already full. Glycogen can

be stored in the adult liver in amounts up to about 6 percent of that organ's weight. Glycogen synthesized by the liver does not enter the bloodstream.

Lipogenesis (Synthesis of fat) Part of the extra glucose is converted to triglycerides by the liver. Some is stored as fat in the liver. The remaining endogenous triglyceride is combined with protein to form lipoproteins which transport fat to body cells. (These lipoproteins differ in size and composition from chylomicrons.) High carbohydrate intake stimulates hepatic lipogenesis. The hepatic processes of glycogenesis and lipogenesis can significantly reduce the blood sugar level, but not enough to be adequate as the only means of control.

INSULIN

An increased level of glucose in the blood stimulates production and release of the hormone insulin by the beta cells of the pancreas. Insulin circulates in the blood throughout the body and has several effects on fuel levels. It (1) stimulates entry of glucose into body cells; (2) retards the release of free fatty acids into the blood, thus favoring the utilization of glucose rather than fat for fuel; (3) promotes the formation of glycogen and triglycerides; and (4) stimulates entry of amino acids into the cells, thus reducing the amount of amino acid available for gluconeogenesis (the formation of glucose from amino acids). Once glucose has entered any type of cell other than hepatocytes (liver cells) it is "captured" and cannot leave again as glucose.

PHYSICAL ACTIVITY

Physical activity increases the fuel requirement of muscle tissue and increases the speed with which glucose enters muscle cells. Exercise is sometimes described as having an insulin-like effect because it acts to reduce blood glucose levels.

KIDNEYS

If the above means are inadequate to keep the amount of glucose in the blood below about 140 to 180 mg. percent, the kidneys excrete glucose in the urine. The

TABLE 14.1 *Entry of fuels into the blood and tissues*

DIET	FORM IN WHICH FUEL ENTERS BLOODSTREAM	ORGAN OR TISSUE WHICH FIRST PROCESSES THE FUEL
Carbohydrate	Monosaccharides	
Protein	Amino acids, dipeptides	LIVER (all are carried
Alcohol	Alcohol	via the portal vein)
Fat	Short- and medium-chain fatty acids	
	Chylomicrons	Adipose tissue

blood sugar level at which glucose appears in the urine is called the renal threshhold for glucose. The kidneys may be viewed as a second line of defense to protect the body from damage caused by high levels of glucose in the blood. They function to maintain normal blood glucose levels only when there is a defect in one of the other means of control.

Fat

Following a high fat meal there may be so much fat in the blood in the form of chylomicrons that the plasma appears "milky." This situation is corrected gradually as fat is deposited within the adipocytes. Insulin acts in several ways to promote a net uptake of fat by cells.

The kidneys cannot excrete chylomicrons, triglycerides, or free fatty acids. There is no second line of defense to protect the body from elevated blood lipid levels.

The slowing of digestion which results from eating a high fat meal slows the rate of entry of fat into the bloodstream.

Amino Acids

A high protein meal results in a large "dose" of assorted amino acids in the portal blood. The supply is apt to be much greater than the demand for these building blocks of protein. The liver responds by removing the nitrogen from some of the amino acids and changing them into compounds which can be utilized for energy.

> **POINTS OF EMPHASIS**
> *Regulation of fuel levels following a meal*
>
> • *The liver is a major controlling center which can quickly reduce blood levels of glucose and amino acids.*
> • *The hormone insulin stimulates uptake of glucose, amino acids, and fat by cells.*
> • *Exercise speeds removal of fuels from the blood.*
> • *The kidneys excrete sugar if blood levels become excessively high.*
> • *No mechanism exists for rapid clearing of alcohol from the blood.*

Alcohol

There is no mechanism to closely control the level of alcohol in the blood. If alcohol is ingested and absorbed, it is cleared from the blood at a slow, reasonably constant rate by the liver. Alcohol is not utilized directly by muscle tissue. It takes more than 10 hours to clear all of the alcohol from the blood of someone who is intoxicated (150 mg. alcohol per dl blood). The level of physical exercise does not affect the rate at which alcohol is removed from the bloodstream. Most of the alcohol is partially oxidized and then used for the synthesis of fatty acids. The fatty acids in turn are combined with glycerol to form fat. A significant amount of this fat is deposited in the liver. The rest is handled just like endogenous triglyceride synthesized from carbohydrate.

REGULATION OF FUEL LEVELS DURING SHORT TERM FASTING

Normally during the day there are periods of time when there is no dietary supply of fuel to meet continuing body needs. During these periods, notably during a night's sleep, the individual can be said to be fasting or abstaining from food. The principal fuels used during fasting are glucose, free fatty acids, and ketones. (Ketones are intermediate compounds formed during the breakdown of fat by the liver.) Until food arrives, fuels are introduced into the bloodstream as described in the following section.

Glucose

The liver is the only organ that can release glucose into the bloodstream. This release of glucose is stimulated by glucagon, a hormone produced by the alpha cells of the pancreas. Glucagon stimulates glucose release no matter what the insulin level is. The entry of glucose into the blood is also promoted by a decrease in circulating insulin levels.

Glycogenolysis in the liver   Glycogenolysis is the hydrolysis of glycogen to form glucose. When glycogenolysis takes place within hepatic cells, glucose can be released into the blood. (Glucose released by glycogenolysis within muscle cells is used directly within the cells and does not enter the blood.)

Gluconeogenesis in the liver   Gluconeogenesis is the synthesis of glucose from noncarbohydrate substrates. The substrates used are amino acids or the glycerol portion of triglycerides.

An average of 58 percent of the amino acids released into the blood from body protein can be converted to glucose in the liver. (Some types of amino acids cannot be converted to glucose.) A series of enzyme reactions is required. When the glucose level of the blood is low, there is less uptake of amino acids by the cells because of the low insulin levels. This makes more amino acids available for gluconeogenesis.

Glycerol, which ordinarily is obtained from the breakdown of triglycerides, can also be converted to glucose by a series of enzyme reactions. The amount of blood glucose formed in this way is very small since glycerol accounts for only about 10 percent of a fat molecule.

Free fatty acids

Free fatty acids are released into the bloodstream following lipolysis of fat contained in adipose tissue. Lipolysis is accelerated when glucose and insulin levels are low.

Ketones

The partial oxidation of free fatty acids by the liver results in the formation of substances called ketones, ketone bodies, or ketoacids. These include the chemical substances acetoacetic acid, beta-hydroxybutyric acid, and acetone. As long as glucose is present, ketones are quickly metabolized by muscle tissue so that ketone levels of the blood remain relatively unchanged.

POINTS OF EMPHASIS
Regulation of fuel levels following short term fasting

- *The liver forms glucose from its stored glycogen and from amino acids; this glucose is released into the blood.*
- *Adipose tissue releases free fatty acids into the blood.*
- *Physiological symptoms of hunger prod a person to replenish the fuel supply.*

FUELS UTILIZED BY SPECIFIC TISSUES

Tissues differ to some extent in their ability to utilize different fuels, depending primarily on whether or not they have mitochondria (Table 14.2).

Muscle tissue of all types (smooth, cardiac, and striated) can utilize available glucose if insulin is present to facilitate transport of glucose into the cells. Muscle tissue can readily utilize free fatty acids and ketones, even when insulin levels are low. Tissues use amino acids as an energy source only after they have been converted to products which can be metabolized as carbohydrate or fatty acids.

Under normal circumstances, the brain and other nervous tissue can use only glucose as an energy source. In addition to the controls of blood sugar level, there are special safeguards for the adequacy of the fuel supply to the brain—insulin is not required for transport of glucose into nerve or brain cells, and the central nervous system can utilize ketones as a supplemental energy source when the glucose supply is low. Ketones cannot completely eliminate the brain's requirement for glucose, and free fatty acids cannot be used by the brain for fuel.

REGULATION OF FUEL LEVELS DURING STARVATION

When food is unavailable for a prolonged period of time, survival depends on the body's ability to maintain a supply of fuel for essential body functions.

Since the amount of glycogen stored in the body is limited, the supply of glucose from glycogenolysis is rapidly depleted during starvation. Nonetheless the central nervous system continues to require glucose. This is supplied at the expense of muscle tissue by the process of gluconeogenesis. Initially the amount of body protein which is used for fuel is high, about 40 to 60 gm. or more daily.[2,3] This is equivalent to loss of about 160 to 240 gm. of muscle tissue and partially accounts for the rapid weight loss seen in starvation.

Adaptation gradually occurs, favoring preservation of body protein and utilization of fat as the principal source of fuel. Adaptation occurs in the following manner:

1. Insulin levels remain low. This helps save glucose for use by nervous tissue.
2. Muscle cells adapt to the use of free fatty acids as their principal fuel.
3. The liver accelerates synthesis of ketones from free fatty acids and releases them into the general circulation.
4. Blood ketone levels rise, favoring their utilization by the central nervous system and reducing the amount of glucose required by the brain.
5. More of the available glucose is recycled. The glucose is only partially broken down to supply fuel and the metabolites are resynthesized into glucose. Although this cycle is wasteful of energy, it conserves body protein by conserving glucose.
6. The basal metabolic rate gradually decreases (measured by a decrease in the thyroid hormone triiodothyronine [T_3]), reducing the overall energy requirement. In prolonged starvation or semi-starvation the BMR can decrease by one third or more. This reflects an overall slowdown in body processes which will also be indicated by a decreased pulse and body temperature.[4]
7. A feeling of weakness and lethargy results in reluctance to engage in physical activity, thus tending to keep the energy requirement low.
8. Linear growth of children ceases.

As a result of these adaptations energy required for

TABLE 14.2 *Fuels utilized by selected tissues*

TYPE OF TISSUE	FORMS OF FUEL
Muscle tissue (all types), other types of cells which have mitochondria	Glucose
	Free fatty acids
	Ketones
Nervous tissue, other types of cells which do not have mitochondria	Glucose
	Ketones (for part, not all, of energy requirement)

survival is provided and body protein is preserved for a longer period of time. The breakdown (wasting) of muscle tissue which occurs during starvation provides visible evidence that much body protein has been used for fuel despite the adaptations mentioned.

If a starving individual is provided with enough protein (about 1.5 to 1.7 gm. protein per kg. ideal body weight) to cover nitrogen losses, lean body mass may be better preserved despite continued severe caloric deficit. This is the basis for protein-sparing therapy (or protein-sparing modified fast) which is sometimes used for hospitalized clients who cannot eat and for severely obese individuals who are losing weight under a doctor's supervision. Adaptations to starvation occur during protein-sparing therapy, at least in healthy individuals.

Semi-starvation

If an individual experiences prolonged caloric deficit while ingesting a well-balanced diet, he is undergoing the stress of semistarvation. Since there is a continuing supply of glucose, some of the adaptations seen in complete starvation may not occur. Even if the diet contains what is usually an adequate amount of protein, considerable amounts of muscle tissue will be used for fuel. This was clearly demonstrated in the Minnesota Starvation Studies[5] in which healthy active men consumed diets (averaging 1570 kcal.) designed to be deficient primarily in calories. (The normal caloric requirement of these men was approximately 3500 kcal. daily.) By the end of 6 months the men had lost approximately one fifth to one fourth of their muscle mass and a much larger fraction of their adipose tissue, equalling a total average weight loss of 17 kg. (37 lb.). Similar undesirable loss of lean body mass can be expected in individuals experiencing famine, very low-calorie reducing diets, or other forms of caloric deprivation. Obese individuals may adapt more successfully to the stress of semistarvation, losing relatively little muscle mass.

Some of the physiological responses to caloric deficit are common to all types of starvation. A typical complaint is intolerance to cold. Starving or semistarving individuals usually feel the need to wear extra clothing and use extra blankets even when the environmental temperature is warm. A decrease in basal metabolic rate is also typical.

Some physiological discomforts depend on the type of starvation. The rise in blood ketone levels which develops in complete starvation and protein-sparing therapy tends to dull the appetite and sometimes to cause nausea. A marked rise in blood ketone levels can often be detected without the aid of laboratory testing by presence of unusual breath odor similar to the odor of nail polish remover. (The odor is due to the exhalation of acetone.)

Although many of the changes occurring in response to starvation and semistarvation appear to be "unhealthy," they actually are adaptations which help to maintain essential body processes.

POINTS OF EMPHASIS
Regulation of fuel levels during starvation or semistarvation

• *Body fat, carbohydrate, and protein are all used to supply energy.*
• *Ketones become an important source of fuel for the brain when carbohydrate levels are low.*
• *Metabolic adaptations occur to reduce fuel requirements and to conserve body protein and glucose.*
• *Unpleasant symptoms such as intolerance to cold, fatigue, and hunger or nausea are associated with protective adaptations.*

RELEASE OF ENERGY FROM FUEL

When carbohydrate, protein, and fat are oxidized, energy released must be harnessed. Part of the energy released is trapped in a chemical compound called adenosine triphosphate or ATP. ATP is a high-energy phosphate compound that provides usable energy for muscle contraction, nerve impulses, active transport of substances across cell membranes, anabolism—in fact for each and every body process. It provides the link between the breakdown of fuel and the utilization of the energy produced for useful work. ATP cannot be stored, but it can transfer its energy to form another high-energy compound called creatine phosphate. Some creatine phosphate can be stored so that usable energy will be immediately available in time of emergency.

ANAEROBIC METABOLISM

The initial steps in the breakdown of glycogen and glucose do not require oxygen for the generation of ATP. Because oxygen does not participate, this process is called anaerobic metabolism. When the supply of oxygen is low, glucose or glycogen are the only fuels that can be metabolized to produce ATP. Muscle glycogen is the preferred fuel for anaerobic metabolism since it can release more ATP than can an equivalent amount of glucose from the blood. The amount of ATP produced in anaerobic metabolism is small compared to potential ATP production when oxygen is present, but anaerobic metabolism greatly increases the ability to adapt to temporary oxygen deficits. Anaerobic metabolism allows an athlete to race his fastest even though he can't breathe hard enough to supply his tissues with all the oxygen they need to completely oxidize glucose or fat. Anaerobic metabolism is of importance in very strenuous exercise and in certain disease conditions that limit the supply of oxygen to the tissues.

The end product of carbohydrate metabolism under anaerobic conditions is lactic acid. As lactic acid accumulates it diffuses from the cells into the bloodstream and most of it is eventually reconverted to glucose in the liver.

AEROBIC METABOLISM

Aerobic (oxygen-requiring) metabolism takes place in the mitochondria of cells and is the principal means of generating ATP. When oxygen is present, carbohydrate metabolism results in the formation of pyruvic, but not lactic, acid. Pyruvic acid is further broken down and enters a metabolic pathway called the tricarboxylic acid cycle or Krebs' cycle. This aerobic cycle is described as a common metabolic pathway. This is because metabolites of *all* of the major energy nutrients can be completely *oxidized* via this cycle. The points at which specific compounds enter the cycle differ, but the end result is the same. The compounds are all oxidized to carbon dioxide and water and much ATP is produced.

HEAT

A large fraction of the energy produced during both anaerobic and aerobic metabolism is not captured in the form of ATP but instead is dissipated as heat. This heat production can be just as important to the body as is ATP production, since it is vital to be able to maintain body temperature. The fraction of energy dissipated as heat varies among individuals.[6] The greater the fraction lost as heat the more fuel required for doing a given amount of work.

Fuel in relation to physical activity

Athletes are particularly interested in having available an adequate supply of the right type of fuel to meet their energy requirements during competition. Maximal physical work and athletic performance depend, of course, on a well-nourished body and therefore on a diet which provides the needed amounts of all nutrients. If the training program is quite vigorous, energy expenditure will be high, requiring a high caloric intake. Contrary to popular belief, the protein requirements is not significantly increased by exercise nor does extra protein improve athletic performance. In fact, a high protein meal eaten before an athletic event might produce undesired results; it would probably be high in fat as well as protein and, therefore, would remain in the stomach for a long time.

Glucose and/or fatty acids are excellent fuels for aerobic exercise such as jogging, swimming, and bicycling at a comfortable pace (Appendix 4F). Glucose, however, is the only fuel which can be used for an-

aerobic exercise (e.g., during a race). Glycogen stores help maintain an adequate supply of glucose for prolonged very strenuous activity.[7,8]

Oxygen supply   Maximal utilization of fuel depends on an adequate supply of oxygen. This can be provided only if blood hemoglobin levels are normal, since hemoglobin is needed to transport oxygen to the cells. Diet can affect hemoglobin level.

POINTS OF EMPHASIS
Release of energy from fuel

• *Part of the energy from fuel is transferred to adenosine triphosphate (ATP), a compound which harnesses the energy in a usable form.*
• *ATP provides the energy for energy-requiring body processes (e.g., anabolism, movement).*
• *The remaining energy from fuel is dissipated as heat.*
• *Carbohydrate is the only fuel which can be used for anaerobic metabolism (the type of metabolism occurring when the supply of oxygen is low).*
• *Anaerobic metabolism is a less efficient form of energy production than is aerobic metabolism. An excess amount of lactic acid is produced during anaerobic metabolism.*
• *Glycogen stores facilitate continued anaerobic exercise; adipose tissue can supply the fuel for aerobic exercise.*

Energy value of nutrients

Fortunately when consumers and health professionals try to find out the energy value of foods, they don't need to determine how much ATP is produced by an orange or a slice of bread. The numbers involved would be so large as to be confounding. Instead they find the caloric value or energy equivalent of foods by means of nutrition labeling, nutrition books, or other sources of calorie lists. Sometimes it is helpful for the health professional to be able to estimate the caloric value of foods or diets when only the approximate composition is known. This can be done by making use of numbers called "physiological fuel values." Physiological fuel values are *average* values for the number of calories per gram provided by carbohydrate, protein, fat, and alcohol. The physiological fuel values are carbohydrate 4 kcal. per gm.; protein 4 kcal. per gm.; fat 9 kcal. per gm.; and alcohol (ethanol) 7 kcal. per gm. (recent research indicates that this value may be too high[9]).

Sugar of any type is essentially 100 percent carbohydrate. Therefore 4 gm. (1 tsp.) sugar provides approximately 16 kcal. Vegetable oil is 100 percent fat. Five gm. (1 tsp.) of any type of vegetable oil provides about 45 kcal.—more than twice as many calories as the same weight of sugar. Many foods contain a significant amount of water, which provides no calories. Thus a water-containing high protein food such as fish provides much less than 4 kcal. per gm. of fish.

Since no nutrient provides more calories per gram than does fat, fat is described as the most *concentrated* source of energy.* Pure ethanol comes in a fairly close second, with 5 cc. providing nearly 35 kcal. Since available alcohol contains some water (100 proof liquor equals 50 percent alcohol and 50 percent water), the caloric value is diluted. Nevertheless, the addition of even small amounts of hard liquor to a soft drink sharply increases its caloric value.

Physiological fuel values make it apparent that no food can provide significantly more than 900 kcal. per 100 gm. A 30 gm. candy bar provides much less than 270 kcal. since a large fraction of its weight is contributed by carbohydrate. The more water a food or beverage contains, the lower is its caloric value for a given volume. Thus, even if the caloric value of a food is not known, useful rough estimates may be made.

In order to provide energy, nutrients must enter the body and be utilized by the cells. Differences in digestion, absorption, or metabolism of nutrients affect the amount of calories a food actually provides. For example, the amount of calories obtained from raisins or nuts will be greatly decreased if they are not well-digested as a result of incomplete chewing. Persons who are lactase deficient obtain fewer calories from milk than do individuals who can digest lactose. The amount of calories actually provided by carbohydrate is decreased by lack of insulin, as in the disease diabetes mellitus, since glucose can be oxidized only if it can enter the cell.

In most normal circumstances, the actual caloric value closely parallels the value found from calorie lists or from calculation, but the possibility of differences should not be overlooked.

---

* A distinction should be made between the "most concentrated" and the "quickest" source of energy. The latter term is often applied to sugar because of its rapid digestion and absorption and its role in anaerobic metabolism.

STUDY QUESTIONS

1. Can eating a lot of high protein food make a person become fat? In general terms, what is the metabolic explanation for your answer.
2. Why may a woman have more fuel reserve than a man even if she weighs somewhat less?
3. How does the brain obtain a supply of glucose during long term abstinence from food? What fuel reduces the brain's demand for glucose during fasting?
4. Why does the rate of weight loss decrease after a period of dieting or shortage of food?
5. What compound directly provides energy for synthesis of body tissue and for muscle work?
6. What fuels can be used by exercising muscle when there is no shortage of oxygen?
7. Why is fat correctly described as the most concentrated source of energy?

References

1. Lieber, C. S.: Alcohol and nutrition. *Nutr. News* 39:9, 1976.
2. Albanese, A. A., and Orto, L. A.: The proteins and amino acids. in R. S. Goodhart and M. E. Shils (eds.): *Modern Nutrition in Health and Disease.* Philadelphia: Lea & Febiger, 1973, p. 74.
3. Morgan, A., Filler, R. M., and Moore, F. D.: Surgical nutrition. *Med. Clin. North Am.* 54(6):1367, 1970.
4. Bistrian, B. R.: Biochemical and medical aspects of a protein sparing modified fast. In G. L. Blackburn (ed.): *Obesity.* Boston: Center for Nutritional Research, 1977.
5. Keyes, A., et al.: *The Biology of Human Starvation,* Vol. 2. Minneapolis: University of Minnesota Press, 1950.
6. Hegsted, D. M.: Energy needs and energy utilization. *Nutr. Rev.* 32:33, 1977.
*7. Smith, N. J.: *Food for Sport.* Palo Alto CA: Bull Publishing Co., 1976.
8. Review. Diet, exercise and endurance. *Nutr. Rev.* 30:86, 1972.
9. McDonald, J. T., and Margen, S.: Wine versus ethanol in human nutrition. *Am. J. Clin. Nutr.* 29:1093, 1976.

---

* Recommended reading

15

The role of nutrients in regulation

Regulation of body processes makes it possible for the human body to operate as an integrated whole, to maintain a stable internal environment, to grow at appropriate times, and to repair itself as needed. Eating, drinking, abstaining from food or water, exercising—in fact, all aspects of life itself—make this regulation necessary. Nutrient levels need to be regulated, but nutrients also provide the components from which regulatory substances and structures are made. Many nutrients actually function as regulators of specific body processes, while the presence of certain nutrients has indirect effects on regulation.

This chapter describes some of the ways in which nutrients are involved in maintenance of fluid and electrolyte balance, hydrogen ion balance, enzyme activity and other selected chemical reactions, functioning of the nervous system, and hormonal activity. Identification of factors which influence recommended intake of nutrients is included in Tables 16.2 to 16.6, pages 181 to 183.

Dynamic equilibrium

In humans, as in all mammals, the interior* of the body has specific characteristics which tend to remain constant despite outside influences. Characteristics of the internal environment (e.g., temperature, pH, osmolarity, and water content) must be maintained if cells are to retain their integrity and their ability to function normally. The fact that the internal environment is stable does not mean that the situation is static. On the contrary, the body continually undergoes change even though no change can be readily observed.

* The contents of the alimentary tract are not considered to be part of the interior of the body.

MAINTENANCE OF FLUID AND ELECTROLYTE BALANCE

A major aspect of the internal environment is the state of fluid and electrolyte balance. The fluid involved is water. All but one of the major electrolytes are ionic forms of essential minerals, specifically sodium (Na^+), potassium (K^+), magnesium (Mg^{++}), calcium (Ca^{++}), and phosphorus (the phosphates HPO_4^{--} and $H_2PO_4^-$). The exception is the electrolyte bicarbonate (HCO_3^-), which is a product of metabolism rather than a nutrient. Electrolytes are unevenly distributed throughout the body. Some ions are more prevalent in the *intracellular* fluid (fluid contained within cells) and others are more concentrated in the *extracellular* fluids (fluid found between cells, also called the *interstitial* fluid, and specialized fluids such as blood plasma, cerebrospinal fluid, and vitreous humor). Figure 15.1 illustrates differences in chemical composition of intracellular fluid, interstitial fluid, and blood plasma. Interstitial fluid and blood plasma are so similar in composition that they are often considered together.

Even though there are marked differences in composition of the intracellular and extracellular fluid compartments, the osmolarity of both fluid compartments is essentially the same. The normal osmolarity of the interstitial and intracellular fluid is about 281 milliosmoles per liter. (That of the blood plasma is slightly higher.) This means that the total number of dissolved particles per unit of fluid on the inside of a cell membrane equals that found on the outside of the membrane. Water moves freely through cell membranes to achieve this equilibrium.

If the osmolarity of the extracellular fluid increases, water moves out of the cells by osmosis, causing the

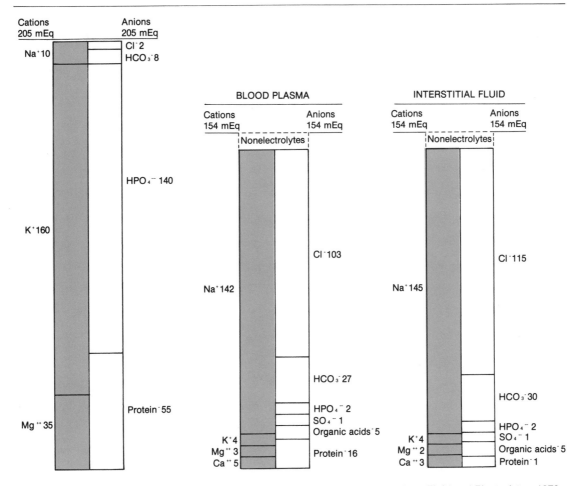

FIGURE 15.1. Electrolyte content of fluid compartments. (Adapted from *Fluid and Electrolytes*, 1970, pp. 10, 11, Abbott Laboratories)

cells to shrink. If the osmolarity of the extracellular fluid decreases, water moves into the cells, causing them to swell. Excessive movement of water either into or out of cells can damage the cells.

Water

Water serves as a solvent, a component of all cells and body fluids, a means of regulating body temperature, and a lubricant. Fifty to seventy percent of adult body weight is water; the amount varies inversely with the proportion of body fat. The water content of the body, expressed as percent of body weight, falls with age. This holds true for adults even if they do not gain adipose tissue.

Water cannot be stashed away in the body for future use; that is, output of water balances input. If someone drinks extra water, urinary output increases to maintain a steady state.

Thirst usually serves as a reliable guide to the need for water. This is fortunate since the minimum requirement for water is highly variable. It depends on the amount of water required to rid the body of wastes via the urine, and it also depends upon losses of several other types. There is an obligatory but variable loss of

water in insensible perspiration (perspiration unnoticed because it evaporates before it has a chance to accumulate), the breath (as water vapor), and feces. Sweating, the key means of cooling the body, can greatly increase fluid loss. Other types of fluid loss can be associated with disease conditions and injury (e.g., due to watery diarrhea or blood loss respectively). Table 15.1 summarizes typical daily fluid losses.

Specifically, the need for water depends upon (1) solids present in the diet (because of their effects on body wastes), (2) environmental temperature, (3) humidity, (4) type of clothing worn, (5) state of health, (6) amount and type of exercise, and (7) respiratory rate.

There are more sources of water available to the body than many people recognize. Beverages of any

TABLE 15.1 *Typical daily fluid losses in an adult*

Urine*	1500 ml
Perspiration† (mainly insensible)	450
Respiration	350
Feces	200–250
	Total about 2500

* Amount can greatly increase or decrease according to need
† Amount can greatly increase, especially if engaged in strenuous physical activity in hot weather

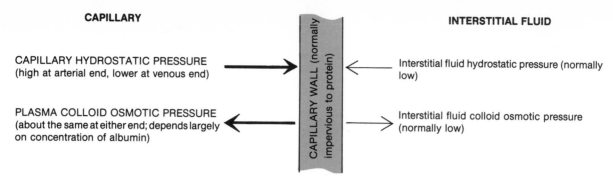

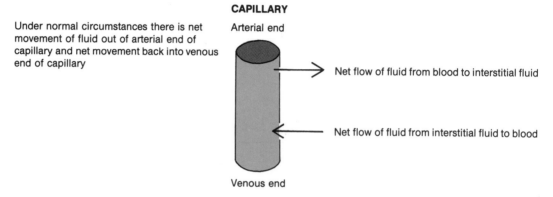

FIGURE 15.2. Serum proteins influence fluid balance by their osmotic effect.

kind have a high water content. Most foods contain a high percentage of water, including some foods which appear quite dry such as bread and meat. Melons, celery, and many other fruits and vegetables contain about as much water as does milk, or sometimes more.

Metabolic breakdown of food for energy is an even less obvious source of water. The end products of the oxidation of energy nutrients are carbon dioxide and water. The amount of water produced endogenously (within the body) is small compared to that consumed in the diet, but it gains significance when the intake of water must be limited.

The amount of water produced by oxidation of energy nutrients depends on the nutrient involved, as follows: 100 gm. fat produce 107 ml. water (and 900 kcal.); 100 gm. carbohydrate produce 56 ml. water (and 400 kcal.); 100 gm. protein produce 41 ml. water (and 400 kcal.). If a person's daily energy expenditure is 2000 kcal., his endogenous water production would be in the vicinity of 230 ml. (nearly 1 c.).

Desirable intake of water exceeds the minimum required for replacing obligatory losses. An ample water intake helps maintain normal water content of the feces. (When in short supply, extra water is absorbed from the colon.) In this way adequate fluid intake promotes regular bowel movements. Moreover, by increasing the flow of urine, a generous water intake may help to prevent urinary tract infections and kidney stones.

Individuals normally experience little day-to-day variation in water content. The body cannot tolerate much fluctuation since change adversely affects the concentration of dissolved substances and the integrity and functioning of cells.

Diet can cause small but measurable changes in water content of the body for reasons unrelated to the amount of water contained in the foods consumed. The following features of the diet have a significant effect on fluid balance.

SODIUM

The human body tolerates a wide range of dietary intakes of sodium. However, when there is extra sodium present in the body, the sodium tends to "hold" water with it. Thus extra sodium (salt) may increase the water content of the body. Although fluid retention may not be noticeable, cutting down on salt intake causes many people to lose a little weight (fluid).

High intake of sodium is common in the U.S., most of it supplied in the form of salt (sodium chloride). Most individuals do not develop noticeable fluid retention.

CARBOHYDRATE

Carbohydrate content of the diet affects sodium and fluid balance. A net loss of sodium and fluid occurs when carbohydrate is absent from the diet or in low supply, as during starvation or adherence to a low-carbohydrate reducing diet. Adding carbohydrate back to the diet leads to regain of fluid and sodium. Similar responses have been reported when carbohydrate levels are changed without changing caloric intake.[1]

PROTEIN

Normal distribution of water between the blood plasma and the interstitial fluid requires a normal level of serum protein, particularly the protein called albumin. In turn a normal serum level of albumin depends upon an adequate dietary intake of protein and calories.

Serum proteins influence fluid balance by their osmotic effect. They tend to draw water back into the blood from the interstitial fluid. This may seem surprising since proteins are such large molecules. Actually the large size of the molecules is responsible for protein's powerful effect on fluid balance. A simplified explanation of the process is given in Figure 15.2.

A very low protein diet could cause the serum albumin level to fall so much that fluid would collect between the cells, increasing total body water. However, changes in dietary intake of protein may not cause observable changes in water balance for weeks or months, while changes in sodium and/or carbohydrate intake cause shifts in water content of the body within a matter of hours.

POINTS OF EMPHASIS
Fluid balance

• *Water, the most abundant compound in the body, is needed for all physiological processes.*
• *The percent of water in the body normally decreases with age.*
• *A healthy person's need for water varies greatly, depending mainly on obligatory urinary losses and losses via perspiration.*
• *Water is obtained from beverages, food, and the oxidation of energy nutrients.*
• *Extra sodium intake tends to result in a small amount of extra fluid retention in healthy individuals.*
• *Low carbohydrate intake results in loss of body fluid.*
• *Adequate intake of protein and calories helps to maintain normal fluid balance by helping to maintain a normal serum albumin level.*

Electrolytes

Electrolytes are involved in a number of regulatory processes in that they influence nerve and muscle irritability, cellular activity, and hydrogen ion balance. Table 15.2 lists functions of each.

TABLE 15.2 *Functions of major nutrient electrolytes*

ELECTROLYTE	FUNCTION
Sodium (Na^+)	Hydrogen ion balance
	Maintenance of osmotic pressure of extracellular fluid and movement of fluid from one compartment to another
	Gastrointestinal absorption of specific monosaccharides and amino acids
	Normal muscle irritability and contractility
	Normal cell permeability
Potassium (K^+)	Normal excitability of nervous tissue
	Contractility of muscles (cardiac, skeletal, and smooth)
	Intracellular osmotic pressure and hydrogen ion balance
	Anabolism of muscle tissue, lean body mass
Chloride (Cl^-)	Maintenance of osmotic pressure, especially of extracellular fluid
	Hydrogen ion balance
	Component of hydrochloric acid of gastric juice
	Chloride shift
Magnesium (Mg^{++})	Cofactor for many enzymes, especially those involved in the formation of ATP
	Normal cardiac contraction
	Normal functioning of muscle and nervous tissue
	Mineralization of skeleton and teeth
	Normal calcium metabolism
Calcium (Ca^{++})	Muscle and nervous tissue function
	Blood clotting
	Strength and rigidity of skeleton, mineralization of teeth
Phosphate (as $H_2PO_4^-$ or HPO_4^{--})	Component of high energy compounds such as ATP (Storage and transfer of energy)
	Buffer system to help maintain normal H^+ balance
	Component of certain coenzymes (joined with a vitamin as in pyridoxal-phosphate)
	Nervous tissue metabolism
	Component of phospholipids: transport of lipids, structural component of cell membranes
	Component of nucleic acids (DNA and RNA) needed for cell protein synthesis
	Mineralization of bones and teeth

When discussing electrolytes it is convenient to divide them into cations (positively charged ions) and anions (negatively charged ions). Sodium, potassium, calcium, and magnesium are all cations. They influence nerve and muscle irritability in an interdependent fashion. Chloride and phosphates are among the anions in body fluids. In conjunction with bicarbonate, chloride and phosphates serve to maintain electroneutrality and help regulate hydrogen ion concentration.

Potassium, magnesium, and phosphate are noted for being *anabolic* electrolytes. They move into cells when needed for anabolic purposes (such as protein synthesis) and are released from cells during catabolic activity.

The concentration of each electrolyte in each fluid compartment must be maintained within its own narrow range. Abnormal change in concentration of any one ion adversely affects the integrity and functioning of cells, tissues, and organs. Change in concentration of one electrolyte upsets the delicate balance existing among the ions. Diet influences the amount of each electrolyte available.

A proper concentration and balance of electrolytes in the various fluid compartments is so important that the body has a number of mechanisms for their regulation. These are described briefly here.

SODIUM, POTASSIUM, AND CHLORIDE

The initial mechanisms for controlling the level of *sodium* in the plasma include (1) stimulation (or lack of stimulation) of thirst, (2) rapid diffusion of sodium through capillary membranes, and (3) shift of water between intracellular and extracellular space (osmosis).

Hormonal controls are of utmost importance in the regulation of the serum concentration of both sodium and potassium ions.

Antidiuretic hormone (ADH) This hormone, which is released by the posterior pituitary gland, helps correct high osmolarity of the extracellular fluid. Antidiuretic hormone facilitates renal reabsorption of water while allowing sodium (and other ions and small molecules) to be excreted in the urine. Increased osmolarity of the blood, most commonly resulting from increased sodium content, promotes release of ADH.

Aldosterone Aldosterone, a hormone secreted by the adrenal medulla, promotes reabsorption of sodium by the renal tubules and promotes excretion of potassium in the urine. Levels of circulating aldosterone rise and fall primarily in response to rise and fall of the serum potassium level.

Mechanisms for controlling serum sodium levels are so effective that a healthy person can tolerate a wide range of sodium intake. Potassium is poorly conserved when in short supply. An ample daily supply is desirable for maintaining normal potassium levels. Serum chloride levels are regulated by the kidneys. Table 16.2 (p. 181) provides information about factors influencing the need for these and other electrolytes.

CALCIUM, PHOSPHORUS, AND MAGNESIUM

Several mechanisms regulate serum levels of calcium, phosphorus, and magnesium. Less is known about control of magnesium levels than about control of the other two cations.

Bone If the serum calcium level is high, passage of the blood through the bone normally removes much of the excess calcium, leaving it deposited within the ends of bones. These calcium deposits are readily available for raising the serum calcium level if it should start to fall.

Solubility product The solubility product of serum calcium and phosphorus (the result obtained by multiplying the concentration of calcium times the concentration of phosphorus) normally remains about the same in blood serum. Thus, if the serum concentration of calcium increases, the serum concentration of phosphorus normally decreases.

Kidneys If serum levels of phosphorus, magnesium, or calcium are high, there will be increased excretion of the ion present in excess. There is some evidence that the serum level of calcium inversely affects the urinary excretion of magnesium. That is, if the serum calcium level is high, magnesium excretion will be depressed.

pH If the pH of the blood falls, calcium tends to be released into the blood. (Calcium becomes more soluble when exposed to more acidic solutions.) If the blood becomes more alkaline, pH of the blood rises and calcium deposition tends to increase, decreasing serum calcium level.

Hormones Hormones which influence serum levels of calcium and phosphorus are released or withheld in response to changes in serum calcium but not the serum phosphorus level.

Active Vitamin D (1,25-dihydroxycholecalciferol or 1,25-DHCC). Vitamin D in its active form, 1,25-DHCC, is considered to be a hormone and is often called vitamin D hormone.[2] However, vitamin D resulting from the action of sunlight upon the skin and that obtained from fortified foods and vitamin pills is the chemical cholecalciferol and is not vitamin D hormone. To become active, vitamin D (cholecalciferol) must undergo chemical changes. The first step in the activation of vitamin D takes place in the liver, where the vitamin is changed to 25-hydroxycholecalciferol (25-HCC). This is the normal circulating form of the vitamin. It can undergo further change in the kidneys to produce 1,25-dihydroxycholecalciferol (1,25-DHCC), which is the form of the vitamin that promotes calcium and phosphorus absorption and, thus, increases serum levels of these nutrients. Active vitamin D also initiates bone mineral mobilization.[3] If the precursor is available, the supply of vitamin D hormone is closely regulated according to need. More vitamin D is converted to the active form whenever the serum calcium level starts to fall.

Parathyroid Hormone. Increased amounts of parathyroid hormone (parathormone) are secreted by the parathyroid glands when the serum calcium level falls. Parathyroid hormone stimulates the following changes: (1) release of calcium and phosphorus from the bone into the blood; (2) increased renal tubular reabsorption of calcium and magnesium; (3) increased urinary loss of phosphate, which promotes increase in serum calcium; and (4) increased formation of active vitamin D (1,25-DHCC) from circulating 25-HCC, which promotes intestinal absorption of calcium. The primary purpose of parathyroid hormone is to maintain an adequate supply of calcium in the blood. If serum calcium level falls because of inadequate calcium intake or absorption, demineralization of bone provides the needed calcium. Since a variety of mechanisms are involved in restoring serum calcium level, demineralization of bone is usually of short duration. Serum phosphorus level is controlled only indirectly.

Calcitonin. Increased amounts of calcitonin are secreted by the thyroid glands when the serum calcium concentration rises. This temporarily favors reduction of serum calcium levels by increased mineralization of bones.

POINTS OF EMPHASIS
Nutrient electrolytes

• *Sodium, potassium, chloride, magnesium, calcium, and phosphate are the major nutrient electrolytes. They participate in many body processes in an interdependent manner.*
• *Electrolytes are distributed unevenly between intracellular and extracellular fluid. Different concentrations of electrolytes in intracellular and extracellular fluids are vital to normal physiological processes.*
• *Mechanisms for maintaining proper concentration and balance of electrolytes vary depending on the electrolyte. They include shifts of water and ions; hormonal regulation of excretion by the kidneys; thirst or lack of thirst; and changes in bone mineralization/demineralization due to hormones, pH, solubility product.*
• *Sodium can be well conserved by the body.*
• *Potassium is poorly conserved by the body.*
• *Serum levels of calcium and phosphate are normally maintained within normal limits even if the dietary supply is low since these ions can be released from the bones.*

Changes in dietary intake of calcium and phosphorus have relatively little effect on *serum* levels of these electrolytes. In contrast, decreased dietary intake of magnesium is apt to result in decreased serum magnesium level.

MAINTENANCE OF HYDROGEN ION BALANCE

Maintenance of normal H^+ balance is essential for correct distribution of electrolytes and for enzyme activity. The small size of hydrogen ions contrasts sharply with their potency. People become vividly aware of the power of infinitesimal hydrogen ions when they drink or eat something quite acidic— lemonade, perhaps, or a sour pickle. The mouth and stomach can tolerate fairly acidic substances, but enzymes, cells, and tissues within the body cannot. The body functions properly only within a very narrow pH range. Therefore, elaborate regulatory mechanisms act to keep the concentration of H^+ within a *very* narrow range. This range is represented by a blood pH between 7.35 and 7.45.

The principal regulatory mechanisms for controlling blood pH fall into several categories: dilution by water, buffer systems,* and excretion.

Organic acids resulting from metabolism

CARBONIC ACID

The catabolism of carbohydrate, fat, and/or protein for energy results in the production of large volumes of the gas carbon dioxide (CO_2). For example, one molecule of glucose produces 6 molecules of carbon dioxide. The CO_2 readily diffuses out of the cell and into the bloodstream. A small amount of CO_2 dissolves in the interstitial fluid and plasma, producing the weak organic acid called carbonic acid:

$$CO_2 + H_2O \rightleftharpoons H_2CO_3$$
(Carbon dioxide + water $\rightleftharpoons$ carbonic acid)

Carbonic acid partially ionizes, forming hydrogen ions and bicarbonate ions:

$$H_2CO_3 \rightleftharpoons H^+ + HCO_3^-$$

The reaction is reversible, as indicated by the double arrows. The amount of free H^+ formed in this way is very small because so little CO_2 dissolves in extracellular fluid.

Blood doesn't bubble like a carbonated beverage, so what happens to all of the carbon dioxide? Much of it

---

* Buffer systems are combinations of substances which react with acid or base to resist a change in pH.

diffuses into the red blood cell where an enzyme called carbonic anhydrase (C.A.) catalyzes the reaction:

$$CO_2 + H_2O \underset{C.A.}{\rightleftharpoons} H_2CO_3$$

The red blood cell can handle the resulting hydrogen ions nicely because reduced hemoglobin (hemoglobin not carrying oxygen) neutralizes the acid.

The reaction is reversed in the lungs, allowing the excretion of carbon dioxide. This, in turn, reduces the concentration of carbonic acid and hydrogen ions. As long as the lungs are functioning normally, there should be no accumulation of acid produced as a result of metabolic reactions yielding carbon dioxide. A husky, active male exhales more carbon dioxide than does a petite older woman. This compensates for his higher metabolism and carbon dioxide production.

LACTIC ACID

Lactic acid can accumulate during periods of anaerobic metabolism of carbohydrate. Normal functioning of the lungs allows the situation to be quickly corrected, but in a different manner. When heavy breathing continues after strenuous exercise has ceased, extra oxygen is used to help clear the blood of lactic acid. Diet has no direct effect on this reaction.

KETOACIDS

Metabolism of fatty acids by the liver produces acidic substances called ketoacids, sometimes known as ketones or ketone bodies. These circulate in the bloodstream and are quickly metabolized by muscle cells to carbon dioxide and water. When the ketoacids produced are quickly used, there is no net effect on hydrogen ion balance.

Diet can affect this balance. If the dietary supply of carbohydrate is limited, the catabolism of fatty acids increases to meet energy needs. This occurs during starvation and during dieting with any of the popular low carbohydrate diets. If the rate of production of ketoacids exceeds the rate at which they are utilized, the extra H^+ needs to be buffered to prevent dangerous decrease in body pH. The kidneys eliminate some of the excess ketoacids, also helping to keep blood pH within normal limits. As long as there are no related disease conditions (such as diabetes mellitus or renal disease), accumulation of ketones resulting from diet should not cause serious alteration in the pH of the blood.

URIC ACID

Small amounts of purines—components of high energy compounds, DNA, RNA, and certain other vital chemicals in the body—are regularly catabolized to a weak organic acid called uric acid. Uric acid is also produced by the catabolism of purines obtained from foods such as liver, sardines, flesh foods, and certain vegetables. (Purines are not essential nutrients.) Uric acid has little effect on blood pH since it is a very weak acid which is not very soluble in water. When the serum concentration of uric acid rises there is no worry about its causing the blood pH to fall. Rather, there may be concern that crystals of uric acid will precipitate out and damage tissues such as the joints. The kidneys normally excrete excess uric acid so that uric acid level is maintained within a normal range.

Metabolizable acids supplied by the diet

A variety of organic acids are either present in foods or are released by digestive processes. Most of them can be oxidized rapidly via normal metabolic pathways so that they normally have no significant effect on the pH of blood. Amino acids and fatty acids are the most prevalent, but they are only weakly acidic. Citric acid from citrus fruits or processed foods is metabolized to carbon dioxide and water. Acetic acid (from vinegar), malic acid (from apples), fumaric acid (a commonly used food additive), and lactic acid (from yogurt) are other examples of organic acids which humans metabolize completely.

Nonmetabolizable organic acids

Two organic acids that cannot be metabolized by humans are sometimes supplied by the diet. These acids (benzoic and quinic acids) are found in plums, prunes, and cranberries. Because they cannot be converted to carbon dioxide and water, they contribute H^+ to the blood. These acids can be cleared from the body only by excretion in the urine. Therefore, ingestion of these acids results in a reduction of the pH (increase in acidity) of the urine.

Ascorbic acid (vitamin C) taken in excess contributes H^+ to the blood and to the urine. The effect of ascorbic acid is marked only when pharmacological doses of the vitamin are ingested.

Inorganic acids

Catabolism of protein produces two strong inorganic acids—sulfuric and phosphoric. The sulfuric acid is derived from the sulfur-containing amino acids and the phosphoric acid from phosphoproteins and phospholipids. These powerful acids are not allowed to circulate "as is." Instead, the hydrogen ions are immediately combined with bicarbonate or another basic compound so that the pH of the blood and other body fluids is minimally affected.

Sulfate, acid phosphate, and hydrogen ions from the

catabolism of protein are eventually excreted in the urine if present in excess. Consequently most high protein foods (eggs, meat, poultry, fish, legumes) tend to lower the pH of the urine.

Milk products, although high in protein, tend to increase the pH of the blood and urine. The protein in milk and cheese produces considerable acid; however, this is offset by the large amount of calcium and other basic minerals. The net effect of eating dairy products is to decrease the acidity of the urine.

Chloride is considered to be an acidic ion—a part of the strong inorganic hydrochloric acid—but it is normally balanced by the basic sodium ion.

POINTS OF EMPHASIS
Maintenance of hydrogen ion balance

• *Concentration of hydrogen ions in blood must be carefully regulated within a narrow pH range (pH 7.35 to 7.45) for normal body function.*
• *Control mechanisms include dilution, buffering, and excretion of acid or base.*
• *Acids are introduced into the body by anaerobic and aerobic metabolism of energy nutrients, incomplete oxidation of fatty acids, and ingestion of foods containing nonmetabolizable organic and inorganic acids.*
• *Most high protein foods tend to decrease pH of the blood; increased urinary excretion of acid is the principal means of compensation.*
• *Bases are introduced primarily by ingestion of foods containing basic minerals. Ingestion of excess base results in rise in pH of urine.*

ENZYME ACTIVITY

Enzymes might be viewed as "sparks" of life. An enzyme increases the rate at which a specific chemical reaction takes place. Two chemicals might be together in the same solution for hours with no apparent reaction but, add the right enzyme(s), and that specialized protein causes marked chemical changes to occur. (This assumes that conditions such as pH and temperature are favorable for enzyme activity.) Many enzyme reactions proceed only in combination with certain vitamins and minerals.

Vitamins as coenzymes

Many of the vitamins from the B complex have been found to function as *coenzymes* in metabolic reactions. A coenzyme is an organic molecule which, when attached to an enzyme, enables the enzyme to catalyze a given reaction.

The B vitamins differ considerably in structure. Each has its own specific role as a particular coenzyme; however, the actions of coenzymes are inter-related. A sampling of the roles of B vitamins as coenzymes follows.

Vitamin B_{12} and folic acid act as two distinct coenzymes in the formation of molecules of deoxyribonucleic acid (DNA). DNA is a complex chemical compound which is commonly called a gene. Each gene (DNA molecule) controls the formation of another type of nucleic acid called ribonucleic acid (RNA). Folic acid also acts as a coenzyme in the formation of RNA. RNA controls protein formation and, thus, controls enzyme formation and cell structure. Therefore, folic acid and vitamin B_{12} indirectly affect essentially all body processes.

Five of the B vitamins—thiamine, niacin, riboflavin, pantothenic acid, and biotin—all act as distinct coenzymes which make possible the use of fuels for the production of ATP.

More than one vitamin participates in the metabolism of a given energy nutrient. Each vitamin functions at different steps, in combination with different enzymes. Since the catabolism or anabolism of a body compound occurs in a series of steps, a lack of one of the coenzymes interferes with the entire process. This situation can be likened to a plugged drain. No matter where the obstruction occurs, it causes backup and eventually interferes with the movement of material along the entire length of pipe. Thus, if even one of these coenzymes is lacking, ATP production is impaired. Decreased ATP production may have undesirable effects since it limits the supply of energy needed for anabolic and regulatory purposes.

Vitamin B_6 (pyridoxine) serves as a coenzyme for a number of reactions essential to the metabolism of amino acids. Certain other B vitamins are required as coenzymes for synthesis of compounds such as fatty acids, cholesterol, and proteins.

For most clinical purposes it is not necessary to know the names of each coenzyme and specifically how each functions in metabolism. Table 15.3 is included for reference. It gives a general idea of the functions of B vitamins as specific coenzymes.

One B vitamin, niacin, can be synthesized within the body if there is an adequate supply of the essential amino acid tryptophan. This reaction requires vitamin B_6 coenzyme. From 60 mg. tryptophan about 1 mg.* of niacin is synthesized. The remainder of the tryptophan is used for other purposes. Nevertheless, dietary protein of high biological value can be a very significant source of niacin because of the tryptophan it contains.

Table 16.3 (p. 182) lists factors influencing requirement and supply of B complex vitamins.

Minerals and enzyme activity

A myriad of enzyme-catalyzed reactions depends upon minerals as well as on vitamins. This is most evident for the *metalloenzymes* (enzymes in which a "metallic" mineral is an integral part of the enzyme itself). Among

---

* 1 mg. niacin equals about 5 percent of an adult's RDA for this vitamin.

TABLE 15.3 *Functions of B vitamins*

VITAMIN	COENZYME	GENERAL FUNCTION
Thiamine (B_1)	Thiamine Pyrophosphate (TPP or cocarboxylase)	Plays a key role in carbohydrate metabolism, allowing conversion of pyruvic acid to a 2 carbon compound that can enter Krebs' cycle. Participates in reactions in Krebs' cycle
Riboflavin (B_2)	Flavin mononucleotide (FMN) and flavin-adenine dinucleotide (FAD)	Hydrogen acceptors. Required for the generation of ATP in aerobic metabolism. Also involved in amino acid and purine metabolism
Niacin	Nicotinamide adenine dinucleotide (NAD), nicotinamide adenine dinucleotide phosphate	Hydrogen acceptors. Required for aerobic metabolism, synthesis of fatty acids and cholesterol, conversion of the amino acid phenylalanine to tryptophan.
Pyridoxine (B_6)	Pyridoxal-phosphate	Amino acid metabolism: (1) decarboxylation (removing carbon dioxide) of amino acids to form other compounds (as tryptophan → the vasoconstrictor serotonin); (2) transamination; (3) transferring sulfur from amino acids to other compounds; (4) converting the amino acid tryptophan to the vitamin niacin
Pantothenic acid	Coenzyme A	Entry of carbohydrate into Krebs' cycle. Synthesis of acetylocholine, a key chemical in the transmission of nerve impulses. Oxidation of energy nutrients. Synthesis of fatty acids, cholesterol, and related compounds and of porphyrin (a component of hemoglobin)
Biotin	No common name for the coenzyme	Decarboxylation. Metabolism of energy nutrients in the Krebs' cycle. Carboxylation reactions (addition of CO_2). Synthesis of fatty acids, purines (needed for DNA and RNA). Deamination of specific amino acids
Cyanocobalamin (B_{12})	No common name for the coenzyme	Synthesis of DNA
Folic acid	Tetrahydrofolates	Synthesis of DNA and RNA
Choline*		Donates methyl (CH_3^-) groups needed for many reactions, helps prevent deposition of fat in liver (lipotropic action), is a component of phospholipids and of acetylcholine (needed for transmission of nerve impulses)

* May not be a dietary essential. Can be synthesized in the body.

the minerals functioning in this way are iron, zinc, copper, manganese, and molybdenum, all of which are present in the body in exceedingly small concentration (trace elements).

Several types of enzymes contain iron, including the respiratory* enzymes called *cytochromes*. The cytochromes are part of the respiratory chain which allows the production of ATP during aerobic metabolism of energy nutrients.

Copper is a second metal which is required for the functioning of cytochromes. Copper is a part of numerous other metalloenzymes as well. The trace minerals zinc and molybdenum compete with copper for enzyme sites. If they are successful in displacing copper, the activity of the metalloenzyme is impaired. Because of this, high levels of zinc or molybdenum increase the requirement for copper.

Zinc alone is a part of more than 40 different metalloenzymes, including carbonic anhydrase. Zinc is needed for synthesis of both DNA and RNA and, therefore, for protein synthesis.[4]

Specific minerals, including some of those mentioned previously, form metalloenzyme complexes. In these complexes there is a loose association between

* In this case "respiratory" refers to oxidative reactions occurring within cells.

POINTS OF EMPHASIS
Role of nutrients in enzyme activity

- *Many enzymes must combine with a specific coenzyme in order to function as biological catalysts.*

- *B complex vitamins serve as coenzymes involved in both anabolic and energy-releasing reactions.*

- *Several B complex vitamins may be involved in the synthesis or breakdown of any one compound.*

- *One B vitamin, niacin, can be synthesized in the body if there is an adequate supply of the precursor tryptophan (an essential amino acid).*

- *Some trace metals are an integral part of metalloenzymes and, therefore, are necessary for catalyzing some metabolic processes.*

- *Some minerals activate enzymes by forming metalloenzyme complexes.*

- *Trace minerals function in an interdependent manner, e.g., excess of one may result in undesirable displacement of another.*

- *Need for any one trace element varies with composition of the diet.*

TABLE 15.4 *Functions of trace elements*

ELEMENT	FUNCTION
Iron	Oxygen transport and utilization: component of hemoglobin, myoglobin, cytochromes, and certain other enzymes
	Normal blood platelet production
	Normal growth and appetite
	Integrity of mucous membranes
Copper	Synthesis of hemoglobin and cytochromes
	Component of certain metalloenzymes including cytochrome oxidase
	Maintenance of bones and neurological function
	Formation of myelin
	Constituent of the connective tissue called elastin
	Melanin pigment formation
	Normal sense of taste
Zinc	Component of more than 30 metalloenzymes, including carbonic anhydrase
	Synthesis of DNA and RNA, catabolism of RNA
	Normal growth and strength of bone
	Normal sexual maturation and reproduction
	Integrity of skin; wound healing
	Normal sense of taste and smell, normal appetite
Manganese	Activator of several enzymes
	Metalloenzyme involved in formation of urea
	Functioning of the central nervous system
	Component of bone
	Carbohydrate and lipid metabolism
	Synthesis of mucopolysaccharides of cartilage
	Normal reproduction
Iodine	Component of thyroid hormones thyroxine and triiodothyronine; therefore important for normal metabolism, growth, neuromuscular function, normal reproduction, skin integrity
Molybdenum	Component of at least 2 metalloenzymes
	Catalyzes oxidation of fatty acids
Selenium	Component of metalloenzyme that protects hemoglobin and some other body compounds from oxidative damage
	Normal growth and fertility in animals
Fluoride	Optimal mineralization of teeth and bones
	Helps prevent dental caries and may help protect against development of osteoporosis
Chromium	Component of glucose tolerance factor; needed for normal insulin activity
	Normal growth
Tin Nickel Silicon Vanadium Arsenic Others?	Essential in one or more mammals. Role in human nutrition requires further clarification

the mineral and the enzyme. The effect of the mineral is to activate the enzyme. Nutrients which function in this way are sometimes called cofactors. Magnesium activates a number of enzymes. In some metalloenzyme complexes manganese can substitute effectively for magnesium.

There is incomplete data regarding how many trace elements are actually essential in enzyme reactions in humans. It is assumed that a number of trace elements essential for experimental animals are also essential for man. Included among these minerals are some notorious for their toxicity. (Arsenic is an example.) Trace minerals may perform vital functions when present in minute concentration, whereas in increased amounts they may displace other minerals to the body's detriment.

Some of the known functions of selected trace minerals are presented in Table 15.4. All but two of these functions involve enzyme reactions.[5]

The actions of trace minerals are intricately inter-twined. Some of the mysteries concerning them may never be untangled. In fact, it may be more important to recognize that trace minerals function in an inter-dependent fashion than to be able to identify specific functions of each. Information about factors influencing recommended intake and dietary supply of trace minerals is summarized in Table 16.5 (p. 183).

OTHER SELECTED CHEMICAL ACTIVITIES

ACTIVITY OF VITAMIN E AND SELENIUM

There is some lack of agreement as to just how vitamin E functions in the body. Coenzyme activity has been suggested but not documented. However, vitamin E is well-known for its antioxidant properties.[6] By reacting with oxygen, vitamin E can prevent the oxidation of other nutrients such as vitamin A and polyunsaturated fatty acids. Vitamin E is inactivated in the process, but it serves to protect less expendable components of the body such as cell membranes. Vitamin E may also cause the inactivation of very reactive particles called "free radicals" which are formed when polyunsaturated fatty acids are oxidized. The importance of this reaction with free radicals in the human body has not been determined.

Vitamin E appears to work synergistically with a selenium-dependent enzyme system in preventing certain undesirable oxidation reactions.[7,8] In animals a small amount of selenium greatly reduces the requirement for vitamin E.

Selenium and vitamin E both appear to independently protect the body against certain pollutants, namely mercury and cadmium. In addition, vitamin E appears to afford some protection against lead toxicity (toxicity increases if the body is deficient in vitamin E).[5]

ACTIVITY OF VITAMIN C

Vitamin C (ascorbic acid) is a powerful chemical *reducing agent*. This chemical property no doubt is responsible for many of the metabolic functions of vitamin C. Vitamin C participates in a number of synthetic reactions, including hormonal synthesis. It is probably best known for its role in the synthesis of the structural protein called collagen.

POINTS OF EMPHASIS
Other selected chemical activities of micronutrients

- *Vitamin E and selenium function as antioxidants, retarding undesirable oxidation of polyunsaturated fatty acids and other substances.*
- *Vitamin C functions as a chemical reducing agent needed for synthesis of collagen.*

ACTIVITY OF THE NERVOUS SYSTEM

The dietary supply of nutrients affects the functioning of the nervous system. Activity of the nervous system depends on an adequate fuel supply. Glucose and ketones are the only substances known to penetrate the blood brain barrier for use as fuels. If for some reason the blood glucose level falls sharply, behavioral changes and impaired body function quickly develop. Drowsiness following overeating is commonly observed, but not well explained.

Neurotransmitters are chemical compounds released from nerves which cause biological responses in adjoining cells. The concentration of neurotransmitters in the brain has been found to vary with the diet. It has been suggested that these changes may influence hunger, sleep, body temperature,[9] and sensitivity to painful stimuli.[10] This is an active area of research which may result in important findings related to diet.

The vitamins which are most obviously related to functioning of the nervous system are vitamin B_6, thiamine, and niacin, although other vitamins certainly participate. Vitamin B_6 serves as a coenzyme in reactions necessary for the formation of neurotransmitters and neurohormones. The explanation for the relationship of thiamine and niacin to neurological function is less clear. The brain's dependence on glucose as a fuel is no doubt involved since these vitamins are required for utilization of glucose. Deficiency of these three B vitamins results in neurological changes. Severe lack of niacin can actually cause dementia, and lack of vitamin B_6 may cause convulsions. Vitamin B_{12} helps maintain the integrity of nerves.

Nerves can function properly only if the body's electrolyte balance is maintained.

HORMONAL ACTIVITY

Hormones, specific organic compounds secreted by endocrine glands, perform a wide variety of regulatory functions. Some types of hormones are proteins or much smaller compounds which are synthesized from animo acids. Examples include the protein insulin, the polypeptide glucagon, and the amino acid derivative epinephrine. A temporary lack of dietary protein does not noticeably interfere with synthesis of hormones.

Other types of hormones are synthesized from cholesterol, a lipid which is not an essential nutrient because it can be synthesized endogenously. Hormones derived from cholesterol include any vitamin D synthesized by the body, corticosteroids, mineralocorticoids, and sex hormones.

Production of thyroid hormones, insulin, glucose tolerance factor, and prostaglandins may be linked to the diet.

THYROID HORMONES

Iodine is an essential constituent of the thyroid hormones thyroxine and triiodothyronine (T_3). Hence normal production of thyroid hormones depends on an adequate intake of iodine. If there is a continued dietary lack of iodine, the thyroid gland enlarges as a means of compensation. This condition is called simple goiter (see Fig. 2.7, p. 22). Excessive iodine intake can also result in alterations in production of thyroid hormone and enlargement of the thyroid gland.

Normal production of thyroid hormones, especially T_3, depends on an adequate caloric intake. T_3 level falls during starvation or other forms of caloric deprivation including dieting. This causes the basal metabolic rate to decrease.

INSULIN

Insulin production varies in response to changing fuel levels in the blood. The amount of body fat also appears to influence insulin production, e.g., insulin production tends to increase with increase of adipose tissue.

The effectiveness of insulin at the cellular level is potentiated by an essential micronutrient called glucose tolerance factor (GTF). GTF acts like a hormone in that it is released in response to increased levels of insulin in the blood and exerts its effect when it reaches the target cells.

Glucose tolerance factor is an unusual micronutrient which might be classified as an essential mineral or as a vitamin.[11] GTF contains the trace mineral chromium. Apparently some individuals can synthesize active GTF from chromium, niacin, and amino acids. For these individuals GTF is not a dietary essential but chromium is. Other individuals appear to require a dietary source of preformed GTF. For them GTF might be called a vitamin.

POINTS OF EMPHASIS
Nervous and hormonal activity in relation to diet

• *An inadequate or overabundant fuel supply can interfere with normal functioning of the brain.*

• *Diet can influence the supply of neurotransmitters in the brain.*

• *Electrolyte balance and an adequate supply of B vitamins are required for normal functioning of the nervous system.*

• *Normal production of thyroid hormones requires iodine and adequate caloric intake.*

• *Chromium is required for formation of glucose tolerance factor, a hormone-like substance which improves effectiveness of insulin.*

• *Linoleic acid is required for formation of prostaglandins (local hormones).*

PROSTAGLANDINS

Prostaglandins (PGs) are a group of organic compounds which exert hormone-like activity in regulating body processes. They differ from hormones in that they are synthesized within cell walls and exert their influence locally. They are sometimes called local hormones.

Linoleic acid, the essential fatty acid, is a precursor for prostaglandin formation. PGs are unstable compounds which retain their original structure and ac-

tivity for only a few minutes.[12] Biosynthesis of prostaglandins may be dependent upon the availability and, hence, on the dietary supply of linoleic acid.

STUDY QUESTIONS

1. What factors increase a healthy individual's need for water?
2. How may a sharp decrease in carbohydrate intake affect fluid balance?
3. What is the principal force that draws water back into the capillary at the venous end?
4. Why is vitamin D considered to act like a hormone?
5. What types of nonmetabolizable acids are provided by foods? Do meats tend to produce acid or base?
6. What is meant by the statement, "Many B complex vitamins serve as coenzymes in energy metabolism"?
7. What is the precursor of niacin? What types of foods are good sources of this precursor?
8. In what way are the functions of most trace elements similar?
9. What happens to vitamin E when it serves as an antioxidant in the body?
10. What nutrients are involved in the formation of glucose tolerance factor? What is the role of this hormone-like substance?

References

1. Randall, H. T.: Water, electrolytes and acid-base balance. In R. S. Goodhart and M. E. Shils (eds.): *Modern Nutrition in Health and Disease.* Philadelphia: Lea and Febiger, 1973, p. 360.
2. DeLuca, H. F.: Vitamin D: A new look at an old vitamin. *Nutr. Rev.* 29:179, 1971.
3. DeLuca, H. F.: Metabolism of vitamin D: Current status. *Am. J. Clin. Nutr.* 29:1258, 1976.
4. Prasad, A. S.: Nutritional aspects of zinc. *Diet. Currents* 4(5):27, 1977.
5. Mertz, W.: Trace elements. *Contemp. Nutr.* 3(2) Feb. 1978.
6. Review. The function of vitamin E as an antioxidant, as revealed by a new method for measuring lipid peroxidation. *Nutr. Rev.* 36:84, 1978.
7. Roe, D. A.: *Drug Induced Nutritional Deficiencies.* Westport CT: Avi Publishing Co., 1976.
8. Levander, O.: Selenium and chromium in human nutrition. *J. Am. Diet. Assoc.* 66:338, 1975.
9. Wurtman, R. J., and Fernstrom, J. D.: Effects of the diet on brain neurotransmitters. *Nutr. Rev.* 32:193, 1974.
10. Fernstrom, J. D., and Lytle, L. D.: Corn malnutrition, brain serotonin and behavior. *Nutr. Rev.* 34:257, 1976.
11. Mertz, W.: Effects and metabolism of glucose tolerance factor. *Nutr. Rev.* 33:129, 1975.
12. Vergroesen, A. J.: Physiological effects of dietary linoleic acid. *Nutr. Rev.* 35:1, 1977.

16
The role of nutrients in maintenance, repair, and growth

Growth, maintenance, and repair of the body require nutrients which can be used for structural purposes. This chapter focuses attention on (1) protein, the primary structural component of protoplasm, and (2) the minerals making major contributions to body structure. Consideration is also given to nutrients which play supporting roles in synthesis of particular proteins, cells, and body structures.

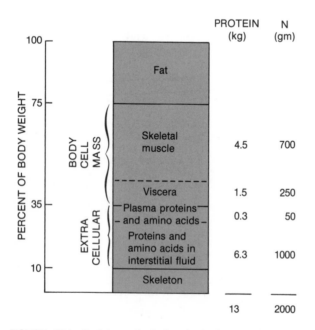

FIGURE 16.1. Protein content of major body compartments in normal adult male weighing 72 kg. (Drawn from Blackburn, G. L., Flatt, J. P., and Hensle, T. E.: Peripheral amino acid infusions. In J. Fischer [ed.]: *Total Parenteral Nutrition.* Boston: Little, Brown, & Co., 1975, p. 365)

Body compartments

For purposes of better understanding the roles of nutrients in growth, maintenance, and repair, it is useful to think of the body as divided into four compartments: adipose tissue, body cell mass, extracellular fluid, and skeleton (Fig. 16.1).

Adipose tissue Adipose tissue plays a minor role in this discussion, since its major function is storage of fat for energy. The fatty deposits surrounding the kidneys and certain other vital organs might be viewed as serving a structural function because they provide some support and protection against injury.

Body cell mass (BCM) Body cell mass refers to the metabolically active intracellular substances comprising skeletal muscles, viscera, and red blood cells. Body cell mass accounts for approximately 35 to 45 percent of normal weight in males and 30 to 40 percent in females. Since body cell mass does not include fat, the term lean body mass (LBM) is a frequently used synonym. Figure 16.1 indicates the approximate amount of protein contained in the body cell mass of an individual who weighs about 70 kg. Most women contain proportionately less protein because of their smaller body size, but it is similarly distributed.

Extracellular fluid (ECF) Extracellular fluid includes all body fluid *outside* of the cells, namely interstitial fluid, blood plasma, fluids of the alimentary canal, and other specialized fluids (cerebrospinal, intraocular). The adult female has approximately 12 to 13 L. of extracellular fluid; the adult male has an average of about 15 L. All extracellular fluids contain proteins (such as albumin, enzymes, certain hormones) which serve transport and/or regulatory purposes. The plasma and interstitial fluid also contain amino acids which can move into the cells to be used for protein synthesis.

Skeleton Because of its hardness, the skeleton is often incorrectly viewed as a group of inert bones made principally out of minerals. Actually bone contains bone cells (osteocytes) which are metabolically active. An organized arrangement of osteocytes forms and maintains the protein matrix of bones. Minerals are incorporated into the matrix, contributing hardness and rigidity. Neither the protein nor the mineral content of the bone is static.

Cartilage is another type of skeletal tissue, found in the ear, nose, and certain other parts of adults. It is softer and more flexible than bone because it has a lower mineral content. Cartilage comprises a large percentage of the skeletal tissue of infants. Much of this cartilage is gradually mineralized to form bone.

DYNAMIC EQUILIBRIUM OF BODY PROTEINS

Protein is an integral component of all cells. All body protein is in a dynamic state of breakdown and renewal. The rate of turnover varies with the type of tissue. Hepatocytes (liver cells) have a long life, but half of the proteins within these cells turn over within four days or less. Protein turnover is much slower within the osteocytes.

Normal turnover of body protein in the adult amounts to approximately 240 gm. daily, an amount greatly in excess of usual daily protein intake. Each day some cellular protein is hydrolyzed to amino acids which are then released into the plasma. Conversely, new cellular proteins are synthesized from amino acids obtained from the plasma. The cells do not distinguish between amino acids provided by the diet and those released from the body's own cells. The ability to reuse amino acids makes it possible for one tissue to supply the amino acids needed to repair damaged tissue.

The amino acid pool

The free amino acids which are present in the liver and plasma comprise an amino acid pool. The amino acid pool provides a supply of essential and nonessential amino acids which can be used for protein synthesis in any part of the body. The supply of amino acids in the pool is maintained by dietary intake of protein and by catabolism of body protein.

INFLUENCE OF HORMONES

Certain hormones influence the rate of anabolism or catabolism of body protein. Hormones promoting anabolism include growth hormone, insulin, andro-

gens, and a normal level of thyroid hormones. Hormonal states which promote catabolism are increased levels of glucocorticoids or thyroxine and low levels of insulin. (A summary of hormonal effects on body protein is found in Table 27.1, Page 293.) Depending on hormonal levels, there can be net gain, net loss, or maintenance of body protein.

METABOLISM OF AMINO ACIDS

Synthesis of protein Both essential and nonessential amino acids serve as building blocks for body protein. RNA directs protein synthesis, serving as a template on which essential and nonessential amino acids are arranged and joined in a precise pattern. Each amino acid must be available in the correct amount or the protein cannot be made. The essential amino acids are the specific amino acids which must be included in the diet. Nonessential amino acids are also essential for anabolism of protein. They can, however, be synthesized in the body when they are needed if there is an adequate supply of a usable form of nitrogen.

Synthesis of nonessential amino acids Endogenous formation of amino acids involves two general processes: (1) synthesis of the carbon skeletons of the amino acids (α-ketoacids) and (2) addition of an amino ($-NH_2$) group to the α-ketoacid, usually by the process of transamination.

The body can synthesize the α-ketoacids of nonessential amino acids but cannot synthesize the α-ketoacids of essential amino acids.

Transamination In transamination, the amino group from an existing amino acid is transferred to an α-ketoacid, forming a new amino acid. Transamination can be represented by the following word equation:

amino acid A + α-ketoacid B $\rightarrow$ α-ketoacid A + amino acid B

In other words, one amino acid donates its amino group so that a different amino acid can be made. The amino group is transferred, not actually lost.

CATABOLISM OF AMINO ACIDS

The liver is the principal site of amino acid catabolism. Every day amino acids are destroyed primarily via the activity of hepatic enzymes. Total loss (catabolism) of amino acids varies depending on diet and state of health. When the protein content of the diet is increased, more amino acids are catabolized in the liver. (Normally this is not harmful but might be considered to be a waste of protein.) Breakdown of amino acids may increase dramatically when a person is injured or ill. Some amino acid catabolism occurs even under ideal circumstances. There is a daily obligatory loss of amino acids as a result of catabolism. *Deamination* is the process initiating the catabolism of amino acids.

Deamination When an amino acid is deaminated, its vital amino group ($-NH_2$) is removed. The remaining carbon skeleton of the amino acid, an α-ketoacid, is either oxidized for energy or converted to a carbohydrate or fat. Deamination always precedes gluconeogenesis, the endogenous formation of glucose. If the amino group which was removed from the amino acid is not used to form a nonessential amino acid, it becomes a part of a nitrogenous waste product called urea. The kidneys excrete urea in the urine. In simplified form, the reaction is as follows:

$$\text{amino acid} \xrightarrow[\text{enzymes}]{} \text{ketoacid} + \text{urea}$$

Urea production varies greatly with diet and state of health but never falls to zero, even during fasting.

Loss of protein-containing substances from the body

Small amounts of protein-containing substances are lost from the body each day. Hair, nails, sloughed-off (exfoliated) epithelial cells, and menses all contain protein. A daily intake of protein is required to cover these losses plus the losses caused by deamination of amino acids. The protein ingested must include adequate amounts of each of the essential amino acids if it is to be used for anabolic purposes.

Maintenance of vital body protein in the absence of dietary protein

If there is no dietary supply of amino acids, breakdown of protein in muscle tissue releases amino acids into the blood, temporarily maintaining the amino acid supply in the amino acid pool. When there is a shortage of amino acids, visceral and plasma proteins are maintained at the expense of the muscle. Use of muscle as a source of amino acids is an inefficient process. A significant proportion of the three branched-chain amino acids (leucine, isoleucine, and valine—all essential amino acids) are oxidized in muscle tissue. This prevents them from being released into the bloodstream. A relative lack of these branched-chain amino acids limits the use of the other amino acids for anabolism. The all-or-none law always applies to protein synthesis, namely: all essential amino acids must be present at the same time and in the proper proportion for protein synthesis to occur.

Collagen formation

Collagen is an *inter*cellular protein which is a major structural protein of the body. There are several ways in which it contributes structure to tissues: (1) the protein matrix of bone and cartilage is made of collagen, (2) collagenous fibers are arranged in an organized

fashion in connective tissues such as tendons, and (3) in certain tissues, such as the dermis of the skin, collagen fibrils extend in all directions forming a kind of network which helps to hold cells together. Collagen is often called a cementing substance since it helps to hold cells together. Vitamin C is a key nutrient required for the formation of collagen from amino acids.

POINTS OF EMPHASIS
Dynamic equilibrium of body protein

• *Body protein is in a state of dynamic equilibrium in which synthesis and breakdown (anabolism and catabolism) are ongoing processes.*
• *The body requires a supply of amino acids to allow for continual synthesis of proteins for maintenance, repair, and replacement of body cells and tissue.*
• *A growing body has increased need for amino acids.*
• *Amino acids released from one body protein can be reused to form a different protein.*
• *Nonessential amino acids can be synthesized in the body if there is a supply of nitrogen in the form of amino groups.*
• *Amino acids can be used for energy after they are deaminated.*
• *Urea is the nitrogenous waste product produced when amino acids are catabolized.*
• *Collagen is a specialized intercellular structural protein which can be formed and maintained only if vitamin C is available.*

The state of protein nutrition

NITROGEN INTAKE VERSUS OUTPUT

The state of protein nutrition is usually called the state of *nitrogen balance*. Nitrogen is dealt with rather than protein for reasons of simplicity. Nitrogen is the element which distinguishes protein from carbohydrate and fat. Practically all the nitrogen ingested is in the form of protein, but most of the nitrogen lost from the body is in the form of nitrogen-containing end products of catabolism. These include urea, creatinine, uric acid, and ammonium salts.

Protein-Nitrogen Conversions

Protein contains 16% nitrogen by weight
Gm. of N in food consumed
    = Gm. of dietary protein $\times$ 0.16
Gm. of protein lost
    = Gm. of nitrogen lost $\times$ 6.25

The state of nitrogen balance is the *net result* of intake and loss of nitrogen. This is influenced by the relative rates of anabolism and catabolism of nitrogen-containing substances (amino acids, protein, and related compounds). It is possible to make some reasonable predictions about the state of nitrogen balance in a variety of conditions, without resorting to laboratory tests and calculations.

Nitrogen balance (input equals output) Adults are usually in nitrogen balance. That is, their output of nitrogen equals their dietary intake of nitrogen. Anabolism of nitrogen-containing compounds keeps pace with catabolism and loss of nitrogen-containing compounds, preventing net gain or loss of nitrogen from the body. One can accurately assume that a person is in nitrogen balance if he is ambulatory, healthy but not growing or replenishing body tissue, and if he is consuming a diet adequate in essential amino acids, total protein, calories, and micronutrients. Regular consumption of a high protein diet *does not* produce a state of positive nitrogen balance in healthy adults, but it can lead to a state of positive calorie balance (weight gain). Extra nitrogen intake is balanced by increased nitrogen excretion in the form of urea. The more protein eaten the higher the production and excretion of urea.

POINTS OF EMPHASIS
Nitrogen balance

• *When lean body mass (LBM) remains the same, as is normal for adults, an individual is in nitrogen balance.*

• *When LBM increases as a result of growth, pregnancy, repletion of muscle tissue, or body-building exercise, nitrogen balance is positive.*

• *When LBM decreases owing to lack of food, inadequate protein intake, illness, injury, or immobilization, nitrogen balance is negative.*

• *Eating more protein than is necessary to meet body needs does not result in increase in LBM or in positive nitrogen balance.*

• *If a healthy individual follows "A Daily Food Guide" and meets caloric requirements, he should be in the type of nitrogen balance appropriate for his stage of development (in balance or positive).*

Positive nitrogen balance (input exceeds output) Positive nitrogen balance means that nitrogen intake *exceeds* nitrogen loss. When total anabolism of protein and other nitrogenous substances exceeds catabolism and loss, a person is in a state of positive nitrogen balance. Positive nitrogen balance is present during periods of growth and during periods of tissue repletion. *Growth* includes (1) normal increases of height and lean body mass occurring during childhood and adolescence, (2) increases in maternal and fetal tissues during pregnancy, and (3) muscle growth occurring in the initial phases of physical conditioning.

Repletion includes (1) rebuilding of body tissue occurring during convalescence from an illness which caused protein depletion and (2) rebuilding of tissue

following a period of fasting or inadequate intake of protein and/or calories. An ample supply of calories, protein, essential amino acids, and micronutrients is required to achieve a state of positive nitrogen balance.

Negative nitrogen balance (output exceeds input) When catabolism exceeds anabolism, an individual is in a state of negative nitrogen balance. Negative nitrogen balance means that loss of nitrogen from the body is greater than the amount of nitrogen consumed. The imbalance may result from an increased rate of catabolism, a decreased rate of synthesis or an increased loss of body protein. Negative nitrogen balance occurs if (1) the diet is inadequate in essential amino acids, total protein, calories, or any combination of these, (2) an individual is immobilized (on bedrest) for any reason, or (3) an individual is exposed to unusual stress as a result of trauma (including surgery) or a variety of disease conditions.

DYNAMIC EQUILIBRIUM OF THE SKELETON

Bones are metabolically active tissues containing live cells called osteocytes. Osteocytes must be provided with energy, structural materials, and other nutrients if the bones are to be strong and rigid. Bone and teeth are distinguished from other kinds of tissue by their high mineral content.

The minerals present in bone in the largest quantity are calcium and phosphorus. Minerals incorporated into bone in smaller amounts but which are no less important are magnesium, zinc, manganese, sodium, and chloride. Proper amounts of fluoride have recently been found to contribute to the strength of bones.

A number of nutrients facilitate the growth and/or mineralization of bone without actually being incorporated into the skeleton. Among them are vitamin D, vitamin C, and vitamin A.

The calcium and phosphorus content of bone is in a state of flux. These minerals are continually being taken up by or released back into the blood in order to maintain normal serum calcium and phosphorus levels. Adults turn over approximately 600 to 700 mg. calcium daily—several times more calcium than is ordinarily absorbed from food in a day. Turnover of phosphorus occurs at the same time because calcium salt deposits are made of both calcium and phosphate ions. In children the turnover rate of calcium (and phosphorus) is much higher than in adults, sometimes approaching 5000 mg. calcium or more daily.

STRESS OF WEIGHT BEARING

The stress of weight bearing helps to maintain the strength of bone. Weight bearing stimulates the activity of osteoblasts, bone-forming cells which deposit strong new bone. Other bone cells, the osteoclasts, cause absorption (loss) of bone. This absorption process (sometimes also called resorption of bone) accelerates when the stress of weight bearing is absent. Prolonged bedrest, immobilization by a cast, and space travel all cause a decrease in bone deposition and an increase in bone absorption. Bones gradually demineralize if not under stress.

Remodeling　In healthy ambulatory adults consuming adequate diets, the mass of bone remains quite constant, but bones continually undergo remodeling or change. Osteoblasts build or renew the bone and osteoclasts remove undesirable bone. The action is similar to having a house remodeled by tearing it down and rebuilding it bit by bit. Effective remodeling of bone takes place only if there is an adequate supply of nutrients to meet anabolic requirements.

LOSS OF MINERALS

Bone is vulnerable to slow demineralization and degeneration unless provided with an adequate supply of nutrients. Calcium and phosphorus can be reused, but there is a daily obligatory loss of these minerals. Each day small amounts of calcium and phosphorus are lost via the urine, sweat, skin, and secretions into the digestive tract. If these losses are not replaced by dietary intake, serum calcium level starts to fall and the calcium and phosphorus content of the bone gradually decreases to maintain the serum calcium level. Zinc and magnesium appear to remain as an integral part of bone.[1,2]

POINTS OF EMPHASIS
Dynamic equilibrium of the skeleton

• *Bones require a continuous supply of nutrients since they are metabolically active tissues.*
• *Calcium and phosphorus are readily taken up and released from bone.*
• *Other minerals incorporated into bone (zinc, magnesium, manganese, sodium, chloride, fluoride) are firmly held by bone.*
• *Vitamins (especially A, D, C) are not a part of bone but are essential for its formation and maintenance.*
• *Diet alone is insufficient to maintain bone strength. Weight bearing is also needed.*
• *Bones are gradually remodeled (changed) according to need; the process is aided by an adequate supply of nutrients.*

The state of structural mineral nutrition

Nutritional status of calcium and phosphorus is often described by referring to the state of balance of these minerals, that is, how intake compares with loss. The state of calcium balance can usually be predicted based on information about a person's state of health, exercise level, age, and diet.

INPUT VERSUS OUTPUT— CALCIUM AND PHOSPHORUS

Balance (input equals output)　A person is in calcium and phosphorus balance if his intake of these minerals equals his output of them. It is normal for input of calcium and phosphorus to equal output in healthy ambulatory adults ingesting a diet which contains adequate amounts of calcium, phosphorus, and vitamin D.

Positive balance (input exceeds output)　Positive balance means that intake of calcium and phosphorus is greater than loss of these minerals. Mineralization of the growing skeleton (including that of the fetus) requires a state of positive mineral balance. This occurs when the bones are lengthening, and also during the period of strengthening which follows. Adults experience a period of positive balance when bone is remineralized following immobilization, dietary inadequacy, and certain illnesses.

POINTS OF EMPHASIS
Calcium and phosphorus balance

• *When there is no net change in mineral content of bone, as is normal for young adults, a person is in calcium and phosphorus balance.*
• *When the mineral content of the skeleton is* increasing, *as during lengthening or strengthening of bones, calcium and phosphorus balance is* positive.
• *When the mineral content of bones is decreasing as a result of immobilization, aging, or an inadequate intake of calcium and/or vitamin D, calcium and phosphorus balance is* negative.

Negative balance (output exceeds input)　An inadequate intake of minerals obviously results in negative mineral balance. Immobility causes loss of calcium and phosphorus from bone and a corresponding state of negative balance, even when the dietary intake of these minerals is high. After about 40 years of age, individuals may experience chronic slight negative calcium balance owing to gradual bone demineralization —even if diet is adequate. This occurs more commonly in women than in men. Physical activity helps to retard bone demineralization.

CELL FORMATION AND PROLIFERATION

This section identifies a few of the myriad ways in which nutrients participate in cell formation and proliferation. These are highlights which are most apt to be useful in clinical practice.

CELL PROLIFERATION

Nucleic acids (DNA and RNA) are intimately involved in cell proliferation because of their roles in directing protein synthesis. Folic acid and vitamin B_{12} are both needed for formation of nucleic acids. This is especially important when there is rapid turnover of cells, as in the maintenance of the gastrointestinal tract and during times of growth.

Cellular and subcellular membranes

Cellular and subcellular membranes are specialized structures which provide a barrier to the entry and exit of ions and molecules. They allow controlled passage of certain particles through their pores. The major constituents of cell membranes are protein and lipids, particularly phospholipids. Phosphorus and *linoleic acid* are needed for the biosynthesis of phospholipids. Arachidonic acid is another polyunsaturated fatty acid needed for synthesis of cell membranes and is sometimes called an essential fatty acid. It can be made in the body if there is an adequate supply of its precursor, linoleic acid. Phospholipids apparently help to regulate cell permeability. Normal cell function and integrity depends on an adequate supply of both phosphorus and linoleic acid.[3] The integrity of cell membranes may also depend upon an adequate supply of *vitamin E*, since this vitamin helps prevent breakdown of unsaturated fatty acid.

Myelin Myelin, often referred to as the myelin sheath, is a specialized thick cell membrane covering some nerves. The composition of myelin is different from that of other cell membranes. The lipid to protein ratio in myelin is very high—about six times higher than that of other cell membranes. Galactolipids (compound lipids containing galactose) are abundant in myelin but not in other cell membranes.

The rate of myelination of nervous tissue is high prior to and shortly after birth. Normal development of the brain and nervous system depends on an adequate supply of nutrients during this critical period.

Vitamin B_{12} and *linoleic acid* are among the nutrients which must be provided by the diet if normal myelination is to take place.

Turnover of myelin is very slow but does occur. Thus vitamin B_{12} must be supplied to maintain the integrity of the nervous system. Continued lack of vitamin B_{12} eventually results in lesions of myelinated peripheral nerves, lesions of the myelinated posterior and lateral cords of the spinal column, and/or cerebral damage. Once the lesions occur, they respond poorly to improved diet.

Blood

THE RELATIONSHIP OF BLOOD TO NUTRITION

Blood is the vehicle which allows cells and tissues to be nourished. Blood transports absorbed nutrients to the cells and also shuttles amino acids and fatty acids from one part of the body to another. Metabolic waste products do not have a chance to accumulate and damage cells because blood whisks them away for eventual excretion.

Adequate transport of oxygen to the cells and of carbon dioxide away from the cells requires an adequate supply of red blood cells (erythrocytes) and of hemoglobin (the red-colored protein contained in erythrocytes). Normal transport of some micronutrients depends upon the presence of other types of proteins (e.g., albumin transports free fatty acids; retinol binding protein transports vitamin A). Of the many components of blood, only red blood cells are covered in this section.

RED BLOOD CELLS

Red blood cell formation is an ongoing process which is performed by cells in the bone marrow. There is a continual turnover of red blood cells. Their average lifespan is about 120 days. Hemoglobin is incorporated into the cells at the time they are formed. Specific nutrients make it possible to maintain a desirable level of healthy red blood cells with a normal hemoglobin content.

Maturation Vitamin B_{12} and folic acid, because of their role in DNA formation, are essential for normal rate of production and *maturation* of erythrocytes. If the dietary supply of these vitamins is inadequate, fewer erythrocytes are produced and they become abnormally large in size. If released into the bloodstream when still immature, the large cells are called megaloblasts. Mature large cells, called macrocytes, are fragile and have a shorter life than do normal red blood cells. Macrocytes may be destroyed within a few weeks rather than functioning for several months as do normal red blood cells. A normal lifespan for erythrocytes also depends on an adequate supply of magnesium[4] and probably of vitamin E and linoleic acid.

Hemoglobin Hemoglobin, a specialized protein, is an essential part of the red blood cell. It gives blood two of its unique properties: (1) the ability to transport large volumes of oxygen and release it easily to the cells and (2) the ability to transport large amounts of carbon dioxide safely away from the cells and release it readily in the lungs.

A number of nutrients are needed for hemoglobin formation: (1) amino acids are required to build up the protein molecule; (2) iron is the crucial part of the molecule allowing hemoglobin to transport oxygen; (3) copper is not a part of hemoglobin but is required for a normal rate of hemoglobin formation; (4) vitamin B_6 promotes hemoglobin formation; and (5) fuel supplies energy for hemoglobin formation, as for all anabolic processes.

If all nutrients are present in adequate amounts, the size and hemoglobin content of the red blood cells should be normal. Nutritional deficiencies, specific genetic defects, and certain disease conditions interfere with erythropoiesis (red blood cell formation).

Maintenance of an adequate supply of iron The body avidly holds (conserves) iron which has been absorbed. Iron is not excreted in the urine. Only very small quantities of iron are lost when cells are shed from the skin and mucous membranes. Hair contains only a tiny amount of iron. Losses of this sort normally total about 1 mg. daily.

Females in the childbearing years, however, lose iron regularly in the menses. Menstrual losses amount to about 0.5 mg. per day when averaged over a month's time.[5] If the menstrual flow is heavy, iron loss from the menses alone may exceed an average of 1.4 mg. daily. Thus even among menstruating women, need for iron varies considerably.

Blood loss is the major way in which iron can be lost from the body. For many healthy people, blood loss is common. Those who donate blood, whether male or female, lose a significant amount of iron each time they donate (about 250 mg. iron).

Individuals who suffer frequent cuts and scrapes as a result of their occupation also may lose considerable amounts of iron. Persons infested with hookworms lose large amounts of blood daily; this is a common occurrence in many parts of the world.

Twenty to twenty-five mg. of iron are used daily within the body to meet the usual need for synthetic purposes. Five times this much iron can be used in a day if this much iron is available and if there is an increased demand for red blood cells. The amount of iron used can greatly exceed the amount absorbed because iron is continually recycled. Iron is released when erythrocytes and the hemoglobin they contain are broken down. This iron is picked up by a plasma protein called transferrin, the same protein which picks up iron after it is absorbed from the intestinal tract. Transferrin takes iron directly to the bone marrow for red blood cell production or to the liver or other tissues for storage in the form of ferritin.

When bleeding occurs within a tissue, as when a muscle is bruised, iron is not lost from the body[*]; however the rate of production of red blood cells must accelerate to make up for loss of erythrocytes.

It can be very beneficial to have a supply of *stored* iron to use for erythropoiesis following blood loss (hemorrhage). Stored iron can be quickly mobilized for this purpose. A dietary supply of iron is less effective for meeting immediate needs than is stored iron because of the limited capacity to absorb iron.[5]

Epithelial tissue

Epithelial tissue (skin and mucous membranes) serves as a principal means of protecting the body from external injury. Much synthetic activity is required to maintain the skin and mucous membranes since they are rubbed, scraped, bumped, pierced, and generally assaulted in the normal course of daily living. Countless epithelial cells are shed each day even under the best of conditions. Because of the body's remarkable ability to replace lost cells, changes in the skin and mucous membranes are seldom noticed. An adequate nutrient intake supports this high rate of turnover and, thus, allows maintenance of healthy epithelial tissue.

It is not really accurate to single out one or two nutrients as the key elements in maintaining the integrity of the epithelium. Appendix 4G indicates that lack of practically any nutrient is reflected in changes in the skin and/or mucous membranes. After all, many nutrients must work together in any synthetic process. The role of a few nutrients in the formation and maintenance of epithelial tissue are pointed out below, by way of example.

POINTS OF EMPHASIS
Cell formation and proliferation

• *Every essential nutrient may affect cell formation and proliferation either directly or indirectly.*

• *Folic acid and vitamin B_{12} are crucial to proliferation of all types of cells because of their roles in nucleic acid (DNA and RNA) formation.*

• *Linoleic acid is needed for cell proliferation and renewal since it is an integral part of all cell membranes.*

• *Iron is an integral part of the hemoglobin molecule and must, therefore, be available for formation of red blood cells. Many other nutrients participate as well.*

• *Vitamin A allows normal differentiation of epithelial cells in the presence of an adequate supply of other nutrients.*

---

[*] This statement does not hold true if bleeding occurs from mucous membranes, as within the lumen of the intestinal tract.

Vitamin A Vitamin A plays a crucial role in *differentiation* of epithelial cells. The outcome of cell differentiation depends on the amount of vitamin A available. If vitamin A is lacking, the cells are apt to take on an abnormal shape (such as squamous cells instead of goblet cells). Vitamin A permits the formation of smooth skin and moist, healthy mucous membranes.

Linoleic acid Linoleic acid facilitates the maintenance of smooth, healthy skin which is impermeable to water.[6]

REPAIR AND PROTECTIVE MECHANISMS

The body has a number of means of protecting itself from injury and disease and of repairing damage to cells and tissues. Those repair and protective mechanisms most closely tied to nutritional status are now discussed. They include barriers to injury and to entry of antigens (foreign materials), prevention of blood loss, wound healing, and immunological competence.

BARRIERS TO INJURY AND ANTIGENS

The first barriers to the entry of antigens include (1) physical integrity of the skin and mucous membranes, (2) the layer of mucus, and (3) specific mucosal immunity. Any nutrients essential to the building and maintenance of epithelial tissues and to their secretory function, therefore, are important for resistance to injury and penetration by foreign materials.

Vitamin A comes to mind immediately because of its role in epithelial tissue formation. In fact, vitamin A has sometimes been called an "anti-infective" vitamin. This label is misleading, however, since extra vitamin A does not confer extra resistance to infection.

PREVENTION OF BLOOD LOSS

A complex series of reactions must quickly take place to prevent excessive blood loss should injury cause a blood vessel to be severed. An adequate supply of specific nutrients must be available for this process. Very shortly after the blood vessel is injured, blood platelets aggregate in an attempt to plug the opening. A normal *supply* of blood platelets requires adequate dietary intake of iron.[7] Studies suggest that *activity* of blood platelets requires vitamins A and C. The next step in staunching the flow of blood is clot formation.

Blood coagulation Blood coagulation is a complex process which must be carefully regulated in the body so that it will occur only at appropriate times. The factors needed for blood coagulation must all be present in the blood, ready to act in emergency situations.

Vitamin K acts to regulate hepatic synthesis of four blood clotting proteins, the most well known of which is prothrombin.[8] By promoting normal blood levels of these clotting factors, vitamin K promotes a normal blood coagulation time. For this reason vitamin K is sometimes called the antihemorrhagic vitamin. Unlike other fat-soluble vitamins, little vitamin K is stored in the body. For this reason any interference with vitamin K nutrition will quickly be followed by interference with blood coagulation. It is important to remember that lack of vitamin K is not the only cause of bleeding tendencies.

Calcium is also required for blood coagulation. It apparently binds to prothrombin, allowing formation of the enzyme thrombin. Calcium also acts in the formation of fibrin threads, which make up the clot.

WOUND HEALING

Permanent closure of a wound is necessary to restore the protective barrier of the skin and to permit rejoining of other injured tissues. A key element of this wound healing process is collagen, that cementing substance previously mentioned.

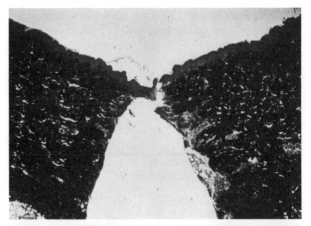

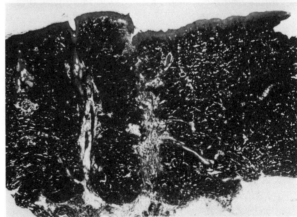

FIGURE 16.2. Role of vitamin C in wound healing. *Above,* Biopsy 10 days after a wound was made in a man who had not consumed any vitamin C for 6 months: no healing is evident except of the epithelium (gap in tissues was filled with a blood clot). *Below,* After 10 days of treatment with vitamin C, another biopsy of the wound shows healing with abundant collagen formation. (From *The Vitamin Manual.* Upjohn Co., Kalamazoo)

It has long been known that ascorbic acid is needed to promote normal healing of wounds. It does this by promoting the formation of collagen. The role of vitamin C in wound healing is illustrated in Figure 16.2. An adequate supply of amino acids from dietary protein and an adequate caloric intake promote the healing process. Recently it has been found that normal levels of zinc facilitate wound healing and that other trace elements and linoleic acid are also involved.[9] Certainly a broad spectrum of nutrients is needed for such a complex process.

IMMUNOLOGICAL COMPETENCE

Immunological competence is the ability of the body to detect and respond appropriately to microorganisms and other foreign materials which have managed to penetrate the body. If the immune system is competent, an array of cells and chemical substances collaborate in destroying and ridding the body of the "enemy." A well-nourished individual is likely to have powerful immunological defenses but will not necessarily be able to withstand any and all assaults.

There are two general types of immunity: humoral and cell-mediated. Humoral immunity arises primarily from B lymphocytes (the specialized white blood cells which produce antibodies). T lymphocytes are the white blood cells responsible for cell-mediated immunity (CMI), sometimes called delayed hypersensitivity or cellular immunity.

POINTS OF EMPHASIS
Repair and protective mechanisms

• *An adequate supply of all essential nutrients is necessary for protecting the body from injury and illness and for repairing any type of tissue damage.*

• *Nutrients are involved in several of the steps necessary to prevent blood loss. Blood coagulation itself requires vitamin K for prothrombin formation and calcium for thrombin and fibrin formation.*

• *Wound healing is a specialized process which requires a good supply of vitamin C and zinc.*

• *Wound healing involves renewal of cells and, therefore, makes use of a full range of nutrients.*

• *Immunological competence involves both humoral and cell-mediated immunity (CMI). CMI, in particular, requires an adequate supply of nutrients.*

The ability to make most immunoglobulins tends to be retained even if the diet lacks protein and calories. However, normal production of another protective humoral substance called complement appears to depend on adequate nutrient intake.[10, 11] T lymphocyte production is reported to be sensitive to nutritional status.[12-14] Thus a loss of ability to defend against cancer cells, viruses, and slowly developing bacteria may accompany malnutrition, especially protein-energy malnutrition.

Other aspects of immunological function have been found to depend on adequate nutrient intake and absorption. The ability of leukocytes to destroy organisms (bactericidal activity) is diminished by malnutrition.[15] Malnutrition may result in decreased production of interferon, a protein that inhibits replication of viruses.[16] It appears that iron nutrition affects resistance to infection; the relationship is complex. Bacteria sometimes grow better when more free iron is available to them,[17] but consuming recommended amounts of iron may positively affect an individual's defense mechanisms.[18,19]

ROLE OF NUTRIENTS IN VISION

Nutrients are intimately involved in maintenance of vision. Vision is dependent on the structure of the eye and on specific chemical reactions which allow messages to be sent to the brain. The effectiveness of vision depends to a great extent on genetic factors, but an adequate intake of vitamin A, or its precursor carotene, is required for achieving ones genetic potential. Thus the common expression "Eat your carrots— they'll help you see better," although inaccurate, is not without truth.

Vitamin A is directly involved in chemical reactions required for the visual process and is essential to the integrity of the eye.

Visual process   Vision involves (1) photoreceptor (light receiving) systems, called cones, which perceive high intensity light and color and (2) rods, which perceive low intensity illumination. Vitamin A participes in both of these systems, but its effect is most noticeable with regard to functioning of the rods.

The rods contain a pigment called rhodopsin or visual purple. Rhodopsin is made up of a specific protein and a chemical form of vitamin A called retinal. A supply of vitamin A is necessary to maintain dark adaptation (normal vision in dim light following exposure to bright light). Lack of dark adaptation, commonly called night blindness, is an early indication that the dietary intake of vitamin A is inadequate.

Integrity of the eye   Mucous secretions, distributed by blinking, keep the conjunctiva (the mucous membrane lining the eyelids and the exposed portion of the eyeball) moist and clean. Since vitamin A is essential for both secretory function and normal growth of epithelial cells, this fat-soluble vitamin helps maintain the integrity of the eye. Thickening, drying, and more

TABLE 16.1 *Factors influencing recommended intake of energy nutrients and water*

NUTRIENT	FACTORS INFLUENCING AMOUNT NEEDED BY HEALTHY INDIVIDUALS*	COMMENTS
Protein	Need somewhat smaller than RDA if biological value of the protein is high rather than intermediate Inadequate caloric intake increases the protein requirement If very heavy physical activity results in profuse sweating, need for protein increases somewhat; otherwise exercise has little effect	RDA is based on 0.8 gm/kg of desirable adult body weight. Adjustments for protein quality are unnecessary for adults, since this RDA assumes that efficiency of utilization is relatively low Typical American diets contain more than the RDA for protein. (A diet which just meets the RDA for protein is viewed as restrictive)
Carbohydrate	Increased energy expenditure increases need	A minimum of 50 to 100 gm daily is recommended to avoid ketosis and other undesirable metabolic responses
Fat	Increased energy expenditure increases need	15 to 25 gm of appropriate food fats can meet minimum need (See linoleic acid, Table 16.4)
Water	Physical activity, a high environmental temperature, and/or a high renal solute load can greatly increase need. Kidneys conserve water if necessary	Thirst is ordinarily a good guide to need. In extreme situations thirst may not stimulate adequate intake

References for this table are listed at the end of chapter references.
* In all cases, need is increased by growth (including pregnancy), lactation, and by increased (non-obese) body size.

serious changes occur in the conjunctiva when vitamin A intake is inadequate.

Riboflavin is another vitamin which is essential to the integrity of the eye, the cornea in particular. A number of eye complaints, including photophobia, de-velop after a prolonged dietary lack of riboflavin, a B vitamin.

Zinc is normally present in high concentration in the retina of the eye and appears to be necessary for normal visual function.[20]

TABLE 16.2 *Factors influencing recommended intake of nutrient electrolytes*

NUTRIENT	FACTORS INFLUENCING AMOUNT NEEDED BY HEALTHY INDIVIDUALS*	COMMENTS
Sodium	Kidneys conserve sodium if necessary Perspiration increases requirement	Usual dietary intake is 2.5 to 7 gm or more If fluid intake exceeds 4 L. per day due to heavy sweating, increase salt (sodium chloride) intake by 2 gm (about ½ tsp) for each additional L of water
Chloride	Losses usually parallel sodium losses	Intake usually ranges between 4.9 and 21 gm daily[2]
Potassium	Kidneys' ability to conserve potassium is limited Low carbohydrate or low calorie diets may accelerate loss Profuse sweating increases losses[1]	A diet which overemphasizes highly processed foods may be low in potassium Deficiency may develop during fasting, on low carbohydrate or low calorie diets, or due to strenuous physical activity in hot weather. Supplemental potassium may be recommended
Calcium and Phosphorus	A low protein intake may reduce the calcium requirement Vitamin D is needed to promote calcium absorption Bioavailability of these minerals differs in different foods	RDA assumes protein intake is high Phosphorus intake usually exceeds calcium intake, especially if foods high in phosphate additives are used Concern has been expressed that calcium-phosphorus imbalance may contribute to development of osteoporosis[3,4] Vitamin D may help offset an imbalanced intake[4]
Magnesium	Need may be influenced by intake and utilization of calcium and phosphorus Heavy alcohol use increases requirement	American diets may be low in magnesium compared to RDA,[5] especially if low in calories[6] or if they overemphasize highly refined food

References for this table are listed at the end of chapter references.
* In all cases, need is increased by growth (including pregnancy), lactation, and by increased (non-obese) body size.

TABLE 16.3 *Factors influencing recommended intake of water-soluble vitamins*

NUTRIENT	*FACTORS INFLUENCING AMOUNT NEEDED BY HEALTHY INDIVIDUALS**	*COMMENTS*
C (ascorbic acid)	Cigarette smoking appears to decrease absorption in proportion to the number of cigarettes smoked (serum vitamin C levels of smokers may be reduced 25 to 40%[7])	RDA allows maintenance of a body pool which is at or near its maximum[8] Some nutrition experts recommend that all individuals exceed the RDA for vitamin C to achieve tissue saturation Smoking habits were not considered when RDA was established
B_1 (thiamine)	Increased energy utilization increases requirement	Intake is likely to fall below RDA if diet is high in "empty calories" (e.g., alcohol, sugar) Few unfortified foods are excellent sources of thiamine
B_2 (riboflavin)		Intake may be low relative to the RDA if products from the milk group are not used
Niacin	Increased energy utilization increases requirement High protein intake reduces requirement Niacin can be synthesized from tryptophan, an essential amino acid	Typical American diets are so high in protein that deficiency is unlikely
B_6 (pyridoxine, -al, -amine)	Requirement increases with increasing protein intake Requirement may increase with use of oral contraceptive agents	RDA assumes protein intake is high. Most high protein foods are good sources of B_6
B_{12} (cyanocobalamin)	Lack of intrinsic factor (a substance normally produced by the stomach) prevents intestinal absorption	Customary intake by meat eaters is higher than RDA Vegans are susceptible to deficiency unless they use a B_{12} supplement
Folacin	Bioavailability of folacin varies in different foods Requirement may increase with use of oral contraceptive agents	If pure forms of folic acid are used, recommended intake is only about a fourth as high. The Food and Nutrition Board of the National Research Council has stated that intake of 300 μg folacin daily is ample for meeting usual needs[9] Improper handling of food may lead to serious losses of folacin, thus increasing the chance of inadequate intake

References for this table are listed at the end of chapter references.
* In all cases, need is increased by growth (including pregnancy), lactation, and by increased (non-obese) body size.

TABLE 16.4 *Factors influencing recommended intake of fat-soluble vitamins and linoleic acid*

NUTRIENT	*FACTORS INFLUENCING AMOUNT NEEDED BY HEALTHY INDIVIDUALS**	*COMMENTS*
A (retinol), precursor: carotene	Proportion of retinol and carotene affects amount needed (bioavailability of carotene is lower than that of retinol) Stores in liver reduce need for a daily supply	RDA allows for some storage of the vitamin in the liver. Significant fractions of the American (and world) population have low liver stores[2] Excessive intake is potentially harmful
D (calciferol)	Exposure to sunshine decreases need for dietary supply Stores in liver reduce need for a daily supply	Adults who are not regularly exposed to the sun should have a dietary supply Excessive intake is potentially harmful
E (tocopherol)	Need for vitamin E relates to polyunsaturated fatty acid intake (i.e., low when diet is consistently low in fat) High need for vitamin E persists for a while if polyunsaturated fat intake is sharply reduced; vitamin E supplements may be recommended[2]	RDA assumes moderate intake of polyunsaturated fat Evidence indicates that the American population ingests sufficient vitamin E[2]
K	Synthesis by bacteria in intestinal tract provides much of adult need Fasting or use of broad spectrum antibiotics may decrease this source	Deficiency in adults rare except in disease conditions or with certain types of drug therapy It is recommended that newborn infants be given vitamin K intramuscularly to prevent hemorrhage due to vitamin K deficiency (They initially have no supply from intestinal synthesis)
Linoleic acid	Stores in adipose tissue reduce need for a daily supply	Deficiency in adults has been seen only with intravenous feeding

References for this table are listed at the end of chapter references.
* In all cases, need is increased by growth (including pregnancy), lactation, and by increased (non-obese) body size.

TABLE 16.5 *Factors influencing recommended intake of trace elements*

NUTRIENT	FACTORS INFLUENCING AMOUNT NEEDED BY HEALTHY INDIVIDUALS*	COMMENTS
Iron	Amount needed by women varies according to menstrual losses, i.e., need is greater if menstrual flow is heavy, as for some women who use IUDs (intrauterine devices) Other forms of blood loss increase need (e.g., donating blood 5 times a year increases average need by 3 to 4 mg daily, and occult (invisible) bleeding within the GI tract due to aspirin use increases need) Improved iron absorption follows blood loss of any kind, making it difficult to predict how much extra dietary iron is needed to compensate for losses Bioavailability varies greatly; less is needed if iron is supplied by meat rather than by plant foods	Significant incidence of deficiency is reported in surveyed populations 18 mg/day for menstruating women allows for storage to help meet needs of pregnancy Stored iron is definitely an asset following blood loss since limited ability to absorb iron limits supply of iron for production of hemoglobin Meat, fish, poultry, and/or vitamin C improve the absorption of nonheme-iron
Iodine	Need increases with increased need for thyroid hormones	Intake in the U.S. is highly variable and difficult to estimate Incidence of iodine deficiency has dropped to very low levels in the U.S.
Zinc	Bioavailability varies widely; less is needed if zinc is supplied by meat rather than by unleavened whole grain products	Diets low to moderate in calories may fall well below RDA for zinc[10-12] Children from low socioeconomic backgrounds in America have been reported to have physical and biochemical indications of zinc deficiency[13] Intake by vegans is apt to be lower than RDA
Copper, chromium, manganese, others	Bioavailability varies widely. Intake of one trace metal may be influenced by intake of other trace minerals or other nutrients	Adequate intake is most likely if a variety of lightly processed foods are chosen from the four food groups

References for this table are listed at the end of chapter references.
* In all cases, need is increased by growth (including pregnancy), lactation, and by increased (non-obese) body size.

STUDY QUESTIONS

1. How is the amino acid pool maintained in the absence of a dietary supply of amino acids (protein)?
2. A healthy adult who regularly eats a high protein diet is likely to be in what type of nitrogen balance? A pregnant woman who meets her nutrient requirements is likely to be in what type of nitrogen balance?
3. Name several nutrients essential to normal bone formation even though they do not contribute to the structure of bone.
4. When are adults likely to be in negative calcium balance?
5. In what ways does linoleic acid contribute to the integrity of cells?
6. Why is it better to have a supply of stored iron than to depend on iron supplements when you need to replace blood lost as a result of hemorrhage?
7. Some people say that vitamin A is an anti-infective vitamin and that it also gives you good vision. What is correct and what is misleading about these statements?

References

1. Review. Relation of zinc to calcium in bone. *Nutr. Rev.* 34:294, 1976.
2. ——— Magnesium in human nutrition. *Dairy Counc. Dig.* 42(2):7, 1971.
3. Vergroesen, A. J.: Physiological effects of dietary linoleic acid. *Nutr. Rev.* 35:1. 1977.
4. Elin, R., and Alling, D. W.: Survival of normal and magnesium-deficient erythrocytes in rats: Effect of magnesium-deficient diet versus splenectomy. *J. Lab Clin. Med.* 91:666, 1978.
5. Finch, C. A.: Iron metabolism. *Nutr. Today* 4(2):2, 1969.
6. Review. Essential fatty acids and water permeability of the skin. *Nutr. Rev.* 35:303, 1977.
7. Review. The relation of iron to blood platelets. *Nutr. Rev.* 34:25, 1976.
8. Review. The functional significance of vitamin K action. *Nutr. Rev.* 34:182, 1976.
9. Briggaman, R. A., and Crounse, R. G.: Skin. In H. A. Schneider, C. E. Anderson, and D. B. Coursin (eds.): *Nutritional Support of Medical Practice.* Hagerstown MD: Harper & Row, 1977, p. 268.
10. Review. Immune deficiency in malnutrition. *Nutr. Rev.* 33:334, 1976.
11. Suskind, R., et al.: Complement activity in children with protein-calorie malnutrition. *Am. J. Clin. Nutr.* 29:1089, 1976.
12. Review. Lymphocyte function in malnutrition. *Nutr. Rev.* 33:110, 1975.
13. Review. Immunocompetence in adult malnutrition. *Nutr. Rev.* 32:201, 1974.
14. Review. Lymphocyte number and function in protein malnutrition. *Nutr. Rev.* 34:208, 1976.
15. Review. Nutrition and the body's defense mechanism. *Nutr. Rev.* 31:115, 1973.
16. Schlesinger, L., et al.: Decreased interferon production by leukocytes in marasmus. *Am. J. Clin. Nutr.* 29:758, 1976.

17. Review. Mucocutaneous fungal lesions and iron deficiency. *Nutr. Rev.* 34:203, 1976.

18. Chandra, R. K.: Iron and immunocompetence. *Nutr. Rev.* 34:129, 1976.

19. Review. The relationship between infection and the iron status of an individual. *Nutr. Rev.* 33:103, 1975.

20. Prasad, A. S.: Nutritional aspects of zinc. *Diet. Currents* 4(5):27, 1977.

References—Tables 16.1 through 16.5

1. Lane, H. W., and Cerda, J. J.: Potassium requirements and exercise. *J. Am. Diet. Assoc.* 73:64, 1978.

2. *Recommended Dietary Allowances,* ed. 8. Food and Nutrition Board, National Research Council. Washington DC: National Academy of Sciences, 1974.

3. Bell, R. R., et al.: Physiological responses of human adults to products containing phosphate additives. *J. Clin. Nutr.* 107:42, 1977.

4. Raper, N. R.: Calcium and phosphorus: Dietary concerns. *Nutr. Program News.* USDA Washington DC, Jan.–Apr. 1977.

5. Marshall, M. W., et al.: Composition of diets containing 25 and 35 percent calories from fat. *J. Am. Diet. Assoc.* 66:470, 1975.

6. Ohlson, M. A., and Harper, L. J.: Longitudinal studies of food intake and weight of women from ages 18 to 56. *J. Am. Diet. Assoc.* 69:626, 1976.

7. Pelletier, O.: Vitamin C and cigarette smokers. *Ann. N.Y. Acad. Sci.* 258:156, 1975.

8. Hodges, R. E., and Baker, E. M.: Ascorbic acid. In R. S. Goodhart and M. E. Shils (eds.): *Modern Nutrition in Health and Disease,* Philadelphia: Lea & Febiger, 1973.

9. *Folic Acid: Biochemistry and Physiology in Relation to the Human Nutrition Requirement.* Food and Nutrition Board, National Academy of Sciences. Washington DC: National Academy of Sciences, 1977.

10. White, H. S.: Zinc content and the zinc-to-calorie ratio of weighed diets. *J. Am. Diet. Assoc.* 68:243, 1976.

11. Greger, J. L., and Sciscoe, B. S.: Zinc nutriture of elderly participants in an urban feeding program. *J. Am. Diet. Assoc.* 70:37, 1977.

12. Sandstead, H. H.: Zinc nutrition in the United States. *Am. J. Clin. Nutr.* 26:1251, 1973.

13. Hambidge, K. M., et al.: Zinc nutrition of preschool children in the Denver Head Start program. *Am. J. Clin. Nutr.* 29:734, 1976.

17

The role of nutrients in dental health

Nutrition plays a key role in the development and maintenance of strong healthy teeth and gums. Attention to nutrition and to oral health measures is beneficial to all of the oral structures. It can significantly decrease the incidence of dental caries and periodontal disease, both of which are painful destructive diseases of the teeth and their surrounding structures. In the case of oral health, sound nutrition means much more than just meeting nutrient requirements. It means practicing sound eating habits which promote and maintain the integrity and optimal functioning of all the structures in the oral cavity.

The oral cavity consists of teeth, gums (gingival tissue), tongue with taste buds, palate, salivary glands, mucous membranes, and the alevolar (jaw) bones. When these structures are functioning together in an optimal manner an individual can comfortably ingest food to supply his body with nutrients. The integrity of each tissue in the oral cavity is partially dependent on (1) the health of each of the other oral tissues and (2) the normal functioning of the mouth. For example, chewing stimulates salivation; saliva participates in remineralization of tooth enamel; and intact teeth facilitate chewing. Even the trace minerals zinc and copper may have an indirect effect on oral health. A normal sense of taste depends on an adequate supply of zinc and copper.

Adequate nutrition is important to promote and maintain the integrity of the oral structures for two reasons: (1) the turnover of the cells in the oral cavity is rapid, except for those comprising teeth and alveolar bone, and (2) the oral cavity is continuously exposed to a variety of mechanical, thermal, chemical, and microbiological stresses because of its location and function. Nutrients exert both a *local* and a *systemic* effect on oral structures. Nutrients supplied systemically are important in tooth formation and in the development, maintenance, and repair of other oral tissues. Nutrients in food and saliva exert a local or topical influence on oral tissues when they pass through the mouth.

Teeth

Teeth are composed of the hardest material in the body. Each tooth has a crown which protrudes through the gum into the oral cavity and a root which fits into the bony socket of the jaw. Teeth consist of one highly vascular tissue and three calcified tissues: (1) dental pulp, (2) dentin, (3) enamel, and (4) cementum, as illustrated in Figure 17.1.

The main body of both the root and crown of a tooth is composed of *dentin*. Dentin is similar to bone in composition. It consists primarily of a calcified protein

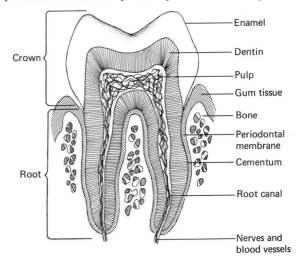

FIGURE 17.1. Cross section of a normal tooth and its supporting tissue.

matrix and hydroxyapatite crystals. The hydroxyapatite crystals form prisms which increase the tooth's ability to endure the mechanical stresses of chewing and biting. Dentin is traversed with dentin tubules. These tubules radiate from the dental pulp to the junction of the dentin and tooth enamel. Dentin does not have a direct blood supply and does not remodel as bone does. However, some limited systemic exchange of nutrients probably occurs via the dentin tubules.

Enamel covers the crown of the tooth and is the hardest, most dense of the calcified tissues. Enamel also contains hydroxyapatite crystals which contribute to its strength and make it resistant to breakdown by enzymes and other corrosive agents. Enamel does not have a direct systemic contact with the body's internal environment.

Cementum, the most bone-like of the calcified tissued, covers the root portion of the dentin. The periodontal ligament, which is composed of collagen fibers, passes from the jaw bone into the cementum to hold the tooth in place.

Inside each tooth is *dental pulp*, a soft connective tissue that contains blood vessels, lymphatics, and nerves.

Each person has two sets of teeth during a lifetime, a primary (temporary) set and a permanent set. Although specific teeth do not appear for months or years after birth, they begin to form shortly after conception. The primary teeth, also called deciduous or baby teeth, begin to form between the sixth and eighth weeks of gestation. The permanent teeth begin to form later, at about 30 weeks of gestation.

The first primary teeth usually begin to emerge from the gum about the sixth month of life; all 20 primary teeth erupt by about age 2. Between ages 6 and 12 years the roots of primary teeth are reabsorbed and the teeth are shed. Permanent teeth replace each of the primary teeth and an additional 8 to 12 molars also develop. The 28 to 32 permanent teeth are fully erupted by approximately 18 to 21 years of life.

Periodontium

Periodontium is a general term used to describe structures surrounding teeth, namely, cementum, periodontal ligament, alveolar bone, and gingiva. These structures support the teeth and hold them firmly in place.

NUTRIENTS AND ORAL HEALTH

Some of the ways nutrients affect oral health are similar to those seen in other tissues. The roles of nutrients in growth, maintenance, and repair of alveolar bone are similar to their roles in relation to other bones of the body.

Vitamin C is important for collagen formation in the gingival tissue and oral mucosa. In general, a balanced varied diet promotes development and maintenance of healthy oral tissues.

Prior to eruption a tooth has contact with the body's internal environment through vascular and neural pathways. Pre-eruptively, nutrients provided via systemic routes critically influence tooth development. When a tooth erupts in the oral cavity, several changes occur in the tooth's environment. The blood and nerve supply to the dentin and enamel of a tooth is severed. After eruption a tooth does not have a systemic source of nutrients to repair major structural defects which might have occurred during development or to repair damage caused by injury.

Upon eruption, a tooth is exposed to a new environment, the oral cavity. Contents of the oral cavity such as saliva, food, fluids, and other substances exert local effects on the teeth. Normally the tooth's enamel is continuously bathed in saliva. Evidence suggests that there is an exchange of nutrients, particularly minerals, between the enamel and the saliva.[1] Mineral exchange between saliva and enamel upon tooth eruption may contribute to the enamel's resistance to tooth decay. For this and for other reasons adequate saliva production is essential to maintain integrity of teeth as well as other oral structures.

Laboratory studies have shown that the type of food in the oral cavity after teeth erupt may affect the enamel. A high intake of cariogenic (decay promoting) carbohydrates at this time interferes with tooth mineralization and decreases the tooth's resistance to decay.[2]

Ingesting food promotes sucking, chewing, and muscular activity, all of which influence the direction in which developing teeth erupt. These activities contribute to alignment of the jaws. Proper alignment of teeth and jaws is essential for their optimal functioning.

Tooth development

Oral tissues undergo the same stages of growth as other tissues and organs in the body. The systemic influence of nutrients is most important in utero and in early and middle childhood before teeth have erupted.

There is still little concrete evidence identifying the specific effects of a mother's nutritional state on tooth development in a fetus. In many instances deficiencies must be severe before obvious changes in tooth formation are noted. However, slight deficiencies may cause subtle changes in structural integrity, leaving the erupted teeth more vulnerable to decay. During pregnancy, nutritional deficiencies at critical periods of tissue growth are probably a factor in the development of cleft lip, cleft palate, or other congenital anomalies of oral tissues.

Some nutrients are particularly involved in promoting the development of healthy teeth. During the initial stage of tooth development a matrix of protein is laid down. The matrix is gradually calcified. During matrix formation there is a need for collagen-forming nutrients such as protein and vitamin C. Calcium, phosphorus, and vitamin D are other nutrients needed during the initial period of calcification. Fluoride functions mainly during the period of final crystallization and maturation of tooth enamel. The integrity of the tooth enamel is enhanced by the presence of fluoride. Fluoride seems to strengthen enamel by promoting the conversion of hydroxyapatite to fluorapatite crystals. The fine, stable fluorapatite crystals are more resistant to the action of microbial acids than are hydroxyapatite crystals.

The dentin and enamel of teeth develop from epithelial tissue. Thus vitamin A and other nutrients participating in epithelial tissue formation contribute to tooth formation. Young children whose diets are severely lacking in vitamin A and other nutrients have been noted to have tooth malformations.[3]

After a tooth has erupted, the presence of some nutrients in the oral cavity is beneficial while the presence of other nutrients may actually be harmful. This becomes more apparent when related to disorders commonly occurring within the oral cavity.

POINTS OF EMPHASIS
Nutrition and oral health

- *The integrity of the oral cavity is promoted when all its structures are functioning together in an optimal manner.*
- *An adequate supply of nutrients and sound eating habits promote oral health.*
- *Nutrients affect teeth both before and after eruption.*
- *Nutrients exert a systemic effect on teeth before they erupt. After eruption only dental pulp maintains direct systemic contact with the body.*
- *Upon eruption the contents of the oral cavity (including nutrients) exert a local effect on teeth. Local effects may be helpful or harmful.*

Dental caries

Dental caries, an infectious disease frequently called tooth decay, is characterized by localized destruction of the enamel and dentin of teeth. The term *rampant caries* means that caries are numerous and worsen rapidly. If the caries process is not arrested, bacteria may invade the dental pulp and form an abscess (a pocket of infection). Dental caries constitute a major public health problem, particularly in children and young adults. It has been estimated that the annual cost of treating dental caries in the U.S. exceeds 2 billion dollars.[4] Untreated tooth decay causes pain, tooth loss, malalignment, malocclusion, and an unsightly appearance. Missing or malaligned teeth may contribute to the development of speech defects in young

children. An individual with rampant dental caries may develop nutritional deficiencies if pain keeps him from chewing and ingesting adequate amounts and kinds of food. It is certainly less painful and more economical to prevent dental caries than it is to treat them.

The process of tooth decay involves demineralization of the outer surface of the tooth by organic acids. These acids are produced by fermentative action of bacteria in dental plaque. Dental plaque is generally considered to be a sticky, colorless, gelatinous material which is very densely populated by bacteria. Plaque adheres to the surface of teeth and can only be removed by mechanical cleansing.

The initiation of caries depends on the interaction of several factors, including (1) a susceptible host, (2) cariogenic bacteria, (3) a suitable substrate for bacterial action, and (4) a sufficient period of time.

The integrity of a host (tooth) and its susceptibility to tooth decay are influenced by many factors. Nutrition certainly plays a significant role. Probably the single most effective nutrient for prevention of dental caries is fluoride. Foods rich in proteins and phosphates also may have a cariostatic (decay retarding) influence on teeth. Genetic factors and environmental stressors may increase or decrease a host's susceptibility to decay.

Cariogenic plaque bacteria produce lactic and other acids when they are supplied with a suitable substrate, such as sugar. These acids lower the pH of the plaque. When the pH drops to 5.5 or less, demineralization of susceptible tooth enamel begins. The longer the pH remains low, the greater the demineralization is. Demineralization allows proteolytic (protein decomposing) bacteria to invade the dentin and destroy it.

The nutrients a person ingests influence the types of bacteria present in the oral cavity, their proliferation in dental plaque, and the resistance of teeth to decay.

Fermentable carbohydrates are the necessary substrate for the development of dental caries. Sucrose has been identified as the most cariogenic carbohydrate. Other sugars such as fructose, lactose, and glucose support the growth of cariogenic bacteria. Complex carbohydrates such as starch are less cariogenic.

Sugars are present in many different foods. The most obvious sources are refined sugar (table sugar), corn syrup, honey, molasses, and dextrose. It is important to note that these sugars appear in a wide assortment of food products. Prepared foods such as candies, sweet baked goods, and soft drinks contain a high percent of sugar. Less obvious is the high sugar content in many ready-to-eat breakfast cereals, catsup, canned and frozen fruits, noncarbonated soft drinks, fruit yogurt, and many other highly processed foods.

Some "natural" foods are potentially cariogenic, especially foods like honey, sweetened granola, and dried fruits. Even fresh fruits and vegetables contain sugar in varying amounts. However, fresh fruits and vegetables are low in cariogenicity.

The frequency and form of carbohydrate ingestion affect the time required for oral clearance, that is, for food to be completely removed from the mouth. It takes approximately 20 minutes after food is cleared from the mouth for the acidic pH of dental plaque to return to neutral. This means *each time* a sugar-containing food is ingested teeth may be exposed to decalcifying acids for 20 minutes or longer. Figure 17.2 shows two graphs: one depicts the pattern of acid production when three daily meals are eaten without snacks; the other shows the pattern of acid production when three small snacks are eaten in addition to three daily meals.

Brushing the teeth immediately following a meal or snack is an effective way to clear the mouth rapidly. Foods having a long oral clearance time are more cariogenic than those rapidly cleared from the mouth. Children who suck lollipops or sip soft drinks expose their teeth to sucrose for a long time. The greater a food's stickiness, the longer the oral clearance time and the greater the cariogenicity. Sticky solids such as dates, raisins, or caramels adhere to the surfaces of teeth and remain in cracks and crevices of teeth for a long period of time. On the other hand, fibrous foods such as raw fruits and vegetables have a short oral clearance time and exert a natural cleansing activity by promoting the flow of saliva as they are chewed. Raw apples, for example, contain sugar but are not very cariogenic since chewing the fiber in them helps to clear sugar and food debris from the mouth. This partially explains why fresh fruits such as grapes and plums are less cariogenic than their dried counterparts, raisins and prunes.

Sugar eaten between meals in the form of a snack or dessert probably remains in the mouth longer than sugar ingested with meals. At mealtime the mechanical action provided by chewing foods such as meat and vegetables may serve to clean the teeth. Liquids taken with a meal probably help to wash sticky carbohydrates away from teeth. Also brushing is more commonly practiced after meals than after snacks.

Limiting both the amount and frequency of cariogenic carbohydrate ingestion has been shown to decrease the incidence of dental caries. From the standpoint of dental health it is better for a child to eat a bowl of presweetened cereal with milk for breakfast than to munch on the same cereal throughout the morning. It is better still for children to eat unsweetened cereals. A list of relatively noncariogenic snack foods is presented on page 91.

Nutritive sugar substitutes such as sorbitol, mannitol, and xylitol are being used in "sugarless" products such as gum and candy. Although they taste sweet, they are less readily fermented by plaque bacteria than are the previously named sugars. Initial evidence suggests that xylitol has anticariogenic properties.[5]

NURSING-BOTTLE SYNDROME

The relationship between the length of tooth exposure to carbohydrates and destruction of the teeth is vividly seen in children with nursing-bottle syndrome. This condition is characterized by rapid extensive loss of the upper deciduous teeth and occasional loss of the lower molars as pictured in Figure 17.3. This extensive tooth destruction occurs in some young children (18 months to 4 years) who are fed carbohydrate-containing beverages in a nursing bottle. A child who drinks from a bottle at bedtime and naptime is particularly at risk of developing the nursing-bottle syndrome. A baby who is drowsy or asleep seldom sucks and swallows; his saliva flow is minimal. The sugar-containing solution remains in contact with the teeth for long periods of time.

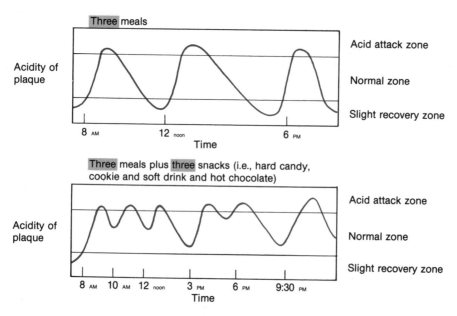

FIGURE 17.2. Pattern of plaque acid production after eating. (Adapted from Truuvert: How to avoid the high cost of dental work. *J. Can. Dental Assoc.* 39:779, 1973.)

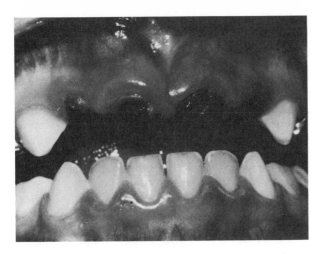

FIGURE 17.3. A child with tooth loss (upper incisors) resulting from "nursing bottle syndrome." The lower teeth are as yet relatively unaffected. (From Fomon, S. J.: *Infant Nutrition.* Philadelphia: W. B. Saunders Co., 1974, with permission.)

While the tongue offers some protection to the lower incisors, the upper incisors are bathed in cariogenic liquid and, thus, are vulnerable to caries formation. Beverages such as noncarbonated soft drinks, sweetened fruit drinks, and infant formulas containing sucrose and corn syrup are of more concern than are plain milk or formula sweetened with lactose. Some research has indicated that lactose, the sugar in milk, is not particularly cariogenic. In fact, milk and milk-saliva mixtures may prevent decalcification of enamel.[6]

POINTS OF EMPHASIS
Dental caries

• *Dental caries is a major public health problem.*
• *Severe dental caries may interfere with adequate food intake.*
• *Caries process is initiated by the formation of acid in dental plaque, a gelatinous material comprised primarily of bacteria.*
• *Acid production occurs when fermentable carbohydrates are eaten.*
• *The longer food remains in the mouth, the longer teeth are exposed to decay-producing acids.*
• *Some foods, such as raw fruits and vegetables, are less cariogenic than others, such as candy, cake, and soft drinks.*
• *Parent education can help prevent nursing-bottle caries, rapid extensive decay, and loss of teeth in early childhood.*

Nursing-bottle caries are preventable. Parents who are aware of the problem and its cause can take several steps to prevent its occurrence. Parents can be encouraged to use a nursing bottle only to provide food (infant formula, unsweetened juices, and water) when the in-fant is awake and actively sucking. This assures that the oral clearance time will be fairly rapid. Parents also can be discouraged from (1) offering cariogenic beverages in a nursing bottle and (2) offering a bottle as a pacifier at bedtime or naptime. If parents cannot be dissuaded from offering a bottle at these times, then only water should be used. Toward the end of the first year a baby can be gradually weaned from a bottle to a cup.

Periodontal disease

Periodontal disease, an inflammatory process involving the supporting structures of teeth, affects about three fourth of the world's population. Periodontal disease rather than tooth decay is a major cause of tooth loss in middle age; the disease, however, often begins in adolescence.[7] In some cases periodontal disease is the result of an infectious process. In most cases, however, the exact cause of the inflammatory process is not clear. Local irritants probably play a role. When the teeth are not cleansed properly, dental plaque begins to harden, forming a material called calculus or tartar on teeth. The calculus, if not removed, continues to accumulate, particularly near the gum line. Calculus may extend toward the roots of the teeth, forming pockets between teeth and the gums. Plaque, food, and other debris collect in the pockets and irritate the gum tissue. The ensuing inflammation of the gums is a form of gingivitis. Initially the only indication of this painless process is bleeding and a reddish, slightly swollen, appearance of the gum tissue. If allowed to progress, the inflammation gradually spreads to the bone and other supporting structures of the teeth. Bone loss may occur and the fibers holding the teeth in place may become infected. Teeth loosen and are eventually lost.

The type of food an individual ingests has been shown to influence the amount and composition of plaque and calculus. It is also likely that systemic factors, including hormonal and nutritional status, play a role in the development of periodontal disease. The results of one study showed a decrease in gum bleeding and tooth mobility in individuals with periodontal disease whose diets were supplemented with 1 gm. of calcium daily for 6 months.[8] The role of calcium in periodontal disease needs further investigation.

Thorough brushing and flossing of the teeth every day help remove plaque and prevent calculus from developing. If calculus has formed it must be removed by a dentist or hygienist. *Keeping teeth clean* is the primary method of prevention and treatment for this disorder. Decreasing between-meal snacks of carbohydrate-containing food helps keep the teeth clean.

Aging

Several factors related to aging affect the health of the oral cavity. As an individual ages, cells in the salivary glands atrophy, resulting in decreased salivary flow and changes in the composition of saliva. *Xerostomia* is the term used to denote decreased salivary flow. Lack of saliva causes the oral mucosa to dry, makes chewing and swallowing more difficult, and may increase the incidence of dental caries. Encouraging chewing moist foods to stimulate salivary flow helps alleviate xerostomia. Some researchers in dentistry recommend chewing sugarless gum to relieve this problem.[9]

Aging affects the surface of the tongue and mucous membranes lining the oral cavity. The tongue gradually loses papillae, small projections in which taste buds are located. This gradually reduces a person's sense of taste. The mucous membrane thins with age, making it more susceptible to injury.

In response to changes in the oral cavity, people often modify the consistency of their diet, eating non-abrasive, nonirritating, and easily chewed foods. This method of adaptation can lead to several problems. First, there may be inadequate stimulation for saliva production. Secondly, gingival circulation may diminish. Thirdly, the balance between alveolar bone formation and absorption may be unfavorable.

Edentulism (loss of teeth), although not specifically a result of aging, is more prevalent in older age groups. Without teeth the mouth takes on a purse-string appearance. Loss of teeth may contribute to absorption of alveolar bone since the bone is no longer necessary for tooth support. Bone changes, in turn, cause the face to appear shortened.[9] Edentulism interferes not only with mastication but also with proper closure of the jaw.

Early replacement of missing teeth with a properly fitting dental prosthesis is recommended to facilitate the process of eating, to maintain alveolar bone alignment, and to enhance a person's appearance and self-image. Improperly fitting dentures may interfere with eating. Since dentures are expensive, many people cannot afford to buy them; persons who have dentures may delay replacing them when they begin to cause problems. If an individual's financial resources are limited, he should be helped to locate and use government resources or medical insurance to cover the cost of purchasing dentures.

Wearing dentures is not quite the same as having one's own teeth. Learning to eat with dentures is simplified by progressing from swallowing to chewing and finally to biting. This means initially consuming foods liquid in consistency, progressing to soft foods, and finally returning to a regular varied diet.[9]

Mouth care after meals and proper handling of dentures promotes oral health. Many fundamental nursing texts provide guidelines for care of dentures.

Nutrients with special roles

FLUORIDE

Fluoride has been identified as one of the most significant factors in determining an individual's resistance to tooth decay. The incidence of dental caries is re-

duced by about 60 percent in communities where drinking water is fluoridated.[10] Ingestion of fluoride is most important when teeth are forming (6 months to 12 to 18 years of age).

Fluoridation of drinking water is an effective, safe, economical public health measure to decrease the incidence of dental caries. Many Americans drink water which naturally contains fluoride or which has been fluoridated to the recommended level of 1 ppm. (approximately 1 mg. of fluoride per L. of water). However, many people do not have access to fluoridated water. An alternate means of providing fluoride is in drops or tablets. These are available by prescription only. If tablets are used for children over 3 years, chewing and swishing them before swallowing results in topical as well as systemic benefits. Topical benefits can also be increased by giving a fluoride supplement after a meal or at bedtime. One limitation of drops or tablets is that parents must remember to give them.

Parents must also take precautions to store the tablets in a place where children do not have access to them. Children usually enjoy the taste of fluoride tablets and might eat them like candy, if the opportunity arose.

Before fluoride supplements are prescribed a child's fluoride intake from all sources should be considered to avoid giving too much. Foods are generally an insignificant source of fluoride. Tea, however, contains a significant amount of fluoride. Some children are allowed to drink several cups of tea daily; in this case fluoride supplements may not be desirable. If water is fluoridated, it is important to determine how much water a child drinks, as well as how much he ingests via foods prepared with water, such as infant formula, reconstituted frozen juice, and soups. If water is not used, supplementation may be desirable.

Fluorosis If too much fluoride (more than 2 parts per million) is ingested when the teeth are forming (up to about age 12 to 18) fluorosis of the enamel may occur. The enamel becomes roughened, mottled, and discolored. If fluorosis is of a minor degree, the teeth remain strong and caries-resistant but appear less attractive. If the mottling is severe, enamel may have a chalky consistency which crumbles easily. Some dentists recommend use of nonfluoridated water for infants under 6 months of age to reduce the chance of fluorosis.

PHOSPHATES AND OTHER NUTRIENTS

McBean and Speckman suggest that phosphates have cariostatic (decay retarding) properties.[11] The results of various studies have, however, produced some conflicting results.[12,13]

Dietary proteins and fats may actually be cariostatic. A diet high in protein increases the level of urea in the saliva. The urea, in turn, acts as a buffer, neu-

Forbidding children to eat between meals might decrease tooth decay but may not be the best way to meet a child's energy and nutrient needs.

POINTS OF EMPHASIS
Food habits to promote oral health

- *Food habits which promote oral health should begin in infancy and continue throughout life.*
    - *Guidelines for infants:*
        1. *Feed solid foods free of added sugar.*
        2. *Use a nursing bottle only when an infant is wide awake.*
        3. *Offer unsweetened fruit juices in a cup.*
        4. *Provide an opportunity for the infant to chew on foods such as zweiback, rusk, and dry toast when the teeth are erupting.*
        5. *Clean teeth gently with gauze after feedings.*
    - *Guidelines for young children (ages 2–5 yrs.):*
        1. *Provide snack foods low in refined sugar and/or sucrose content (see page 91).*
        2. *Restrict the intake of sweets. If sweets are eaten, encourage prompt thorough tooth brushing.*
        3. *Encourage frequent use of foods which require chewing such as raw fruits and vegetables.*
        4. *Teach children to brush their teeth right after eating and snacking. Supervise and assist children with brushing. Disclosing tablets which color plaque are helpful when children are learning to brush their own teeth.*
        5. *Teach the child to rinse the mouth thoroughly with a "swishing" motion if brushing is not possible.*
        6. *Take the child to the dentist twice a year.*
    - *Measures for older children and adults:*
        1. *Continue to encourage use of fibrous foods and avoidance of highly cariogenic foods.*
        2. *Teach children to use dental floss in conjunction with tooth brushing. (By age 7–9 it is reasonable to expect a child to effectively brush and floss his teeth.)*
        3. *Capitalize on concerns about self-image and economy to promote dental health.*

STUDY QUESTIONS

1. Why is adequate nutrition important for dental health both before and after tooth eruption?
2. In addition to avoiding pain and financial expense, why should an effort be made to maintain the health of the temporary (baby) teeth?
3. List several reasons for recommending that a local community fluoridate its water supply. What arguments are frequently raised in opposition to fluoridation and how can they be refuted?
4. List several relatively noncariogenic snacks appropriate for:
    a. toddlers
    b. school age children
5. From the standpoint of dental health, explain why it is preferable to eat a large chocolate bar at dinner rather than to eat small caramels at frequent intervals during the day?
6. How does brushing teeth immediately after eating help decrease the process of tooth decay?
7. List several measures to help prevent the development of periodontal disease.

References

1. Shaw, J., and Sweeney, E.: Nutrition in relation to dental medicine. In R. Goodhart and M. Shils (eds.): *Modern Nutrition in Health and Disease,* ed. 5. Philadelphia: Lea and Febiger, 1973.
2. Shaw, J.: Preventive Nutrition. In J. Bernier and R. J. Muhle (eds.): *Improving Dental Practice Through Preventive Measures.* St. Louis: C. V. Mosby Co., 1976.
3. Sweeney, E. A., Saffir, A. J., and DeLeon, R.: Linear hypoplasia of deciduous incisor teeth in malnourished children. *Am. J. Clin. Nutr.* 24:29, 1971.
4. Rowe, N., et al.: The effect of age, sex, race and economic status on dental caries experience in permanent dentition. *Pediatrics* 57:457, 1976.
*5. Bowen, W.: Dental Caries. *Contemp. Nutr.* 2:8, 1977.
6. Jenkins, C., and Ferguson, D. B.: Milk and dental caries. *Br. Dent. J.* 120:472, 1966.
7. Stahl, S. S.: Nutritional influences on periodontal disease. *World Rev. Nutr. Diet.* 13:277, 1971.
8. Krook, L., et al.: Human periodontal disease morphology and response to calcium therapy. *Cornell Vet.* 62:32, 1972.
*9. Nizel, A.: Role of nutrition in oral health of the aging patient. *Dent. Clin. North Am.* 20(3):569, 1976.
10. Shaw, J.: Diet regulations for caries prevention. *Nutr. News,* 36:1, Feb. 1973.
*11. McBean, L., and Speckman, E.: A review: The importance of nutrition in oral health. *J. Am. Dent. Assoc.* 89:109, July 1974.
12. Halifax, D.: Phosphates and dental caries. In H. Myers (ed.): *Monographs in Oral Science,* Vol. 6, Basel, Switzerland: S. Karger, 1977.
*13. Nizel, A.: Preventing dental caries: The nutritional factors. *Pediatr. Clin. North Am.* 24(1): 141, 1977.

* Recommended reading

tralizing acids formed by bacterial fermentation. It has been suggested that fats may form a protective coating on the tooth surface or that they may exert some antimicrobial action.[9]

Health care providers need to consider all the nutritional needs of individuals when making recommendations to promote oral health. A diet which is helpful for preventing one disease may contribute to the development of another. A diet high in fat and protein, while it may be cariostatic, is certainly not prudent.

18

Evaluation

The field of nutrition is permeated with misinformation and controversy. Nutrition is a young science which retains an aura of mystery and magic. The idea that people are what they eat prods lively imaginations. Many people who have little or no formal education in nutrition devise new ideas for improving health or curing disease by changing eating habits. Even among experts there is disagreement about nutritional matters. This provides lively debate but does little to help the man on the street make decisions relating to food and nutrition.

When an individual considers nutritional messages that appear in the media, he should remember that freedom of speech and freedom of the press are fundamental rights guaranteed by the Constitution. These freedoms give people the opportunity to express themselves as they wish. There is nothing illegal about anyone communicating misleading or incorrect information about nutrition (or other topics); exceptions are made with regard to special forms of communication such as labeling and "truth in advertising." If the use of the media were stringently controlled, the rights of freedom of speech and freedom of the press would be lost. However, these rights do give citizens access to many points of view, enabling them to consider both sides of a problem before making decisions. Therefore, consumers must make the choice of relying on the integrity of communicators or on their own ability to determine the reliability of sources of information and/or the reliability of the information itself.

Unfortunately many people are gullible and assume that whatever appears in print is true. The impact of books, articles, and television talk shows upon peoples' actions should not be underestimated. After the book *Vitamin C and the Common Cold* was published,[1] drug companies had to temporarily import Vitamin C until they could step up their own production to meet greatly increased demand for the vitamin.

Health care providers render a service by helping consumers develop a questioning attitude toward the nutritional messages they receive. This chapter attempts to provide some insight into interpretation of nutrition information appearing in the media. General guidelines are presented, followed by discussion of some controversial issues.

INTERPRETATION OF MESSAGES APPEARING IN THE MEDIA

When trying to interpret or evaluate nutritional messages it it helpful to ask a series of questions.

WHAT IS THE SOURCE OF THE INFORMATION?

Scientific journals Articles submitted to scientific peer-reviewed journals are reviewed by experts in the field prior to being accepted for publication. A method of determining if a journal is peer-reviewed is perusal of the contents page of the journal to learn the composition of the editorial board. Students learning to use scientific journals could look at the listing of periodicals abstracted in the "New in Print" section of *The Journal of the American Dietetic Association*. (The listing appears regularly in the June and December issues of the journal.) The periodicals named there are considered to be generally reliable sources of nutrition information.

Errors which appear inadvertently in peer-reviewed scientific journals are corrected in subsequent issues. Letters to the journal editor raise questions about the validity of some articles or may offer additional support of new findings.

Even very factual reports of scientific investigations may be misleading. The design of an experiment may be faulty or the conclusions drawn may be based on insufficient evidence. Terms which refer to some commonly used test methods are briefly defined below:

Clinical trials. The study of effects of a change upon a given group of individuals.

Matched groups. The control and experimental groups are selected so that they are very similar (or identical) in age, sex, smoking habits, and/or other characteristics which might influence the results of the study.

Randomized trial. Division of subjects into control and experimental groups is done according to rules of chance (that is, on a random rather than a systematic basis that might introduce a bias).

Double-blind. Neither the subjects nor the investigators know who is receiving the test substance or test diet and who is in the control group. (Special codes are used to make this possible.)

Crossover study. After a specified interval the control group and the experimental group are reversed.

Placebo. A tablet, capsule, formula, or the like which contains only an inert substance (such as sugar) having no physiological effects in the form and amount given.

New findings in scientific investigations are usually not accepted as fact until they are verified by other investigators.

There are some quasi-scientific journals which do not require qualified peer review prior to publication and which publish papers of questionable validity. The book *The Dynamics of Clinical Dietetics*[2] provides detailed guidelines for evaluating scientific articles.

Textbooks by reputable publishers　Prior to publishing a text, reputable editors send out chapters for review by qualified professionals. Textbooks occasionally contain inadvertent errors. Material included in textbooks is less up-to-date than most journal articles published the same year.

News articles　Ideally, news articles such as appear in newspapers, news magazines, or on radio or television are accurate, concise reports of statements made by individuals, groups, agencies, and so forth. Accuracy of the information itself depends on both the accuracy of the original source of the information and the quality of the reporting. Exaggeration may creep into an article in the interest of increasing sales or attracting listeners/viewers. When validity of information is questioned and a consumer wants to look into the matter further, a media representative (e.g., editor, TV news manager) can usually provide additional details regarding the original source of the material.

Popular press　Popular press includes feature articles in newspapers and magazines and books for the general public. Accuracy of information appearing in the popular press varies with the expertise and integrity of the author. According to Deutsch ". . . Not one major national magazine has failed to use a kind of nutrition sensationalism, whether taken from books or not, to boost its sales."[3] When not constrained by facts, authors can make nutrition more interesting than it otherwise might be. Some unreliable nutrition books have sold millions of copies.

Talk shows, interviews, and other non-news features on radio and television　The preceding comments under "Popular Press" apply to this category as well.

WHAT QUALIFICATIONS DOES THE ORIGINATOR OF THE INFORMATION HAVE? ARE ANY SPECIAL INTERESTS INVOLVED?

The qualifications and special interests of the originator can often be more difficult to determine than appears to be the case. Educational preparation in the specific field of nutrition is desirable; nontheless, some science writers produce very accurate nutrition books and articles by working in close collaboration with nutritionists. The title "doctor" or a PhD after a name does not necessarily mean a person is a reliable source of nutrition information. At least one well-known radio personality who has been promoted as a "leading nutrition consultant" reportedly has no formal nutrition or health care background.[4] However, the term "Doctor" in front of his name lends an air of authority to his statements.

Even some publications by physicians and nutritionists have not been accepted as reliable. The late Adelle Davis, author of many popular nutrition books, earned degrees in dietetics and biochemistry at reputable universities. She has been criticized with sprinkling facts liberally with misleading information.[4,5] While her books remain popular, health care providers should be familiar with her work, especially *Let's Get Well*.[6] That volume might lead a person to try to treat himself for a serious condition such as heart disease, cancer, burns, or kidney stones.

Public interest groups and "watchdog" agencies currently provide considerable amounts of nutrition-related information. Because of the nature of their work, they sometimes focus on only one or two sides of a many-faceted issue, taking the part of the consumer against "big business." Often they publicize information seldom mentioned by other sources.

Industry has become actively involved in disseminating nutrition information. This is most commonly seen in the form of advertisements (many of which could be described as containing an "anti-nutrition" message). Since most Americans can easily satisfy their hunger, advertising is commonly directed toward the meeting of higher needs (e.g., esteem or love and belongingness). This approach can make the nutritional value of a product seem unimportant.

In addition to advertising directly, many food companies design pamphlets, posters, and booklets for use in school classrooms and adult education programs. Quality of presentation of nutrition messages is highly variable.

Nutritionists who work for a food company or a product-related association are likely to marshall arguments in support of their employer's interests. Sometimes close examination is needed to detect that a nutrition article might be slanted because of a link to a special interest group.

Agencies of the federal government, especially within the U.S. Department of Agriculture (USDA), produce many publications regarding food and nutrition. These publications generally are quite reliable, being written by people trained in the field. To date, however, most government publications omit information that would help Americans achieve a more prudent diet.

Since it is difficult to give lay people foolproof advice about how to determine reliable sources of information, consumers can be encouraged to consult organizations such as the American Dietetic Association, the American Medical Association, the American Public Health Association, and the American Home Economics Association for their lists of recommended books and articles on nutrition. Universities having a nutrition department or the county extension service

can also provide this type of information. Book reviews which comment on the accuracy and usefulness of new publications appear in health-related journals such as The *Journal of the American Dietetic Association*, the *Journal of Nutrition Education*, the *American Journal of Nursing*, and *Nursing*.

WHAT DEVICES ARE USED TO PROMOTE A PRODUCT OR AN IDEA?

Numerous devices can be used to make a food product appear more healthful or a better source of nutrients than it actually is. Comparisons or other carefully chosen descriptive statements are frequently capable of fooling the public. When evaluating claims about the nutritive value of foods the following points might be used in conjunction with points covered in Table 18.1.

1. Portion sizes. Are equal weights compared? Is the portion size the amount customarily eaten?
2. Role of the food in the diet. Is it eaten often (more than once daily), occasionally, or infrequently?
3. Omitted information. Does the product contain or lack nutrients or other components or characteristics which affect its nutritional role?

TABLE 18.1 *Analysis of advertising claims*

EXAMPLE	ANALYSIS	TYPE OF CLAIM
"X contains 5 times as much fiber as white bread."	A true statement which implies that X is much richer in fiber than is actually the case	Spurious—(1) the food is compared to another food recognized as a poor source of the nutrient
"30 gm. of Crunchy-O's contain no more sugar than an apple, orange, or banana."	A true statement which disregards potential disadvantages of feeding children sugar-coated cereal. The statement makes the product look good by comparison with widely respected foods	Spurious—(2) different portion sizes are compared
"Crackle-sweet breakfast bites contain as much protein and energy as a fried egg, a slice of buttered toast, and a glass of orange juice—without the cholesterol."	Statement implies that the breakfast bites would be a nutritionally sound substitute for the more traditional breakfast. The value of other nutrients and the enjoyment afforded by the variety of color, flavor, texture, and temperature are overlooked. The final phrase tries to take advantage of the current concern about cholesterol	Engineered or fortified food compared with a natural food (i.e., a basic food not highly processed)
"Y breakfast drink is richer in vitamin C."	A meaningless statement which, nonetheless, suggests that the drink is valuable because of its vitamin C content	Dangling comparison—the food is compared to an unspecified food
"Blue araucana eggs are low in cholesterol."	A claim that could not be checked by using a table of food composition. At the time this claim was first made the cholesterol content of blue araucana eggs had not been analyzed. Subsequent analysis, in response to numerous inquiries by consumers and health professionals, revealed that the eggs are higher in cholesterol than are ordinary eggs[7]	Lack of comparison—a descriptive statement (which might be vague or specific) is made about the food

4. Is the food worth the cost or can the same nutrients be provided in a more economical manner?

Misleading advertisements deserve more criticism than they ordinarily receive since these messages help to shape the eating habits of Americans.

Perhaps one of the most powerful tools for putting food products in a favorable light is associating them with something else which is highly desired. Words and/or pictures are used to associate foods with health, happiness, esteem, or youth.

There are a number of other cues which signal misleading, incorrect, or dangerous information. These include:

1. Offering easy solutions to difficult problems. This is exemplified by "painless" weight loss schemes which promise freedom from hunger.
2. Using fear arousal techniques. Using strong language to alarm the public about dangers in the food supply is common and tends to discourage consideration of both sides of a question.
3. Recognizing only one problem at a time. Plans suggesting bizarre, unbalanced diets as a means of relieving arthritis or other disease conditions overlook the need to nourish the body adequately.
4. Suggesting that only one factor is involved in the development of an undesirable condition. Suboptimal intake of vitamin E has been indicted as the cause of aging. Lack of pantothenic acid has been blamed for the greying of hair.
5. Making blanket statements. Statements such as "All food additives are dangerous," should make a person question the reliability of the nutrition information.
6. Referring to studies or cases which involved a very limited sample or were otherwise poorly designed or controlled. Emotional personal testimonials attract attention and are a very persuasive means of gathering a following for a product or an idea. Documented "successes" should not be used as the basis for abandoning a well-balanced diet or professional medical care. Temporary improvement in disease conditions often results from a placebo effect—a belief that the new treatment will be beneficial. Some diseases typically have periods of spontaneous temporary remission which may happen to coincide with a new treatment.
7. Using excessive criticism of the medical profession or "the establishment." Blaming others for being closed-minded is a convenient means of sidestepping issues such as lack of a scientific basis for an idea or failure of controlled studies to produce the desired result.

PROTECTION AGAINST FALSE ADVERTISING OR LABELING

Three federal governmental agencies have power to enforce specific regulations designed to help protect consumers from fraudulent practices involving foods,

nutritional supplements, drugs and devices to promote weight loss, and nutrition-related books. Their roles are summarized briefly.

FOOD AND DRUG ADMINISTRATION (FDA)

The FDA enforces labeling regulations which prohibit false nutritional claims. For example, the word "health" cannot be used on a label in connection with foods since this could mislead consumers to believe that the food has special curative properties or other unusual health benefits. However, the FDA cannot necessarily prevent labels from stating correct but misleading information. The FDA also enforces laws regarding the labeling and safety of drugs, including those promoted for weight control purposes.

Some products sold in health food stores to be ingested do not come under the legal classification of either food or drug. Bone meal (a nutritional supplement made from finely ground bone) is an example. The FDA cannot regulate such products even if they travel across state lines.

The FDA investigates "medical" devices such as those promoted as a means of ridding the body of fat or of inches. The Medical Device Amendments of 1976 have strengthened FDAs authority to remove defective and fraudulent devices from the market and to require premarket approval of *some* kinds of medical devices. Unfortunately, unless a device is clearly dangerous, it usually can be promoted and sold until all court proceedings have been completed. This can take a very long time.

FEDERAL TRADE COMMISSION (FTC)

The FTC is involved in establishing food advertising trade regulation rules. The agency is empowered to act in cases of deceptive advertising. The procedure is cumbersome and allows an advertiser considerable time to continue to promote a product dishonestly, as illustrated in Figure 18.1.

POSTAL SERVICE (PS)

The Postal Service enforces laws against mail fraud. This has been an important means of removing fraudulent and dangerous weight-reducing or spot-reducing products from the market. These laws apply only to products distributed via the mail.

Protection offered by these government agencies is limited. Just because a product is on the market, is advertised, or travels through the mail, it is not necessarily legitimate or healthful. Total protection is not possible without infringement of rights guaranteed by the Constitution. Consumers are protected most effectively if they themselves are both knowledgeable and

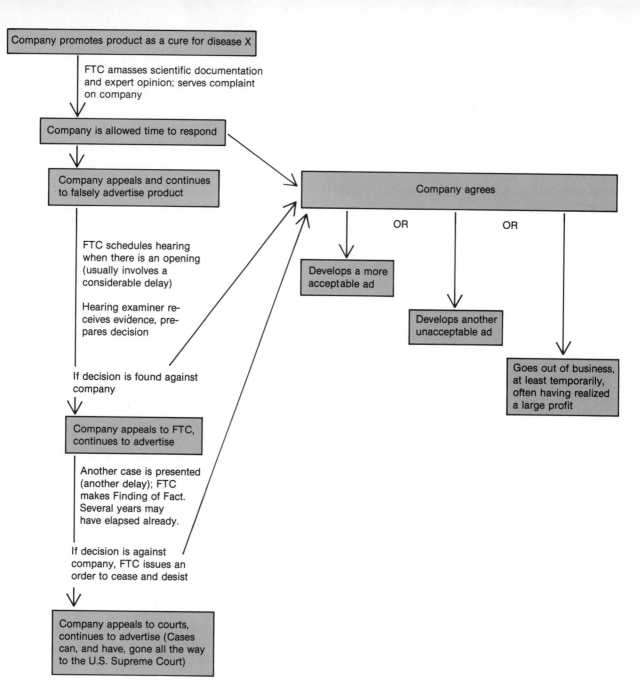

FIGURE 18.1. Possible results of FTC action to halt false advertising.

skeptical. Wise consumers investigate questionable claims before making a purchase or trying a new food product or diet.

UNORTHODOX USES OF DIETS, FOODS, AND GADGETS

Health professionals should be aware of the roles unorthodox ideas about diets, food, nutrients, and gadgets may play in the lives of their clients. Over the ages, diets and food-related products have been promoted as capable of solving many of mankind's problems—disease, tiredness, aging, hair loss, impotency, and many others.

Curing disease

The number of diseases toward which nutrition claims are directed has dwindled in correspondence with advances in medicine. Today most people who are out to make a profit gear their sales pitches toward curing *chronic* diseases such as arthritis, cancer, atherosclerosis, and multiple sclerosis.

People who are afflicted with these chronic diseases are sometimes desperate. When medical science cannot ethically promise a cure or offer treatment acceptable to the client, even the most intelligent person may be susceptible to the allure of "nutrition quackery."

Health professionals should be concerned about nutrition-related schemes promoted for curative purposes when (1) self-treatment delays or interferes with sound medical/surgical treatment and/or (2) there are adverse effects of the unorthodox treatment method. It has been suggested that health care providers can help to offset the allure of the "quack" not only by providing clients with factual information about orthodox and unorthodox treatment but also (and more importantly) by *paying more attention to meeting their emotional needs.*[8]

Clients who continue with prescribed medical treatment may want to simultaneously try one or more of the current nutritional "cures." If this is the case, health care providers should review the proposed plan for nutritional adequacy and make suggestions for adjusting the plan if necessary.

An example of a "diet cure" is briefly described and discussed in Figure 18.2.

Another substance which has been widely heralded as a "cure" for cancer, despite good evidence to the contrary, is laetrile. It is mentioned here because it is sometimes called vitamin B_{17} by its promoters. There is absolutely no evidence that it is a vitamin. It is a cyanide-containing compound that is potentially toxic to humans in relatively low doses.[9,10]

Weight loss

Despite abundant claims to the contrary, there is no easy way to lose weight and keep it off. Nevertheless, unrecommended weight loss schemes flourish; they include fad reducing diets, pharmacological agents, and gadgets.

FAD DIETS AND REDUCING SCHEMES

Fad diets and reducing schemes have more appeal than well-balanced, safe reducing diets because of novelty, quick initial weight loss, peer influence, and/or false promises. Some may be dangerous. Liquid protein diets, which were widely promoted in 1977, have been closely linked to a number of untimely deaths.

A Diet Evaluator (Table 18.2) can serve as a guide for assessing the safety and potential effectiveness of popular weight reduction schemes. Use of this evaluator reveals that many fad diets have potentially serious shortcomings.

CLAMS AS A SOURCE OF MERCENENE

...In the research of the past twelve years she has isolated this anti-tumor agent, the liquid mercenene from the edible ocean clam. — Suggests that mercenene can destroy cancer cells

Dr. _____'s discovery has received confirmation from various parts of the world. (Dr. _____ has developed an oral clam diet which has shown remarkable results in several cancer patients), one of them being Dr. _____'s own mother. Having undergone two operations for cancer, Mrs. _____ refused chemotherapy and cobalt treatments. _____ put her on the clam diet. She recovered—and seven years later is well and active.

— No information on the type of doctor is given
— Vague claims
— Testimonial approach
— Invites self-treatment

The clam diet consists of one to twelve "shucked, drained clams daily" from unpolluted water.

(From the directions):

1. Upon arrival, scrub shells to remove sand, store 3–7 day supply in the refrigerator. The remainder place in the freezer *in the shell.* — Length of time exceeds the usual safe storage time

2. Remove the daily number of clams to be eaten.

We cannot recommend a specific quantity. This can vary from one to a half-dozen or more. — Vagueness

FIGURE 18.2. Excerpts from an unsolicited mailing sent to a diagnosed cancer patient in 1978.

TABLE 18.2 *Diet evaluator*

	YES	NO	LACK INFORMATION
1. Diet is realistic.	——	——	——
2. Suggests your doctor be consulted.	——	——	——
3. Foods used instead of vitamin and/or diet pills	——	——	——
4. Forbidden foods at minimum.	——	——	——
5. Meets nutritional needs for all nutrients.	——	——	——
6. Exercise recommended.	——	——	——
7. Weight loss no more than 1–2 lbs. per week.	——	——	——
8. Long-term possibilities.	——	——	——
9. Sensible balance protein/ fat/carbohydrate.	——	——	——
10. Allows healthful snacks.	——	——	——
11. Emphasizes portion control.	——	——	——
12. Establishes good food habits for permanent weight control.	——	——	——

YOUR COMMENTS

1. What is your personal reaction to this diet?

_____

2. What additions or modifications would improve this diet?

_____

_____

From Mapes, M. C.: *A Fad Dieting Resource Portfolio*, Div. Nutritional Services, Cornell University, with permission.

PHARMACOLOGICAL AGENTS

A variety of types of pharmacological agents are promoted for weight reduction, some of which are described here.

Prescription drugs Prescription drugs include the following:
1. Amphetamines (including dextroamphetamine and phenmetrazine). These compounds temporarily result in mild suppression of the appetite. They are addictive drugs with potentially dangerous side effects and been grossly misused. The short-lived effect on appetite (which has been called trivial in controlled trials) does not appear to offset the serious risks involved with their use.
2. Nonamphetamines with activity similar to the amphetamines (such as phentermine hydrochloride, phendimetrazine tartrate, diethylpropion-hydrochloride, fenfluramine hydrochloride). Like the amphetamines, these drugs have minimal appetite-depressing effects and have potentially danger-

ous side effects. Drug literature advises doctors to weigh the limited usefulness of these agents against possible risk factors.
3. Human chorionic gonadotropin (HCG). This drug is an expensive hormone which has been given by injection 6 days a week in conjunction with a 500 kcal. diet. Controlled double-blind clinical trials have failed to demonstrate any significant beneficial effect from HCG.[11]

Nonprescription drugs The following are nonprescription drugs:
1. Bulking agents. Inert substances that swell when mixed with liquid have been promoted as appetite suppressants. (They are more commonly used as a means of relieving constipation.) Carboxymethyl cellulose and psyllium hydrophilic mucilloid (Metamucil) are examples. If taken before a meal, bulking agents produce a temporary sensation of fullness. Regular use of bulking agents seldom results in significant decrease in food intake.
2. Fortified candy promoted as a diet aid. The idea be-

hind this type of product is that eating a piece of the "diet-aid" about half an hour before each meal will take the edge off of the appetite so that less food will be eaten. Those who believe that the product is an appetite suppressant may benefit temporarily from a placebo effect.

3. Mild diuretics. These produce temporary weight loss caused entirely by fluid loss. Certain herbs are promoted for their diuretic effect. Misuse of any diuretic can cause disturbances in fluid and electrolyte balance.

GADGETS

All gadgetry promoted for weight reduction or "spot reducing" should be viewed with suspicion. The FDA states that all of the following are fakes: (1) "passive" or "effortless" exercise machines, (2) "body-wraps" and other sweat-inducing garments, (3) massagers promoted as spot reducers, and (4) any other gadget represented as capable of changing one's figure or physique without proper diet and active exercise.

Retarding aging

In a search for the fountain of youth, many have put their faith in health foods and diet supplements. Among the schemes promoted in the popular press and by commercial interests are eating yogurt, taking vitamin E or selenium, and eating a diet rich in nucleic acids.[12] Proponents of these and other plans for retarding aging often use a limited piece of scientific information to back up their claims, making the schemes appear reasonable to many consumers. For example, proponents of vitamin E say that it intercepts free radicals, preventing these active particles from causing chemical changes responsible for aging. Animal studies do not support this claim. Consumers who testify to the effectiveness of vitamin E (or of other supplements or health foods) are no doubt enjoying the benefits of a placebo effect or of wishful thinking.

PHARMACOLOGICAL USE OF NUTRIENTS

MEGAVITAMIN THERAPY

Megavitamin therapy refers to continued administration of very high doses (usually ten times the RDA or more) of one or more vitamins. Megavitamin therapy has been widely promoted for correction of certain psychiatric disorders.[13] Except for the correction of vitamin deficiency diseases, megavitamin therapy is actually a pharmacological rather than a nutritional use of vitamins. (For example, giving large doses of B vitamins does not increase coenzyme activity since vitamins function as coenzymes only when combined

with an enzyme.) A second term has been coined for this type of treatment, namely *orthomolecular* medicine. This refers more broadly to the use of substances that are normally present in the human body—so-called "right" (ortho) molecules.[14]

Several points are pertinent with regard to the safety of megavitamin therapy:

1. Any substance, even water, is potentially toxic if taken in excess. People vary in their susceptibility to adverse reactions. Table 18.3 summarizes some of the problems which may result from excessive intake of vitamins.

2. High doses of vitamins A and D pose serious health hazards. Since the body has no mechanism for excreting these vitamins, they can rapidly accumulate to toxic levels. Giving infants and children 20,000 IU of vitamin A daily may produce symptoms (hypervitaminosis) within 1 to 2 months.[15] Smaller doses for a longer time could also be harmful.

3. High dosages of vitamins can be obtained without a prescription. Examples include 50,000 IU vitamin A per capsule, 50,000 IU vitamin D per tablet, and 500 mg. vitamin C per tablet.

4. A high intake of water-soluble vitamins and of vitamin E is accompanied by increased loss of the respective vitamins. This is due to increased breakdown and urinary excretion or to decreased percent absorption of the vitamins. Even though increased excretion helps to prevent accumulation of vitamins, toxic effects are possible. The kidneys require time to remove substances from the blood.

5. Although many benefits of specific types of megavitamin therapy have been claimed, few have been substantiated by controlled clinical trials.

The usefulness of megadoses of vitamin C in prevention and treatment of the common cold has been investigated in a wide variety of controlled clinical trials. Results remain inconclusive because of lack of agreement among different experiments. One particularly interesting co-twin* double-blind study found no overall significant difference between the vitamin C treated groups and controls but did note that younger children who were given megadoses of vitamin C appeared to have significantly milder symptoms than their identical twin controls.[17] This study might have been influenced by the mothers' knowledge of which children were receiving vitamin C and which were receiving placebo. Four mothers admitted having distinguished the placebo from the vitamin C by tasting the contents of the capsules.

If there is any benefit from megadoses of vitamin C in the prevention and treatment of the common cold, it appears to be of a minor nature. Some investigators have likened the effect of vitamin C to that of a mild antihistamine.[18] Against a possible mild benefit should be weighed possible side effects of megadoses of vita-

---

* Sets of identical twin children were used in the study; one twin served as a control, the other was in the experimental group.

TABLE 18.3 *Potential toxic effects of acute overdose or of chronic ingestion of excessive amounts of vitamins*

VITAMIN	POSSIBLE EFFECTS OF EXCESS
A	Fatigue, malaise, headache, loss of hair and/or nails, bone pain, cerebral edema, vomiting, skin changes, fever, enlarged liver
D	High blood calcium level, kidney damage, growth retardation
E	Headache, nausea, fatigue, dizziness, blurred vision, changes in epithelial tissue
K	Menadione, a synthetic compound which has vitamin K activity, has produced irritation of the skin and respiratory tract, hemolysis of red blood cells in individuals with an uncommon inborn error of metabolism called glucose-6-phosphate-dehydrogenase deficiency. (This condition is occasionally found in Sephardic Jews, blacks, and Orientals.) Menadione may contribute to hemolytic anemia and other problems of the newborn, especially the preterm infant
C	Nausea, diarrhea
	Excessive absorption of iron, especially in males
	Uric acid kidney stones, especially in people who have gout or a high uric acid level; cystine kidney stones in predisposed individuals
	Scurvy in infants born to women who took high doses during pregnancy
	Hemolysis of red blood cells in individuals who have glucose-6-phosphate-dehydrogenase deficiency
Thiamine	None reported owing to high doses administered by *mouth*
Riboflavin	*
Pantothenic acid	*
Biotin	*
Folic acid	*
Vitamin B$_{12}$	*
Niacin	Flushing, itching, persistent skin changes, tachycardia (rapid heart beat), liver damage, high blood sugar, high blood uric acid
Pyridoxine	May produce liver disease[16]

* None reported in normal individuals who were not on drug therapy

min C, especially the higher dosages up to about 10 gm. daily. For example, does excess circulating vitamin C favor bone demineralization because the pH of the blood is maintained on the low side of normal?

Although a well-balanced diet may provide more than the RDA of vitamins, including vitamin A, eating nutritious foods is not comparable to megavitamin therapy. Consuming a moderate excess of vitamins from whole foods is not ordinarily a matter of concern. Vitamin toxicity caused by unfortified food has only been associated with eating large quantities of polar bear liver.

LARGE DOSES OF MINERALS

Large doses of minerals have also been promoted commercially, as illustrated by the following excerpts from an advertisement:

National newspapers and magazines are now carrying news of the enormous potential benefits of selenium.
Science doesn't yet know how this essential nutrient works for us. Only that it does. It functions as a powerful antioxidant (anti-aging) nutrient to protect each of the sixty-trillion cells in the body.[19]

For some minerals, including selenium, the margin between nutritional effect and toxicity is relatively narrow. Selenium toxicity in animals was discovered long before selenium was found to be an essential nutrient.

The Food and Nutrition Board of the National Research Council was sufficiently concerned about selenium supplementation that they issued a detailed statement in 1977 which included the following warning:

There is reason, however, to suspect that indiscriminate selenium supplementation of the diet is potentially hazardous.[20]

Other minerals may also cause problems if taken in excess. The FDA is taking action to warn about hazards associated with overuse of potassium supplements. Their action followed the death of an infant who was given an overdose of potassium chloride. Accordingly to a report in *FDA Consumer*, "The mother was following the advice of a book by the late Adelle Davis entitled *Let's Have Healthy Children*."[21]

VITAMINS AS INSURANCE

Even more popular than megavitamin therapy is the daily use of a standard strength multivitamin tablet as a kind of nutritional insurance, just in case the diet is inadequate. (A standard strength multivitamin provides the U.S. RDA for most, but not necessarily all, of the vitamins.) Promotion of highly fortified foods, such as some ready-to-eat cereals, often draws attention to this same idea. The "just to be sure" attitude contributes to an unfounded lack of confidence in the nutritional quality of a well-balanced diet.

"Stress vitamins" have been highly promoted recently. These actually may contain megadose levels of some of the vitamins. The implication is that these high levels are needed by people under everyday stress (such as that associated with a hectic schedule, using oral contraceptives, or eating "on the run"). The names of some of the products are suggestive of therapeutic or other highly beneficial effects, e.g., Fortespan and Stress-tabs.

There is certainly no danger of toxicity with the use of one *standard strength* multivitamin daily. However, it seems that many parents do not recognize that vitamin supplements are potentially dangerous; they may fail to keep them out of reach of young children. Approximately 4000 cases of vitamin poisoning are reported each year, more than three fourth of which involve children.[22] Some parents may think vitamins are so harmless that they fail to seek immediate medical attention if a child takes an overdose of vitamins. Iron supplement poisoning is also a potential problem.

NATURAL VERSUS SYNTHETIC VITAMINS

Natural vitamins, that is, vitamins extracted from plants or animals, have been widely promoted as being very much more beneficial than synthetic vitamins. Actually the chemical structure of the two kinds of vitamins is nearly always the same. The value of synthetic vitamins in correcting vitamin deficiency diseases has been amply documented. Natural vitamins are more expensive and offer no clear advantage to the consumer. In fact, natural vitamins are not always what they seem—they may be mixed with synthetic vitamins.

A study of bioavailability of natural versus synthetic ascorbic acid revealed that the *synthetic* form resulted in slightly *higher* serum ascorbic acid than did natural vitamin C (from orange juice).*[23] This does not mean that people should use a synthetic vitamin C tablet instead of drinking orange juice. Neither should they use a natural vitamin C supplement instead of a food source of vitamin C. Whenever possible a well-balanced diet should be the source of vitamins.

Food additives

The general public tends to feel comfortable using food additives with which they are familiar, for example, salt, herbs and spices, and vitamins. In response to consumer concern about the safety of less familiar food additives, industry has launched numerous efforts to put food additives in a more favorable light. Many organizations and companies produced booklets, advertisements, and pamphlets designed to educate the public about the safety of food additives and the reasons why they are used.

Some purposes of food additives are listed in Table

---

* Since a bioflavonoid called rutin (a substance found in citrus fruit) is often promoted as necessary for optimum vitamin C absorption, it was also tested in the same study. Rutin failed to increase bioavailability of synthetic ascorbic acid in man.

18.4 accompanied by examples and related comments. Food additives have been developed for other purposes not listed in Table 18.4, most of which are meant to improve the appearance, texture, or storage life of convenience foods. Many convenience foods would be unavailable without the use of food additives.

RISK VERSUS BENEFIT

A number of intentional food additives have recently been the subject of intense investigation and debate, much of which revolves around considerations of benefit versus risk.

Since the Delaney clause (the amendment prohibiting use of any amount of a carcinogenic additive in food) allows no consideration of benefit versus risk, some individuals and groups have urged repeal of this law, calling it unduly restrictive. They often mention that some carcinogenic substances are naturally present in the food supply. The best example is the carcinogen aflatoxin, traces of which may contaminate peanut butter or milk.[25] Other individuals and groups firmly back the Delaney clause, fearing that the FDA will lose authority needed to assure food safety if the clause is repealed.

The issue of benefit versus risk and the Delaney clause became particularly heated when the FDA announced a ban on saccharin in March 1977. The FDA reported on the results of a well-controlled Canadian study which demonstrated beyond reasonable question that saccharin causes bladder tumors in test animals and that the effect is magnified in the second generation. Apparently in the interest of avoiding unnecessary panic, the FDA tempered its remarks.[26] The result was that many people thought the study was ridiculous and risk nonexistent. Letters and calls of protest poured into the FDA and Congress. Many claimed that the benefits of saccharin in weight control far outweighed what they understood to be the risks. In November 1977, Congress imposed a moratorium on the saccharin ban (Saccharin Study and Labeling Act). During this time there was to be further study of existing information on the carcinogenicity of saccharin, gathering of new information, and consideration of the probable impact of a ban. To warn consumers of the potential hazard, foods containing saccharin were required to be clearly labeled with the words:

Use of this product may be hazardous to your health. This product contains saccharin which has been determined to cause cancer in laboratory animals.

If saccharin is banned, it is expected that it will still be available in plain form in drug stores. Anyone choosing to use it, whether it is banned or not, should understand the degree of risk involved. No matter what the final outcome of this issue, there are some points regarding cancer-testing technology which health professionals should be able to explain to consumers.

TABLE 18.4 *Some purposes of intentional food additives*

PURPOSE	EXAMPLES	VALID POINTS WHICH MIGHT BE RAISED BY NATURAL FOOD ENTHUSIASTS	OTHER CONSIDERATIONS
Improve nutritive value	Iron and vitamins B_1, B_2, and niacin added to refined grain products	Whole grain products are better balanced nutritionally than are enriched refined grain products	The enrichment program has helped eliminate pellagra in the U.S.
	Potassium iodide added to table salt	Iodine can be obtained from kelp and seafood	Iodized salt has greatly reduced the incidence of endemic goiter
Enhance flavor	Natural herbs, spices, and essential oils	(Usually no objection)	
	Aromatic chemicals such as artificial strawberry or grape flavor	These are most commonly used in fabricated products (such as fruit-flavored soft drinks or gelatin desserts) which are poor substitutes for fruits	Artificial flavors such as vanillin are less costly than their natural counterparts and are more consistent (not always better) in flavor
Maintain appearance, palatability, and wholesomeness	Antioxidants and chelating agents in vegetable oil or products containing vegetable oil, such as crackers, mixes for baked products	Use of fresh ingredients or foods eliminates the need for preservatives EDTA (a chelating agent) may reduce intestinal absorption of trace metals	Antioxidants protect against destruction of vitamin E in vegetable oil Decreased loss owing to retardation of spoilage may help keep down costs to the consumer BHT, one of the antioxidants whose safety is questioned, is not essential even in convenience foods. Several brands do not contain it.[24]
	Mold inhibitors in bread such as calcium propionate		Calcium propionate increases the calcium content of bread. Propionate is a normal metabolite in the body
	Sodium nitrate and sodium nitrite in cured meats	May cause formation of carcinogens in meat	Helps protect against development of the toxin botulin by suppressing growth of *C. botulinum*
Control pH	Phosphoric acid in cola	Many foods containing added acid are high in sugar	Essential to the soft drink industry
Add color	Artificial color in soft drinks, frozen desserts, maraschino cherries, sauces, puddings, prepared mixes	Pleasing colors are available in natural foods, especially if they are properly prepared	Coloring agents may be particularly helpful in promoting adequate food intake by individuals who must limit intake of natural foods because of abnormal conditions such as chronic renal failure or phenylketonuria
	Orange coloring applied to the outside of oranges	Norway and Sweden have banned the use of synthetic dyes in food products because of concern about potential hazards[24a]	The FDA banned Red Dye No. 2 because safety had not been proven even though potential harm had not been proven either
Impart and maintain desired consistency	Emulsifiers in margarines; stabilizers in ice cream, soft drinks; thickeners in sauces		Some of these additives might be considered to be "natural" substances. The emulsifier lecithin is a popular "supplement" sold in health food stores

CANCER TESTING AS RELATED TO FOOD ADDITIVES

There are several methods of testing substances for potential carcinogenicity.[27]

Short term tests, which require only a few weeks, may be used for screening purposes. In short term tests, specific microorganisms are exposed to the test chemical and the organisms are later investigated for mutagenic changes. (Mutagenic changes are changes in DNA. Such changes are thought to be involved in carcinogenesis.) Short term tests are not definitive but are very suggestive. Results of some of the screening tests for saccharin have been positive.

Animal tests are more expensive than short term tests and require a much longer period of time but are the best method currently available for predicting whether a substance will be carcinogenic in man. Any substance which is carcinogenic in any test animal is presumed to be a potential human carcinogen. There is no scientific reason to think otherwise.[27]

The method of testing a substance in animals requires some explanation. A substance either is or is not carcinogenic. A high dose of a carcinogen hastens the process of carcinogenesis and increases the incidence of overt cancer. A low dose over a long period could also cause cancer. When testing for carcinogenesis, it is necessary to use high doses of the chemical in question in order to produce measurable results using a reasonable number of test animals in a reasonable period of time. In the Canadian tests, saccharin accounted for 5 percent of the total diet fed to the rats. Relatively few chemicals fed at a level of 5 percent or more cause tumors. A 5 percent level is needed to be able to statistically predict if a more moderate dose of a substance might cause cancer in at least one of every 20,000 people. Unfortunately there is no experimental or theoretical basis for believing that there is a level below which a carcinogenic substance is harmless.[28]

On the basis of the results of the animal tests with saccharin, statistical methods have been used to estimate that moderate intake (one large diet soft drink daily) over a lifetime by each American might result in an extra 1200 extra cases of bladder cancer each year.[29] Unquestionably, saccharin is a weak carcinogen, but "weak" refers to the number of cancers caused, not to the seriousness of the condition if it develops.

Epidemiological tests have been briefly described in Chapter 5. Currently there is scanty epidemiological evidence regarding a positive association between saccharin and human bladder cancer. Studies are underway to collect additional data.

More about saccharin The large number of people exposed to saccharin and the amount of saccharin to which they are exposed increases the concern about the potential danger from this artificial sweetener. An annual intake of about 6 million pounds of saccharin is reported, three fourths of it in the form of diet soft drinks.[30]

There are a number of unresolved questions regarding the degree of risk associated with saccharin. Among the most significant of these is whether maternal use of saccharin during pregnancy and lactation results in greater risk to the baby. (The increase in incidence of bladder cancer in rats exposed to saccharin from the time of conception and throughout life makes this a concern.)

Canada has successfully banned saccharin despite public outcry.

NITRITES

In a few instances, safety benefits of food additives have caused governmental agencies to give more heed to benefit-risk considerations. The use of nitrites provides a good example. Nitrites have been used for centuries in curing meats such as ham, bacon, corned beef, and smoked fish and poultry. Nitrites are definitely beneficial in that they retard growth of *C. botulinum*, thereby helping to prevent formation of a potent neurotoxin. Nitrites also impart an attractive color which consumers have come to expect in some cured meats. The danger lies primarily in compounds called nitrosamines which may be formed when nitrites are present in meat. Some nitrosamines are carcinogenic in laboratory animals. USDA has taken steps to reduce (not completely eliminate) the amount of nitrite used in bacon, a food which is particularly susceptible to nitrosamine formation. (A different additive is substituted to retard growth of botulism organisms.)

Because food additives are prevalent in the food supply, consumers are exposed to them unless they make a conscious effort to purchase additive-free food. In most cases there appears to be very little risk associated with any one additive. Unanswered questions remain regarding (1) possible synergistic effects of additives (the increased physiological activity of combinations of additives) and (2) cumulative effects resulting from high intake of many additives for a prolonged period of time.

Organically grown food

Animal products may contain residues of animal drugs (hormones and antibiotics in particular) and of pesticides. Plant foods may be contaminated with traces of pesticide residue. Concern about use of animal drugs and pesticides largely accounts for increased interest in using organically grown foods. These concerns have some basis in fact. (1) Pesticides are particularly dangerous to the many people *who work directly with them.* Lack of knowledge or carelessness make use of pesticides particularly dangerous for home gardening. (2) The National Advisory Food and Drug Committee of the FDA "Affirmed that the long-term goal of the FDA should be to eliminate from animal feed the use of any antibiotic drugs used to treat disease in people."[31] The threat involves the development of antibiotic-resistant strains of bacteria rather than the residue in food.

Economic considerations are a major reason for using pesticides and animal drugs. These substances promote increased production at relatively low cost. Environmentalists are promoting adoption of farming methods which would reduce pesticide use without excessive sacrifice of profit.[32]

Another aspect of organic farming is using organic fertilizers and soil conditioners such as compost, manure, and bone meal rather than artificial fertilizer. Probably the most valid reasons for preferring use of organic fertilization methods are ecological, but large scale farmers choose chemical fertilizers because they are cost effective. Many large scale farmers use some organic methods in combination with chemical fertilization.

". . . carefully controlled experiments have failed to show consistent differences in favor of either form of fertilization."[33] Chemical fertilizers do not have any harmful effects on plants or on people who eat fertilized plants. The plants themselves primarily utilize inorganic forms of minerals from the soil. Organic mineral complexes from organic fertilizers are broken down to inorganic forms before the plant can benefit from them. There is no test which can distinguish an organically grown plant from a chemically fertilized one. For either fertilization method used (for plants of the same species and variety) nutritive value is the same with the possible exception of trace mineral content.

MAINTENANCE OF FOOD SUPPLY

Discussion of the value of food additives, animal drugs, and agricultural chemicals often draws attention to maintenance of an adequate supply of nutritious foods. This can be illustrated by the following quote:

ARE ADDITIVES NECESSARY?

Commercial additives are essential for our coast to coast food distribution system and for feeding our ever expanding population. With only 5% of the U.S. population growing food for the remaining 95%, much of the food would spoil before reaching the dinner table if it were not for additives.[34]

Those who are most strongly opposed to use of food additives and agricultural chemicals are likely to question the soundness of the above argument for ecological reasons. After all, a move toward vegetarianism would change the character of the needed food supply and would reduce the need for agricultural chemicals, animal drugs, and food additives. However it appears that many Americans place a high value on the types of foods which these controversial substances make possible. Once again health care providers need to try to keep an open mind, to view the issues from a broad perspective, separate facts from fallacies and unresolved issues, assess risks versus benefits, and help others do the same.

STUDY QUESTIONS

1. While listening to a talk show on the radio you hear someone state that taking vitamin A supplements helps to keep the skin soft and supple. How could you verify whether this statement is accurate or not? In either case would there be any danger in taking vitamin A supplements? Explain.

2. Look in newspapers and magazines for nutritional statements included in news items or feature stories. Determine whether they are factual, misleading, or dangerous.

3. Find examples of several advertisements or commercials giving a "counter-nutritional" message (a message conflicting with sound nutrition).

4. In what ways are the FDA and the FTC limited in their ability to prevent fraudulent labeling and advertising of foods?

5. Identify some reasons why people may be vulnerable to false claims for diets, health foods, and nutritional supplements. How can health professionals help to counteract this situation?

6. When testing food additives for carcinogenicity, why are very high levels of the substance fed to test animals?

7. Examine an article or other publication which gives industry's view of food additives. What valid points are made? Are any important facts overlooked?

References

1. Pauling, L.: *Vitamin C and the Common Cold.* San Francisco: W. H. Freeman, 1970.
*2. Mason, M.: *The Dynamics of Clinical Dietetics.* New York: John Wiley & Sons, 1977.
*3. Deutsch, R. M.: *The New Nuts Among the Berries.* Palo Alto CA: Bull Publishing Co., 1977. p. 274.
4. Rynearson, E. H.: Americans love hogwash. *Nutr. Rev.* Special Supplement: 1–13, July 1974.
5. Rynearson, E. H.: Adelle Davis' books on nutrition. *Med. Insight* 15:32, 1973.
6. Davis, A.: *Let's Get Well.* New York: Harcourt, Brace, Jovanovich, 1965.
7. Peterson, S. W., et al.: Composition of and cholesterol in Araucana and commercial eggs. *J. Am. Diet. Assoc.* 72:45, 1978.
8. Bruch, H.: The allure of food cults and nutrition quackery. *J. Am. Diet. Assoc.* 57:316, 1970.
9. —— Laetrile (Vitamin B₁₇)—A statement by the National Nutrition Consortium (Commentary) *J. Am. Diet. Assoc.* 70:354, 1977.
10. Lehmann, P.: Laetrile: The fatal "cure." *FDA Consumer.* 11(8):10, 1977.
11. Stein, M. R., et al.: Ineffectiveness of human chorionic gonadotropin in weight reduction: A double blind study. *Am. J. Clin. Nutr.* 29:940, 1976.
12. Frank, B., and Miele, O.: *Dr. Frank's No-Aging Diet.* New York: Dell, 1977.
13. Megavitamin therapy for childhood psychoses and learning disabilities. Committee on Nutrition, American Academy of Pediatrics. *Pediatrics* 58:910, 1976.
14. —— To dose or megadose. A debate about vitamin C. *Nutr. Today* 13(2):6, 1978.
15. Nutritional aspects of vegetarianism, health foods, and fad diets. American Academy of Pediatrics Committee on Nutrition. *Nutr. Rev.* 35:153, 1977.
16. Herbert, V. D.: Megavitamin therapy. *Contemp. Nutr.* 2(10), Oct. 1977.

17. Miller, J. Z., et al.: Therapeutic effect of vitamin C: A co-twin control study. JAMA 237:248, 1977.

18. Coulehan, J. L., et al.: Vitamin C and acute illness in Navajo school children. *New Engl. J. Med.* 295:973, 1976.

19. ——— The news is out. SELENIUM! *Bestways* 6: 63, July 1978.

20. Are selenium supplements needed (by the general public)? Food and Nutrition Board, Division of Biological Sciences, Assembly of Life Sciences, NRC. *J. Am. Diet. Assoc.* 70:249, 1977.

21. ——— Warning planned on potassium chloride! *FDA Consumer* 12(6):22, 1978.

22. Heenan, J.: Myths of vitamins. *FDA Consumer.* HEW Publication No. FDAt6-2047, March 1974.

23. Pelletier, O., and Keith, M. O.: Bioavailability of synthetic and natural ascorbic acid. *J. Am. Diet. Assoc.* 64:271, 1974.

24. Jacobsen, M.: BHT: Weighing the benefits and risks. *Nutr. Action* 4(9):6, 1977.

24a Jacobsen, M.: Tips on labeling from abroad. *Nutr. Action* 5(6):6, 1978.

25. Rodricks, J. V.: Hazards from nature. Aflatoxins. *FDA Consumer* 12(4):16, 1978.

26. ——— The great saccharin snafu. *Consumer Reports* 42:410, 1977.

27. *Cancer Testing Technology and Saccharin.* Office of Technology Assessment. Washington DC: U.S. Govt. Printing Office, October 1977.

28. ——— Animal tests and human health. *FDA Consumer* 11(7):12, 1977.

29. Pines, W. L., and Glick, N.: The saccharin ban. *FDA Consumer* 11(4): 10, 1977.

30. ——— Saccharin: Where do we go from here? *FDA Consumer* 12(3):16, 1978.

31. Larkin, T.: Using drugs in food animals. *FDA Consumer* 11(3):6, 1977.

32. Jacobsen, M.: Agriculture's new hero: IPM. *Nutr. Action.* 5(10):3, 12, 1978.

*33. Soil fertility and the nutritive value of crops. Food and Nutrition Board, Division of Biological Sciences, Assembly of Life Sciences, NRC. *J. Am. Diet. Assoc.* 70:469, 1977.

34. Consumer Relations Department. Additives and our food heritage. Chicago: Kraft Food Co. HS-8154.

* Recommended reading

Part 2

Bibliography and Additional Recommended Readings

Anderson, L., et al.: *Nutrition in Health and Disease,* ed. 16. Philadelphia: J. B. Lippincott Co., 1976.

Bhagavan, N. V.: *Biochemistry,* ed. 2. Philadelphia: J. B. Lippincott Co., 1978.

Chaney, M. S., Ross, M. L., and Witschi, J. C.: *Nutrition,* ed. 9. Boston: Houghton Mifflin, 1979.

DePaola, D., and Alfano, M.: Diet and oral health. *Nutr. Today* 12(3):6, 1977.

Evans, E., and Miller, D. S.: Slimming aids. *J. Human Nutr.* 32:433, 1978.

Fomon, S. J., et al.: *Recommendations for feeding normal infants.* DHEW Publ. No. (HSA) 79-5108. Washington DC: Superintendent of Documents.

Glick, N.: Low-calorie protein diets. *FDA Consumer* 12(3):7, 1978.

Goodhart, R. S., and Shils, M. E. (eds.): *Modern Nutrition in Health and Disease,* ed. 5. Philadelphia: Lea & Febiger, 1973.

Guyton, A. C.: *Textbook of Medical Physiology,* ed. 5. Philadelphia: W. B. Saunders Co., 1976.

Johnson, N.: Teaching dental health to children. *Pediatr. Nurs.* 4:20, 1978.

Jukes, T. H.: All additives are not bad. *N. Engl. J. Med.* 297:427, 1977.

Lehmann, P.: More than you ever thought you would know about food additives . . . Part I. *FDA Consumer* 13(3):10, 1979.

Megavitamin therapy. *Am. J. Clin. Nutr.* 31:1712, 1978.

Nutrition Reviews' Present Knowledge in Nutrition, ed. 4. Washington DC: Nutrition Foundation, 1976.

Smith, N. J.: *Food for Sport.* Palo Alto CA: Bull Publishing Co., 1976.

Sodium-Restricted Diets and the Use of Diuretics. Committee on Sodium-Restricted Diets, Food and Nutrition Board, National Research Council. Washington DC: National Academy of Sciences, 1979.

The saccharin question re-examined: An A.D.A. Statement. *J. Am. Diet. Assoc.* 74:544, 1979.

Vitamin-Mineral Safety, Toxicity, and Misuse. National Nutrition Consortium. Chicago: The American Dietetic Assoc., 1978.

Providing Nutritional Care

19

Health maintenance and nutritional care

Health professionals use three broad approaches to assist people to maintain their health. Nutritional care is an integral part of each of these approaches. *Promoting health* is aimed at motivating individuals and assisting them to utilize their resources to adapt effectively to the environment. *Preventing disease* focuses on teaching individuals about the causes of disease and ways to avoid and protect themselves from those causes. This also involves eliminating from the environment factors which cause disease. *Treating disease* involves specific measures to assist an individual to recover from an illness and to prevent future illnesses.

THE HEALTH TEAM

The health team consists of health professionals, other health care workers, and the client. All of these people work together to provide nutritional care to clients. Health professionals function independently, dependently, or collaboratively according to the circumstances. Each group of professionals has a distinct role which is defined by law and based on educational preparation.

Some health care functions may be delegated from one discipline to another. The health team member who performs a delegated assignment functions dependently. Certain areas in which health professionals are competent overlap. When this is the case both groups can work collaboratively, sharing in decision making. Through cooperative efforts team members gain more insight about the client's nutritional needs. This enables professionals to formulate and implement a more comprehensive plan of care for the client.

Various team members formulate their own plans of care, each of which contributes to the total plan for the client. A health team member should know how each member functions.

The *physician* is responsible for management of the client's medical-surgical problems. She diagnoses and treats disease. She must consider how nutritional status and diet are related to disease and its treatment. Frequently the physician must obtain data from the nurse and dietitian in order to accurately identify the client's special nutritional needs.

The *nurse* assists clients to meet their basic needs, one of them being the need for food. She provides direct care to clients and encourages and teaches clients to better care for themselves. Her close and frequent contact with clients, both in the hospital and in the community, places her in an excellent position to identify some of their nutritional needs and to determine problems with which they need assistance. The nurse may then call upon other health team members to provide specific kinds of care for clients. The nurse often coordinates activities of various health team members, promoting and facilitating communication among them. The *nurse practitioner* is prepared in a special program and assumes an expanded role in nursing. She acts as a primary health care agent; she assesses clients' needs and implements a therapeutic plan through independent action, referral, counseling, and collaboration with other health professionals.

The *dietitian/nutritionist* is the nutrition specialist on the health team. She assesses the nutritional status of clients and identifies nutritional needs. She utilizes this information to develop an individualized diet plan conforming to the client's diet orders and reflecting his usual eating pattern. She works closely with the physician and recommends changes in diet order and/or method of feeding when indicated. In some agencies the dietitian writes diet orders. A major responsibility of the dietitian is teaching clients about special diets and about prudent eating to promote health.

The *social worker* is concerned with the psychosocial and economic aspects of client care. She works closely

211

with the client's family, identifying resources available to them. She helps family members utilize these resources to assist and support their family member. The social worker evaluates the family's economic resources and assists families to obtain various forms of financial assistance, such as helping them make arrangements for obtaining food stamps.

The *occupational therapist* and *physical therapist* are team members who have a role in helping clients with activities of daily living. The occupational therapist might teach the client to use assistive devices for cooking or eating; the physical therapist might assist a handicapped client learn to chew and swallow food.

The health team members described thus far are professionals who have the responsibility for planning and directing client care. Other health care providers (such as dietetic technicians and licensed practical nurses) work with them. These individuals usually have two years of education past high school. The dietetic technician is a new member of the health team who works directly with clients in health agencies. One of her functions might include maintaining a file of client food preferences and dietary requirements.[1] A variety of aides assist in giving care. Aides complete a short inservice program in order to learn to perform their various tasks. Nurse's aides and dietary aides work in hospitals and other health care agencies. They provide direct client care such as feeding individuals and assisting clients to fill out menus, respectively.

Sometimes clients are confused by the array of health team members who provide health care. Often the client is uncertain about where to turn for assistance. It is helpful if each client has a primary care provider who is responsible for overall planning and coordination of the client's care. Health team members have a responsibility to inform the client of the kinds and types of service each provides.

The client and his family are central members of the health team. Health professionals who attempt to form a "therapeutic alliance" with the client and his family may be more successful in providing health care than those who do not.

Health professionals and paraprofessionals working in community agencies provide many kinds of supportive services for clients. Public health nurses can do much to facilitate or promote development of sound eating habits; when requested they provide follow-up nutritional care. Most state, county, or city health departments have one or more nutritionists who can discuss or send information about the state's nutrition programs and services, provide direct services to clients, work with community groups, set up exhibits, and provide other nutrition services for both consumers and health professionals.

Many large cities have a service called Dial-a-Dietitian. (It is listed by that name in the white pages of the telephone directory.) This service provides accurate answers to clients' questions about food and nutrition. The dietitians who provide this service *do not prescribe* modified diets.

The local field office of the State Department of Public Welfare offers in-home supportive services, including some related to nutrition and food preparation. These services are directed toward the aged, blind, disabled, and families receiving Aid to Families with Dependent Children (AFDC). Home health aides may assist homebound, ill, and handicapped persons with shopping, meal preparation, and cleanup.

High quality nutritional care requires the health professional to possess competencies in several areas, namely: (1) knowledge of nutrition facts, principles, and concepts; (2) ability to identify the need for nutritional care; (3) commitment to her professional role; (4) ability to utilize concepts from the behavioral sciences; and (5) skill in utilizing tools and resources to provide nutritional care.

SCIENCE OF NUTRITION

Nutrition is an applied science. It incorporates both scientific aspects and aspects of the arts. As a discipline it has evolved from and integrated knowledge from several other sciences, including chemistry, anatomy, physiology, psychology, and sociology. As an art it has developed from both intuitive personal behavior and actions based on personal experience. It is often tempting to initiate a specific action because "it sounds good" or because it worked before; however, the necessity of providing nutritional care based on sound scientific information cannot be overemphasized.

Although there have been tremendous advances in knowledge about food and nutrition, there seems to be a lag in utilizing this knowledge. For example, the value of fluoridated water in prevention of dental caries is well documented, yet many communities have refused to let fluoride be added to their water supply. Through education and appropriate action individuals must be encouraged to use scientific knowledge for their benefit.

Since new discoveries are continually being made competent health professionals keep their knowledge current and apply this new knowledge to their practice.

IDENTIFICATION OF NEED FOR NUTRITIONAL CARE

Perhaps one of the most significant changes affecting the delivery of nutritional care is a shift in focus concerning the concept of *health*. In the past health was seen as merely the absence of disease; currently, health is seen as high level wellness. The World Health Organization gives the following definition: "Health is a state of complete physical, mental and social well-being and not merely the absence of disease and infirmity." Initial studies suggest that the health of many individuals can be improved through educating people about how to protect and maintain their own health.

The rising cost of health care is another item directing attention to health maintenance. As greater shares of health care financing come from government sources, more concerted efforts will be directed toward controlling cost. Maintenance of health has been proposed as one possible way to decrease medical bills.[2] Proper nutritional care is an essential component of health maintenance.

If nutritional care is to be a major component of health maintenance, a change from the traditionally disease-oriented delivery system to a health-oriented system is necessary. Health professionals need to shift from being authoritarian directors of care to being *facilitators* of care, encouraging clients to assume responsibility for their own health and nutritional status. More emphasis must be placed on nutrition education. This means relating nutrition to health, translating nutrition knowledge into everyday food practices, and encouraging clients to eat prudently.

COMMITMENT TO PROFESSIONAL ROLE

Commitment to provide high quality nutritional care is based on values and beliefs about fellow human beings. Values and concepts shared by many health professionals include (1) respect for the individual and (2) the belief that health is the right of every individual. Many values differ from person to person. Thus, it is important for health professionals to identify how they utilize their own values and beliefs when implementing care and to be sensitive to the impact their values have on others.

Committed health professionals are willing to assume responsibility for the services they provide and are accountable for their actions. They possess necessary skills and use tools competently to provide quality nutritional care to clients. Much diligent practice is necessary to develop skill in using tools. For example, to interview clients effectively, a health practitioner acquires knowledge of the communication process. She learns how to apply this knowledge to her practice and then works to develop expertise in interviewing. The quality of interpersonal relationships health professionals establish with clients influences outcomes of care. Effective health care workers identify and cultivate behaviors which positively influence the outcomes of client care.

Professionals assume many different roles when delivering health care. Four roles for providing nutritional care are advocate, motivator, teacher, and provider.

Professionals, as *advocates*, act for or in behalf of other people. Inherent within the role is the concept of helping. Advocacy may have slightly different meanings to different members of the health care professions. However, a few generalizations can be made. Advocates possess knowledge and expertise in specific areas. They have an attitude of concern for the welfare of others and they are willing to publicly put themselves forth to help others. Because of their competencies and beliefs they can (1) assist people to identify and define problems, (2) establish mutual goals with people, (3) initiate action for people who are not able to do so themselves, and (4) encourage people to act on their own behalves. Professionals assume the role of advocate in a variety of settings and situations.

Professionals can act as advocates for individuals when they are providing direct client care. The hospital nurse who notes a client has eaten very little for several days may initiate action to increase the client's nutrient intake.

As *motivators*, health professionals encourage clients to strive for goals. Inherent within the role of motivator are the concepts of hope and self-worth. To strive to make changes in one's lifestyle an individual must have hope of success and feel that he has self-worth. While many of the complexities of motivation are yet to be unraveled, motivators can base many of their activities on knowledge from the behavioral sciences. Once the health care worker has identified dominent motives which influence the way a person acts she can (1) present him with more healthful alternatives, (2) help him weigh the risks involved in making change against the benefits to be gained, and (3) provide him with support and encouragement to make the change.

Characteristics which may help the professional act as a motivator include sensitivity, honesty, warmth, acceptance, positive regard, empathy, and belief in the client's ability to change.

As *teachers*, health professionals work to change clients' behavior. Both formal and informal teaching are an integral part of nutritional care.

Recently, emphasis has been placed on the concept that a teacher facilitates learning. The word educator comes from the Latin word *educare* meaning to lead, to guide. The teacher not only provides knowledge and information but she (1) shares some of herself, her enthusiasm, interest, and involvement in the subject matter, (2) focuses her attention on the learner, establishing a cooperative climate of inquiry, and (3) encourages the client to apply his newly acquired knowledge.

When clients are not able to carry out activities of daily living to meet their own needs, health professionals may act as *providers* of care. They perform a variety of activities to support and supplement the client's ability to meet his basic needs. The concept of caring (concern for the welfare of another) is inherent in providing care. Clients who are ill often look to professionals for comfort and protection.

Providing food is an important activity which should meet not only the client's nutritive needs but also a variety of his psychosocial and safety needs. Quality care requires interpersonal and technical skills. For example, safely administering a tube feeding requires knowledge of anatomy and physiology of the gastrointestinal tract, correct application of principles of physics, and appreciation of and empathy for the client's reactions to this method of feeding.

CONCEPTS FROM THE BEHAVIORAL SCIENCES

Health professionals acquire knowledge of human behavior to improve their effectiveness in working with people. Although human behavior is often elusive, theories of behavior suggest factors which influence behavior and predict how individuals behave in various situations. These theories help provide a basis for determining desirable methods of changing a person's behavior. However, each person's heritage and individuality must be recognized and considered when planning for change.

Behavioral concepts useful for working with clients include (1) communication, (2) teaching and learning, and (3) change and compliance. These concepts are interrelated and overlap.

Communication

Communication is the process of sharing information, feelings, and ideas. It takes several forms: verbal, nonverbal, and written. Communication is essential to the formation of relationships among individuals. An individual's self-concept, his relationship to others, and his perceptions of the world and his place in it are developed primarily through communicating with others. Communication is necessary for much of learning to occur. Via the communication process people receive information, clarify problems, and formulate plans for adapting to internal and external changes. *Feedback,* a form of communication in which a person receives information about himself and his actions, helps him realistically perceive himself, others, and his environment.

Teaching and learning

Learning is often described as consisting of two phases. First an individual acquires information, and then he changes or modifies his behavior as he applies his newly acquired knowledge. Learning may occur in three general domains—cognitive, affective, and psychomotor. The *cognitive* domain relates to the acquisition of knowledge, understandings, and skill in using them. The *affective* domain pertains to the acquisition of attitudes, appreciations, and interests. The *psychomotor* domain relates to development of motor activities and skills. Professionals consider the domain in which learning is to occur when planning learning experiences and selecting teaching materials.

Teaching is a process of providing knowledge and insight. Recently the term *counseling* and, specifically, nutrition or diet counseling is being used in reference to the teaching-learning process. It is a broader term than teaching. It incorporates the idea of working with a client, encouraging him to make changes in his pattern of living which he sees as desirable and attainable, and supporting him throughout the process. Counseling is based on two premises: (1) each person controls his own life and behavior and (2) each individual has a background of personal interactions, socialization, and education that he uses to make choices about his behavior. The health professional uses her knowledge and skills to assist clients to identify problems, discover and list possible solutions, consider the consequences of each alternative, choose a solution, and incorporate that solution into his activities of daily living.[3]

Change and compliance

Theories of change attempt to describe how and when change will occur. Change may occur within an individual or within a group. Health professionals may promote change in an individual, such as helping him alter his eating habits. In addition they might promote change within the social and cultural environment such as supporting legislation to promote health and optimal nutritional status of the elderly. An individual who promotes or facilitates change is referred to as a change agent.

The change process   Change is a process involving not a single incident but, rather, a series of events. A description of the change process useful to health professionals is as follows:

State of compliance. Initially an individual identifies a problem and recognizes that change is desirable. He allows himself to be influenced because he sees new behavior as a way of obtaining something he wants. The change agent (person trying to initiate change) acts as a motivator.

Stage of identification. An individual identifies behaviors he wishes to imitate or add to his own. A conflict of values may occur at this point as an individual looks at how he was and considers the risks and advantages of change. The intervention of a change agent may assist the individual to successfully integrate the new behavior with existing behavior.

Stage of internalization. During this stage an individual actually believes new concepts, integrating them into his own value system. The internalized behavior becomes self-rewarding and external support is no longer necessary.

Change may occur slowly or quickly. When change is slow health professionals can support individuals by pointing out to them any changes which have occurred.

Facilitators of change   Several elements facilitate change. These include trust, tolerance, mutual appreciation, involvement of the client in planning and decision making, informing the client of the reason for change, assisting the client to perceive rewards to be obtained from the changes, and providing the client with support during the change process. When making

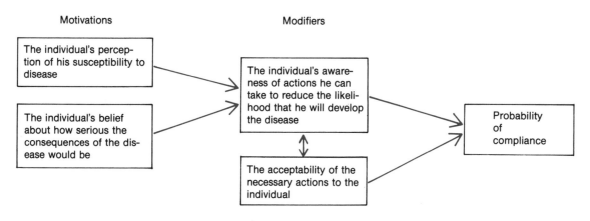

The individual's percep-
tion of his susceptibility to
disease

The individual's belief
about how serious the
consequences of the dis-
ease would be

The individual's aware-
ness of actions he can
take to reduce the likelihood that he will develop
the disease

The acceptability of the
necessary actions to the
individual

Probability
of
compliance

FIGURE 19.1. A health belief model.

a decision to change or modify behavior, people weigh the gains derived from the change against the losses which may result.

Compliance   Compliance is the degree to which an individual is willing to make and sustain changes in his behavior. An individual's beliefs about health and the impact a health crisis (illness) makes on him are two factors influencing whether or not a person will comply with health care recommendations. A *Health Belief Model* is a tool which helps predict whether or not an individual will take action to maintain or promote his health.[4] The tool may be useful to distinguish areas where health professionals may intervene to promote compliance. Figure 19.1 shows a Health Belief Model.

TOOLS FOR PROVIDING NUTRITIONAL CARE

Good tools are essential to provide quality nutritional care. Just as it is not possible for a mechanic to maintain or repair an automobile without specific tools, it is not possible for the health professional to accurately identify client needs and implement an appropriate plan of care without appropriate tools.

There are many tools available for providing nutritional care. Three general types of tools described in this chapter are (1) the clinical care process, (2) the problem-oriented medical record, and (3) quality assurance control. There are also many specific tools, such as food composition tables, height and weight charts, and food exchange tables.

The clinical care process

The clinical care process serves as an excellent tool for identifying and meeting clients' needs. The process involves a logical series of activities to approach and solve problems. It is based on scientific problem-solving methodology and is flexible and adaptable for use by various health care providers.

The organized and systematic framework of the clinical care process provides for identification of client problems, planning and implementation of care, and evaluation of outcomes.

Although the clinical care process has been characterized in a variety of ways, the process and its component parts are similar whether it is described as a three, four, or five step plan. The process discussed and utilized in this text includes four elements: (1) assessment, (2) planning, (3) implementation, and (4) evaluation. An overview of the clinical care process is presented on page 216. Details for implementing the process are discussed in subsequent chapters in this part of the book.

The problem-oriented medical record

The problem-oriented medical record (POMR) is a valuable communication tool. Information about all aspects of client care including nutritional care is recorded according to client problems. The POMR has several advantages over the traditional medical record (which many health agencies still use). In the traditional record, client data is recorded according to its source. Results of laboratory tests are recorded in one section, physician's notes in another, nurse's notes in still another, and so on. Health professionals may have to look through an entire source-oriented record to review all data pertinent to a particular client problem. The POMR was developed by Dr. Lawrence Weed so that client data would be recorded according to client problems. Since the basic components of the POMR closely parallel the steps in the clinical care process, the POMR facilitates systematic delivery of health care.

The POMR emphasizes assessment by clearly identifying the data which is to be collected about the client. From this data the client's problems are identified. Initial plans for and outcomes of care are clearly stated. This facilitates evaluating the client's response to care and the quality of care given. Ideally, all health team members work with the same problem list and record progress notes in an integrated manner. Thus health professionals can be more cognizant of what each team member is doing; duplication and fragmen-

CLINICAL CARE PROCESS

ASSESSMENT

Purposes:
• *to identify areas where nutrition intervention is required*
• *to provide a baseline for later evaluation of client's progress*

Components:
• *data gathering: purposeful, structured, systematic collection of data*
• *data analysis: classifying, synthesizing, and making inferences based on all available relevant data, scientific knowledge, and expertise*
• *diagnosis of problem (actual or potential): statement identifying a condition which is interfering with or is likely to interfere with nutritional needs*

PLANNING

Purposes:
• *to determine what can be done to achieve and maintain an optimal nutritional state for the client*
• *to identify specific criteria for evaluation of care*
• *to select appropriate methods for intervention*
• *to guide health team members in implementing care*

Components:
• *client-oriented goals: measurable, realistic outcomes of care (evaluation criteria)*
• *nutritional care plan: specific measures to be implemented in caring for the client, including ongoing assessment activities, direct care activities, and client education*

EVALUATION

Purposes:
• *to identify the extent to which objectives have been met*
• *to promote provision of quality nutritional care*

Components:
• *ongoing measurement of client's progress toward stated objectives (criteria)*
• *evaluation of effectiveness of plan: analysis of all steps in the clinical care process*
• *revision of the plan: reordering priorities, restating objectives, reformulating plan*

IMPLEMENTATION

Purpose:
• *to carry out activities identified in the nutritional care plan*

Components:
• *provision of care: giving supportive care*
• *coordination of care: providing for consistency of approach, cooperation, and communication among health care workers*
• *teaching and counseling clients: assisting clients to make necessary modifications in their activities of daily living*

tation of care can be minimized. POMR is also useful as an educational tool and as a means for audit to control the quality and cost of care.

COMPONENTS

The manner in which the POMR is utilized varies from one health agency to another; in fact, many health agencies use only part of it. The four basic components of the POMR, as described here, are based on the work of Dr. Weed.[5] They are (1) a defined data base, (2) a client problem list, (3) an initial plan of care, and (4) progress notes.

The data base The data base consists of a predefined amount of information which a health care agency designates is to be completely and accurately collected from each of its clients. In some settings, such as a clinic for the treatment of persons who have diabetes mellitus, the data base might include a complete history and physical examination, results of a nutritional assessment, and several laboratory studies. In other health agencies, such as a maternity clinic, the type of care being provided and the goals of each facility are different. The data base is most effective if it reflects these differences.

The data base is the pool of information from which initial client problems are identified. It serves as a yardstick against which to measure the client's progress and the outcomes of care. Since the data base is predefined it promotes consistency in the quality of care being given. When problems need further clarification, additional data are collected and recorded in progress notes.

The problem list   A problem is defined to exist if the client requires assistance in meeting a basic need. A problem may threaten an individual's health and well-being or interfere with his ability to function at his optimum level. Problems may range from lack of ability to prepare food to lack of interest in eating or lack of appetite to cancer of the small intestine which interferes with digestion and absorption of nutrients. Initially, problems are identified from and supported by information in the data base. The initial problem for a client who enters the hospital with an unexplained weight loss may simply be "unexplained weight loss." Later if it is determined from physical findings and laboratory studies that the client has a problem, such as protein-energy malnutrition, the initial problem may be redefined or a second problem added to the list.

Each health professional diagnoses problems within her realm of practice. The doctor diagnoses particular diseases such as "coronary artery disease." The nurse or the dietitian on the other hand may note that the client "does not follow his sodium and cholesterol restricted diet."

The problem list serves as a table of contents for the client's medical record. Problems are numbered and dated. The list is usually placed at the beginning of the chart. Health professionals wanting information about a particular problem can note the number, then quickly thumb through the chart looking only at notes with that number.

Initial plans for care   An initial care plan is formulated for each problem. It should specifically outline (1) further data which need to be collected, (2) therapeutic measures to be implemented, and (3) education of the patient and his family to be carried out.

Progress notes   Progress notes are narrative notes describing the progress the client is making with each of his problems. They are often referred to by the acronym SOAP (Subjective, Objective, Assessment, and Plan).

The following are guidelines for charting using the SOAP format
S. Subjective data: record how the client feels, his concerns and his description of his symptoms.
O. Objective data: record observable verifiable data, specific care treatments and client education provided, and the client's response to treatments and education.
A. Assessment: state your impression of the client's progress and response to care based on analysis of subjective and objective data. Identify suspected causes of the client's problem.

P. Plans: formulate new plans or revise existing ones according to the data collected and assessment made. Head each progress note with the date and the name and number of the problem.

Chart on problems only when new data is available, the client's condition has changed, or specific care has been provided. Read the notes written by other health professionals to be aware of and use the data they have collected and to facilitate teamwork in providing client care. Write brief concise notes, avoiding duplication of material.

Flowsheets. In some instances, flowsheets are used to record specific measurements over a period of time. The results of laboratory studies, vital signs, calorie counts, intake and output, and daily weights are examples of parameters which may be recorded on flowsheets.

Discharge summary. At the time of discharge a summative progress note is written for each of the problems identified on the client's problem list; resolution or disposition of each problem is stated.

Quality assurance control

Professional review is one tool which can be used to monitor and improve the quality of health care rendered to clients. Professional review of nutritional care is an important aspect of quality assurance control. Several groups have been pressuring health professionals to institute quality control. In 1972 the United States Congress passed an amendment to the Social Security Act which provided for Professional Standards Review Organization (PSRO).

PSRO

The purposes of the PSRO are (1) to provide for systematic professional review of the necessity and appropriateness of medical care services and (2) to assure the quality of the care provided.[6] The PSROs are in the process of being developed and implemented.

At present PSROs are required to carry out three functions, primarily in short-stay general hospitals. One of these functions, medical care evaluation studies, should include evaluation of the nutritional care provided to clients. Retrospective studies are one form of review which are usually carried out after the client has been discharged from the health agency. The focus is primarily on evaluation of medical care through patient care or medical audits. These retrospective audits are specifically designed to focus on potential problem areas. Outcomes of audit may identify the need for a change in the organization and delivery of nutritional care. For instance, if the dietitian does not have sufficient time to do nutritional assessments of all clients, some of her other more routine tasks may be reassigned to paraprofessional personnel.

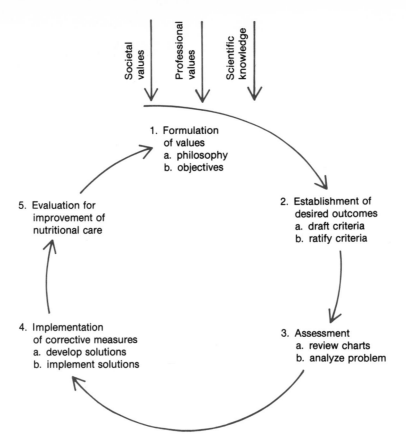

FIGURE 19.2. The process of quality assurance.

After corrective action is taken, a follow-up study should be done to determine whether or not the desired change has occurred.

IMPLEMENTING QUALITY ASSURANCE

Quality assurance is carried out in several ways, as illustrated in Figure 19.2.

Well-written audit criteria are an essential component of a quality assurance program. There are three types of criteria: (1) structure criteria, (2) process criteria, and (3) outcome criteria. Structure criteria describe the organizational, physical, and fiscal aspects of care. A specific structure criterion might state that a diet teaching plan is included in the client's nursing Kardex. Process criteria identify specific activities which health professionals carry out for the client, such as recording food intake. Outcome criteria identify measurable changes in the actual health state of the client. Losing a specified number of pounds of body weight is an example of outcome criteria.

The following are guidelines for writing criteria:
1. Start with simple problems.

TABLE 19.1 *Possible audit criteria for adult clients who have undergone surgery for the construction of a colostomy in the descending colon*

ELEMENTS	EXCEPTIONS	INSTRUCTIONS
(1) Client is provided with information about foods which may cause excessive gas formation or stimulate excessive peristalsis		(1, 2, 3, & 5) See progress notes written by nurse or dietitian
(2) Client identifies foods which are gas formers for him	(1, 2, & 3) The client who is being fed parenterally	
(3) Client identifies food which cause him excessive peristaltic stimulation		
(4) After 6–8 days client has 2–3 semi-soft stools per day	(4 & 5) The client who is receiving high doses of antibiotics	(4) See graphic chart
(5) After 7–9 days client has flatulence no more than 1–3 X/24 hr	(5) The client who swallows large amounts of air	

2. Write 10 to 15 criteria which are aimed at ensuring adequate care.
3. Write criteria which are realistic, understandable (by nonprofessionals), measurable, and achievable.
4. Identify exceptions when criteria cannot be met.
5. List instructions for measuring the criteria along with where to obtain data necessary to carry out the evaluation process.
6. Share the criteria with both colleagues in the same health profession and those belonging to other health disciplines. Criteria must be acceptable to and ratified by the health professionals using them.

Table 19.1 presents some specific examples of audit criteria.

Initial audits of records using newly developed criteria often give the impression that care has been poor. After the need for accurate documentation of activities has been pointed out, re-auditing records often shows improvements.

When an audit identifies specific problems, alternative approaches to providing nutritional care are selected and implemented. Solutions should identify *who* is going to carry them out, *when* and *how* they will be implemented, and *when* a re-audit will be conducted.

STUDY QUESTIONS

1. Why is it important that the client and his family be included as members of the health team?
2. Why is it desirable for health professionals to act as *facilitators* of health care?
3. How does diet counseling differ from diet teaching?
4. List several advantages of using the problem-oriented format for recording data about a client.

References

*1. Davis, P. B.: Using supportive personnel to improve patient care. *Hospitals* 51:62, 1977.
*2. Kristein, M. M.: Health economics and preventive care. *Science* 195:457, 1977.
*3. Danish, S.: Developing helping relationships in dietetic counseling. *J. Am. Diet Assoc.* 67:107, 1975.
4. Becker, M., Drachman, R, and Kirscht, J.: A new approach to explaining sick-role behavior in low-income populations. *Am. J. Public Health* 64:205, 1974.
5. Weed, L.: *Medical Records, Medical Educations and Patient Care.* Cleveland: Press of Case Western Reserve University, 1970.
*6. Zimmer, M.: Quality assurance outcomes. *Nurs. Clin. North Am.* 9(3):305, 1974.

* Recommended reading

20
Data gathering

Giving a client nutritional care without first collecting data about his nutritional and health needs is much like sailing a ship in the fog without a compass, charts, and information about the weather and currents. It is difficult if not impossible to correctly determine what direction to take. Data collection provides a baseline of information from which nutritional needs can be identified and plans for care established. Data which may be useful in identifying nutritional needs of an individual includes information about the client's physical and psychosocial status, the influence of his lifestyle on his pattern of food consumption, and his views of nutrition, health, and illness.

Since the needs, concerns, and perceptions of the client vary from time to time, data collection and analysis of data are an ongoing process. The focus is on both day-to-day nutritional needs of the individual and long term overall needs. Ongoing assessment (i.e., data collection and analysis) is an important part of the evaluation process. Identifying the client's response to care is a necessary step in determining the effectiveness of care provided.

Nutritional assessment aids in identifying (1) overt malnutrition, (2) covert nutritional deficiencies, (3) individuals at risk of developing malnutrition, (4) individuals at risk of developing nutrition-related diseases, and (5) resources available to individuals to assist them in overcoming nutrition problems. Collecting and analyzing data conveys to the client that someone is taking a personal interest in him, his problems, and his needs.

WHO SHOULD BE ASSESSED

Nutritional assessment is one aspect of the total health assessment of individuals. It should be included as part of periodic health evaluations of "well" individuals. At particular stages in the life cycle and under certain circumstances individuals are at risk of developing specific nutrition-related problems. Increased attention should be given to identifying individuals within high risk groups. Table 20.1 lists clients who are most likely to benefit from nutritional assessment and care.

Certainly a client who requires care in a health care facility needs to have his nutritional status evaluated. The client's disease and treatments, especially surgery, drugs, and radiation therapy, affect his nutritional status. It is particularly important to check for protein-energy malnutrition. It is essential to identify needs and institute therapy promptly since nutrient stores of a sick individual may be rapidly depleted. This is particularly likely to occur if a client is under great stress or is unable to eat for a period of time (10 days or more).[1]

The client who is comatose or who is not able to communicate effectively cannot indicate his needs and concerns. Health professionals have added responsibility for seeing that this client's nutritional needs are identified and met.

TYPES OF DATA

There are two major types of data which can be obtained about a client: subjective data and objective data.

Subjective data includes information which the client verbally conveys to health professionals. Information is subjective if it can be directly felt or perceived only by the individual who has experienced it. The client who says he hasn't eaten very much today because he feels nauseous is relating subjective data. Family, friends, or other health professionals may contribute subjective data about a client. They may state their

TABLE 20.1 *Clients who are likely to benefit from nutritional assessment and care*

PRENATAL CLIENTS
A. Factors involved in nutritional risk
1. New clients
2. Teenagers 19 years of age or less
3. Low hematocrit/hemoglobin (<34% or <11)
4. Underweight before pregnancy (10% or more below standard weight for height)
5. Inadequate weight gain* (<2 lb per month after the first trimester)
6. Obesity** (20% or more above standard weight for height or excessive weight gain >7 lb per month)
7. Medical conditions requiring a special diet
8. Frequent conceptions (<24 mo between conceptions)
9. Multiple birth
10. High parity (>3 live births)
11. Previous premature births
12. Previous stillbirth, spontaneous abortions, etc.
13. Low income
14. Excessive smoking, alcoholism, drug addiction
B. Any client with detected poor eating habits or inability to manage food resources

CHILDREN
A. Factors involved in nutritional risk
1. Underweight (<tenth percentile of weight for height by NCHS Growth Chart)
2. Low stature (<tenth percentile by NCHS Growth Chart)
3. Overweight (>90th percentile of weight for height by NCHS Growth Chart)
4. Low hematocrit/hemoglobin (<31% or <10 6–23 mo)
5. Failure to thrive (height and weight below the 5th percentile coupled with a hemoglobin less than 9 gm/100 ml or hematocrit less than 28%)
6. Specific diseases requiring a special diet
7. Physical or mental handicaps affecting feeding
8. Rampant caries (more than 1 DMF† per year of life)
9. Low income
B. Any client with detected poor eating habits or inability to manage food resources

AMBULATORY CLIENTS
A. Clients with prescribed special diets who are having difficulty understanding or following them
B. Clients whose eating habits result in poor nutrition and who could benefit from supportive help from the nutritionist
C. Clients recently released from a long hospital stay because they may be nutritionally depleted
D. Conditions in the elderly which may also result in poor nutrition
1. Ill-fitting dentures or no dentures
2. Diminished sense of taste and smell resulting in decreased appetite
3. Digestive changes resulting in increased digestive time, impaired fat digestion, increased constipation,
4. Decreased kidney function
5. Living alone
6. Reduced income

FAMILY PLANNING CLIENTS
A. Factors involved in nutritional risk
1. Obesity
2. Underweight

(Table continued next column)

TABLE 20.1 *Clients who are likely to benefit from nutritional assessment and care (continued)*

3. Low hematocrits/hemoglobins (<35% or <12)
B. Clients on special diets for a medical condition, e.g., diabetes, kidney conditions
C. Clients with detected poor eating habits or inability to manage food resources
D. Clients who have family members with nutrition or special diet problems
E. Clients who have been on the oral contraceptive for 2 or more years (since the "pill" may cause nutrient depletion)

MENTAL HEALTH AFTERCARE CLIENTS
A. Factors involved in nutritional risk
1. Underweight or unwanted weight loss
2. Unwanted weight gain
B. Clients with detected poor eating habits or inability to manage food resources
C. Groups of clients who could benefit from sessions on general good nutrition, meal planning, food buying, weight control, etc.

ALL OTHER CLIENTS
A. Any client with conditions as above who could benefit from nutrition counseling

Adapted from *Who Needs Nutrition Counseling?* Bureau of Nutrition, Virginia State Health Department, Richmond, rev. 1978.
* The *American College of Obstetrics and Gynecology* recommends a woman gain 10–12 kg (22–27 lb) throughout the course of pregnancy
** The *National Academy of Sciences* recommends that the curve of "normal" weight gain related to duration of pregnancy developed by them be used to assess the pattern of weight gain during pregnancy
† DMF: decayed, missing, or filled teeth

feelings, ideas, and observations about a client. Unless the health professional can validate this data it is subjective. Much of the information included in a health history is subjective. The diet history is a collection of data about the client's dietary practices. It may include information about the client's actual food intake; cultural, social, economic, and family factors affecting food intake; and methods of food procurement and preparation.

Objective data is factual information obtained during the health professional's observations and measurements of the client. Objective data can be directly supported and validated by another person. A food intake record (calorie count) is one type of objective data. The health professional observes what the client eats for a day and records the quantity and a description of each food eaten. If it is a small amount, the record supports the client's subjective statement that he hasn't been eating very much. A client's statement about feeling nauseous, however, would remain subjective data. This symptom cannot be measured by the health professional. Anthropometry, biochemical measurements, and the physical examination are other examples of objective data. Anthropometric measurements are measurements of various body parts, such as height, weight, and arm circumference. Biochemical measurements are tests which indicate the amount of various substances in body fluids or tissue. The number of grams of hemoglobin per 100 ml. of blood is a biochemical measurement.

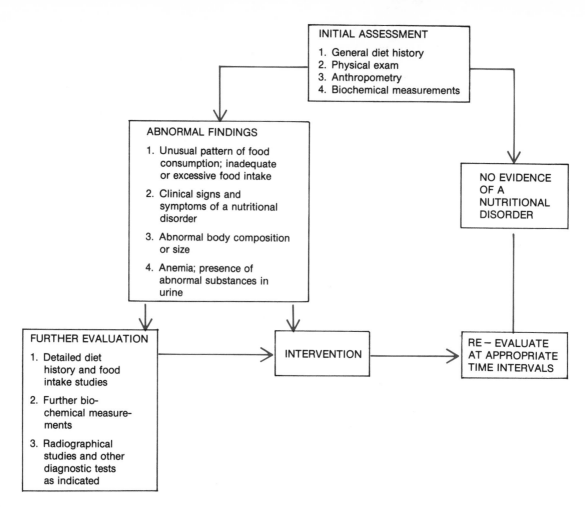

INITIAL ASSESSMENT

1. General diet history
2. Physical exam
3. Anthropometry
4. Biochemical measurements

ABNORMAL FINDINGS

1. Unusual pattern of food consumption; inadequate or excessive food intake
2. Clinical signs and symptoms of a nutritional disorder
3. Abnormal body composition or size
4. Anemia; presence of abnormal substances in urine

NO EVIDENCE OF A NUTRITIONAL DISORDER

FURTHER EVALUATION

1. Detailed diet history and food intake studies
2. Further biochemical measurements
3. Radiographical studies and other diagnostic tests as indicated

INTERVENTION

RE – EVALUATE AT APPROPRIATE TIME INTERVALS

FIGURE 20.1. Nutritional screening process.

Identifying priority information

The health professional collects selected data in a systematic, purposeful manner. Probably the most efficient way to initially obtain data pertinent to nutritional status is to use a screening process. A screening process identifies what data is to be collected and suggests actions to be implemented depending on the findings. Analysis of the data may reveal no specific problem, one or more specific problems, or abnormal findings which require further investigation as outlined in the next chapter. Figure 20.1 illustrates the screening process.

When possible, health professionals initially collect data directly from the client. He is, in most instances, the expert on himself. However, referring to the client's medical record, the diet Kardex, or the nursing Kardex may save time and avoid duplication of work if the client has already had contact with other health professionals.

USE OF MEDICAL RECORDS

The client's medical record often provides valuable information about his nutritional status. Medical records vary in specific types of data included. A medical

history, social history, and physical examination are usually obtained and recorded by the physician when a client initially receives health care. Other health professionals such as the nurse, dietitian, and social worker may each obtain subjective and objective data from the client. This information is recorded along with an assessment and plan for dealing with specified client problems. If the hospital has a clinical nutrition team there may be a nutrition assessment and summary sheet in the record. Data about drugs the client has or is taking, results of laboratory tests, and reports of electrocardiogram and radiographic studies may be found in the client's record. Progress notes are written by various health team members. They list data collected on an ongoing basis, changes in the client's condition, the client's response to therapy, and changes and additions to the plan of care.

Medical history Among points to look for in the client's medical history and physical exam are those factors which alter the ingestion, absorption, utilization, or excretion of nutrients. The most obvious of these are recent or previous diseases or surgery of the gastrointestinal tract, and metabolic diseases such as diabetes mellitus. Examples of other conditions which cause alterations in nutritional status include chronic heart, renal, liver, and lung diseases; psychiatric disorders; neurological diseases; and trauma. It is important to note disease in which inappropriate nutrition is an etiological factor, such as cardiovascular disease.

It is helpful to look for information about the client's activities of daily living. The medical history includes information about whether or not a client smokes or uses alcohol and the amount and frequency of use. A client's activity level may be described. To estimate energy expenditure it is necessary to know the frequency of, duration of, and seasonal variations in exercise. Elimination patterns, including bowel habits, use of laxatives, and urinary frequency are usually indicated. Excessive loss of nutrients may be related to abnormal elimination patterns.

Drugs Many drugs interact with nutrients in ways which affect the client's nutritional status. It is important to identify all drugs (both over-the-counter and prescription medication) the client is currently using and has used in the recent past. The amount, frequency, duration, and reason for taking should be ascertained. A list of drugs a client in a health agency is receiving may be found on a nursing or medication Kardex.

Social history The client's social history often gives information about the client's role in his family, his role in the community, his home and community environment, and educational background. These data frequently provide insight about why the client eats what he eats. Social and cultural factors which influence food selection and preparation may be noted as well as economic and community factors influencing food availability.

Diet Kardex A diet Kardex may contain helpful data which the dietitian has collected. This may include a diet history, estimate of energy requirement, and identification of possible nutrient deficiencies. Complete data are not always recorded on the client's record; some may be found instead on a diet Kardex.

Nursing Kardex The nursing Kardex often contains a summary of the nursing history obtained from the client, a list of client problems, and a plan of care. The type of diet, method of feeding (whether by mouth, tube, or intravenously) and treatments the client is receiving are usually recorded in the nursing Kardex.

OBTAINING DATA FROM THE CLIENT

Specific skills are necessary in order to obtain accurate data. The interview is the primary method used to obtain subjective data from the client and other individuals. Observation and inspection skills are used to obtain objective data. Often a variety of health professionals work together in collecting data about a client. All the pertinent information obtained should be recorded in the client's health or medical record. The data then become a valuable resource to all team members.

Interviewing

Interviewing is a specialized pattern of verbal interaction. It may be directed toward obtaining specific information, ideas, and feelings from an individual. The interview is also a method of giving information and influencing an individual's behavior. The health care professional can more accurately identify the client's immediate and long range nutritional needs if she can conduct an interview in which the client states facts and expresses feelings about relevant aspects of his life. The interview gives the professional an opportunity to establish with the client a sense of mutual trust and respect. Establishing rapport and maintaining it through an interview contributes to the development of a relaxed, comfortable climate. This kind of climate enhances exchange of information.

The health care professional structures the interview in a manner which facilitates the collection of essential data. While it is necessary to ask specific questions in order to obtain relevant information, it is also important to recognize and respond to cues given by the client.

GENERAL FORMAT OF THE INTERVIEW

Particularly when a health professional first begins to conduct interviews it is helpful to follow a general format. The format should serve as a guide and does not need to be rigidly followed. As the professional becomes more comfortable and experienced, the interviews may become more individualized. Guidelines for interviewing are the following:

1. Introduce yourself by name and title. It is important to be certain the client knows the kind of health care he can expect to receive from you.
2. Explain the purpose of the interview. The client needs to know why information is being obtained and how it will be used to help him.
3. Define the limits of the interview. Identify how much time you are planning to spend with the client now and in the future.
4. Use an appropriate form as a guide, for example, a diet history form. The form serves as a reminder to obtain all essential data.
5. Be familiar with the questions on the form. Frequently referring to the form detracts from the flow of conversation.
6. Jot down only pertinent comments. Often interviewers are concerned that they will not be able to remember all pertinent data when recording them later. To the contrary, if the interviewer listens carefully, gives the client his full attention, and records the data immediately following the interview, complete recall usually results.

7. Avoid social "chit-chat." Social responses tend to avoid or cover up feelings.

The client should have an opportunity to answer each question completely, before moving to the next question. This does not mean allowing the client to digress to a variety of other topics. Open-ended questions such as "What kinds of vegetables do you like?" require the client to give some information. Closed questions often result in an answer of yes or no. Little data is obtained if the client is asked "Do you eat breakfast?" On the other hand, asking the client to describe what he does after he gets up in the morning will elicit information about his morning activities. He may indicate whether or not he eats breakfast and perhaps even the value he places on eating breakfast. Asking an open-ended question avoids biasing the client's response. If the client is asked, "What nutritious foods do you eat for breakfast?" he may feel that eating a good breakfast is important to the interviewer. This might influence his answer. Questions beginning with *how*, *what*, *where*, *when*, and *who* encourage the client to explain and clarify data. *Why* should be avoided in an interview of this type as it often implies to the client that he is being asked to justify what he has said or done.[2]

POINTS OF EMPHASIS
General ideas for interviewing

• *Encouraging the client to express his thoughts keeps the interview focused on his concerns.*
• *Using nonverbal activities such as nodding encourages the client without interrupting the flow of the interview. (Nodding should be used with care since it may be interpreted by the client to mean approval of what he has said.)*
• *Responding nonjudgmentally conveys acceptance to the client.*
• *Conveying acceptance to the client reduces his need to be defensive.*
• *Focusing on significant leads and cues keeps the interview moving.*

LISTENING

Listening is an essential component of the interviewing process. It requires active work on the part of the health professional to avoid some common pitfalls, such as hearing only the things she wants to hear or thinks are important.

To facilitate listening, Van Dersal, a psychologist, suggests keeping three key questions in mind: (1) "What does the speaker mean?" Individuals often use simple nontechnical words differently. The client may say "I don't want *hot* food." He may mean that he does not want highly spiced food, he may be referring to the temperature of the food, or he may hold a cultural belief that he has a "hot" disease which should be treated by eating only "cold" foods. It is important to be sure the meaning is clear. (2) "How does the speaker know?" The basis for his statements should be determined if possible. (3) "What is the speaker leaving out?" It often becomes apparent when listening that the speaker is leaving out important facts and details.[3] This information may be too emotionally charged for the client to discuss.

Another important concept in listening is to listen for themes in what the client is saying. Identifying themes or patterns may provide the health professional with insight about the client's behavior and clues useful in motivating the client.[4] Relevant themes include:

1. Attitudes toward food and eating. (These have been discussed in Chapter 6.)
2. Concepts of health and illness. Does the client relate his nutritional status to his state of health? What value does he place on health? Is the client seeking health care or is he simply looking for a cure for his current ailments?
3. Factors motivating his lifestyle. What things does the client value? Money, possessions, power, friends, family, health, good looks?
4. Strengths and assets of the individual. What personal behaviors does the client view favorably? What aspects of his life does he feel especially competent to handle?
5. Previous experiences with diet modifications. Have the client's attempts to modify his diet been successful or not? What criteria indicated success or failure to the client? How was the client's self-esteem affected?

VALIDATING DATA

A short little old lady who supposedly weighs 160 lb. states she only eats small amounts of food. Since excessive caloric intake is necessary for excessive weight there appears to be a discrepancy in the data. When a discrepancy occurs the data need to be validated. In this instance the lady's current weight can be rechecked. Her previous weight must be compared to her current weight to determine if there has been a recent weight change. Her intake could be observed, or what she means by "small amount" can be clarified to determine which data are accurate.

It is desirable to confirm or verify data if there are unusual discrepancies or if data lack clarity. This is especially important if data are to be used to make judgements. The purpose of validating data is to keep them free from error, bias, or misinterpretation.

RECORDING DATA

For data to be useful and available to others, they must be recorded in a systematic objective manner. Making inferences and judgments should be avoided. For instance, recording the statement "Mother is doing fine with her baby" could mean almost anything. The interviewer should ask herself "What data led me to draw this conclusion?" In this case perhaps the mother stated that she is feeding her infant approximately 3 oz. of formula every 4 hours. She doesn't encourage the baby to finish the whole bottle if he seems full. She describes how to correctly prepare formula, using the aseptic technique. (This is the information which should be recorded.)

Information is recorded clearly and concisely but without sacrificing essential facts. Professional jargon should be avoided. When an opinion is expressed a statement is made which indicates it is the opinion of the recorder.

The diet history

The diet history is a useful tool for collecting data about the client's recent food and fluid intake and eating habits. An individual's food intake may vary somewhat from day to day in both amount and type of food consumed. The intake record should be an accurate reflection of foods consumed during a representative period of time. There are a variety of formats which can be utilized to determine intake and food habits. These include the diet recall and the food diary.

DIET RECALL

The diet recall provides a brief general record from the client's memory of food and fluid intake. It can serve as a basis for diet instruction. It can also be used to readily identify individuals who follow an unusual food pattern or fad diet or who exclude important foods or food groups from their diets. A client's recall can be facilitated by asking the client to relate food intake to his activities during the past 24 hours, indicating what time and what amounts of food he has eaten. Visual aids which show common serving sizes of the foods may help the client give a more accurate response. Alternately, the client might be asked to compare the portion size he usually uses to amounts served on his tray. Another way to obtain the same type of information about food intake is to present the client with a list of foods grouped into major food categories (a food frequency list). The client indicates the number of times per day or week that he eats these foods and the amounts usually eaten. To validate data, the health professional can compare the results of the 24-hour recall with the food frequency list. The fewer discrepancies there are, the more reliable the data are likely to be.

Studies have shown that the accuracy of the 24-hour recall does vary. Intake as determined by 24-hour recall tends to be higher than that reported in a 7-day record. Women and younger people tend to report more accurately than men and elderly people.[5]

FOOD DIARY

A written food diary provides more specific information than the diet recall or diet history. The client writes the specific types and exact amounts of food eaten as soon as possible after they have been consumed. He may also be asked to comment about his feelings, behaviors, and particular habits related to his food consumption. To keep this record the client must be able to write and measure or estimate food quantities accurately. The food diary is useful when the health professional wants to carefully analyze calorie and nutrient intake. It is useful, too, in analyzing patterns of behavior related to eating. The client may deliberately or unconsciously modify his intake during the assessment period. These modifications will influence the results obtained.

A 3-day diary provides fairly accurate information for the client whose intake does not vary significantly from day to day. Infants, school-aged children, and most adults fall into this category. A 7-day or longer term diary may be used for clients whose intake is more variable or for whom more extensive data is desired. Nutritional assessment of the toddler, preschooler, and adolescent, whose appetites and intakes fluctuate widely, or persons with specific eating problems (e.g., obesity) occasionally requires this longer form. It should be kept in mind that keeping a diary for any length of time requires motivation and discipline on the part of the client or his family.

The form shown in Figure 20.2 indicates many of the kinds of information which could be included in a food diary. Many forms are not as detailed as this. Along with the food diary form, the client should be given suggestions that will increase the chance that he will record data completely and correctly. The following are guidelines for the client who is keeping a food diary:

1. Keep the food record sheet with you.
2. Record amounts of all foods eaten immediately following the meal or snack, using household measures or weights, i.e., ½ c. fresh cooked carrots, 3 oz. hamburger fried.
3. Indicate the specific type of food. For example: skim milk or whole milk, fresh fruit or fruit canned in heavy syrup.
4. Indicate how the food was prepared: baked, broiled, fried, boiled, etc. Special recipes should be attached.
5. Be sure to include condiments used, such as butter, jelly, salad dressings, and whipped cream.
6. Include between-meal snacks.

Eating habits

Interviewing is probably the most convenient method of determining the client's eating habits and attitudes toward food. A general form and some specific modifications which can be made depending on the age of the

FOOD	HOW MUCH?	TIME?	WHERE ARE YOU? Home (specify room) Work Restaurant Recreation Activity Engaged In	WHO IS WITH YOU?	HOW DO YOU FEEL? A– Anxious F– ____ B– Bored G– ____ C– Tired D– Depressed E– Angry

FIGURE 20.2. Food intake inventory form. (Reprinted from Extension Bulletin E-781: "Behavioral Control—A New Self-Help Approach to Weight Control." Cooperative Extension Service, Michigan State University, East Lansing, Michigan, 48824)

client are presented in the box on page 227. Incorporating questions about eating habits into assessment activities directed toward other aspects of a client's life may be a helpful strategy to obtain accurate information. For example, in her article, "Food becomes fun for children," Wills describes how health care workers can obtain useful information about a child's food habits while administering the Denver Developmental Screening Test (a standardized test used to assess the development of children between birth and 6 years of age).[6]

OBSERVATION AND INSPECTION

Observing and examining the client provides information about overt behavior and physical signs. This objective data may further help determine the client's nutritional status and identify nutrition-related problems. Each individual makes observations through "glasses" constructed of expectations, past experiences, and values. These glasses distort what is seen.

Skillful, unbiased observation demands diligent practice and discipline. Observation involves describing what has been seen, touched, and smelled. Observations should be recorded in a manner which provides the reader with a mental picture of what has been seen. Descriptors related to shape, size, contour, activity, movement, expression, texture, and odor should be used. Phrases such as the client's skin felt "doughy" or the oatmeal was "gluey" give the reader an objective picture of what has been observed.

General appearance

Inspection of general appearance, behavior, and observable body tissues such as skin and mucous membrane provides clues regarding the client's concern for himself and his nutritional status. Observation of the environment surrounding the client and how he fits into it provides useful data. Does the client appear to be comfortable? ill-at-ease? out of place? Sometimes inspection can be carried out in a systematic manner. It is desirable to first observe the client's general appearance, then inspect specific tissues. A systematic inspection follows a planned sequence of observation, such as face, head, neck, upper extremities, chest, abdomen, lower extremities, and back. Table 20.2 presents a guide for observation of general appearance.

It is not always possible or appropriate to conduct a formal head-to-toe inspection. When it isn't, observations can be made in an informal manner. When meeting the client some of his features may be noted imme-

QUESTIONNAIRE I. ADULTS
(directed to client or primary caretaker)

Background information:
  Name, age, sex, family and occupational roles, general health status, dietary restrictions (past or present)

Food Purchase and Preparation:
  Who purchases and prepares food?
  What factors influence kinds of foods purchased?
  Is budgeting a matter of concern when buying food?
  Where is food purchased?
  How often do you shop?
  What facilities are available for food storage and preparation?
  What foods are served most frequently?
  Do you participate in community food programs?

Relationship of Food to Lifestyle:
  Food likes and dislikes
  Favorite foods when growing up
  Special family foods for celebrations
  Atmosphere at mealtime
  Foods your body needs
  Food supplements (vitamins, minerals)
  Sources of information about nutrition

QUESTIONNAIRE II. INFANT/TODDLER
(directed to parents or primary caretaker)

Who feeds? What foods does an infant need?
Breast or formula feeding—approximate amount and frequency?
If breast feeding—pattern and duration of feeding?
If formula, type? iron fortified? preparation?
Supplemental feedings—fluids, solids, preparation? how liked?
Weaning? Teething? Self-feeding?

QUESTIONNAIRE III. YOUNG CHILD
(directed to parents or primary caretaker)

What foods does your child need? When does he eat?
Appetite? Likes, dislikes? Food jags?
Frequency of snacking? Types?
Vitamin and mineral supplements?
Method of rewarding and punishing child?
Who child eats with?
Arrangements for eating away from home (school)?

QUESTION IV. ADOLESCENT
(directed to adolescent)

What is nutritious? Foods body needs?
Where are meals eaten? When is food eaten?
How much snacking?
How does eating affect appearance?
What do you do when you're unhappy or upset?
Does anyone comment about your eating habits?

QUESTIONNAIRE V. ELDERLY
(directed to client or primary caretaker)

Amount of income budgeted for food?
Where client lives? Where he eats?
Who he eats with?
Who prepares meals? Purchases food?
Dentures or own teeth? Effect on eating?
Recent changes in food habits?
How does food taste?
Likes, dislikes?
Use of alcohol?
Dietary restrictions?
Amount of normal activity?

diately. His posture, body size, motor activity, facial features, the condition of skin and hair, and body and breath odors can usually be ascertained. The condition of the client's clothing is easily observed also. There may be dried food on it or he may be wearing a sweater on a hot day. By shaking hands with the client it is possible to inspect the condition of his nails and the strength of his hand grip. Getting the client to smile provides an opportunity to inspect the condition of his mouth. The tissues of the mouth are one of the first areas to exhibit signs of nutritional deficiencies. These features provide the examiner with data from which an overall impression of the client's state of health can be determined.

Nutrient intake in a health care facility

Observing what and how the client eats when he is in a health care facility is particularly important considering the high incidence of malnutrition in hospitals. Accurate information about food intake and eating behavior makes it possible to identify potential and actual nutritional problems. This, in turn, can result in the implementation of measures to improve the client's nutritional state. It is important to document occurrences such as refusal of a meal or of all solid foods. Missing one meal usually doesn't have serious

TABLE 20.2 *Observation of general appearance*

CHARACTERISTIC	DESCRIPTORS
Body size and stature	Large or small frame Thin, obese, muscle wasting Symmetry in size and shape of body parts
Posture	Erect, rigid, slumping, stretched out
Body movements	Strength of movement, speed, symmetry of movements, tremors, twitching, purposefulness
Skin	Color, luster (dull, shiny), turgor, sags, wrinkles, lesions, edema, perspiration
Tongue, gums, and mucous membranes	Edema, lesions, raw, red or pale color, changes in papillae on tongue
Teeth	Missing, caries, grey or white spots on enamel (mottled enamel)
Hair	Distribution, density, luster, grooming, color
Nails	Length, grooming, thickness, ridging, color of nailbed, spoon shaped
Clothing	Appropriate for age and climate, cleanliness, neat or disheveled
Speech	Clarity, speed, loud or soft, hoarse, whining, halting, stuttering
Mental status	Alert, responsive, lethargic, listless, apathetic
Mood	Smiling, frowning, presence of anxiety indicated by tapping fingers or feet, wringing hands, cold moist palms, furrowed brow
Presence of discomfort or pain	Moaning, writhing, guarding of a body part

consequences, but a pattern of inadequate intake may go unnoticed if isolated instances are not reported. Documentation of intake should serve to validate data from the client. It may provide information about the client's actual intake and eating behavior, which will be needed to identify realistic ways to improve these in the health agency. The following questions provide a guide for making pertinent observations of the client's nutrient intake and eating behavior:

1. Is the client on a regular diet or a special diet?
2. Who is selecting his menu?
3. How does he accept suggestions about what to order?
4. Has he commented about the food selection available?
5. When the meal comes does he remark about the choices he made?
6. Does he feed himself or require assistance?
7. What kind of appetite and interest in food does he display?
8. What kinds of comments does he make about the food and eating? (e.g., "That looks good." "I don't feel well enough to eat." "Did I order that?")
9. How conducive is the environment to enjoyable eating? Consider client's personal comfort (position, state of his mouth), lighting, noise, smell.
10. Is the opportunity present for the client to socialize while eating? Does he do so?
11. Does he engage in any other activity while eating such as watching television or reading?
12. How fast or slowly does he eat?
13. How well does he chew his food?

24-HOUR FOOD-INTAKE RECORDS

The dietitian sometimes initiates 24-hour food-intake records, also called calorie counts, to be kept for a client residing in a health care facility. This is usually done over a period of days. The data obtained are useful to help (1) determine the value of initiating alternate feeding methods, (2) estimate the client's state of nitrogen balance, or (3) accurately estimate the client's intake of particular nutrients and/or calories. This record can be an invaluable tool for monitoring nutritional status. A detailed record is vital if the data are to be useful.

Recording intake The amount of food the client actually consumes may be determined by looking at his tray and subtracting the amount of each item left from the amount he was initially served. In order to accurately identify fluid volumes, it is necessary to know the capacity of various containers. A variety of foods which have a solid appearance in reality are primarily liquid and are usually measured as such. Included among these items are ice cream, sherbet, popsicles, and gelatin desserts. Foods and fluids should be described as accurately as possible by volume (such as 90 ml. of vanilla custard) or by estimated amount (such as ½ hamburger patty—45 gm. with 30 ml. of gravy).

Between-meal feedings and food from other sources Obtaining the cooperation of the client and his family will help assure that the intake record is accurate. The client should understand the importance of accurately recording *everything* he consumes. He may be asked to report all between-meal snacks and food he has obtained from other sources. If appropriate he may be taught to record his own intake. If food was brought in from home it needs to be described accurately. The description should list the brand name of the food or list the ingredients and method of preparation.

Intravenous feedings and nutrient supplements Some clients receive intravenous feedings and nutritional supplements during their hospitalization. Vitamin and mineral supplements and protein supplements may be listed with the medications the client is taking. Clients may receive dextrose, amino acids, or a fat emulsion intravenously. The amount of calories the client is getting can be easily calculated if the health professional

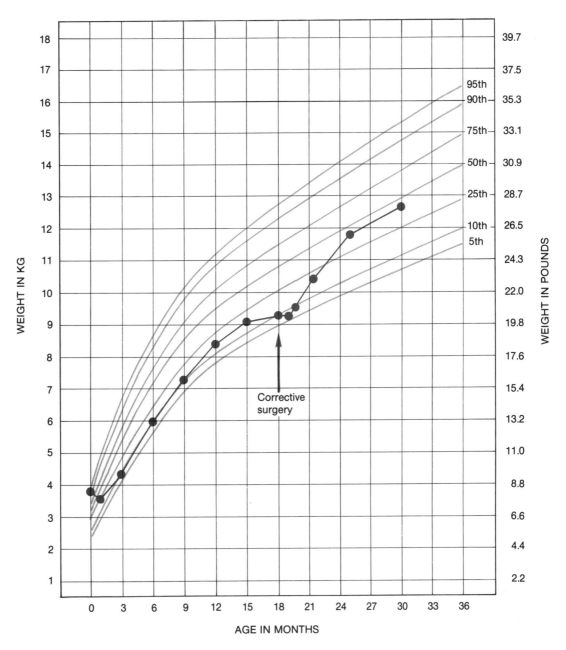

FIGURE 20.3. Plotted on this chart is the growth of an infant girl who had corrective surgery for a congenital heart defect when she was 18 months old. Note the effect of undernutrition in early infancy and the catch-up growth exhibited following cardiac surgery. (Plotted on a NCHS physical growth percentiles chart for girls, birth to 36 months. Monthly vital statistics report of National Center for Health Statistics. Health Resources Administration, Rockville MD. [HRA] 76-1120)

knows the type of solution and rate of infusion. Chapter 32, page 372 shows how some of these calculations are made.

Anthropometric measurements

Anthropometric measurements are measurements of body size and composition. This information is needed for assessing nutritional status and for planning diets.

Height, weight, and skinfold (fatfold) thickness are anthropometric measurements frequently obtained. Collecting measurements such as height and weight over a period of time is particularly useful in assessing growth. Various body circumferences such as midarm circumference, head circumference, and abdominal girth provide useful data about muscle mass, brain growth, and fluid retention respectively. Close attention needs to be paid to following proper technique when obtaining each of these measurements. For the measurements to be meaningfully compared to reference standards they must be obtained in the manner prescribed for the reference standards used.

HEIGHT AND WEIGHT

Height and weight are two of the most important parameters of nutritional status. It is, therefore, particularly important that they be obtained accurately.

In the case of children, pregnant women, and individuals who are overweight, a record of weight over time provides more useful information than a single measurement. Daily weights may be taken when it is desirable to monitor a client's fluid balance. If sequential measurements are taken it is important to use a procedure minimizing the effects of external variables. Some of the external variables influencing an individual's weight include the amount of clothing worn, the time of day the measurement is taken, the scale used, and the individual making and recording the measurements. To minimize these variables the client should be consistently weighed on the same scale, with the same amount of clothing, at the same time of day, by the same individual, if possible.

Growth charts For data to be clinically useful they must be compared to a standard or reference, such as a growth chart. Data are commonly plotted directly on growth charts to facilitate assessment of a child's physical growth. The most up-to-date growth charts for infants, children, and youth are those compiled by the National Center for Health Statistics (NCHS). One set of these charts is for boys and girls from birth to 36 mo. of age and shows (1) weight, length (recumbent), and head circumference for age and (2) weight for length. The other sets, for boys and girls 2 to 18 yr. of age, show (1) weight and stature (standing) for age and (2) weight for stature. Specific directions for obtaining these measurements in the same way the reference measurements were obtained are described in the **DHEW** publication *Nutritional Disorders of Children: Prevention, Screening and Follow-up.*[7]

Chronological age is a significant variable in comparing a rapidly growing child to a reference standard. It is essential that the child's exact age in years and months be determined and plotted correctly on all the growth charts except weight for length or weight for stature charts. If the child's birth date and the current date are also recorded, then a second individual can double check the accuracy of the plotting on the graph. Major events influencing food intake should be noted on the child's growth chart or in the child's medical record. Illness, the end of breast feeding, the birth of a sibling, a move, the death of a parent, divorce, and a significant change in family income are events having an impact on a child's nutritional status and growth. The NCHS growth charts overlap from age 2 to 3. During this age interval the amount of clothing the child should wear and his position (recumbent or standing) depends on which chart is used. Figure 20.3 shows one of the NCHS growth charts.

Prenatal weight gain Weight gain during pregnancy can be charted on a graph to aid in identifying a pregnant woman's pattern of weight gain. If gain varies from the standard pattern further data should be collected to help determine the cause.

SKINFOLD THICKNESS

Skinfold thickness is a useful measure to assist in determining the degree of body fat. Many different skinfolds such as subscapular and abdominal can be measured, but the triceps skinfold is most frequently obtained, as illustrated in Figure 20.4.

MID-UPPER ARM CIRCUMFERENCE

Mid-upper arm circumference can be easily measured using a tape measure snugly wrapped around the nondominant upper arm at the midpoint. The mid-upper arm muscle circumference can be estimated from the arm circumference using a special formula.[8] This can be used to estimate the area of the triceps muscle which is representative of the person's muscle mass.

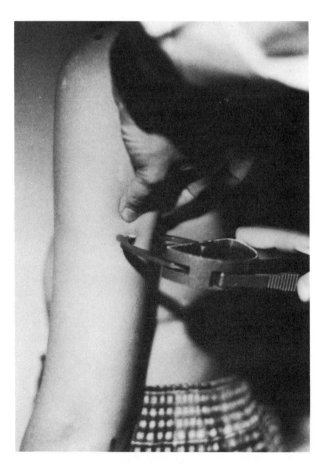

FIGURE 20.4. Measuring the triceps skinfold. (Courtesy of Samuel J. Fomon, Iowa City IA)

HEAD CIRCUMFERENCE

Head circumference correlates with the amount of brain growth and the size of the brain. It is helpful in identifying microcephaly or macrocephaly (small or large brain size). To obtain the measurement a flexible tape is placed over the most prominent part of the occiput and just above the ears and the supraorbital ridge. The hair should be compressed as much as possible.

Radiological studies

Bone age can be estimated by taking roentgenographic pictures of ossification centers at the epiphyses of long bones such as at the wrist. This may provide useful data about the child whose linear growth is very slow or extremely rapid. Bone age also correlates with sexual maturation and provides data relevant to assessment of an adolescent with growth and maturation problems. Radiological studies may be useful to detect specific nutrient deficiency diseases such as rickets and scurvy, which cause bone deformity.

Laboratory data

There is a wide array of laboratory tests. Some are routinely obtained, others are not. Usually, hospitalized clients will have a complete blood count and urinalysis done on admission.

Identifying pertinent laboratory data Laboratory data can often indicate potential nutritional problems before clinical manifestations develop.

Tests which may be relevant to assessing nutritional status include (1) concentrations of protein in the blood or urine, (2) vitamin, lipid, and mineral (including electrolytes) concentrations in the blood or urine, (3) tests of enzyme functions, (4) tests on stool for guaiac (occult blood), fat, and parasites, and (5) tests of immunological function. Results of laboratory studies are usually recorded in the client's medical record. A guide identifying useful laboratory data and giving suggestions for interpretation is presented in Appendix 4G.

OBTAINING SPECIMENS

Samples of various substances must be carefully obtained in order for results to be accurate. The time of day, the container, the actual method of procuring the specimen, and storage may influence test results. If a 24-hour urine sample is necessary, having a complete collection is essential to insure accurate results. Sometimes blood and urine samples are tested simultaneously or sequentially. These samples must be collected on time. The client will be more cooperative and less anxious if the purpose of the test and method of collection are explained to him.

STUDY QUESTIONS

1. From the following list identify subjective data. Suggest one way of validating each piece of subjective data.
   missing teeth
   painful gums
   edema of extremities
   poor appetite
   vomiting
2. List kinds of information which might be obtained from a medical record pertinent to assessing a client's nutritional status.
3. Why is it important to correctly and concisely record in a client's medical record data obtained about him?
4. Discuss several useful techniques to encourage a client to share information about his eating habits with a health care worker.
5. Describe one method of validating data about a client's food intake as determined using a 24-hour diet recall.

References

*1. Butterworth, C., and Blackburn, G. I.: Hospital malnutrition. *Nutr. Today* 10(2):8, 1975.
*2. Edinburg, M., Zinberg, N., and Kelman, W.: *Clinical Interviewing and Counseling, Principles and Techniques.* New York: Appleton-Century Crofts, 1975.
*3. Van Dersal, W. R.: How to be a good communicator and a better nurse. *Nursing 74* 4:57, 1974.
*4. Hein, E.: Listening. *Nursing 75* 5:93, 1975.
5. Madden, J., Goodman, P., and Guthrie, H.: Validity of 24-hour recall. *J. Am. Diet. Assoc.* 68:143, 1976.
6. Wills, B.: Food becomes fun for children. *Am. J. Nurs.* 78: 2082, 1978.
*7. Fomon, S. J.: *Nutritional Disorders of Children: Prevention, Screening and Follow-up.* Public Health Services Administration. DHEW Publ. No. (HSH) 76-5612. Washington DC: U.S. Govt. Printing Office, 1976.
8. Gurney, J., and Jelliffe, D.: Arm anthropometry in nutritional assessment: Nomogram for rapid calculation of muscle circumference and cross-sectional muscle and fat areas. *Am. J. Clin Nutr.* 26:912, 1973.

* Recommended reading

21

Comparison with standards to aid in identification of needs

After initial data are collected health professionals continue assessment activities, analyzing the data and identifying nutrition-related problems. Health professionals use data analysis and problem identification as a basis for establishing objectives and planning care. Nutritional problems may be actual or potential, overt or covert. Health professionals also analyze data for factors which appear to influence clients' behavior. With this information they can more effectively identify methods of intervention.

STEPS IN THE ANALYSIS PROCESS

In order to be comprehensive and complete, analysis of data should be carried out in a systematic manner. Steps in the analysis process include (1) grouping similar kinds of data, (2) correlating data to scientific knowledge of nutrition, (3) comparing collected data to appropriate norms or reference standards, (4) looking for patterns in the data, (5) identifying the client's health related values and behaviors, and (6) identifying the problem.

Grouping data

Grouping similar kinds of information facilitates data analysis. Four groupings helpful for analyzing nutritional data are (1) food intake, (2) physiological, (3) behavioral, (4) socioeconomic data. Food intake data include information obtained from dietary histories about what the client actually eats. Food intake data allow identification of adequacy, deficiency, or excess nutrient intake. Physiological data include results of the physical examination, anthropometric measure-

ments, biochemical tests, and other diagnostic studies. Physiological data give an indication of the client's body composition, structure, and function, all of which are related to the body's utilization and stores of nutrients. Behavioral data include information from food habit questionnaires; from medical, nursing, or dietary histories; from nurses' notes, or from consultations written by social workers. From behavioral data, health professionals can often identify factors which motivate a client or influence his behavior. Socioeconomic data describe the client's environment including where the client lives geographically, his social and cultural domain, family setting, and economic status. These data suggest factors affecting selection, procurement, and preparation of food.

Correlating data to scientific knowledge

Data analysis requires scientific knowledge. Problems may be identified more accurately if the health professional knows (1) the kinds of nutrients the body needs, (2) how to estimate the amounts of nutrients needed by an individual, (3) how the body obtains and maintains adequate supplies of nutrients, (4) the function of various nutrients in the body, and (5) relationships between adequate nutrition and health and inadequate nutrition and illness.

DEVELOPMENT OF MALNUTRITION

To analyze and interpret data correctly the health professional utilizes knowledge of how malnutrition develops and what forms it may take.

Malnutrition is a general term indicating an excess, deficit, or imbalance of one or more essential nutrients. The term malnutrition is also used to describe an excess or deficit of calories. Psychosocial, economic, geographic, and physical factors can contribute to the development of malnutrition.

When a healthy individual habitually eats in such a way that his nutritional needs are not properly met, the type of malnutrition he develops is *primary* malnutrition. Primary malnutrition is due to poor food choices or to an inadequate supply of food.

When malnutrition is the result of faulty body function, *secondary* malnutrition results. This is sometimes referred to as conditioned malnutrition. Altered body function may interfere with (1) ingestion, (2) digestion, (3) absorption, (4) transport, (5) utilization and/or (6) excretion of nutrients. Secondary malnutrition may also result as a side effect of certain medications and medical or surgical treatments. It is important to differentiate between primary and secondary malnutrition in order to treat the condition correctly.

Two other terms used to describe a malnourished individual are undernutrition and overnutrition. *Undernutrition* applies to an individual who does not ingest an adequate supply of nutrients. *Overnutrition* applies to the individual who eats more food than he needs. Either type may interfere with body processes.

Malnutrition may develop gradually or rapidly. The speed with which nutrient deficiencies develop depends on the severity of nutrient deprivation, the extent of the body's reserves, and the body's need for nutrients. With either decreased intake or increased utilization of nutrients the body draws on nutrient stores. Nutrient reserves dwindle, tissues become "desaturated," cells are deprived of essential nutrients, and biochemical disorders appear if the nutrient deficit persists. Early biochemical disorders are characteristic of *subclinical* malnutrition, that is, malnutrition presenting no clinical symptoms. Review of data obtained by biochemical analysis of body fluids, cells, or tissues may reveal subtle early changes in nutritional status.

Biochemical disorders gradually upset body physiology, including such diverse processes as transmission of nerve impulses and immunological function. As deficiencies become more severe, cell structure as well as function is impaired. At this time clinical manifestations (lesions) or overt signs and symptoms appear. Figure 21.1 illustrates the steps in the progression of a nutritional deficiency and types of data used in assessing each of these.

Deficiency of a single nutrient, such as a vitamin, rarely occurs. More often an individual is deficient in several nutrients. Therefore a variety of conditions can occur.

Protein-energy malnutrition Protein-energy malnutrition (PEM) is probably one of the most serious nutritional problems in the world. Often infants and young children in developing nations suffer from a lack of protein and/or calories. Some form of PEM probably affects a fourth to a half of the clients in acute care facilities.[1,2] Clients residing in other types of facilities may also be vulnerable to this form of malnutrition.

There are three main types of "hospital" malnutrition as described here. These are not completely distinct categories. Rather, there is an overlap of signs and symptoms from one type to another.

Protein deficiency state. People who are deficient in protein often appear well nourished or even overnourished. Their anthropometric measurements are usually within normal limits. Certain biochemical measurements, however, reveal marked changes. Since the visceral proteins are acutely depressed this disorder is sometimes called acute visceral attrition.

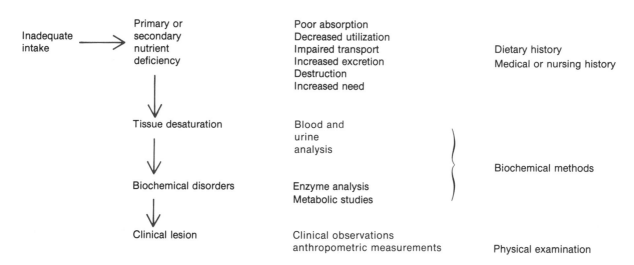

FIGURE 21.1. Progression of a nutritional deficiency. (Redrawn from Kamath, Savitiri: Nutritional assessment. In Malasanos, L., et al.: *Health Assessment*. St. Louis: C. V. Mosby Co., 1977, with permission)

The condition is similar to kwashiorkor in children. A diet providing calories but completely or partially lacking protein leads to this condition. Some vulnerable individuals end up with a severe protein deficiency if their intake (oral or by other means) is limited to carbohydrates for a number of days. For example, a client who undergoes major surgery and is fed an intravenous solution of dextrose and water (D_5W) for about 10 days may develop this form of malnutrition. Persons who have biochemical signs of protein deficiency tend to be quite vulnerable to infection.

Marasmus. People who have marasmus appear malnourished. They look cachectic, that is, they have severe muscle wasting and almost no subcutaneous fat. They have decreased anthropometric measurements; however, the results of certain biochemical studies are usually within a normal range. A diet chronically inadequate in protein, calories, and other nutrients leads to the extensive loss of muscle, fat, electrolytes, and vitamins which characterize this condition. A hospitalized client may develop marasmus if fed an insufficient quantity of a nutritionally complete diet, such as a tube feeding, for a prolonged period. Individuals under severe emotional stress may become anorexic, limit their food intake, and develop this condition. Individuals who have cancer accompanied by anorexia, nausea, and vomiting may become marasmic. Marasmic individuals are at increased risk of developing complications because of their lack of nutrient reserves.

Mixed State. If a person has marasmus and then is subjected to stress, a very serious mixed form of PEM may develop. Depressed anthropometric and biochemical measurements reflect the severe depletion of nutrient reserves. These individuals may be so vulnerable to any form of catabolic stress that aggressive nutritional support may be needed to save their lives.

The individual who has PEM of any type may have multiple nutrient deficiencies also. Several B complex vitamins, iron, and zinc are particularly likely to be lacking since certain high protein foods are important sources of these micronutrients. Even if stores of iron or vitamin A are not depleted, the individual with PEM may be unable to mobilize and utilize them owing to lack of the necessary transport proteins. PEM may cause physiological changes which impair nutrient absorption, further aggravating the malnutrition.

Consequences of protein-energy malnutrition Health professionals should be geared toward early identification and correction of PEM since the effects of PEM are serious, even life threatening. Prevention of serious forms of PEM is less costly, less time-consuming, and much more advantageous for the client than is correction of PEM and its many consequences.

Nutrient deficits may cause breakdown of both nonspecific and specific protective mechanisms against infection and injury. Cells and substances making up the defense systems are constantly being lost or destroyed. An adequate nutrient supply is needed to replace them. Nonspecific protective mechanisms provide general kinds of protection against all types of microorganisms and against mechanical injury. Examples of nonspecific defenses include body secretions, such as mucus and digestive juices, and intact skin and mucous membranes. These substances and structures form a barrier to the entry of infectious organisms and interfere with their growth and proliferation. They also provide protection against chemical injury.

Nonspecific defenses protect tissue from breakdown caused by mechanical insults such as chafing or constant pressure. The risk of developing decubitus ulcers appears to be greater in persons with PEM because of their decreased tissue integrity and lack of nutrients for repair.

Specific defense mechanisms include humoral immunity and cellular immunity. Cellular immunity may fall rapidly with the development of PEM. Less is known about changes in humoral immunity. The net effect of PEM is a greatly increased susceptibility to infection.

If an infection should develop in the individual with PEM, the original nutritional deficits may be compounded by deficits resulting from anorexia, nausea, vomiting, diarrhea, and/or increased metabolic rate owing to fever. This, in turn, further decreases resistance to infection in an ever-worsening cycle.

The lack of nutrient reserves in PEM may interfere with the healing of surgical or other wounds. Wounds may not heal at all; rather, they may increase in severity.

ENVIRONMENTAL AND CULTURAL FACTORS INFLUENCING THE DEVELOPMENT OF MALNUTRITION

A variety of environmental and cultural factors leaves some people especially vulnerable to malnutrition or nutrition-related disorders. Community nutrition surveys may identify some of these factors. If possible the health professional should be familiar with results of community nutrition studies when analyzing data about a specific client.

Community nutrition survey A community nutrition survey may provide information about the nutritional status and nutritional resources of a given community and its members. Ideally, such a study includes data regarding prevalence of malnutrition, levels of income, types of housing, the prevalence of disease, the food supply, cultural practices, and the kinds of health care available.

Cultural Influences. The cultural practices of certain communities may lead to specific kinds of nutritional deficiencies. It is particularly useful for health professionals to note the main staples in the diets of various cultural groups and whether or not there is sufficient variety in typical diets to provide adequate nutrition.

Environmental Factors. The food supply in a community may greatly influence the risk of developing certain types of malnutrition. For example, the health professional should know if there are desirable amounts of iodine and fluoride in the local food and water supply. If not she should determine whether the client's intake of these micronutrients is adequate or excessive and institute corrective measures.

Studies have shown that individuals in lower socioeconomic groups are at greater than average risk of developing nutritional deficiencies. Poverty limits the kinds, amounts, and quality of food which may be purchased. Inadequate housing limits the family's ability to safely store and prepare food. On the other hand, individuals with adequate socioeconomic resources may indulge in fad diets, limit the variety of food in their diets or go on crash reducing diets. Thus a higher socioeconomic level does not preclude the possibility of malnutrition.

The health professional has a responsibility to find out what government nutrition intervention programs are locally available to particular socioeconomic groups and whether or not they are being effectively utilized by individuals (Appendix 2).

POINTS OF EMPHASIS
Malnutrition

• *Malnutrition is a general term referring to a number of conditions characterized by an excess or deficit of nutrients and/or calories.*
• *Initially malnutrition may only cause biochemical disorders. The more severe and prolonged nutrient and/or calorie deficiencies are, the more overt clinical manifestations become.*
• *Malnutrition frequently occurs in clients who reside in health care agencies.*
• *Anthropometric and biochemical measurements are useful to identify specific forms of protein-energy malnutrition.*

Using reference standards

Health professionals use reference standards or appropriate norms to determine how selected client data compare to the same type of data collected from a group of people. Reference standards usually denote an average for a particular population group. They should be used with care since the average is not always what is desirable. For example, the average weight for an adult American is probably 4.5 to 6.8 kg. (10 to 15 lb.) heavier than the desirable weight. Values falling outside a normal range do not always indicate that the client has a problem. In some instances abnormal values are merely suggestive of a problem. Further investigation may be required to more clearly identify the significance of the finding. Norms do not take each person's uniqueness into account. It is, therefore, important to consider data in the context of the client's immediate background as well as to compare them to standards.

Health professionals should take into account a variety of variables when using standards. How the reference data were collected, when they were collected, and from whom they were collected may limit the data's usefulness. Several of these limitations are discussed later in the chapter as they apply to specific reference standards.

POPULATION DIFFERENCES AFFECTING USE OF REFERENCE STANDARDS

Anthropometric and biochemical differences have been noted for certain population groups in the U.S. that cannot be accounted for by socioeconomic differences. Garn[3] and Foster[4] identify ways some anthropometric and biochemical data differ for American blacks and American whites. For example, for all age groups the average hemoglobin concentration is lower by about 1.0 gm. per 100 ml. and the average hematocrit is lower by about 3 percent for blacks than for whites.

Looking for patterns in data

After each group of data has been compared to reference standards (where applicable), a series of steps can be taken to help integrate and interpret the data: (1) Find out if there is any evidence that the client has a problem which is prevalent for his community, his age, culture, or socioeconomic group. (2) If one piece of information suggests a problem, try to find other information to help confirm it or rule it out. Review all types of available data pertaining to the problem. (3) If past records are available, determine if current data indicate improvement, lack of change, deterioration, or a fluctuating pattern.

Identifying the client's health-related values and behaviors

One of the major goals of nutritional care is to assist the client to make needed changes in his food habits. Knowledge of factors influencing an individual's usual pattern of behavior with respect to diet is useful to plan care. The health professional should review data about the client's eating habits and shopping, cooking, and food storage practices, identifying the meanings and values the client attaches to these activities. An individual is more likely to modify his food behavior if the plan developed is congruent with the meanings and values he attaches to food.

When possible the health professional develops a plan of care which encourages the client to actively participate in his care. Most people have faced problems. Some they have dealt with successfully; others they have handled less well. Once the professional has identified resources the client has previously used, she can work to mobilize these in the client's behalf. Often clients can be helped in effectively organizing and utilizing their own resources. When assessing the client's own resources consider the following points:

1. Physical functioning. What is the client's general health status? Does he have reserves with which to withstand stress? How has he physically tolerated and adapted to stress in the past? Is he able to carry out activities of daily living independently? How do food and eating fit into his activities of daily living?
2. Emotional functioning. What is the client's general mood? What are his feelings about dependence and independence? What does he value? What kinds of things motivate his behavior? How does he relate food and nutrition to health?
3. Intellectual capacity. What kind of food knowledge and skills does he possess? Can the client understand recommendations? Can he follow directions? Can he make appropriate choices and judgments?
4. Spiritual, social, and economic resources. Does the client have and/or derive support from religious beliefs? How do his religious beliefs relate to his health status? What family and community resources does the client have available to him? Does the client have adequate financial resources to meet his basic needs?

Identifying the problem

Whether or not the specific problem and its cause can be definitely stated (diagnosed) it soon becomes necessary to start planning and implementing care. In some cases the client is referred to one or more other health team members for more in-depth assessment and expert care. In other cases the health professional needs to make a clinical judgment about the client's nutritional needs and how to best meet these needs. There are several steps involved in making a clinical judgment: (1) The health professional weighs data suggesting a particular problem against those which do not. (2) She determines the benefits and risks the client will derive from care. (3) She considers past experiences with similar problems. (4) She takes these into consideration when choosing among possible actions.

When further assessment is deemed temporarily unnecessary or is delayed, nutritional care often serves to confirm or rule out a problem. For example, a nurse practitioner might decide to provide nutrition counseling rather than carry out further assessment based on the following observations: An 11-month-old infant's only food source is milk; his hemoglobin is 9.2 gm. per 100 ml. If the anemia is due to iron deficiency, increasing iron in the infants diet should correct the problem.

SPECIFIC TYPES OF DATA

The remainder of this chapter explains how specific types of data are analyzed to help identify nutritional problems.

Analysis of dietary intake

In order to estimate the nutritional adequacy of a client's diet, it is necessary to compare data on intake to an accepted reference standard. Intake includes food, nutritional supplements, and parenteral nutrients, if applicable. The reference standards most commonly used are food guides and the Recommended Dietary Allowances. Food guides allow *qualitative* analysis of the adequacy of the diet. That is, by comparing actual food intake with a food guide, one can estimate if nutrients appear to be present in amounts sufficient to promote the health of normal persons. Recommended Dietary Allowances are used as a reference standard when the intake of specific nutrients has been estimated *quantitatively* using tables of food composition. Use of Pennington's *Dietary Nutrient Guide* simplifies calculation of a client's intake of seven index nutrients.[5] If intake of the index nutrients is adequate, overall nutrient intake is assumed to be adequate as well.

FOOD GUIDES

Food guides such as the Basic Four provide a simple, practical tool for qualitative dietary analysis even though they were not originally designed for that purpose. Figure 21.2 shows a form which has been used to compare actual food intake to slightly modified Basic Four recommendations.

Guidelines for utilizing the Basic Four as a tool for diet analysis follow:

1. If the diet normally provides the recommended number of servings from each of the food groups, assume that the diet provides the RDA for seven of the eight leader nutrients: protein, vitamins A and C, thiamine, riboflavin, niacin, and calcium.
2. If the number of servings from any food group is below recommendations, identify what should be contributed by that group. Then look to see if anything is eaten which compensates.
3. Determine the sources of iron in the client's diet. If there are no unusually rich sources (liver, highly fortified cereal, food cooked in iron pans) intake is apt to be low. This is particularly important for children and for women during the childbearing years.
4. Determine whether or not good sources of folacin (such as dark-green leafy vegetables, liver, kidney, wheat germ, or bran) are included. Intake of this B vitamin is apt to be low if excellent sources are not included.
5. Identify the specific sources of Vitamin D in the diets of children and pregnant or lactating women. If fortified milk is not used, intake is apt to be below recommendations.
6. Evaluate the amount of variety in the client's diet. Determine the frequency with which special reliance on single food types, cultural foods, and highly processed foods are used. If there is reliance on sin-

Food group	Actual intake number of servings per day			Recommended intake number of servings*				
	Day 1	Day 2	Day 3	Child	Adolescent	Adult	Pregnant adult	Lactating adult
Bread and cereal†				4	4	4	4	4
Vegetables fruits — Green leafy				1	1	1	1	1
Vegetables fruits — Orange (veg.)				1 at least qod if green leafy not used				
Vegetables fruits — Citrus or other vitamin C rich food				1	1	1	1	1
Vegetables fruits — Potatoes and others				To achieve a total of 4 or more servings when added to above				
Milk and milk products				2–3	4	2	3–4	4
Meats Poultry Fish Eggs Legumes				2	2	2	3	2
Others								

FIGURE 21.2. Form for analysis of food intake. See Table 2.1 for serving sizes for adults and teenagers.
† Whole grains provide more fiber and micronutrients.

gle food types or if highly processed foods are used extensively, check carefully for good sources of micronutrients such as zinc, magnesium, or pyridoxine.
7. Consider whether the diet provides an adequate or excessive amount of calories.

FOOD COMPOSITION TABLES

Food composition tables list foods and indicate the amounts of specified nutrients the foods contain. One of many uses of food composition tables is to determine the nutrient contribution of foods eaten by the client. Rarely is it necessary to completely calculate nutrient intake. However, the health care worker may want to utilize food composition tables to determine the adequacy of one or two particular nutrients in an individual's diet. A client's diet, for example, may not include any well-known sources of vitamin C such as citrus fruits. By using food composition tables, it is possible to determine how much vitamin C is obtained from fruits and vegetables which are used and to compare this value to the RDA. Food composition tables can also be used to check whether or not the client's intake meets a diet prescription.

There are a variety of food composition handbooks and tables. Some of those commonly used are:
1. The U.S. Department of Agriculture Handbooks No. 456 and No. 8 (which is currently being revised and published in sections according to food categories).
2. The Home and Garden Bulletin No. 72, *Nutritive Value of Foods*, provides tables of nutritive values in household measures of 730 commonly used foods.

Foods are grouped under ten major headings. Most foods are listed in ready-to-eat form.
3. Church and Church, *Food Values of Portions Commonly Used*, ed. 12, Philadelphia: J. B. Lippincott Co., 1975.

Many of the food composition tables are set up using different formats. A worksheet helps prevent errors and simplifies tabulation of specific nutrients in the client's diet.

POINTS OF EMPHASIS
Use of food composition tables

• *Look closely at the manner in which the food composition table is set up.*
• *Note how the amounts of nutrients are recorded.*
• *Be certain the values are read for the correct form of the food (e.g., dried peas versus frozen green peas).*
• *Double check portion sizes for accuracy. Do not confuse teaspoons (tsp.) with tablespoons (Tbsp.) or metric equivalents.*
• *Double check units used for nutrients. Do not confuse mg. with µg. or gm. or retinol equivalents (RE) with international units (IU).*
• *Round off numbers, especially when nutrient values are multiplied or divided so that they correspond to the quantity of food consumed by the client. Values in food composition tables appear very precise but actually represent averages.*

RECOMMENDED DIETARY ALLOWANCES

In the U.S., the Recommended Dietary Allowances (RDA) are the most commonly used standard to which nutrient intake of an individual is compared, even though they were not designed for that purpose. The definition of the RDA which accompanied the 1974 revision is:

> The Recommended Dietary Allowances are the levels of essential nutrients considered, in the judgment of the Food and Nutrition Board on the basis of scientific knowledge, to be adequate to meet the nutritional needs of practically all healthy persons.[6]

The RDAs represent *recommendations*, not requirements.

The RDA tables indicate the recommended daily allowances of major nutrients according to age group and sex and according to the special needs of pregnancy and lactation. The recommendations are meant to apply to nutrient intake from a varied diet.

The RDAs have been revised approximately every 5 years since they were first published in 1943, with the most recent revision being completed in 1979.

There has been some controversy concerning the recommended levels of nutrients established by the Food and Nutrition Board. Some scientific authorities feel the levels of specific nutrients are too low; others feel they are too high.

The RDA should not be considered to be a guide to the exact and complete nutrient needs of individual Americans for several reasons:

1. Allowances are not definitely stated for all nutrients known to be required by humans. Included among these are water and some of the trace elements. It is possible that there are essential nutrients which have not been recognized.
2. Some of the RDA values are based on limited experimental evidence. This is true for certain nutrients, such as zinc, and for certain age groups, such as adolescents and the elderly.
3. Many factors besides age may influence an individual's nutrient requirements. Variations occur as a result of an individual's genetic makeup, physiologic state, activity level, and environment.
4. The RDA does not make allowances for interactions between nutrients or for the type of food providing the nutrient.
5. The desirability of nutrient stores has been considered in establishing recommended intakes. Thus, for several nutrients the RDA is set at a level which should allow generous reserves to be built up.
6. Diets are more than just combinations of nutrients. The RDA is not a good guide for estimating caloric requirements of individuals. It does not give an allowance for fiber in the diet. A recommended ratio of saturated to unsaturated fats is not identified.
7. Although the RDA have been formulated to cover common mild stresses of daily living, it does not provide coverage for the needs of ill individuals or of persons who are exposed to other severe stresses.

Assessment of dietary intake over a 5- to 8-day period provides a better indication of dietary adequacy of some nutrients than does assessment of a single day's intake. Obviously, the longer the period of time an individual has a suboptimal intake of one or more nutrients, the more he is at risk of developing deficiencies.

When analyzing nutrient intake it is incorrect to assume that a seemingly well person is deficient in a nutrient because his reported intake is, for example, only half of the RDA for that nutrient. Neither is it correct to assume that an ill individual is adequately nourished if he meets the RDA for all nutrients. Such information is suggestive at best. Therefore, it is advisable to look for other evidence to support or rule out such conclusions.

POINTS OF EMPHASIS
Use of Recommended Dietary Allowances

• *Compare the client's intake with the appropriate section of the table for age group, sex, and weight. If the client's weight varies significantly from that designated in the table, adjust values for protein and calories accordingly. If the client is pregnant or lactating, use the section of the RDA providing nutrient guidelines for individuals in these special-needs categories.*

• *Use a rating scale to determine the probable level of dietary adequacy. For example, categories of good (diet contains 100 percent or more of the allowance), fair (67 percent to 100 percent of allowance), and poor (below 67 percent of allowance) could be used.*[7]

• *Base estimates of dietary adequacy on the client's intake over a period of one week, if possible.*

• *Consider variable factors influencing the individual's requirements such as activity level, state of general health, and occupation.*

• *Determine whether nutrient supplements such as vitamin preparations (if used) bring the total intake in line with the RDA or if there is a danger of toxicity.*

• *Even if the calculated dietary intake meets the RDA, review the adequacy of the overall diet with regard to variety of whole foods, fiber content, and fluid intake.*

• *If the calculated dietary intake does not meet the RDA, especially by a large percentage, look for other indications of deficiency.*

Anthropometry

Anthropometric measurements provide data useful for analyzing growth and for determining body composition. Height and weight are commonly employed anthropometric parameters for analyzing growth.

Skinfold and arm circumference facilitate identification of the degree of body fat and the amount of lean body tissue, respectively. They aid in identification of obesity and PEM. To identify the significance of the client's anthropometric measurements, the data must be compared to carefully selected reference standards. For accurate, meaningful analysis of the data the standards should be derived from the client's population group. If this is not possible, adjustments in interpretation of data may be necessary.

ASSESSMENT OF A CHILD'S GROWTH

Assessment of a child's growth is desirable for several reasons. Assessment may assist in identifying whether or not a child is receiving an adequate supply of nutrients. If a child is not growing normally, the health professional further assesses the child, his family, and his environment to try to determine specific causes. Parents may not have adequate knowledge of nutrition and appropriate feeding practices. Many other interwoven factors such as health or illness and genetic potential will have affected growth. Rate of growth tends to change in predictable ways according to season.[8] It is helpful to identify where the child currently stands with respect to growth in order to give parents anticipatory guidance. Anticipatory guidance allows parents to foresee changes that are expected in the normal course of growth and development.

Factors to consider in evaluating a child's growth When evaluating a child's growth the health professional should recognize that each child has an unique set of factors influencing his rate of growth. Children should be compared to their immediate background (parents and siblings) before they are compared to general population standards. A child's small head size may not be significant but, rather, may relate to the fact that he has parents who have small heads. If a child lives in an unsanitary environment it might be appropriate to analyze blood and stool specimens for parasites as a possible cause of growth failure resulting from malabsorption.

Data plotted on growth charts may be used to determine (1) how a child compares in height and weight to the norms for his age and sex, (2) how a child's weight for height compares to the norm for that height (regardless of age) and sex, and (3) how the child's pattern of growth compares to the normal pattern of growth for his sex.

A child who is at the fiftieth percentile for height is of average height. A child who is at the tenth percentile for height is short. Length or height for age is considered to be a good indicator of growth; however, a person's ultimate potential height is genetically determined. Whether or not it is desirable to achieve this potential is debatable.

Weight for age provides less specific information. Weight is more meaningful when the child's height is considered. A child who is at the tenth percentile for weight may or may not be thin. He will weigh less than 90 percent of the children of the same age and sex but, if he is short, his weight for height may be within normal limits. Plotting data on a chart giving norms for weight versus height regardless of age may be helpful.

When possible, health professionals should look at data pertaining to a child's growth over a period of time. Up to age 2, analysis of growth is more meaningful if it is reviewed over a period of months. Older children should be evaluated over a period of 6 months to a year. This allows identification of the overall rate of growth (slow, average, or rapid) and of significant current changes in the growth rate. If a short child is growing at a *normal rate* according to the growth chart, it is likely that this is normal for him.

ANALYSIS OF HEIGHT AND WEIGHT FOR ADULTS

Once an individual has reached adulthood, height should remain fairly constant. Over age 60, height may decrease slightly owing to osteoporotic changes in the bone. Desirable weights for men and women according to frame and height are presented in Appendix 4A. Assessment of weight should include a determination of (1) how the client's weight compares to the desirable range and (2) changes in weight over a period of time.

Weight loss A sudden or unexplained weight loss of 10 percent or more of body weight often indicates ill health. Rapid decrease in weight (more than 1 kg. or 2 lb. per week) usually represents excessive loss of muscle tissue and fluid. The amount of fat lost may be small by comparison. Gradual continuing weight loss generally represents loss of significant amounts of fat tissue.

The individual who has sustained a weight loss should be evaluated to determine the cause. Areas of investigation should identify whether or not (1) food and/or caloric intake equals expected caloric expenditure, (2) digestion and absorption of nutrients are normal, (3) metabolism of absorbed nutrients is normal, and (4) losses of nutrients or body secretions are excessive. Review of fluid intake and output records may reveal that diuresis is the cause of weight loss.

Weight gain Excessive weight may reflect an increase in fat and/or muscle tissue or an excessive accumulation of fluid in the body. Most frequently, gradual excessive weight gain is due to an overgenerous calorie intake which results in accumulation of excess body fat. It is sometimes helpful to analyze body composition to determine whether or not this is the case. Skinfold (fatfold) thickness gives an indication of the amount of subcutaneous body fat. Midarm circumference correlates to muscle mass when adjusted for skinfold thickness. Analysis of fluid intake and output may be useful in identifying fluid retention. An increase in abdominal girth may indicate accumulation of fluid in the peritoneal cavity (ascites).

SKINFOLD THICKNESS, UPPER ARM CIRCUMFERENCE, AND ARM MUSCLE CIRCUMFERENCE

There are a variety of reference standards available for use in analyzing skinfold (fatfold) thickness and mid-arm circumference. Most of the standards currently available have limitations; however, they do suggest the range of variability that can be expected. Average skinfold thickness is not necessarily optimal since it may reflect fatfold of an overweight population. It is important to identify that measurements have been made in the same manner as the standard used.

It is sometimes useful to estimate arm muscle mass as an indicator of an individual's total muscle mass (skeletal protein "reserve"). Arm muscle mass is estimated by an indirect means, using skinfold thickness, upper arm circumference, and a nomogram such as shown in Appendix 4E.

Appendix 4B gives percentiles for triceps skinfolds, midarm circumference, and arm muscle area.

Waist circumference in males is correlated with the degree of body fat. In females the largest circumference of the hip-gluteal region correlates with body fat.[9]

POINTS OF EMPHASIS
Analyzing anthropometric data

- *Use anthropometric data to assess growth and body composition.*
- *Use growth charts to identify a child's pattern of growth.*
- *If a child's growth appears abnormal, look for factors such as genetic potential and state of health which may influence growth rate.*
- *If a client has had a recent unexplained weight loss, review his general state of health.*
- *If a client has sustained a rapid gain in weight, determine whether the gain is due to an increase in body tissue or to excessive accumulation of fluid.*

Analysis of clinical findings

There are numerous clinical findings which may suggest the presence of malnutrition. Many of them are general and nonspecific. However, when they are appropriately assembled and analyzed in conjunction with other assessment data (particularly the diet history and biochemical measurements) they are useful in identifying nutritional problems. Many of the nonspecific signs may be due to disease or other conditions causing metabolic changes. Overt signs indicating specific deficiencies do not usually appear until the deficiencies are quite severe.

Data regarding the client's general appearance may alert the health professional to look more carefully to confirm or rule out a nutritional problem or to help to determine underlying causes of problems. The client who is described as cachectic in the medical record is in an advanced state of malnutrition. The health professional may immediately suspect malnutrition in the child who looks exceedingly small and thin for his age. The individual who is described as large may or may not be obese. Visual inspection can help distinguish between overfatness and an overweight condition which is due to a heavy frame and large muscle mass. Normal body size, however, does not negate the possibility of nutritional problems. Clothing, manner of dress, degree of cleanliness and neatness, and appropriateness of behavior may reflect the client's degree of concern about himself. The individual who is listless and apathetic or slightly disoriented may not be able to look after himself adequately or appropriately. These behaviors are often associated with inadequate nutrition.

Tissues such as skin and mucous membranes have a relatively rapid cell turnover and, therefore, reflect signs of nutrient deficiency sooner than do tissues whose turnover rate is slower.

Data obtained from inspection of the skin and mucous membranes (especially in the oral cavity and eyes) are most likely to be helpful in confirming or ruling out nutritional deficiencies. Changes in hair and nails become apparent more slowly. If the entire nail or hair is affected, a long-standing nutritional problem may exist. Dental caries can often be easily identified during visual inspection. Appendix 4G lists various tissues, the clinical signs often attributed to nutritional deficiencies, and the possible related deficiencies. When two or more physical signs of a deficiency are present simultaneously, it is often advisable to have the client seen by a health professional who has been trained in the diagnosis of nutrition problems. A deficiency state which is so far advanced that it is visible mandates that corrective measures be instituted as soon as possible. The affected person's state of well-being and life is at serious risk should a state of stress develop.

Analysis of diagnostic tests

Laboratory data can be utilized to determine various nutritional problems. Appendix 4G gives values for many of the biochemical tests used to identify nutrition-related problems. Some of the more common tests and their significance are discussed here. Tests are grouped according to nutrients and their function to emphasize their use in identifying nutritional rather than disease-oriented problems.

BIOCHEMICAL ANALYSIS

Analysis of biochemical data may make it possible to detect, rule out, or confirm the presence of certain nutrient deficiencies. A number of biochemical determinations may indicate the presence of marginal or subclinical nutrient deficiencies long before overt signs of malnutrition develop.

Types of biochemical analysis include determination of (1) levels of nutrients, (2) specific types of blood proteins, (3) the activity of specific enzymes requiring vitamins as cofactors, (4) metabolic products (metabolites) of some nutrients, (5) prothrombin time, and (6) hematological studies (these are not strictly biochemical but can be used to screen for certain nutrient deficiencies).

Levels of nutrients or other substances might be determined for whole blood, serum, certain types of cells (such as leukocytes or red blood cells), certain types of tissue (such as bone marrow), urine, hair, saliva, stool, and other test materials.

At present relatively few biochemical tests providing a direct measure of the level of a nutrient in the body are routinely conducted. Direct measurement of the level of a nutrient in the blood or serum may actually provide only an *indirect* measure of the amount of that nutrient in other parts of the body. Therefore, some seemingly direct tests must be interpreted with caution. Indirect measures, such as determination of enzyme activity and load tests, often provide more definitive information about a particular nutritional problem than do levels of nutrients. Changes in enzyme activity may become apparent only if there has been a persistent deficit of the specific nutrient involved. Load tests estimate the levels of certain nutrients in body tissues. The client is given a specified amount (test dose) of a micronutrient. Following this, changes in the nutrient content of the blood and/or urine are measured. The assumption is made that the client who is deficient in the micronutrient would not excrete as much of the test dose as would an individual whose micronutrient level was normal.

Biochemical data may reflect current status but may not indicate how long a deficiency has existed or how severe it is. A few tests, such as hemoglobin and serum proteins, may indicate long term nutrient deficits.

Many biochemical changes indicate either nutritional problems, disease processes, or both. Manuals for the interpretation of laboratory data tend to have a disease orientation and may not specify that certain standard tests can be used as indicators of nutritional status. This complicates accurate interpretation of the data. Nutrition-related data should be analyzed with the client's health status in mind.

The following points should be considered when interpreting biochemical data:

1. Selectivity in using biochemical data is desirable. When possible, health professionals should use test results to answer questions about the client's nutritional status and to support clinical judgements about the client's condition.
2. Biochemical tests provide varying degrees of accuracy. There is some disagreement about when a laboratory value falls outside the normal range. Cutoff points are somewhat arbitrary. Normal values vary from laboratory to laboratory depending on the test methods and the test materials used.

Usually a particular health agency will consistently use the same method of testing and will clearly identify normal ranges for that method. Differences in testing methods should be considered when reviewing data determined for the client by another health agency.

3. The timing of some tests may influence the results because of the relationship of the test to food intake or the body's circadian rhythm (daily rhythmic pattern of some body functions). Some drugs may interfere with testing methods and produce erroneous results.
4. Laboratory values are given primarily for healthy white adults. Many of the normal lab values for infants, small children and pregnant women differ from standard adult values. Pediatric laboratory tables should be used to analyze biochemical data about infants and children.
5. Pathophysiological states such as fever, infection, trauma, malabsorption, and renal impairment influence certain test results.
6. Biochemical data showing either elevated or depressed levels of nutrients or related substances may indicate potential or actual nutritional problems.
7. Laboratory data are often more meaningful if serial testing is done. Determining two or more sequential points gives the health professional an indication of the direction or progression of the disorder.
8. Laboratory data may be useful for determining the client's response to nutritional care.

DIAGNOSTIC TESTS PROVIDING INFORMATION ABOUT PROTEIN NUTRITION

A variety of biochemical tests are useful for estimating protein reserves in the body or for identifying alterations in protein metabolism. These tests are most informative when reviewed in conjunction with anthropometric test data.

Creatinine-height index Creatinine-height index (CHI) provides an indirect estimate of lean body mass (LBM). When renal function is normal, creatinine excretion is primarily dependent upon the individual's muscle mass. CHI is determined by relating actual urinary excretion of creatinine to the amount of creatinine that a well-nourished person of the same height would be expected to excrete in the same period of time. Expected or "ideal" excretion is determined from a reference table (Appendix 4H). Creatinine excretion is subject to some normal fluctuation. For example, a high dietary intake of protein may increase the creatinine excretion.[10]

A CHI of less than 90 percent of standard indicates moderate depletion of muscle mass and, therefore, of protein reserves. CHI should not be used to estimate LBM when renal function is impaired or in catabolic states such as infection or trauma.

Hair Root Diameter Hair root diameter provides an indirect measurement of hair root protein and has been shown to be a sensitive indicator of protein deficiency.[11] Test results which indicate a large number of hair roots have a diameter of 0.06 mm. or less are indicative of protein deficiency.

BLOOD CHEMISTRY

Serum protein levels—albumin Serum albumin levels may be used as a late indicator of PEM. Albumin levels tend to remain stable unless there is a serious protein deficiency or loss of blood protein resulting from certain diseases or hemorrhage. A low serum albumin in the absence of disease, injury, or blood loss points to the possibility that the client is seriously deficient in protein. This requires further investigation. Total protein level is not as valid an indicator of PEM.

Transferrin and retinol-binding protein The levels of both transferrin and retinol-binding protein (RBP) may be used as indicators of PEM. When there is a deficit of amino acids, hepatic synthesis and blood levels of these proteins fall. Levels of these proteins may be decreased in liver disease. Total iron binding capacity (TIBC) may also be used as an indication of transferrin levels. The approximate value of transferrin is [0.8 × TIBC] − 43.[12]

TESTS OF IMMUNOLOGICAL FUNCTION

Skin sensitivity tests Skin sensitivity tests, which reflect the status of cell-mediated immunity (CMI), are used as an indirect indicator of PEM. A depressed skin reaction to test substances such as streptokinase-streptodornase, mumps, and candida antigens is suggestive of protein deficiency. Skin tests are usually read 24 and 48 hours after administration. Some disease conditions such as immunological disorders may result in depressed skin sensitivity.

Lymphocytes The total number of circulating lymphocytes may fall in response to a deficit of amino acids. T lymphocyte levels are particularly likely to fall in PEM of the kwashiorkor-like type. Lymphocyte levels may be depressed in individuals experiencing a stress reaction from burns or trauma. Drugs, such as epinephrine and corticosteroids, and radiation may cause lymphopenia too.

UREA

Since urea is an end product of protein catabolism, it may be used as an indicator of protein metabolism. Blood urea nitrogen (BUN) level or serum urea nitrogen (SUN) and urine urea nitrogen (UUN) level provide different types of information. Impaired renal function causes the BUN and SUN to increase and the UUN to decrease.

BUN If renal function is normal, a significant increase in the BUN may indicate excessive intake of protein and perhaps inadequate fluid intake. If renal function is abnormal, the BUN or SUN is used as one means of monitoring the adequacy of the modified diet in relation to protein and caloric intake.

UUN A determination of the urea nitrogen from a 24-hour urine sample allows a rough estimation of the client's total nitrogen output for the day. This value may be compared to the client's estimated nitrogen intake (determined from food intake records) to identify his state of nitrogen balance. If nitrogen output greatly exceeds nitrogen intake, the client is losing body protein and is at risk of becoming seriously depleted.

If extra-renal nitrogen losses are large (as via diarrhea or fistula drainage) nitrogen content of these secretions can also be estimated to more accurately assess the state of nitrogen balance. The 24-hour UUN is of little use when the BUN is not stable because of renal disease.

LIPIDS (EXCLUDING FAT-SOLUBLE VITAMINS)

Cholesterol and triglycerides Data regarding cholesterol and triglyceride levels in the blood may be analyzed to see if abnormalities are present which might respond favorably to diet modification. In particular there is interest in controlling blood lipid levels as a means of reducing risk of atherosclerosis and coronary artery disease. The data are influenced by a variety of normal body processes as well as by certain disease processes. Whether or not elevated cholesterol level signals a problem depends partly on the way in which the cholesterol is transported in the blood.

Ketones Data regarding ketone levels may provide useful information about fat (and carbohydrate) metabolism. Ketone production increases when there is increased utilization of fatty acids and decreased utilization of carbohydrate as a source of fuel.

A reagent tablet (a tablet which changes color when exposed to ketones) or test paper may be used to test for the presence of ketones in the urine. (Serum plasma or whole blood may also be tested.) The presence of ketones in the urine is indicative of changes in fatty acid metabolism. These changes may mean (1) the client has eaten little or no food and/or received no parenteral glucose for a period of time, (2) the client is following a protein-sparing modified fast or other very low carbohydrate diet, or (3) a diabetic client needs assistance (perhaps urgently) in bringing his disease under control.

Fecal fat   Fecal fat content gives an indication of the client's ability to absorb fat. To be meaningful, fecal fat must be related to fat intake. If, for example, the client ingested 100 gm. of fat daily for a period of days and his fecal fat for the same period averaged 40 gm., the client's fat absorption was only 60 percent, far less than the 96 percent which is normal. A high fecal fat loss indicates that the client is at high risk of a broad spectrum of nutrient deficiencies and of calorie deficiency. The health professional should look for causes of the malabsorption.

CARBOHYDRATE

Blood glucose   Data regarding blood glucose provides information about carbohydrate metabolism. Several different blood glucose determinations may be in the client's record, including the fasting blood sugar (FBS), 2-hour post-prandial blood glucose and random blood glucose. Chapter 30 explains the significance of these tests. Depending on the agency, either plasma blood glucose or whole (venous) blood glucose levels will be measured. A number of techniques might be used for measuring the glucose. Since norms differ considerably for different types of testing, clarification is essential. For rapid estimate of blood glucose level the client's finger or ear lobe may be pricked. A drop of the capillary blood obtained is applied to reagent paper. The color the paper turns depends on how much glucose is present.

Urine glucose   The presence of glucose in the urine usually signals an abnormality in carbohydrate metabolism. The percent of glucose in the urine gives an indication of the severity of the problem. Ordinarily the blood glucose level must be elevated above normal for glucose to spill into the urine. Absence of glucose in the urine does not rule out the possibility of problems with carbohydrate metabolism.

Different types of tests may be used to detect sugar in the urine. Some of these include spot checks, 24-hour collection for glucose, and fractional 24-hour collection. When a spot check is done the results are more accurate if a second voided specimen is used, so the urine used has been freshly excreted by the kidneys. Directions for use of test materials should be read carefully since a variety of substances may give either a false positive or a false negative reading.

FAT-SOLUBLE VITAMINS

Laboratory data indicating abnormalities in the client's levels of fat soluble vitamins may be scarce. The most commonly available data are discussed here.

Tests relevant to vitamin K   Prothrombin time (PT) and blood clotting time both *increase* in response to vitamin K deficiency since vitamin K is needed for synthesis of prothrombin and other blood clotting factors. An elevated PT suggests vitamin K deficiency. However, PT may be elevated if the client has liver disease or is taking the anticoagulant warfarin.

Tests relevant to vitamin D   The level of circulating 25-hydroxy vitamin D can be easily determined. Serum phosphate level is depressed in vitamin D deficiency.

An elevated level of the enzyme bone alkaline phosphatase may help to confirm deficiency of vitamin D.

Tests relevant to vitamin A   The serum level of retinol (vitamin A) provides a clear indication of the client's vitamin A status, but it is seldom determined. A low serum retinol identifies the need for improved nutritional care to prevent progression to overt deficiency disease.

The serum level of beta carotene, a precursor of vitamin A, is *not* a good indicator of vitamin A status, although an abnormally low level may indicate fat malabsorption.

WATER-SOLUBLE VITAMINS

Data on the levels of water soluble vitamins is not routinely available. Serum levels of these vitamins or their metabolites may provide little useful information since they tend to reflect immediate rather than long term intake (see Appendix 4G).

Since water-soluble vitamins are relatively nontoxic (and inexpensive), it may not be essential to confirm deficiency by means of biochemical tests. It is common to give a therapeutic dose if a deficiency is suspected on the basis of medical history, diet history, and/or clinical signs of deficiency and to provide nutritional care directed toward achieving satisfactory intake.

MINERALS

Serum levels   Although data about serum levels of many minerals (Na, K, Mg, Ca, P) are frequently available, its usefulness in assessing nutritional status is limited in a number of ways (see Chapter 28).

Electrolyte imbalances signal serious problems which may require medical or surgical care in addition to appropriate nutritional care.

Urinary levels   Amounts of sodium and potassium excreted in the urine may reflect intake of these minerals or current body levels or may be abnormal owing to a disease process.

Trace minerals   Iron. Hemoglobin level, hematocrit, and red blood cell size are readily obtainable data. Decreased values suggest the possibility of iron deficiency anemia. Total iron binding capacity may indicate the presence of iron deficiency before other changes in the blood are noted. The same type of anemia may be due to inadequate intake or absorption of iron, to blood loss, or to certain other types of stress. Therefore additional data (e.g., food intake, medical-surgical history) should be reviewed to determine the cause. Blood loss from the gastrointestinal tract may be identified by performing a guaiac test on stools to determine the presence of occult blood.

STUDY QUESTIONS

1. Identify several factors which may influence how rapidly an individual becomes malnourished.
2. Mr. S. is suffering from malnutrition despite the fact that he appears obese. What kinds of malnutrition could he be suffering from? Why might his appearance be deceptive in identifying his malnutrition?
3. Which body tissues are likely to exhibit early signs of malnutrition? Explain.
4. List several serious consequences of protein-energy malnutrition.
5. Using the Basic Four Food Guide, a nurse determines that a client's diet contains no obvious sources of vitamin A. What further steps could the nurse take to determine whether or not the client's diet contains adequate amounts of this vitamin?

References

*1. Bistrian, B. R., et al.: Protein status of general surgical patients. *J.A.M.A.* 230:858, 1974.

*2. Bistrian, B. R., et al.: Prevalence of malnutrition in general medical patients. *J.A.M.A.* 235:1567, 1976.

3. Garn, S., and Clark, D.: Problems in nutritional assessment of black individuals. *Am. J. Public Health* 66:262, 1976.

4. Foster, T. A., et al.: Anthropometric and maturation measurements of children ages 5–14 years in a biracial community—The Boglusa Health Study. *Am. J. Clin. Nutr.* 30:582, 1977.

5. Pennington, J. A.: *Dietary Nutrient Guide.* Westport CT: Avi Publishing Co., 1976.

6. *Recommended Dietary Allowances,* ed. 8. Food and Nutrition Board, National Research Council. Washington DC: ACASCI, 1974.

7. Inano, M., and Pringle, D. J.: Diet survey of low-income, rural families in Iowa and North Carolina. I. Research procedures. *J. Am. Diet. Assoc.* 66:356, 1975.

8. Shull, M., et al.: Seasonal variations in preschool vegetarian children's growth velocities. *Am. J. Clin. Nutr.* 31:1, 1978.

9. Björntorp, P.: Exercise in the treatment of obesity. *Clin. Endocrin. Metab.* 5:431, 1976.

10. Forbes, G., and Bruining, G. V.: Urinary creatinine excretion and lean body mass. *Am. J. Clin. Nutr.* 29:1359, 1976.

11. Bregar, R.: Hair root diameter measurement as an indicator of protein deficiency in non-hospital alcoholics. *Am. J. Clin. Nutr.* 31:230, 1978.

12. Blackburn, G., et al.: Nutritional and metabolic assessment of the hospitalized patient. *J. Parent. Enter. Nutr.* 1(1):11, 1977.

* Recommended reading

22

The use of tools in planning for nutritional care

After the client's problems have been identified through assessment, a nutritional care plan is developed. A comprehensive plan of care includes (1) a list of client problems (actual and potential), (2) goals (the desired outcomes) of care, and (3) an outline of actions to be carried out for and by the client. A distinct nutritional care plan may be developed for a client or a nutritional care plan may be part of a nursing care plan or of a medical care plan. The plan of care should reflect the client's individuality; it should be congruent with other plans of care for the client; and it should be based on sound scientific theory (nutritional, physical, and behavioral). Such a plan helps guide health team members to deliver high quality nutritional care. Care plans may be periodically revised to reflect a client's current needs. Revisions should be based on evaluation of the client's progress and response to nutritional care and teaching.

CLIENT PROBLEMS

CLIENT INVOLVEMENT

Health professionals who consider a client's understanding of his problems, his reactions, and his concerns can more easily develop individualized goals of care. A client is more likely to work toward goals if they reflect his beliefs and expectations. Since food habits are so closely entwined with activities of daily living, successful management of nutritional care must involve the client in planning and decision making early and regularly.

In some instances a client may not initially have the desire, skills, or knowledge needed to participate in care. Often trying to motivate a client and supplying

him with information may prod him to participate and gradually assume responsibility for planning and managing his own care. Health care providers should encourage a client to participate as he is able to do so.

FAMILY INVOLVEMENT

When beginning planning care it is usually desirable to discuss a client's problems with him and his family. This should reveal whether or not they are aware of the existence or threat of certain problems. Ideally the plan of care is geared toward the family rather than just toward the individual who was identified to have a nutrition-related problem. The family can then become involved in improving care by measures such as providing needed moral support, encouraging the client to become more independent, assisting with meal preparation or other food-related tasks, or providing health professionals with suggestions for improving the client's food intake. If the family is not involved, the client is less likely to be willing or able to cooperate with the recommended plan. Many people fail to follow through with doctor's recommendations (one review estimates as many as 30 to 60 percent, depending on the client population studied[1]). Enlisting the aid of the family may help to overcome this problem.

If a change in diet is indicated for the client, in some cases it is desirable for the whole family to change its eating habits. A weight control program might benefit the family as well as the client who is being treated.[2] Other diet guidelines which might be beneficial for both the client and his family are those designed to increase dietary intake of one or more micronutrients, to control blood cholesterol levels or hypertension, or to make more economical food choices. It is important to

245

remember, however, that there are instances when some family members should not follow a client's modified diet. For example, it is not desirable for very young children to drink skim milk, because they need linoleic acid and adequate calories to promote normal growth and development. Diets such as a wheat-free diet or a protein-restricted diet would not benefit other family members and would be undesirably restrictive.

There are several reasons for suggesting the whole family follow many of a client's diet guidelines. Here are a few:

1. The potential for risk (as of obesity) may not be limited to just one family member because hereditary and/or environment influence risk factors. Thus, involving all family members may be a sound health promotion measure.
2. It is difficult for one individual to maintain the motivation needed to adhere indefinitely to a diet different from that of other family members. This is especially true if there are no symptoms of disease. Seeing the whole family enjoy well-prepared meals fitting the client's diet modification can be a real morale booster.
3. If only "allowed" foods are on hand, the temptation to stray from the diet is reduced.
4. When family members eat the same kinds of foods, prepared in the same way, meal planning and preparation are simplified.
5. Diet modifications and other recommended changes in lifestyle are measures which allow maintenance or improvement of health.

Health professionals may have to assume a dominant role in planning and implementing care in acute situations, in terminal stages of illness, or in certain other circumstances. Here, it may be beneficial to enlist the help of family members. They can often inform health professionals of the client's nutritional and health status prior to his illness. Family members are often knowledgeable about a client's food preferences and can suggest helpful feeding techniques. They may be eager to participate in care of the client.

CLIENT GOALS

A *goal* is a statement of desired change which is to occur in the client. It may be a physical, psychosocial, intellectual, or spiritual change. In this textbook goals refer primarily to statements of long term accomplishments. Health professionals sometimes interchangeably use a similar term—objectives. In this textbook, however, *objectives* refers to statements of short term accomplishments which enable goals to be reached.

Goals are derived from a client's diagnosis (problem statement). They aim to restore and maintain a balance between a client's needs and a client's coping abilities and resources. For example, a problem such as lack of transportation to the grocery store interferes with the elderly person's ability to provide adequate food for himself. A general goal of care (directed toward increasing resources) would be to enable the senior citizen to meet his need for food by providing him with weekly transportation to and from a grocery store. Goals may focus on maintenance of adequate nutritional status, prevention of decline in nutritional status, and/or promotion of improved nutritional status.

If goals and objectives are well developed and clearly stated they serve the following purposes:

1. Give a sense of purpose and direction. Client, family, and health care workers know what is to be accomplished. A health professional can more easly identify ways to help a client when goals guide their actions.
2. Provide a sense of pacing for activities. Client, family, and professionals know about how long it will take for desired changes to occur.
3. Contribute to a sense of accomplishment. A method of evaluation is clearly identified so client and professionals are aware of how well goals have been met.
4. Provide a means of communication among client and health professionals. Various health professionals can participate in a client's care and maintain a consistent approach when goals are clearly stated.

WRITING GOALS AND OBJECTIVES

Goals are somewhat general; objectives are quite specific. An example of each is given:

Goal   The client will maintain his weight during chemotherapy treatment.

Objective   The client will drink 240 ml. of prescribed high calorie supplement three times daily between meals.

Long term goals provide a sense of direction but need not always contain specific criteria for measurement of achievement. Short term objectives, on the other hand, clearly spell out what is to be achieved. Often health professionals choose to state short term objectives in behavioral terms. Behavioral objectives indicate the performance desired and provide a standard against which to measure outcomes of care. Well-written goals and objectives are realistic and achievable. They are designed to fit the client's level of growth and development, physical status, and psychosocial characteristics. They are written to allow for some flexibility. A health professional who is learning to write behavioral objectives may find Mager's book, *Preparing Instructional Objectives*, to be a useful guide.[3]

Useful goals and objectives are mutually established with the client and other significant persons. Goals should be acceptable to the client and respect his wishes and circumstances. When writing goals the health professional considers factors which may modify goal setting, including (1) client's personality and values, (2) client's and family's expectations, (3) physical and cultural setting, and (4) available resources (human and material).

RESOLVING DIFFERENCES IN GOALS

Clients and health professionals have different values, backgrounds, and experiences. Often the result is that they desire to achieve different goals. For example, a health care worker's goal may be to assist a client to be willing and able to follow a prescribed diabetic diet. The client's major goal may be to get out of the hospital and back to work as quickly as possible. This client may view diet teaching as one of many nuisances delaying his discharge. The client and health care provider each need to learn what the other person's goals are in order to work toward a resolution of differences. In the example given, the client may be more receptive to assuming responsibility for learning about his diet if he recognizes that proper dietary management will prevent him from losing unnecessary time from work and if part of the instruction can be provided after discharge.

Goal differences are not always readily apparent. Often a client's goals are implicit in his actions rather than explicit in his thoughts or words. Trying to identify what the client is really accomplishing by carrying out particular activities may help a health professional resolve goal differences. Behaviors such as the following should suggest to the health professional that a client's goals differ from her own: lack of cooperation, procrastination, preoccupation, anger, withdrawal.

A client who does not follow his diet guidelines despite encouragement, repeated warnings, teaching sessions, and even frequent hospitalizations may be trying to achieve a goal of which the health professional is unaware. An alert health professional might look to see what the client is gaining by not following his modified diet. If, for example, the client gets a lot of attention only when he is sick enough to be hospitalized, then the health professional can try to find ways for the client to get the attention he desires at home.

RANKING GOALS IN ORDER OF PRIORITY

Specific goals for nutritional care can be placed in a sequence to identify a preferred order for delivery of care. These nutrition-related goals may also be ranked with regard to overall goals of health care. Certainly nutritional care would be a priority goal for a severely malnourished client with no other major health problems. However, nutritional care would not need to be stated immediately as a goal for a client who had just sustained a head injury.

When goals are ranked, the most important ones should receive priority attention. Goals to meet basic needs and maintain life generally have a greater priority than goals to meet higher level needs. Except for crisis situations, motivation of a client is usually one of the most important aspects of nutritional care.[4] If beneficial changes are to occur, a client must value his health and must desire to make changes to maintain or improve it.

POINTS OF EMPHASIS
Establishing goals

• *A goal is a general statement describing desired outcomes of nutritional care.*
• *Objectives specifically describe what is to be accomplished and how and when it is to be accomplished.*
• *It is desirable to secure the cooperation of a client and his family in planning and implementing goals of care.*
• *In many instances family and client alike may benefit from achieving the client's goals for nutritional care.*
• *Goal differences between client and professional should be identified and resolved.*

WRITING A NUTRITIONAL CARE PLAN

The purpose of the nutritional care plan is to outline specific actions to meet the client's goals. A well-written nutritional care plan promotes communication among health team members about what the client's needs are, what desired changes are expected, and what measures are being used to achieve those changes. A successful nutritional care plan gears the client's dietary needs to the realities of his life situation. It is coordinated with his overall plan of care. A main goal included in a nutritional care plan might be for the client to be able to select and eat nutritious foods to promote and maintain optimal health.

Nutritional care plans are most often written by dietitians, nutritionists, dietetic technicians, nurse clinicians, nurse practitioners, and staff nurses. They may be shared among members of various health disciplines or they may be constructed primarily for use by members within one health profession. A carefully developed standardized format may be used by an agency to increase consistency and quality of care. Since many health agencies use their own nutritional care plan, it is necessary for health professionals to become familiar with the plan used in the agency where they work. When competent health professionals use a standardized format they take care to gear it toward the unique characteristics of each client.

Selecting actions

After goals have been identified health professionals select specific activities which can be implemented to achieve desired goals. There may be several interventions which can be directed toward the same goal. The measures chosen depend upon the situation. For example, interventions for a client with anorexia might include: (1) Offering pleasantly flavored foods or offering bland foods. Discussion: Some anorexic clients may find their appetite is increased by the smell and taste of pleasantly flavored foods while other clients may find that the same food makes them nauseous. (2) Suggesting that a client eat with his family or that he eat alone. Discussion: A small child may eat more when his mother is present because he feels more secure. A teenager who is struggling to gain independence from his family may become tense and refuse to eat if his family is present.

Goal-directed actions are developed preferably in collaboration with the client and his family. Clients from some cultural groups may be completely unwilling to receive or participate in care without the approval of their family, an older relative, or a "folk healer."

Useful actions support the client in meeting his daily nutritional needs, foster his independence, and encourage his active participation in care. A thorough assessment of a client and his situation and clear definitions of his nutritional problems simplify identification of nutritional care measures.

The selection of actions to achieve goals should be based on logical, scientific rationale such as principles from the biological and behavioral sciences. For instances, a health professional might suggest that a client drink orange juice or grapefruit juice rather than water when he takes his prescribed iron supplement. The rationale for selecting this activity would be that the vitamin C in those juices favors iron absorption.

To select appropriate actions a health professional needs to consider the various resources available for providing nutritional care. The client himself is a primary resource. If the client's knowledge, skills, strengths, and positive coping strategies have been identified during assessment they can be included in the plan of care.

The competent health professional has current knowledge of community and health agency resources providing or supplementing nutritional care services. Community resources are an invaluable aid in both *preventing* and *correcting* nutritional problems. *Community resources* here refers to (1) financial assistance (e.g., food stamps) and federal, state, and local food assistance programs; (2) nutrition education programs; and (3) resource persons and agencies providing assistance to individuals with problems concerning food and/or nutrition.

Features of federal food programs and of some other types of resources are listed in Appendix 2. A call or letter to the city or state health department in some areas will bring a directory listing all the known community nutrition services in the state. The listing might identify types of services provided, eligibility for participation, and a contact person for each program. Local health libraries often have listings of community and health agency resources.

A series of appropriate actions should be outlined to meet each client goal. Well-written plans include specific directions concerning (1) what is to be done, (2) who is to do it, (3) how it is to be done, (4) where it is to be done, and (5) when and how often it is to be done. The written directions for care may be divided among three distinct areas: (1) ongoing assessment, (2) direct care measures, and (3) client education. Each of these components of a care plan is described here.

ASSESSMENT

Further data collection and analysis may be desirable to more clearly identify the client's problem or to evaluate the client's progress. Specific data-gathering activities such as recording a client's food intake, checking relevant laboratory values, or weighing the client might be listed under assessment activities.

DIRECT CARE MEASURES

Direct care measures include activities to provide for an adequate normal or modified diet.

Adequate normal diet   Providing an adequate normal diet, when possible, is a preferred action. Specific measures to promote normal food intake are outlined in relation to the client's needs. For example, measures such as referral to a WIC (Supplemental Food Program for Women, Infants and Children) program might be listed to assist a mother to obtain adequate amounts and kinds of foods during pregnancy. For a client with stomatitis (an inflamed mouth), measures to decrease pain within the oral cavity might be listed.

Modified diet   It may be necessary for a client's diet to be modified in one or more ways. The type and degree of dietary change needed depends on how problems have affected the client's intake, absorption, utilization, and/or excretion of nutrients. Purposes for diet modification usually fall into three categories: (1) providing extra nutrients in times of increased need, (2) reducing the risk of health problems or complications, or (3) alleviating or eliminating symptoms or other problems. Often a modified diet serves more than one purpose. For example, adhering to a low calorie diet for a period of time may reduce the risk of heart disease and alleviate the problem of shortness of breath associated with exercise.

Diet modifications may be of many types. Changes may be made in (1) amounts and kinds of foods eaten, depending on the food's content of specific nutrients or other substances (e.g., sodium restricted diet, high fiber diet); (2) texture and consistency of food eaten (such as liquids, soft solids); or (3) frequency and method of feeding (such as six small meals daily or intravenous or tube feeding). It is possible to alter both the method of feeding and nutrient content in the same diet.

A modified diet should resemble the client's normal diet as closely as possible, with changes kept to a minimum. Modified diets, if used for more than a few days, should usually meet the client's requirements for essential nutrients and calories. The client's food habits, cultural practices, economic status, and relevant family and environmental factors provide a framework for the modifications.

CLIENT EDUCATION

In most instances it is important to outline a plan for providing client education. Some of the areas in which clients can benefit from teaching include (1) reinforcement of sound eating habits, (2) positive suggestions to improve poor food habits, (3) discussion of reasons for diet modifications, (4) guidance and practice in planning meals meeting specific diet modifications, (5) training in various feeding techniques, and (6) explanations of various assessment and treatment activities. Chapter 23 discusses guidelines for nutritional teaching.

Communicating the nutritional care plan

Since various members of the health team may be working with a client in planning and implementing nutritional care, it is essential to maintain open channels of communication.

The client is the person who probably has the greatest interest in his care plan. He can work better with health team members if he is informed about his current nutritional status, about the relationship of his food habits and nutritional status to his health, and about his total nutritional plan of care. He also needs a description of the care various health team members will provide for him and resources available for his use. Sharing goals and plans with family members and other significant persons helps them clarify their role in assisting the client.

Three specific methods of communication among health team members are (1) diet orders, (2) consultations, and (3) referrals.

DIET ORDERS

The diet order is an important component of a client's care plan. Prescribing a diet is usually the physician's responsibility. In some carefully defined situations, dietitians, nurse practitioners, and nurse clinicians who are working in collaboration with physicians may prescribe diets. A diet order may be for a normal diet or for a modified diet. Modified diets are prescribed to promote the client's health, to make him more comfortable, or to facilitate diagnostic testing. Occasionally modified diets are prescribed for clients as part of closely regulated research projects.

A useful diet order is clearly and precisely written. It specifically identifies the *kinds* and/or *amounts* of food or nutrients allowed, restricted, or prohibited. For example, a diet order for a no-added salt or low sodium diet is not very specific. However, an order for a 2 gm.

sodium diet clearly identifies that the intake of the nutrient sodium is to be restricted to 2 gm. per day. The diet order should indicate the route and frequency of feeding when appropriate. If the client is expected to follow a diet prescription by himself an order for dietary instruction should also be written. It is preferable that orders for teaching be written well in advance of the client's discharge. Nurses, dietitians, or nutritionists should feel free to contact the physician if it appears that this step has been overlooked or if they question the suitability of a diet order.

The dietitian is usually responsible for planning food and menu selections which are appealing and palatable to the client and which provide nutritious food. The nurse frequently collaborates with the dietitian to determine ways to improve a client's adherence to a diet. Adjustments in the diet order may be based on ongoing assessment of the client.

CONSULTATIONS

Health professionals may request the opinion or advice of other health professionals either for an individual client or for a group of clients. Within a health agency if a nurse or physician determines that a client might benefit from specific nutritional assessment or counseling, she may request these services for a client via consultation with the hospital dietitian. In this case the dietitian assumes responsibility for overseeing the nutritional care plan. In a community agency such as a maternity clinic, if a nurse or other health care worker notes that a client is not eating a balanced diet, she might consult with a dietitian or nutritionist to develop a care plan to assist the client to make more appropriate food choices. Alternatively she might refer the client to the nutritionist for assistance.

In some health care facilities a dietitian is available only as an outside consultant. An outside consultant can give advice but usually has no direct line of authority to see that a plan of care is implemented for a client.

Under some circumstances, a group of health professionals might request the services of an outside consultant dietitian (such as a public health nutritionist) so that they can learn to improve nutritional care of clients.

REFERRALS

A health professional may request the assistance of other health care providers, health agencies, or community facilities to provide client care. Referrals are often made for (1) a specific kind of therapy (such as to a dentist for treatment of decayed teeth), (2) rehabilitation or retraining (such as to a physical therapist to assist a client to relearn how to swallow food), (3) education (such as to a community nutritionist to teach a client principles of meal planning), or (4) special community services (such as home delivered meals provided by a community Meals on Wheels program).

Name _____

Record # _____

Transfer to: _____

_____

PATIENT CARE PLAN
(Explain details of care, medications, treatments, teaching, habits, preferences, and goals.)

Medications: note time last dose given on day of discharge. *

Date of admission to health care facility: *

Date of Discharge: *

Medical diagnosis: *

NURSING Self Care Status Check Functional Level		Inde-pen-dent	Needs Assist-ance	Unable
Ambulation	Bed-Chair			
	Walking			
	Stairs			
	Wheelchair			
	Crutches			
	Walker			
	Cane			
Activities	Bathe self			
	Dress self			
	Feed self			
	Brushing teeth			
	Shaving			
	Toilet			
	Commode			
	Bedpan/Urinal			

Bowel & Bladder Program	☐Yes	☐No
Incontinence: Bladder☐ Bowel☐ Date of Last Enema		
Catheter: Type Date last changed:		
Weight Height Date Anointed Yes☐ No☐ Date		

Check if Pertinent (describe at right) ⟩

DISABILITIES
☐ Amputation
☐ Paralysis
☐ Contractures
☐ Decubitus
☐ Other

IMPAIRMENTS
☐ Speech
☐ Hearing
☐ Vision
☐ Sensation
☐ Other

COMMUNICATION
☐ Can Write
☐ Talks
☐ Understands Speaking
☐ Understands English
☐ If no, Other Language?
☐ Reads
☐ Non-Verbal

BEHAVIOR
☐ Alert
☐ Forgetful
☐ Noisy
☐ Confused
☐ Withdrawn
☐ Wanders
☐ Other

REQUIRES
Mark "S" if sent; "N" if needed
☐ Colostomy Care   ☐ Dentures
☐ Cane   ☐ Eye Glasses
☐ Crutches   ☐ Hearing Aid
☐ Walker   ☐ Prosthesis
☐ Wheelchair   ☐ Side Rails
☐ Other

Nurse's discharge assessment and recommen-dations for care

INCLUDE INFORMATION PERTINENT TO NUTRITIONAL CARE SUCH AS: *

- ability to select and obtain a nutritionally sound diet
- ability to feed self
- adequacy of client's "normal" food intake
- amount and kind of assistance client needs to feed self
- alternate feeding methods used, type, amount and times of feedings (e.g., tube feedings)
- other special food and nutrition-related needs (e.g., drugs and treatments causing nutrition-related problems)

_____
Signature of Nurse

Telephone _____   Date _____

NUTRITION: (discuss food preferences, understanding of diet, teaching needs and goals)   Diet enclosed   ☐Yes   ☐No

For example: *
- describe special diet modifications, instruction and counseling provided, materials given to client
- need for follow-up teaching
- need for nutrition assessment following discharge, such as client's success in maintaining prescribed diet changes, family and community factors affecting client's food habits
- need for assistance obtaining and preparing food

_____   _____   _____
Nutritionist Signature   Telephone   Date

Referrals may be written or verbal. Sharing pertinent information about the client in a referral promotes consistency of care. The client's problem or need should be identified; the reason for the referral and recommendations or requests for care should be clearly stated. Information about a client's food habits, appetite, understanding of his nutritional needs and diet instruction, and special instructions for feeding should be identified in many types of referrals. In order to insure completeness and continuity of care, many agencies use standardized referral forms such as the one in Fig. 22.1.

STUDY QUESTIONS

1. List several reasons why a whole family might benefit from following diet changes recommended for one family member who has been found to be deficient in folic acid.

2. Write two goals of care for a pregnant woman who has not gained a desirable amount of weight during her second trimester of pregnancy. For each goal write two behavioral objectives identifying specific ways the woman can meet the goals.

3. Why is it desirable to have a modified diet resemble the client's normal diet as closely as possible?

References

*1. Becker, M. H., and Green, L. W.: A family approach to compliance with medical treatment. *Internat. J. Health Ed.* 17(3):1, 1975.

*2. D'Angelli, A. R., and Smicklas-Wright, H.: The case for primary prevention of overweight through the family. *J. Nutr. Ed.* 10:76, 1978.

*3. Mager, R.: *Preparing Instructional Objectives.* Palo Alto CA: Fearon Publishers, 1962.

*4. Sims, L.: Dietary status of lactating women. II. Relation of nutritional knowledge and attitudes to nutrient intake. *J. Am. Diet. Assoc.* 73:147, 1978.

Recommended reading

FIGURE 22.1. Sample of an interagency referral form (partial) (Approved by the Massachusetts Department of Public Health). *Author's addition.

23

The use of tools in providing nutrition education

Nutrition education is a means of helping people to help themselves to improve or maintain their health. It is an important step in the process of providing nutritional care. After a client's nutritional needs have been identified through assessment, a plan of care is developed and implemented. If the client is going to participate in his own program of care, nutrition education is required.

Provision of nutrition education is aided by application of principles of learning and teaching. This chapter describes the teaching-learning process and illustrates ways in which principles of learning and teaching can be applied in nutrition education. The focus of this chapter is primarily on one-to-one teaching.

Health professionals who provide nutrition education help clients to maintain and promote their health in a number of ways including (1) development of positive attitudes about nutrition, (2) provision of knowledge essential to make judicious food choices for health and well-being, (3) provision of information to make economical food choices and to avoid food waste, and (4) promotion of positive food practices in children.[1] Nutrition education is successful when a client has gained specific knowledge of food and of nutrition and then *uses* it in his daily food practices.

Nutrition education may be conducted in formal structured sessions or it may be carried out in an informal manner. Formal teaching is usually based on a structured plan which involves identifying a client's educational needs, stating educational objectives, developing and implementing appropriate content and teaching methods, and evaluating a client's learning. Usually a specific time is set aside for formal teaching.

Informal teaching, on the other hand, may be carried out "on the spot" as the need arises. On-the-spot teaching is useful to reinforce, strengthen, and support

teaching the client has already received. It is also an appropriate way to provide other types of informal nutrition education. For example, a client might ask a question or appear confused after a visit with a health care provider; he may make inappropriate menu selections; or he may give indications that he feels that his diet is not very important. A nurse or other health care worker who recognizes the client's need for teaching can take immediate advantage of opportunities to do on-the-spot teaching. Alternatively, she may plan to meet with the client later to provide teaching in a more structured manner.

When a client who is following a modified diet has a question about whether or not he can eat a certain food, it is desirable for the health care worker to say that she will find out (and for her to then do so). Health professionals may develop slightly different diet plans for the same diet modification. If an overall teaching plan has already been developed for a client and the person providing on-the-spot instruction is familiar with it, that person can provide information consistent with the diet plan.

In either formal or on-the-spot teaching, applying principles of teaching and learning should contribute to the success of the effort.

Health professionals who are acting as diet counselors need to take a number of steps to develop an effective nutrition education program. As with other aspects of nutritional care it is highly desirable to include the family in the teaching-learning process. An initial step in development of a nutrition education program is to determine a client's learning needs. Many of these needs should be apparent from the overall assessment of a client's nutrition-related needs. Goals for nutrition education which are acceptable to both the client and health professional are developed from identified needs. Motivating a client to make needed changes in food-related behavior is often a priority goal.

To meet defined goals, the health professional develops and implements an individualized teaching plan. She tries to locate or make teaching aids she can use to help a client learn. The diet counselor works to become adept at a variety of techniques which will help her to be a skillful teacher. As she implements a teaching plan she evaluates the client's progress. This evaluation guides follow-up instruction, reinforcement, and further attempts to motivate the client.

ASSESSING THE LEARNER'S NEEDS

In order to provide individualized instruction, it is necessary to identify characteristics of the learner which may influence the teaching-learning process. The client's needs for nutrition education must be clearly identified.

Assessing readiness to learn

An initial step in developing a teaching plan is to determine whether or not a client recognizes the need for learning and is, therefore, motivated to learn. If the client is not motivated, the teaching plan should include content to assist him to recognize the need for and value of changing his eating habits. A query such as "Tell me why you think the doctor put you on this diet" sometimes elicits a surprising answer. The answer may point up the need for probing further into conditions which are impeding the client's readiness to learn, or the answer may signal that the client is eager to learn all that he can.

Assessing and dealing with learner characteristics

PHYSICAL AND MENTAL STATUS

A person's physical and mental condition affect his ability to learn. A client who is in pain, tired, or hungry will have difficulty concentrating. Similarly, a client who is worried, distracted, depressed, or anxious cannot easily devote attention to learning. In these instances it might be preferable to delay teaching until the client is in a more favorable physical and mental state.

Planning teaching sessions for a time of day when a client is alert and rested facilitates learning. In a health agency, midmorning or midafternoon may be the most satisfactory times. If possible, it is helpful to let the client choose in advance between two or three different times or at least to let him know when to be ready for the teaching session. In this way distractions

such as visitors or a favorite TV show may be avoided. It is sometimes desirable to refer a client to a community agency or practitioner rather than to attempt to conduct a teaching session when a client is not physically and mentally ready to learn.

If a client is traveling to a community agency for a teaching session, it sometimes aids learning to give him an opportunity to rest in a comfortable location before the teaching session starts. However, if the teaching session does not begin promptly at the scheduled time, the client may become so agitated that his ability to concentrate is greatly reduced. Increasingly, clinics have self-instructional materials available so that learning may begin while the client is waiting to see the health professional. Some clinics such as prenatal, oncology (cancer related), and diabetes clinics provide appropriate snacks for clients. Snacks decrease a client's hunger, help promote adequate food intake, serve to illustrate nutritious food choices, and reinforce the idea that food is an important element of total health care.

In some situations, teaching is necessary despite the fact that physical and/or mental factors interfere with the client's ability to concentrate. A client with severe renal disease, for example, may have difficulty focusing his attention on learning because of the effects of toxic substances in his body. Diet modification is an important aspect of managing renal disease, however, and there are some things the client must know and do to improve his condition. In this situation a teaching plan is modified to fit with the client's current status. For example, teaching sessions can be limited to very short time spans. Frequent repetition may help. The health professional who understands that illness and other stresses can impede learning may have more patience and be more effective in working with clients.

INTELLECTUAL SKILLS, PYSCHOMOTOR SKILLS, PREVIOUS LEARNING, AND ATTITUDES

A client's intellectual skills, psychomotor skills, previous learning, and attitudes influence his approach to learning. Whether content needs to be presented in simple, concrete terms or in depth partly depends on a client's cognitive skills.

Health care providers need to take care not to stereotype a person because of his occupation or educational background. A physician who is ill may need just as much diet instruction as a plumber does. If the plumber is an avid reader who has read reliable books about food and nutrition, he may even be better informed about certain aspects of diet than some health professionals are. However, because there is much misinformation about food and nutrition in books and in the media, it is desirable to find out if the client has acquired misconceptions which may interfere with his learning.

Clients who have a low sense of self-esteem or who have a history of failure in learning situations are likely to underestimate their ability to learn; they may express negative attitudes toward learning. It is particularly important for these clients to be presented with learning tasks with which they can be successful. Differences in people's innate ability to learn may be masked by factors such as motivation to learn and state of mental and physical health.

Cultural beliefs concerning health and diet are likely to influence a client's willingness to learn. A health professional will encounter many persons who regard nutrition instruction as advice which they can choose to follow or disregard. If nutrition "advice" conflicts with a person's cultural beliefs about food and health, he is likely to ignore the advice.[2] To work effectively with clients of different cultural backgrounds, health professionals need to become familiar with and build on a client's folk beliefs concerning diet and health. Since some food beliefs are highly individual, health professionals should try to discuss beliefs about food with each client. It may be helpful to review Chapter 6, pp. 57–63 to identify pertinent topics to discuss.

Some individuals who have limited resources and opportunities may require special consideration if a nutrition education program for them is to be successful. A few people because of their previous experiences and backgrounds are suspicious of health care workers and sometimes question health care workers' motives in offering help. These people may feel that they have little control over most aspects of their lives. They may see their lives as being controlled by others, by God, or by evil spirits. Some of these individuals feel that they are powerless to improve their present condition.[3]

POINTS OF EMPHASIS
Assessing a learner's needs

• Review the assessment of a client's nutritional status to identify a client's potential needs for nutrition education.

• Determine whether the client recognizes his need for learning.

• Identify and deal with learning characteristics which influence a client's ability to learn.

• Plan teaching sessions for times when the client is mentally and physically ready to learn.

• Build on the client's background and previous learning.

Following guidelines such as those suggested here may increase the likelihood of success in working with clients who exhibit these characteristics.

1. Establish a meaningful relationship with the client on a one-to-one basis.
2. Assist a client to deal with the realities of his life and to identify and confront aspects of his life and food behavior which cannot be altered (i.e., economic limitations).
3. Provide emotional assistance. Help the client channel his emotional energy in a constructive manner.

4. Determine areas where changes in food behavior are desirable and can be made.
5. Help a client see how knowledge can give him control over certain aspects of his life.
6. Attempt to provide information to dispel dangerous or self-defeating misconceptions.
7. Encourage the client to help health care workers understand his language (e.g., street talk). In turn, assist the client to learn to use appropriate medical terms as a means of obtaining better health care.

ESTABLISHING EDUCATIONAL GOALS AND WRITING BEHAVIORAL OBJECTIVES

Once the teacher has identified the learner's needs, she and the client mutually establish goals for learning. To facilitate planning, goals are then broken down into behavioral objectives. Jones and Ortel give specific guidelines for developing teaching objectives.[4]

A client's input helps to keep objectives on target. The client's verbal and nonverbal communication can alert the health professional to potential problems (e.g., that the client is overwhelmed by the amount he needs to know or that some of the objectives are irrelevant to his lifestyle).

Objectives are useful for planning teaching strategies when they describe the expected outcomes of teaching and methods for evaluating the learner's progress. Since learning is often a gradual process, objectives may be most realistic and achievable if they specify small changes in behavior.

MOTIVATING A CLIENT AND FACILITATING BEHAVIORAL CHANGE

The importance of client motivation to the success of a nutrition education program should not be underestimated. Even if a person is not resistant to a recommended change, he usually needs to have someone encourage him to value the change enough to take constructive action.[5] A primary goal of nutrition education is to motivate a client to assume positive and responsible attitudes toward establishing sound eating habits and toward necessary diet modifications. Throughout her encounters with a client, the health professional can interact with him in ways which will help him to achieve this goal. The diet counselor knows that specific instructions for actions are also a means of facilitating behavioral change and that these must be compatible with the client's life situation.[6]

A health professional who establishes a trustful, positive relationship with a client has taken a big step toward motivating him to make and maintain necessary changes. When introducing the concept of dietary change, the health professional takes care not to give the impression that the client's past or present dietary habits are bad; rather, the health professional might suggest that certain changes in the client's dietary habits would be beneficial to him at this time.

Health professionals try to increase a client's motivation by identifying reasons why a change in food-related behavior would be desirable. To be effective, the explanation must be presented in terms the client can understand, must be related to his state of well-being, and must fit with his lifestyle. Most nutrition education is directed toward clients who do not experience any immediate distress as a result of their food behavior. Their decision to adopt improved nutritional practices is influenced by cost, effort required, the existence of competing problems, and by what they perceive to be the benefits of taking the recommended action.[7]

When the need for diet change is explained, some clients become afraid. This might be signaled by excessive laughter during a diet counseling session. Too many changes at one time are difficult for a client to accept and handle. Providing stability amidst change helps reassure a client and may increase his willingness to adopt a change.

Stability can be provided in many ways. If one health professional consistently provides counseling for a client, the client is likely to feel more secure than if several persons are all providing instruction one after another. When the expertise of more than one professional is needed, stability can be achieved by having one person coordinate the teaching program. The client should know that he can feel free to contact the coordinator if any problems arise. Keeping the time, place, and length of teaching sessions consistent increases a client's security. The health professional who does what she says she is going to do for or with a client reassures the client, helps him to feel that someone really cares about him, and reinforces a positive sense of self-worth.

Diet counselors may guide clients to think of themselves in positive rather than negative terms. They might, for example, focus on how change will increase the client's assets. This type of help cannot be provided in one brief teaching session. Follow-up is essential. Sometimes referral to a social worker or family therapist is desirable.

Positive experiences encourage a client to develop favorable attitudes and responses. Providing learning experiences with which a client can be successful early in his educational program may encourage him to continue learning.

A diet counselor helps clients have realistic expectations. For example, she lets a client know that lowering his intake of saturated fat will not make him feel better physically but that it should lower his blood cholesterol level and reduce his risk of heart disease. Then she makes sure that he knows when laboratory tests indicate that his cholesterol level has actually fallen.

If there is a need for a change in food-related behavior but the need is not urgent, a diet counselor who is familiar with a client's eating habits may initially suggest one small change which she thinks the client can successfully make. For example, she might see if a mother would be willing to feed her anemic child a bowl of iron-fortified cereal rather than a donut in the morning.

New habits can be designed to fit with current food practices and with economic, social, and physical influences on the client's life in order to successfully change food behaviors. For example, if the client's work requires him to eat out frequently, diet modifications should include suggestions for restaurant dining. It is appropriate for a health professional to help a client who has a low income to obtain financial or food assistance before suggesting changes that impose an additional economic hardship. If certain foods are to be eliminated or restricted, it is desirable to help the client find acceptable substitutes. It is often better to emphasize foods which are *recommended* rather than to list all the things a client "should not" eat.

Some clients are not able or willing to make radical changes in their food practices. Individuals who are rigid in their behavior may fall into this category. Recommendations for these clients might be tailored toward progressive revisions in food behaviors. A client who is unable to give up certain foods may be agreeable to trying to decrease the amounts eaten. A person who insists on letting cooked meat cool completely before refrigerating it may be willing to cut the meat into smaller pieces so that it will cool within a safe period of time. Some persons, however, may prefer to take a chance that they will not be harmed, or they may prefer to suffer ill effects of a poor food practice rather than change their ways. Health professionals who respect their clients allow them the opportunity to decide whether or not to follow recommendations to improve their nutritional and health status. They try to present facts so that clients will make an informed decision. Some clients choose to ignore the health professional's recommendations, even when the consequences are life threatening. These clients still deserve to be treated considerately and in a nonjudgmental manner.

Most clients can make changes in their food behavior in a structured setting where they receive frequent support and guidance. However, when the support and guidance are removed, some clients have a tendency to revert back to their old food habits. These individuals are more successful in achieving desired changes in food behavior if follow-up (reinforcement) instruction and guidance are provided for them. During follow-up they may more fully internalize goals, find answers to previously unanticipated questions, and have help in making the recommended behaviors become automatic. Clients also benefit from having the phone number of a diet counselor they can call for answers to their immediate questions.

When a client receives nutrition or diet instruction in a health agency, it is advisable to remember that the client's life in an agency is not identical to his life at home. Since food usually is provided on a tray ready-to-eat, clients do not always think about where it is coming from, how it is prepared, or how much they are

POINTS OF EMPHASIS
Motivating a client to learn

- *Establish a trustful, positive relationship with the client.*
- *Generate a sense of self-esteem and quiet enthusiasm.*
- *Help the client clearly identify the benefits of changing his food behaviors.*
- *Focus attention on the client's assets and abilities.*
- *Develop realistic expectations for change which are compatible with the client's lifestyle.*
- *Consider and deal with personal, social, cultural, and economic factors which may limit a client's ability to adopt recommended changes.*
- *Assist the client to find acceptable substitutes for food which must be eliminated or restricted.*

allowed to eat. To counteract this situation, nurses and other health care workers can make mealtime be a time for brief and pleasant on-the-spot teaching. For example, they can point out portion sizes, cooking methods, and garnishes which make the food more appetizing, and whether or not any dietetic foods were included in the meal.

If a client is feeling well enough, a health professional can help him anticipate food-related situations that may arise when he gets home. One way to do this is to have the client describe a typical day's activities related to food procurement, preparation, and eating.

PLANNING AND IMPLEMENTING A STRATEGY FOR TEACHING

Knowledge of motivational techniques and of other ways to facilitate a change in behavior should help in planning and implementing a strategy for teaching. Among the activities involved in this part of the teaching-learning process are (1) selecting a method for instructing a client, (2) identifying specific content necessary to meet educational objectives, (3) arranging content in a logical, meaningful sequence, (4) considering available teaching aids and selecting those which will enhance the client's learning, (5) establishing an environment which promotes learning, and (6) identifying ways of evaluating learning.

Writing a teaching plan

A written teaching plan provides guidelines for a teacher to follow during a teaching session. It may also facilitate evaluation of the client's learning. Ideally a written plan identifies objectives for learning, content and skills to be mastered by the learner, and degree of proficiency to be achieved. In some instances, it may be helpful if the teacher specifically identifies teaching methods, teaching tools, and methods of evaluation.

Some health agencies have found that standardized teaching plans are particularly useful when there is a consistent body of knowledge which must be imparted to clients. Standard teaching outlines and guides save teachers time in planning. They promote quality assurance because they facilitate consistent teaching by different health professionals and they help guarantee that certain topics and skills are covered in the teaching sessions.

A few teaching plans are set up so that client progress can be recorded right on the plan.[8] An updated teaching plan is useful even if only one person is responsible for teaching. It is easy to forget just how much a client has already accomplished, especially if the teacher is working with more than one client. Whether or not such a form is available in a health agency, the health professional must document nutrition education in the client's medical record.

Selecting a method for instruction

A health professional selects methods of instruction which she is comfortable using and which she thinks will best meet the needs of the clients she serves. When making a selection of teaching methods she also considers the setting, amount of time, and resources available. She considers whether one-to-one sessions, formal classroom teaching, or facilitated group learning will best meet the needs of the clients she serves.

In many situations it is desirable to provide one-to-one instruction in order to tailor the teaching session to meet a client's unique needs. If stimulating programmed instructional material or other interesting self-instructional aids are available, a teacher might give a client an assignment to complete on his own. The success of a self-instructional program depends upon having teaching materials geared to the client's abilities and upon the client's motivation to complete the assignments.

To help clients learn psychomotor skills a health professional may plan to give demonstrations. She may decide to use role playing as a way to help clients learn to deal with new situations. In many cases a combination of teaching strategies is more effective than using a single method. Varying the form of presentation helps to maintain the learner's interest and may serve different purposes.

Identifying specific content

Content included in the educational program helps a client meet the stated behavioral objectives. Subject matter should be relevant to the client's situation. Well thought-out objectives guide the selection of pertinent content. This point is illustrated by the following example:

Ms. S. was to be discharged from a health agency in a few days on a specified modified diet. She was eager to learn but had a short attention span. The dietitian, therefore, implemented a plan which focused on developing useful skills rather than on mastering specific facts. Some of the points she covered are identified here.

Behavioral objective	Teaching strategy and content	Evaluation
The client demonstrates a desire to learn about her modified diets by asking questions about how she can implement it.	Briefly describe positive aspects of the diet.	Does the client ask pertinent questions?
Using the diet form, the client correctly identifies whether her diet allows specified foods.	Describe format of the diet form.	
	Provide practice in finding out whether specified foods are listed in the "allowed" or "avoid" column. (Focus on allowed foods the client uses frequently.)	Does the client use the form correctly? Does the client give correct responses?
(After the above objective is achieved): Using the diet form, the client identifies ways in which she will change her usual lunch in order to correctly follow her diet.	Show client a menu typical of her usual lunch (based on information obtained from previous diet recall and history).	
	Ask client what substitutions she will make to comply with diet guidelines. Suggest alternatives if necessary. Add helpful notes to diet form (which client can keep).	Does client use the form correctly? Does client correctly identify items needing to be changed? Can she find substitutions acceptable to her?
By the end of the session the client states that she is going to attempt to make recommended changes.		What does client state that she will do?

The dietitian did not assume that Ms. S could use the diet form easily. From experience she knew that many clients have trouble figuring out what group a particular food is in. (Is egg with dairy products or meat? Are potatoes with vegetables, bread, or some other group of food?) The dietitian knew that clients, after locating a food on a chart, are still sometimes unsure whether the food is allowed or whether the amount used makes a difference. This skillful diet counselor found out if Ms. S. needed practice with these skills. By careful questioning and prompting, the counselor guided Ms. S. to success without embarrassing her.

Ms. S. was able to meet behavioral objectives in a short period of time and was relieved to find that she would not have to memorize many facts to be able to manage her diet at home at least temporarily. She was reassured by the fact that a follow-up teaching session was scheduled.

Arrangement of content

Competent teachers try to structure content so it can be easily grasped by a learner. This usually means arranging content so that it builds on the knowledge and skills a client already possesses.

Content often is arranged in a sequence from simple to complex and from general to specific. Instruction might begin with a simple description of how the diet will help the client. This might arouse his interest and motivation. An anxious client may need to have specific information about how to do something before being given an explanation of why the activities are important. Hopefully the explanations will reduce his anxiety and show him that the diet will not interfere with his lifestyle as much as he had anticipated. Since content can be arranged in a variety of acceptable formats, health professionals may want to try different sequences and evaluate the outcomes.

It is important when arranging content to consider the length and number of teaching sessions to be carried out. Keeping sessions short (15 to 20 minutes) helps maintain the client's interest. Ideally, only one subject is covered in a learning session. The client learns best if he is given an opportunity to utilize new knowledge or skills during the teaching session. The health professional tries to avoid overwhelming a client with too much information at once. If the teaching session leaves his head spinning, the client may forget almost everything and develop a negative attitude toward the recommended changes. It is better to make arrangements to continue nutrition education in another session than to try to cram everything into one lesson.

Teaching Aids

Effective use of teaching aids requires careful selection and planning. There are many different types of nutrition education materials available for health professionals to use in carrying out a teaching program.

Health agencies usually have a supply of various nutrition education materials. New teaching aids are regularly reviewed in some professional journals such as the *Journal of Nutrition Education*. Diet counselors may obtain a variety of useful inexpensive teaching aids from federal, local, and private health agencies and consumer groups. A list of resources from which nutrition education materials can be obtained is included in Appendix 1.

Once teaching aids have been located they can be evaluated to determine their appropriateness for a particular client. Some health professionals may choose to develop their own teaching aids or to individualize standardized aids.

Generally, teaching aids fall into two categories: printed and nonprinted (audiovisual) materials.

PRINTED MATERIALS

Among the different kinds of printed nutrition education materials are meal plans, exchange lists, booklets, diet teaching sheets, and directions. An advantage of using printed materials is that they relax the time requirement for learning. Some agencies prepare their own printed teaching aids. These aids often incorporate the schedules and procedures used in the agency to promote consistency in teaching a client.

If printed materials are used during a teaching session the diet counselor should make it clear whether or not the client will be able to keep the learning aid either permanently or temporarily. A client who is placed on a modified diet should always be able to take a written diet plan home with him.

Printed materials should be selected with care—some teaching aids may hinder learning; some actually contain dangerous advice. Several points to consider when reviewing printed materials are listed below:

Is the information correct, easy to read, and easy to understand? Nutrition education material is more motivating if it is clearly understood. Simple vocabulary and short, clear sentences are desirable for most clients. Many teaching materials are written at a fairly high reading level.[9] Often clients read at a lower level than their formal education would suggest. Consequently, many materials may not be appropriate for general use. Some materials may contain questionable suggestions or incorrect information such as an out-of-date exchange list.

Is the information presented in an interesting manner which will hold the client's attention? A pleasing format, easy-to-read print and appropriate use of pictures, tables, and figures attract the client's attention.

Does the material consider and show respect for the client's traditional food habits, meal patterns, and lifestyles? Some teaching aids have been specially prepared for use by individuals of various ethnic backgrounds. Aids should be nonjudgmental. A single woman may not appreciate being given a pamphlet on nutrition during pregnancy which focuses attention on a happy husband and wife.

Are themes or subtle messages present which are incompatible with sound nutrition information? For example, many materials on infant feeding prominently show many appealing pictures of mothers bottle feeding their infants. (Even some pamphlets on breast feeding do this!) Other materials have been criticized for subtly pushing a food group or food product.[10]

Does the teaching aid do what it claims to do? For example, does a pamphlet about successful breast feeding for working mothers devote considerable space to listing reasons why it would be better if the mother did not work?

Are foreign language versions available? If a client does not speak English, an attempt should be made to provide material printed in his native tongue. Health agencies which serve a large non-English-speaking population usually have bilingual teaching aids on hand.

AUDIOVISUAL AIDS

Most audiovisual aids (nonprinted materials) use pictures and sound to present educational material. Some may also appeal to the senses of touch, smell, and taste. Health professionals should try to make use of the fact that involving more than one sense (e.g., sight and hearing) improves initial learning and later retention of content.[11] Visual aids include diagrams, charts, objects, still pictures, and moving pictures. These may be used singly or in combination, with or without sound.

> **POINTS OF EMPHASIS**
> *Factors to consider when selecting teaching aids*
>
> • *Correctness of content.*
> • *Logical, understandable presentation of material.*
> • *Appropriateness of values for client.*
> • *Relationship of content to desired objectives.*
> • *Readability and attractiveness of material.*
> • *Cost of material.*
> • *Availability.*

Audiovisual aids should be evaluated before use for both appropriateness and content. For example, people who are quick to learn and rapid readers may prefer printed materials with added notes over some audiovisual aids such as slide-tapes. The slow pace of a tape may make them impatient. The way color is used in visual aids may influence its acceptability for certain cultural groups.[12,13] Many of the points made previously, relating to evaluation of printed material, can be adapted for evaluating audiovisual aids.

APPROACHING THE CLIENT

Establishing a "therapeutic alliance" with the client sets the stage for a productive teaching session. It is desirable for a diet counselor to clarify her role and responsibilities as a teacher and the client's role and responsibilities as a learner. A teacher can use several techniques such as those which follow to enhance learning:

1. Clarify goals at the beginning of the session.
2. Start instruction in a positive manner.
3. Approach client in a competent, quietly enthusiastic manner.
4. Keep the session client-centered.
5. Focus on the topic to be covered:
   a. Ask the client his opinion about specific content and recommendations.
   b. Encourage the client to practice new skills during the session.
   c. Watch for cues which signal confusion, disinterest, or denial of the need to learn.
6. Adjust teaching approach as the need arises.
7. Find out if the client understands what he is being told by tactfully asking specific questions (not "Do you understand?").
8. Give honest, sincere praise for successes; avoid focusing on errors since that might encourage further errors.

Evaluation of learning

When evaluating a client it is helpful to consider the following points: Has the client's knowledge of a subject changed? Has the client developed any new skills? Does the client express new values or attitudes? Has the client demonstrated ability to apply knowledge?

In a health care agency, evaluation is often informal, perhaps including verbal fedback, observations of changes in a client's behavior, or a client's report about his behavior. A return demonstration is a more formal method of evaluation that should be used to determine if a client has mastered a psychomotor skill. For example, after discussing and demonstrating how to prepare sterile infant formula, a nurse might ask a client to "return the demonstration" by preparing sterile formula. Many clients find formal pencil and paper tests to be threatening. If they are given, they should be designed so that the client can be reasonably successful and feel a sense of accomplishment.

Attitudes are difficult to measure. They may be identified to some degree by observing a client's behavior and his apparent willingness to accept and follow dietary recommendations. Some possible indications that the client's attitude toward diet and nutrition is improving are when he (1) begins to ask questions about his diet, (2) reads a nutrition booklet, (3) agrees to try to follow guidelines at least until the follow-up visit, (4) asks a relative to purchase some appropriate food items, or (5) tells the client in the next bed about what he learned.

Health professionals working in health care facilities must document nutrition education activities in the client's medical record. This information is of most use to others if it includes the following:

S. Client's attitude toward learning.
O. Content covered (e.g., name of modified diet taught, materials given to the client such as names of diet forms and other handouts, particular areas emphasized).
A. Client's response (e.g., ability to answer questions or perform tasks correctly; apparent changes in attitude; need for follow-up).
P. Content to be reinforced, new content to be introduced, and date for follow-up instruction.

Follow-up teaching

After evaluating a client's progress it is highly desirable to plan for follow-up instruction and reinforcement of learning. If a client's knowledge or skills are weak in an area, the material can be presented again. Changing the approach may stimulate the client's interest. Direct contact with the health professional also gives the client an opportunity to ask questions, seek reassurance, and listen to new suggestions related to his nutrition or diet problem. Even clients who have successfully completed a nutrition education program need occasional reinforcement to assure that they retain and correctly utilize newly acquired knowledge and skills. The nurse is often in an excellent position to provide follow-up teaching and reinforcement.

In some situations, visiting the client in his home or calling him may increase his willingness and ability to make recommended modifications in food behavior. Direct contact with the health professional may give him a sense that someone really cares about him and, thus, may help him to feel that it is worthwhile to take care of himself.[14]

Teaching children

Teaching children includes all the steps used in teaching adults, but there are additional points to be considered. The approach to teaching and the content covered are determined with a child's level of cognitive and psychomotor development in mind. (Information about normal child development and how a child learns can be obtained from growth and development texts such as *Childhood and Adolescence: A Psychology of the Growing Person.*[15])

Since children develop at different rates, whenever possible it is wise to assess an individual child's stage of development before teaching plans are detailed. Teaching should be adjusted for a child's dependency needs, his lack of experience, and the developmental tasks he is currently facing. Since children have not developed many ingrained habits, they may learn more quickly and more easily than some adults do. Children often adapt to changes readily. They react positively to a cheerful, enthusiastic approach.

Children usually respond well when they are given opportunities to learn by playing games, painting or using coloring books, reading stories and cartoons, using puppets, handling and tasting food, and by just playing. Since activities of daily living become habits during childhood, health professionals have a special responsibility to help teach children sound eating and health-promoting behaviors.

STUDY QUESTIONS

1. While teaching Ms. T. about her diet, you notice that she is looking around the room and fidgeting. She is scheduled to be discharged to home tomorrow. Discuss constructive actions you might take.
2. Suggest techniques which would help a person who is hard-of-hearing to learn how to follow a diet.
3. While the nurse is helping Mr. A with morning care, he comments that he doesn't understand why health care workers keep telling him that it is important for him to eat his meals. Mr. A states that he thinks he could stand to lose a little weight anyway. What action(s) would it be desirable for the nurse to take?
4. Outline a plan to teach a 10-year-old girl how to increase her intake of vitamin C. Assume that her parents are willing to cooperate and that the girl makes her own lunch.
5. Why is it often desirable to include family members in diet counseling sessions?

References

*1. White, P.: Why all the fuss over nutrition education? *J. Nutr. Ed.* 8:54, 1976.

*2. Snow, L. F., and Johnson, S. M.: Folk lore, food and female reproductive cycle. *Ecol. Food Nutrition,* 7(1):41, 1978.

*3. Suren, J.: Education of the culturally and educationally deprived diabetic. *Nurs. Clin. North Am.* 12(3): 427, 1977.

*4. Jones, P., and Ortel, W.: Developing patient teaching objectives and techniques: A self-instructional program. *Nurs. Ed.* 2(5):3, 1977.

5. Becker, M. H., and Maiman, L. A.: Sociobehavioral determinants of compliance with health and medical care recommendations. *Medical Care* 13:10, 1975.

6. Leventhal, H.: Fear appeals and persuasion: The differentiation of a motivational construct. *Am. J. Public Health* 61:1208, 1971.

7. Kirscht, J. P., Becker, M. H., and Eveland, J. P.: Psychological and social factors as predictors of medical behavior. *Medical Care* 14:422, 1976.

*8. Jones, P.: Patient education—Yes-No. *Supervisor Nurse* 8(5):35, 1977.

*9. Redman, B.: Curriculum in patient education. *Am. J. Nurs.* 78:1363, 1978.

10. ———. The (Nutrition Education) gospel according to NDC. *Nutr. Action* 5(9):3, 1978.

*11. Murray, R., and Zentner, J.: Guidelines for more effective health teaching. *Nursing '76* 6(2):44, 1976.

*12. Redman, B.: *The Process of Patient Teaching in Nursing.* St. Louis: C. V. Mosby Co., 1976.

*13. Kniep-Hardy, M., and Burkhardt, M. A.: Nursing the Navajo. *Am. J. Nurs.* 77:95, 1977.

*14. Winter, J., and Lutz, S.: Cardiac-patient care with heart. *RN* 39(6):45, 1976.

*15. Stone, L. J., and Church, J.: *Childhood and Adolescence: A Psychology of the Growing Person.* New York: Random House, 1973.

*Recommended reading

24

Nutritional care for a client in a health agency

The process of providing nutritional care (assessment, planning, implementation, and evaluation) is similar in most types of health agencies and for most clients. However, details of providing care differ widely from situation to situation, as in a large teaching hospital versus a small nursing home. This chapter deals with providing general types of nutritional care to persons who are residing temporarily or permanently in health agencies.

NUTRITIONAL CARE SERVICES

The focus of nutritional care in health agencies is on providing clients with appropriate kinds and amounts of food (and/or nutrients) and, when possible, on preparing clients to return to the community with satisfactory food behaviors.

Since the severity and frequency of iatrogenic malnutrition (that is, malnutrition resulting from acts or omissions of health care providers) has been recognized, health professionals are directing more attention toward maintaining or improving the nutritional status of their clients. Providing for the client's nutritional health is the mutual responsibility of physicians, dietitians, and nurses. In most health agencies dietitians and the dietary department play a leading role in assuring that quality nutritional care is provided.

Some of the functions of the dietary department include planning regular and modified diets, assessing nutritional needs of clients, and providing individualized nutritional care and counseling.

In small health care agencies such as skilled nursing homes the nursing staff may need to assume much of the responsibility for nutritional care. Small agencies may hire a dietitian on a part-time basis or as a consultant to assist with and approve menu plans, identify clients' nutrient needs, develop nutritional care plans, and provide diet counseling.

Facilities receiving Medicare or Medicaid payments must meet specific requirements with regard to the nutrition services they provide. These requirements motivate participating agencies to provide high quality nutritional care. In certified facilities dietitians meet with clients intermittently to assess their nutritional needs and plan their nutritional care. Health care workers are required to record a client's acceptance and intake of food.

Because a dietitian is only available part of the time in many small agencies, other health care workers must plan carefully to make the best use of her services when she is present. They must also fully understand how to identify problems which should receive the dietitian's attention and how to deliver satisfactory nutritional care in her absence.

In marked contrast to small nursing homes, large teaching hospitals and medical centers are likely to have a multidisciplinary nutritional support service whose function is to serve clients who have special nutritional needs. The goals of a nutritional support service include: (1) monitoring the nutritional status of all clients in a health agency, (2) consulting, (3) supervising the implementation of nutritional support in selected clients, and (4) providing a multidisciplinary approach to nutritional care.[1] Nurses, dietitians, and physicians consult with the nutritional support team when they suspect a client has a serious nutritional problem or when they need assistance handling a client's nutrition-related needs. A protocol may describe the services a nutritional support team provides and criteria used as a basis of determining if the services of the team should be requested.

Health professionals who assist in providing nutritional care should identify who manages the dietary and/or food service departments within the agency. Health care workers need to be familiar with their own responsibilities for meeting clients' nutritional needs and with proper channels of communication to use if a food or food service-related problem arises. It is helpful to know, for example, if the food service administrator is a dietitian or a person who has little educational background in nutrition. Identifying methods of communication is especially important when an outside food service or catering company manages the health facility's food service department. Even if a dietitian is available only on a consultant basis, there should be an efficient method for communicating that problems in food preparation or service are interfering with clients' nutritional care. It is equally important to communicate that a change in food or food service has had a beneficial effect and should be continued.

FOOD DELIVERY SYSTEM

Health care workers need to be familiar with the type of food delivery system in the agency where they work since it affects their food-related responsibilities. A food service system is either centralized or decentralized. With a centralized system a client's food is assembled on a tray in or near the food production area. With a decentralized system food is prepared in large quantities in a central area. Then the prepared food is transported in bulk from the production area to a service kitchen near the client. The client's tray is assembled in the service area.

Both systems require nursing and dietary personnel to coordinate schedules so that clients receive appetizing, attractively served food. Both types also allow for individualized food service, but the manner of achieving this goal is different. For example, if food service is decentralized, a pediatric nurse who knows a child's current appetite and food preferences can assist with assembling a tray to suit the particular child. If service is centralized the nurse must accurately communicate the child's food needs to the food service department in time for changes to be implemented.

Small service kitchens or nourishment centers are located near clients' rooms in many health agencies. These are stocked with foods and beverages for between-meal feedings (often referred to as nourishments) and light meals. Some agencies which have a centralized system for regularly scheduled meals deliver nourishments and late meals to clients from the central kitchen. A few items might be routinely sent via carts to the client area; others must be specially requested. Advance planning helps assure delivery of satisfactory nutritional care when food is not readily available in the client area. Competent health professionals identify the kind of food delivery system a health agency utilizes, who is responsible for delivering meals and nourishments to clients, and what their own role should be in facilitating efficient operation of the system.

MEAL SERVICE PATTERNS

Health professionals who are familiar with a health agency's meal service and nourishment schedule can plan client care with this knowledge in mind. Many agencies serve three meals a day; they may also provide nourishments or snacks between meals as needed or desired by clients.

Recently some agencies have adopted a pattern of serving either four or five meals a day. A four-meal-a-day pattern might be as follows:

    7:00 am light meal (i.e., hot beverage, toast)
    10:30 am brunch
    3:30 pm dinner
    8:00 pm light meal

Agencies using a four- or five-meal schedule have reported that both clients and nurses like the plan and see it as beneficial.[2,3] There were at least three distinct advantages of four- to five-meal patterns: (1) clients were less likely to miss their main morning meal owing to diagnostic tests, (2) clients rested better in the morning, and (3) some clients tolerated small frequent meals better than larger, less frequent meals.

BETWEEN-MEAL NOURISHMENTS AND DIETARY SUPPLEMENTS

Many health agencies offer clients between-meal nourishments and commercial food supplements. These may benefit clients by (1) increasing total nutrient intake; (2) providing extra protein, calories, fluid, and/or micronutrients; and (3) distributing food intake among several small feedings to improve a client's tolerance of food.

Commercial supplements are often used to increase the amount of nutrients and/or calories a client ingests without greatly increasing the volume of food he is asked to consume. Commercial supplements come in many forms and vary widely in energy and nutrient density, palatability, and cost. A dietitian can be of assistance in determining which clients would benefit from use of commercial supplements and which would benefit from between-meal feedings of more traditional foods. For example, some clients might prefer to have a milk shake plus a separate vitamin-mineral supplement instead of a commercial supplement which carries the taste of added micronutrients. Bayless reported that patients accepted nutritional supplements better if they were offered a "taste tray" of suitable nourishments and allowed to select supplements they preferred.[4] Since concentrated or frequent feedings may dull a client's appetite for regular meals, health team members may want to consult with the dietitian about what amount of mealtime food consumption is realistic for a client who is receiving supplements.

NUTRITIVE SUPPLEMENTS GIVEN AS MEDICATION

Nutritive supplements ordered through the pharmacy are usually administered by the nursing staff. These supplements include vitamins, minerals, and intravenous feedings. Sometimes they also include predigested protein concentrates or special oils. If pancreatic enzyme extracts are needed to aid a client's digestion, it is important that the nurse who is responsible for the client's care check to see that the client gets the extract *with* his meals.

Health care workers should determine if maintenance or therapeutic doses of nutrients are being given. Maintenance doses approximately equal the Recommended Dietary Allowances (RDA, see inside back cover). When poorly absorbed nutrients are administered *parenterally* (i.e., by injection), the daily maintenance doses is much lower than the RDA. This is true for minerals (divalent cations) such as iron, calcium, and zinc, and for vitamin B_{12}. Therapeutic doses are at least several times higher than Recommended Dietary Allowances. Since therapeutic doses of some micronutrients carry danger of toxicity if given for a prolonged period of time, steps should be taken to avoid having this occur accidentally.

POINTS OF EMPHASIS
Health agency food services with which health professionals participating in nutritional care need to be familiar

- *The functions of the agency's dietary department.*
- *The agency's food delivery system.*
- *Meal service patterns.*
- *System for between-meal nourishments and for nutrients provided in the form of medicines.*
- *Channels of communication among various health care workers, the dietary and food service departments, and the nutritional support team.*

RESOURCE MATERIALS

Most health agencies have a variety of resources for health professionals to use in planning and providing nutritional care for clients. Resources commonly found in health agencies include diet manuals, diet charts, diet plans, exchange lists, reference texts, and professional journals.

DIET MANUALS

Diet manuals contain practical information about normal and modified diets. Some agency manuals reflect the values and beliefs of a particular health agency or of the people who wrote it. Diet manuals written by an agency's own health professionals generally include information about an institution's food policies such as times and routines in serving regular meals for different age groups, normal portion sizes for different age groups, methods of making diet changes, and procedures for obtaining supplementary and special feedings. If the approved diet manual was developed by another agency or group, food policies may not be stated or may not be applicable. In this case a supplementary set of policies should be provided by the food service or dietary department to facilitate coordination of quality nutritional care.

Diet manuals vary somewhat in their general format and in the specific information they contain. Some of the differences are due to variations in interpretation of theory about diet modifications. Other differences reflect cultural and regional food preferences. A large part of most manuals is directed toward assisting health professionals to implement modified diets. Manuals usually identify conditions for which a modification might be ordered; rationale for the modification; kinds and amounts of foods recommended; listings of foods allowed, restricted, and avoided; explanatory notes about how foods are grouped and comments regarding nutritional adequacy of the diet. Diet manuals are not designed to be used directly for instructing clients about their diets.

Since more than one diet manual may be available in a health care facility, a health professional needs to determine which one, if any, has been approved for use there. (Facilities participating in Medicare must have an up-to-date diet manual approved for use by both the medical and dietary staffs.) Use of the approved manual facilitates consistency in delivery of nutritional care and helps prevent confusion and misunderstanding.

DIET PLANS AND EXCHANGE LISTS

Diet plans and exchange lists are tools which simplify meal planning for both health professionals and clients. They provide easy-to-use information about the kinds and amounts of foods allowed on a specific diet. By using diet plans and exchange lists, health professionals can assist clients to stay within the limits of their diet and still achieve variety and nutritional adequacy using foods they enjoy. A diet plan provides a framework for a diet, helping the health care worker and client to know how many servings of different food groups are recommended each day and how to distribute food among the day's meals. Diet plans usually include lists of allowed and restricted foods. Depending on the reason for the diet modification these guidelines may be very specifically stated or may allow for considerable flexibility.

Guidelines can be individualized to fit a client's special needs. For example, if the plan's usual breakfast pattern would make the client nauseous, the plan might be rearranged to include a light breakfast and a nourishing midmorning snack.

An exchange system is often used in conjunction with a diet plan. An exchange group is a listing of measured foods which are comparable in certain respects. Depending on the diet, foods might be grouped to be similar in sodium content, fat content, or content of other nutrients or calories. Any food in an exchange group can be traded or "swapped" for any other food in that *same* group, as long as the specified amount is used. Thus a health professional can use the appropriate exchange list to make substitutions when a client is dissatisfied with part of his meal. She can also show a client how to do this and encourage the client to practice using the exchange list. This may increase the independence of a permanent resident and may help prepare a temporary resident for discharge.

One of the most widely used exchange lists is the one published jointly by the American Diabetes Association and the American Dietetic Association (Appendix 5I). Each exchange group contains foods which have about the same amount of protein, fat, carbohydrate, and energy if the indicated portion size is used. The lists can be used for planning low calorie, diabetic, and fat controlled diets.

Some clients seem to have difficulty with the concept of exchanges but learn quickly if the term "choices" is used instead. For example, the client might be told that his diet allows him to have any three choices from a specified listing of foods (exchange group).

General diet plans and exchange lists may be found in diet manuals. Sometimes this information is also printed on single sheets of paper for use in teaching clients about their diet modifications. The dietitian can advise other health professionals and clients about what changes can be made in general diet plans without interfering with the therapeutic effect of the modified diet.

When a health professional refers to a general diet plan in a diet manual to identify what foods to offer a client between meals, it is important for her to remember that the number of servings of some allowed foods is carefully controlled and that the dietitian plans the client's meals to include the appropriate amounts. If a client seems dissatisfied with a specified selection of nourishments, contacting the dietitian is recommended. The dietitian can usually plan modified diets to include a wide variety of snack foods. Consultation with the dietitian is particularly beneficial to a client's welfare if he has high caloric requirements but many food restrictions.

PROVIDING GENERAL NUTRITIONAL CARE

Diet orders

In an agency setting some kind of diet must be prescribed for each client in residence. If the facility is a client's permanent home, nutritional care and teach-ing are oriented toward promoting client adjustment to and satisfaction with the food choices provided while allowing him to maintain a sense of independence. If the client is eventually going home, some nutritional care activities are oriented toward preparing him for discharge. Adequate preparation for discharge is particularly desirable for a client who will be following a modified diet at home or who needs to improve the nutritional adequacy of his diet. When a client is familiar with his diet modification and knows *how to* carry it out, the transition from hospital to home is easier.

ASSISTING WITH MENU SELECTION

Many agencies offer a daily menu plan from which a client can select his meals. Clients who have vision problems or difficulty reading or writing require assistance to fill out their menus. An agency which has a selective menu should have routine procedures for assisting clients as necessary with menu selections and for checking the clients' selections for a reasonable degree of nutritional adequacy. Some clients make menu selections which regularly result in low nutrient intake. Occasionally clients check off everything on a selective menu, e.g., two main dishes, three vegetables, soup, salad, roll, and two desserts. A meal such as that contains many more calories than most clients need. Clients who select either too little or too much food or who make unsuitable food selections should receive some guidance.

Health team members need to know who is responsible for assisting clients with menu selection. (Arrangements vary in different health agencies and this important nutritional care measure can be easily overlooked.)

If a nurse or other health professional notices a problem with a client's acceptance of food or overall intake, she should take measures to identify the source of the problem and to deal with it. Some problems may be related to the menu or to procedures used for menu selection.

POINTS OF EMPHASIS

Assisting clients to make appropriate menu selections

• *Determine whether or not clients need assistance to fill out menus.*

• *Check menu selections for reasonable nutritional adequacy.*

• *Help clients anticipate changes in appetite and physical status when making food selections for the next day.*

• *Help clients who are on modified diets to select foods which fit their diet prescription.*

• *Ask the appropriate person in the dietary department to suggest acceptable substitutes if no foods on the menu appeal to a client.*

A selective menu can be used as a teaching aid. After a client has been given information about selecting well-balanced meals appropriate for his diet, menu selection gives him an opportunity to use his new knowledge. Health professionals can evaluate the client's willingness and ability to follow diet guidelines.

If the client is on a modified diet he may or may not be allowed to select his own menu. Some clients are given a selective menu only to find that some of their selections are missing or replaced by other foods. This can be a very frustrating experience. Clients who are on modified diets should have competent health care workers assisting them to choose foods. Explaining which foods are allowed and which foods are restricted and why helps a client learn about his modified diet.

Promoting food intake

When a client receives his tray the food on it should be checked against his diet order, with the selective menu which is usually on the tray, and with the client himself. Usually the person who delivers the tray is responsible for these activities. If not, then the responsibility should be clearly delegated to a specific health care worker.

A client who is in pleasant surroundings and is ready for a meal is more likely to eat well than one who is not. Nursing responsibilities usually include preparing clients for meals and, if necessary, either assisting them with eating or feeding them. If a nurse is not responsible for delivering the tray, channels of communication between dietary and nursing need to be maintained so that the client is ready for his meal when it arrives and he gets assistance if he needs it.

PROVIDING AN ENVIRONMENT CONDUCIVE TO EATING

Many aspects of the environment can be controlled or modified to provide an environment conducive to eating. The spacing of meals, the physical surroundings, the activities occurring at mealtime, and persons present at mealtime all have an impact on how well or how poorly a client eats.

Spacing meals Regular meals contribute to a client's sense of time and its passage. Scheduled meals or feedings may help orient some clients to time and place. This is often an important element in the care of elderly persons in nursing homes or of disoriented clients in intensive care units and elsewhere. An established meal pattern contributes to a client's sense of security.

On the other hand, judiciously providing food for a client when he is hungry, even if it is not a scheduled feeding time, helps assure adequate food intake. It is often possible for a health care worker to fix a nutritious snack for a client in the middle of the night when the client is hungry rather than making him wait several hours until the next scheduled meal.

Creating a pleasant environment The health care worker who carries out some or all of the following measures helps create a pleasant atmosphere for eating:

1. Provide a dining room setting when possible.
2. Involve permanent or long term residents in activities to make the setting cheerful and homelike.
3. Remove any clutter (especially bedpans, urinals, and basins) from the area where clients are eating.
4. Provide adequate lighting and ventilation; maintain a comfortable room temperature.
5. Try to keep the area free from offensive odors and noise.
6. Set table and tray attractively.
7. Arrange utensils and food so client can reach them easily.
8. Take steps to ensure that the food served is fresh and is at the proper temperature.
9. Provide an adequate amount of time for meals; take steps to keep mealtime free from interruptions.
10. Encourage a client to have visitors or to eat with other clients if company makes a favorable impact on food intake.
11. Greet clients in a warm, unrushed manner when delivering their food.

Conditions motivating a client to eat and favoring digestion Adequate nutrition may mean the difference between a speedy recovery and a prolonged illness and hospital stay. Many clients with poor appetites will eat if health professionals take the time and have the patience and creativity to encourage them to do so. Some conditions which help improve a client's appetite are the following: (1) adequate rest, (2) moderate physical activity, (3) relief from pain and discomfort, (4) avoidance of unpleasant treatments preceding or following meals, (5) use of bedpan or urinal before meals, (6) opportunity to wash face and hands and brush teeth or rinse mouth before eating, (7) awakening long enough before eating to be alert and oriented, (8) clean dentures and eyeglasses, (9) comfortable sitting position, (10) appropriately sized portions of attractively served food, (11) foods without strong odors, and (12) catering (within reason) to a client's appetite whims.

Assisting a client to eat

Most individuals prefer to feed themselves if possible. Even when a client appears to be quite ill or handicapped, health professionals should determine whether or not the client actually needs assistance. Allowing an ill or handicapped person to do as much for himself as he can contributes to his sense of independence and self-esteem. Providing unnecessary assistance may offend a person or it may nudge him into a dependent role. If a client needs help to eat it is important for health professionals to determine how to provide it while encouraging maximum client participation in the process.

Occasionally health professionals do not recognize all of a client's capabilities. Persons who have been handicapped even for just a short period of time may be very self-sufficient. Blind clients, for example, can often feed themselves satisfactorily once they know where food, drink, and utensils are placed. Relating placement of food on a plate to the numbers on a clock can be helpful. Handicapped persons may have a special way to have their food and utensils arranged. They may have assistive devices which make it easier for them to feed themselves. It saves time and frustration if the handicapped person is asked how he would like his tray arranged. Clients who are slow, clumsy, or messy should be allowed ample time for meals. A towel under the chin can catch spills and save cleanup time. Steps can be taken to minimize the chance of accidents. For example, if a client's movements are unsteady, it might be appropriate to remove hot coffee from his tray, allow it to cool to a safe temperature, and serve it in a half-full mug rather than a cup.

The type of food served may affect clients' ability to feed themselves. Watery soups, flavored gelatin, and baked custard slip off spoons easily, frustrate a client, and stop him from attempting to feed himself. Firmer foods such as thick cream soup, mashed squash, ground meat, sandwiches cut into small pieces, or other finger foods are easier for a client to handle. However, even foods which end up being messy should be provided if a client prefers them and they are compatible with his diet order.

Persons who are temporarily handicapped may be eager to hear suggestions for ways they can help themselves. Individuals who have an intravenous infusion in an arm or an arm in a sling can often feed themselves if food is cut into bite-sized pieces and containers are opened for them. Occasionally individuals leave food untouched rather than ask for help. Persons who have recently become handicapped and very ill persons require extra support and assistance, but persons who have been allowed to become unnecessarily dependent on others need to be motivated to accept more responsibility for their own care.

Health care workers who are concerned about rehabilitating clients can initiate a self-feeding program. Several factors might be considered when encouraging self-feeding, including alteration of diet (e.g., from puree to soft), providing adequate time to eat, offering foods which are easy for a client to handle and do not require too much energy to eat, proper encouragement of clients, and sincere compliments when clients show even small signs of progress.[5] Elderly should be treated like adults even if they exhibit some childlike behaviors.

FEEDING CLIENTS

When it is necessary to feed a client the health care worker should plan her schedule to allow adequate time for the client to eat in a relaxed, unhurried manner. The client who is sitting comfortably with his tray in front of him feels like he is participating in the meal. The sight and smell of food stimulate the flow of digestive juices. The health professional who talks with a client before feeding him to identify his perferences and who observes the client while he is eating can easily determine what he might like next and the most satisfactory rate of feeding. During the feeding the health care worker can also observe the client to determine whether or not the feeding process is comfortable for the client (e.g., size of bites, placement of utensils when offering food, and temperature of food.) Care must be taken to avoid choking the client or causing him to aspirate food (suck food into his lungs rather than into his stomach). For this reason persons who are unconscious or who do not have a swallowing and gag reflex are not fed orally. Talking with the client while feeding him makes mealtime more pleasant and conveys to a client that he need not feel rushed. Trying to avoid spills and wiping the client's mouth contribute to his comfort.

If an inexperienced person (e.g., a volunteer, friend, or relative) assumes the task of feeding a client, the health professional has a responsibility to tactfully instruct the inexperienced person in safe feeding techniques which are appropriate for the client.

PROMOTING ADEQUATE FLUID INTAKE

Thirst usually regulates a healthy person's fluid intake and assists him to maintain proper fluid and electrolyte balance. However, ill or injured persons may not drink enough fluid unless measures are taken to promote fluid intake. Some individuals may be used to

TABLE 24.1 *Caffeine content of some beverages, foods, and medications*

BEVERAGE OR FOOD	MG CAFFEINE
Brewed coffee	100–150/180 ml (6 oz)
Instant coffee	64/180 ml
Tea made using package directions	24–45/180 ml
Weak tea	18–48/180 ml
Strong tea	70–107/180 ml
Instant tea	Mean 55/180 ml
Instant iced tea	Mean 72/180 ml
Decaffeinated coffee	3/180 ml
Cola	32–72/360 ml (12 oz)
Cocoa	Mean 60/180 ml
Milk chocolate candy	3/30 gm
MEDICATIONS	*MG/TABLET*
APCs (aspirin, phenacetin, and caffeine)*	32
Darvon compound	32
Fiorinal	40
Migral	50

Source: Stephenson, P.: Physiologic and psychotropic effects of caffeine on man. *J. Am. Diet. Assoc.* 7:240, 1977.
Groisser, D. S.: A study of caffeine in tea. I. A new spectrophotometric micro-method. II. Concentration of caffeine in various strengths, brands, blends and types of teas. *Am. J. Clin. Nutr.* 31:1727, 1978.
* Many APC preparations are sold over the counter.

consuming liquids with snacks or during a coffee break. Without these activities their fluid intake may be low. A bedridden client may deliberately limit his intake of fluids so that he won't have to bother the nurse for a bedpan. Some persons feel too ill or are unable to take the initiative to get themselves a drink of water. Offering fluids frequently may be all that is needed to promote adequate intake when fluid requirements are not excessively high.

Clients who are confined to bed often find it is easier to drink cold liquids through a straw. If a client cannot drink from a cup or through a straw, a health care worker can use a small medicine cup, spoon, medicine dropper, or syringe to place liquids in the client's mouth. If there is any question about the client's gag and swallowing reflexes, these should be checked by a competent health professional before offering fluids. Positioning a client with his head elevated or turned to the side minimizes the danger of aspiration. Small amounts of liquid can then be placed on the middle of the client's tongue or off to the side of his mouth. Occasionally, it is necessary to try a variety of approaches to find one that is most appropriate for a particular client.

THE CLIENT WHO REQUIRES AN ALTERNATE METHOD OF FEEDING

Some clients are not able to take foods by mouth, even with assistance. For instance an unconscious client cannot safely swallow food. In a situation such as this it may still be desirable to feed a client enterally (via the gastrointestinal tract). Use of a feeding tube makes this possible. A client whose nutritional needs cannot be met solely by the enteral route (either orally or by tube) can be fed parenterally. Health care providers should be familiar with practical considerations of providing nutritional support via enteral and parenteral routes, so they can carry out these procedures safely. They also need to recognize a client's feelings and fears concerning these methods of supplying food. For example, does the client feel so self-conscious about a procedure that he wants to be fed in privacy?

Common complaints associated with food intake

Some clients have physical discomforts associated with food intake. Frequently people also have these problems at home but they do not think to ask for advice about how to handle them. Observant health professionals detect these problems and help clients relieve them.

For example, if a client complains of feeling jittery and tense (or shows signs that he is), it would be appropriate for the health care provider to find out if caffeine may be contributing to the problem.[6] Caffeine might also contribute to a client's insomnia. Table 24.1 lists the approximate caffeine content of some commonly used beverages, foods, and medications. A dose of 100 to 150 mg. caffeine is reported to be a "physiological dose" which may produce side effects in some individuals.[7] A trial of reduced caffeine intake may be indicated for symptomatic clients whose intake of caffeine equals or exceeds the physiological dose. Health professionals should be aware of the likelihood of caffeine withdrawal symptoms if caffeine is eliminated. Among the withdrawal symptoms are headache and perhaps nausea, vomiting, and irritability.[6]

Some common food-related problems and suggestions for dealing with them are presented here.

Nausea and/or vomiting at mealtime:
1. Eat and drink slowly.
2. Eat small frequent meals to avoid overdistention of the abdomen.
3. Drink fluids between rather than with meals.
4. Eat dry toast or crackers when feeling nauseous.
5. Avoid foods which are poorly tolerated by many clients (e.g., coffee and foods which are spicy), highly acidic foods, and foods high in fat.
6. Stay quiet for an hour or more following a meal.
7. Relax, take deep breaths, and swallow when feeling nauseous.
8. Use prescribed antacids and antiemetics as directed to decrease gastrointestinal symptoms.

Mild diarrhea:
1. Initially limit intake to liquids, gradually add solids as tolerated.
2. Avoid milk and milk products, extremes of temperature, and concentrated sweets.
3. Eat soft foods which contain pectin such as bananas and applesauce.
4. Eat low fiber foods.
5. Participate in quiet pastimes (e.g., reading, listening to music) which promote relaxation.
6. Use prescribed antispasmodics and antidiarrheals as directed to decrease gastrointestinal symptoms.

Constipation:
1. Establish a consistent pattern of food intake and elimination.
2. Eat breakfast or at least take a hot beverage upon arising.
3. Eat foods providing roughage.
4. Eat foods such as prunes which contain natural laxatives.
5. Drink plenty—more than 1000 ml. (1 qt.) of fluids each day.
6. Establish a pattern of fairly regular physical activity.

Gas (Flatus)
1. Avoid food and food-related behaviors which may produce gas (e.g., lactose if lactose intolerant, air swallowing, ingestion of foods with a high air content or of foods which produce gas).[8]
2. Avoid reclining immediately after meals.
3. Decrease fat content of meals.

FEEDING SICK CHILDREN

Children frequently require special attention to meet their nutritional needs whether they are sick at home or are hospitalized. Food intake is especially important for children who have chronic or very severe illnesses or injuries (e.g., cancer, some congenital disorders, or burns). Nausea, vomiting, and diarrhea often accompany a child's illness. This diminishes a child's desire for food and depletes his body stores. Fortunately, most children who were healthy prior to illness recover quickly and can tolerate short periods of inadequate food intake without serious consequences. Parents and health professionals who do not become *overly* concerned about a child's temporary decrease in food intake avoid precipitating food-related problems.

Young children and infants can, however, become seriously dehydrated if they lose body fluids and these are not adequately replaced. For this reason priority attention is given to maintaining a child's fluid intake. Careful documentation of a child's intake and output is important to accurately assess a child's fluid needs. If a child cannot or will not take fluids orally, intravenous therapy may be necessary. Health care workers can try some of the following suggestions to improve oral intake of fluids.

1. Directly approach a child with small amounts (a few sips) of fluid every half hour to hour. Let the child know that you expect him to take at least a little.
2. Determine a child's taste preferences but don't allow him to become manipulative.
3. Offer sherbet, fruit ice, ice cream, frozen fruit juice pops, custard, gelatin, and other foods having a naturally high water content.
4. Add extra fluids to solid foods such as breakfast cereal.
5. If the child is old enough and well enough, encourage him to keep a chart of his fluid intake. The chart might be in pictorial form. For example, each time he finishes a small glass of any beverage, he might put a star (or an X) on a picture of a glass.

Parents and health care workers need to adjust their expectations to realistically fit the situation when a child is ill. Ill children eat better if caretakers are patient and encouraging. Many of the suggestions presented earlier in this chapter to provide nutritional care for ill adults are helpful when working with children. Foods and fluids and mealtime activities are adjusted to the child's level of growth and development as well as to his health condition. Occasionally ill children exhibit retrogressive behavior, such as a toddler asking for a baby bottle. Since food meets emotional and other non-nutritive needs, concerned adults attempt to identify a child's non-nutritive needs and find ways other than food to meet these needs. Ignoring undesirable food behaviors helps to extinguish them. Parents and others who care for ill children may appreciate the many helpful suggestions in the booklet "Feeding the Sick Child."[9]

Hospitalized children frequently refuse food served to them. Several reasons other than likes and dislikes may account for refusal of food. A child may not eat if (1) he doesn't recognize the food, (2) the color, texture, and sweetness are not suitable for him, (3) food portions are large and overwhelming, or (4) there is no friendly face to provide warmth and genuine concern at mealtime. Health professionals who recognize these problems can take appropriate steps to correct them.

Children who continue to refuse to eat adequate amounts of food even when they have apparently recovered do so for many different reasons. Occasionally an unidentified physical problem may exist; however, there are many other possibilities. Some children refuse food to "punish" adults for "letting" them get ill or to try to gain control over one aspect of their lives.

Children readily detect anxiety in their parents and others. Children in turn become anxious and lose interest in eating. Health professionals can help parents and children deal with this type of problem. For example, health care providers may help a child handle his anger or regain control over some aspects of his life. They may help the parents to maintain a positive outlook and to relax.

There are many ways in which health agencies can promote food intake in their young clients. When a child is admitted to a hospital a health care provider should question parents and children carefully to determine a child's food likes and dislikes and "normal" eating behaviors. Often a child benefits if health professionals and parents exchange information about feeding techniques which they have found to be successful. If a change in feeding technique is essential, health care providers enlist the cooperation of the parents to promote a smooth transition.

Offering foods that children like and will usually eat increases their food intake. However, parents should be discouraged from using empty calorie food "treats" as a means of coaxing a child to eat. This invites the child to engage in manipulative behavior.

Some health agencies have kitchens where children and parents can participate in meal preparation or in serving food. When this is the case, it is easier to cater to a child's appetite and to teach parents about modified diets.

Combining eating and play activities helps promote food intake by young children. These activities might include a tea party with real foods, pretending to be cowboys at the chuck wagon, or "play house" activities involving simple food preparation (e.g., making instant pudding, finger sandwiches, and imaginative salads that look like faces or animals). Children enjoy eating at parties such as holiday and birthday celebrations. If none of these apply, health care workers or the children themselves can think up other good reasons for the children to celebrate.

Children benefit from eating together at small tables. A child who is left to feed himself may eat more than a child who is continually coaxed. If it is necessary to encourage a small child to eat, a firm, consistent approach works surprisingly well. Establishing an agreement with a child is another useful technique. For example, a health care worker might say it is time to eat now and that once the meal is finished the child may go to the playroom. When an agreement such as this is established and a child is unable to meet his end of the bargain he should not be punished; rather, emphasis should be placed on the effort he made. Only agreements which are highly likely to be met by both parties should be made. Older children often respond to simple explanations of why food and fluid intake is essential.

Many parents express concern about "spoiling" or overindulging a child. Health professionals and parents can work together to set reasonable limits regarding food and to consistently maintain them. When a child's condition improves, parents should not expect the child to immediately resume "normal" eating habits. The transition from health agency to home is easier if parents are informed that a child may continue to be a fussy eater for awhile after discharge.

STUDY QUESTIONS

1. When a nurse begins working in a health care agency, what kinds of information should she obtain about nutritional care services?
2. An elderly man wants to feed himself but because he is unsteady in his movement he has difficulty doing so without spilling. Suggest specific measures which might help him feed himself more easily.
3. Mr. and Mrs. J. hover over their hospitalized 5-year-old son at mealtime and coax, prod, and bribe him to eat. What action(s) would it be appropriate for a health care provider to take to deal with this situation?

References

1. Blackburn, G. L., and Bistrian, B. R.: Nutritional support resources in hospital practice. In Schneider, H., Anderson, C., and Coursin D. (eds.): *Nutritional Support of Medical Practice.* New York: Harper & Row, 1977.
2. Schultz, H. G.: Hospital patients' and employees' reactions to food-use combinations. *J. Am. Diet. Assoc.* 60:207, 1962.
3. Irwin, E.: Alternate menu patterns—Survey and nutritional guidelines. *J. Am. Diet. Assoc.* 65:291, 1974.
*4. Bayless, E.: Taste tray increases acceptance of nutritional supplements. *J. Am. Diet. Assoc.* 73:542, 1978.
5. Manning, A., and Means, J.: A self-feeding program for geriatric patients in a skilled nursing facility. *J. Am. Diet. Assoc.* 66:275, 1975.
6. Stephenson, P.: Physiologic and psychotropic effects of caffeine on man. *J. Am. Diet. Assoc.* 7:240, 1977.
7. Groisser, D. S.: A study of caffeine in tea. I. A new spectrophotometric micro-method. II. Concentration of caffeine in various strength, brands, blends and types of teas. *Am. J. Clin. Nutr.* 31:1727, 1978.
8. Bond, J. H., and Levitt, M. D.: Gaseousness and intestinal gas. *Med Clin. North Am.* 62(1):155, 1978.
*9. National Cancer Institute of the National Institutes of Health. *Feeding the Sick Child* by Mikie Sherman. DHEW Pub. No. (NIH) 77-795 Washington, D.C. U.S. Government Printing Office.

* Recommended reading.

25

Nutritional care of ambulatory clients

Increasingly the nutritional care process is being applied in the comprehensive health care of ambulatory clients. This care may be effectively and economically provided in hospital outpatient departments or clinics, public health clinics, family and neighborhood health centers, health maintenance organizations, group practice, and rehabilitative and mental health centers.[1] Nutritional care in these settings helps to smooth the transition from health care facility to home. However, emphasis on prevention makes nutritional care an integral part of health maintenance as well. Health care providers in community agencies are trying to better assess nutritional needs of both the well and the ill and to plan realistic means of helping clients meet those needs.

Many skills are required for delivering quality nutritional care to ambulatory clients, including communication techniques, organizational skills, and application of principles from the social sciences. Student health professionals are urged to acquire these skills and to use them when providing nutritional care. Nutritional care for ambulatory clients often involves working with groups and applying principles of behavioral management; these topics are discussed in this chapter. The latter part of this chapter describes how these approaches may be applied in the overall nutritional care of obese clients.

REACHING THE CLIENT IN THE COMMUNITY

To implement nutritional care of ambulatory clients, health professionals develop nutrition education programs for individuals and groups; they also provide supportive services and direct care for clients who cannot completely care for themselves. Outcomes of care are now more frequently evaluated and the findings are used as a basis for improving future care. Careful documentation promotes consistent quality care and aids interagency and intra-agency referral.

By incorporating effective nutritional care into routine health maintenance, dental care, and maternal-child health services, health care workers help clients avoid common but potentially serious nutrition-related problems and they may help improve the quality of clients' lives. Assisting clients to adhere to modified diets or to overcome malnutrition helps to keep ill persons "well" enough to remain with their families or to live independently.

The process of providing nutritional care is the same whether clients are hospitalized or are outpatients; some details of providing nutritional care must be modified, however, when the persons served are living in the community. For example, the content of a teaching session for the same individual may be quite different depending on whether he is hospitalized or not. Effective use of principles of learning and teaching differs in different settings.

Unlike hospitalized individuals, ambulatory clients are not a "captive audience." Many do not recognize when they have a nutrition-related problem. Those who do feel the need for help may find that attendance at clinic is inconvenient or that it interferes with ability to earn a day's pay. Transportation to the meeting place may be an insurmountable problem for a few clients. Activities within and outside of the home tend to divert a person's attention from his own health care, especially if he feels fine. It may be harder to convince ambulatory clients that nutritional care is really worth the expense and effort. Well-organized, high-quality nutritional care needs to be made attractive and easily accessible to clients.

Health care providers can take constructive measures to promote continuing contact with ambulatory clients. Some kind of reminder system (e.g., a post card or telephone call) helps avoid "forgetfulness" on the part of the client and indicates to the client that the visit is important. When it is difficult for a client to come to the health care agency, it may be possible to provide part of the care by telephone or to have the client mail in record sheets or other data. Some health care facilities or communities have a van which is used for clients who need door-to-door transportation. If a client frequently misses appointments, it is usually advisable for the health professional to investigate the reason. The client may need assistance with a practical problem such as babysitting, or the quality of his nutritional care may need to be improved. A home visit, if possible, sometimes uncovers a problem that the client is reluctant to mention.

Health care providers must find ways to make nutritional care cost-effective, that is, to improve results of care and maximize the amount of high quality care that can be provided for a given cost. One program, involving extensive nutritional care as a part of clinic care for diabetics, resulted in several significant benefits to clients and financial savings for the hospital (due to decreased need for drugs and a sharp decrease in diabetic complications requiring hospitalization).[2] Providing quality nutritional care in the community setting has a largely untapped potential for turning back spiraling health care costs.

Clear criteria need to be developed within community health care agencies to indicate types of nutritional care which are to be delivered in different situations. Delivery of this care often depends on the quality of the referral system.[3] Does the primary care provider make nutritional referrals when they are indicated and help the client to arrange for a convenient appointment? Does she follow up to make sure the client has seen a nutritionist and to find out how the nutritionist's recommendations influence the client's overall plan of care? When a primary care provider expresses this kind of concern about an ambulatory client's nutritional care, this may favorably influence the client's attitude toward the value of the nutritional services.

Since most outpatients have to wait for appointments, health professionals may find it useful to develop materials to stimulate clients' interest in nutrition or to increase their knowledge about a particular topic while they are waiting. Brightly colored posters, fast-paced slide-tapes, mini-discussion groups, pamphlets, and displays are all possibilities. Some clinics serving low income groups might find it useful to arouse curiosity by having free samples of a tasty, nutritious low cost homemade soup or other food. Easy-to-follow recipes for that food and for other economical dishes could be offered along with the sample.

Providing nutritional care via group meetings

If a number of individuals have a similar need for nutrition education relating to the same topic, it is reasonable to plan a structured class. If the class is well organized, interesting, and at the level of the audience, it may be an effective way for a health professional to increase the knowledge of a large number of people in the limited time she has available.[4] A class can also be used for motivating clients; however, the lack of individual attention which is characteristic of many classroom encounters tends to limit the ability of this method to promote behavioral change. A nutritional care program which includes both personalized interaction and structured classroom presentations may be a more effective and efficient means of promoting recommended changes in food practices.

Another strategy for helping a group of clients who have similar nutritional concerns is to conduct small group sessions.[5] Group sessions are very different from formal classes. The group leader (who is not necessarily a health professional) acts as a *facilitator* for behavioral change. She encourages full participation by all group members.

A well-led group can provide an environment which fosters "mutual nourishing" of the participants. The group atmosphere is meant to provide support and motivation to members to help them achieve their individual goals. Recommended actions often seem more acceptable when group members tell how they were helped by those actions. Peer pressure encourages an individual to meet established group goals, makes some individuals more willing to assume responsibility for their actions, and helps some members to be more receptive to learning. Learning in groups is sometimes more interesting and "fun" than is independent learning. However, a person benefits from a group only if he can identify with it.

Groups can be disruptive of nutritional care if they are allowed to become negative. In groups that are designed to promote nutritional care, members need to be encouraged by each other's successes rather than to dwell on how difficult it is to overcome some problems.

Behavior modification

Behavior modification (also called behavioral management or behavioral control) is a method of teaching which is beginning to be widely used as a method of changing food-related behaviors.[6] A person who learns to use a behavioral approach learns to promote behavioral change (learning) by rewarding desirable behavior in a planned, effective manner. It can be learned and practiced by health care workers and by lay persons. The person who directs the program is usually called a "behavioral therapist." A behavioral approach is often most useful if applied by family members or by the client himself.

Behavioral control is a particularly valuable technique for promoting weight loss, for promoting the establishment of socially acceptable eating habits (i.e., reasonably good table manners) in developmentally delayed or mentally disturbed persons, and for promoting compliance with modified diets.

Behavior modification strategies are based pri-

TABLE 25.1 *Overview of behavior modification strategies*

ASSUMPTION	GENERAL METHOD TO MODIFY BEHAVIOR	EXAMPLE OF APPLICATION OF METHOD
Learned behavior can be "retrained" (unlearned and replaced by more appropriate responses)	Positive reinforcement is promptly given for desired response; inappropriate response is ignored	Rapid eater agrees to place fork on plate the entire time he is chewing food. He rewards himself in a predetermined way or is rewarded by a companion for successfully meeting this goal X% of the time (The percentage is increased as success is achieved)
Inappropriate behavior can be minimized by avoiding the stimulus that initiates it	Cue avoidance: strategies are used to avoid places, things, smells, sounds, and situations (external cues) which typically elicit an inappropriate response	Obese individual takes a pre-planned low calorie lunch to work to avoid being exposed to inappropriate food choices in the cafeteria
Unlearned behavior can be shaped	Positive reinforcement is given for small changes in behavior so that behavior gradually approaches the final goal behavior	Developmentally delayed child eats cooked cereal with his hands. Step 1: praise (or some other predetermined reward) is given for holding spoon. Step 2: The reward is withheld until spoon is dipped into cereal. Many intermediate steps follow over a period of days or weeks. Late step: reward is given only for successful transfer of cereal from dish to mouth via spoon
Some behaviors are learned by "modeling" (imitation)	Regularly expose individual to an appropriate role model	A parent agrees to act as an appropriate role model for his child's eating behavior. This may mean a parent has to first modify his own behavior. The child may alter his behavior in response to seeing his parent's behavior change
"Prompting" may aid in learning a new behavior	Gentle written, graphic, or verbal reminders	Client places a sign "You are what you eat" on the cookie jar or door of the refrigerator

marily on Skinner's operant conditioning theory. According to this theory, learned behavior can be influenced by environmental stimuli (cues preceding a behavior) and by the consequences of a behavior. It is assumed that learned behavior can be unlearned and replaced by another behavior.

The basic principle is as follows: a stimulus (S) triggers a response (R) which in turn produces consequences (C): S → R → C. If the consequences promptly result in some feeling of satisfaction, they reinforce the response and the chances are good that the stimulus will continue to trigger the same response. The more times the same sequence of events is repeated, the greater the chance that learning will occur.

One of the most important aspects of a behavioral approach is determination of baseline behavior (the individual's usual behavior before treatment). Initially, data must be collected to determine what kinds of activities or other stimuli trigger undesired responses and what outcomes serve to maintain those responses.

Controlling stimuli by removing or avoiding them (often called cue avoidance) is a basic behavior modification technique. Other general techniques used in behavior modification include regularly pairing a stimulus with an activity so that it becomes a new stimulus for that activity (e.g., ringing a bell before meals can become a stimulus to come to the table to eat); and controlling consequences by rewarding desired behavior (positive reinforcement), ignoring undesired behavior (extinction), or punishing undesired behavior (aversive conditioning, the least effective method of controlling behavior). Table 25.1 gives some examples of behavior modification strategies.

Among the different kinds of rewards that might be used in a behavioral approach are praise; a smile or pat; stars or checks on a chart; money; desired objects (e.g., clothes, books, tools); special privileges (perhaps a hike, dance, movie, trip, or visit to friends); and tokens (these can be saved up to be used to purchase special privileges or items in a "token economy"). Depending on the situation, rewards may be self-dispensed, dispensed by another person or persons (e.g., by a family member), or both.

Contingency contracting is a type of reward system sometimes used for clients who can anticipate the future. The behavioral therapist and client set up a contract. In it arrangements are made for the client to receive a specified reward if he meets stated objectives. For example, the client might deposit some money or some other item of value with the therapist; getting it back might be "contingent upon" the client's attendance at 8 out of 10 meetings. Client and therapist would also agree about what is to happen to the valuable if it is not "earned" back.

Resistance to implementing behavior modification techniques is not uncommon among family members and health professionals. Sometimes this may be because they are legitimately concerned about adverse effects of the rewards being used. For example, candy, other sweets, and cigarettes (for adults) have been used in some behavior modification programs. Reluctance to participate in behavior modification may also be due to concern about manipulating another person's life. People who give this argument may not realize how often they use behavior modification techniques but call them by another name.

To be successful in promoting desired behavioral change, the health professional must determine what kinds of rewards are most appropriate for a particular client, how long a delay there can be between the response and the positive reinforcement, and how often rewards should be given. For example, she may plan to give intermittent rather than regular reinforcement as a more effective means of maintaining behavioral change. She also provides assistance with establishing cue avoidance measures and other types of stimulus control. If expected progress is not made, the health professional should assess whether rewards are being given consistently and in the proper manner. In order to foster cooperation of family members in a behavior modification program, a health professional may need to develop a means of rewarding them for their participation.[7] One way of doing this is to encourage the client to praise family members for praising him.[8] Health care providers should also assess for unanticipated effects of behavior modification techniques. For example, a person who is being treated for undereating might start to gain too much weight. Behavior modification is not the best method to use for all situations, but has a useful place in providing nutritional care.

POINTS OF EMPHASIS
General aspects of nutritional care of ambulatory clients

• *Quality nutritional care of ambulatory clients helps prevent disease, reduces the need for hospitalization, and smooths the transition from health agency to home.*

• *Actions should be taken to increase accessibility of quality nutritional care for ambulatory clients.*

• *Well-planned structured classes extend the professional's ability to provide clients with information needed to make changes in food-related behavior.*

• *Group sessions provide a supportive atmosphere which may promote change of attitude as well as enhance cognitive and psychomotor learning.*

• *Behavior modification techniques help change behavior via cue avoidance and other methods of stimulus control and via rewarding of desired actions.*

NUTRITIONAL CARE OF OVERWEIGHT AND OBESE INDIVIDUALS

Obese persons often receive health care for management of their overweight condition in ambulatory care settings. Group work and techniques of behavioral modification can be effective approaches to working with obese clients. Thus a discussion of nutritional management of overweight and obese clients is included in this chapter to illustrate for the student how these approaches to care can be used.

Obesity, one of the most prevalent nutritional problems in the U.S., tends to be extremely resistant to treatment. For this reason emphasis should be placed on prevention. Clients who have already become obese should be carefully screened to determine the likelihood of success of a weight reduction program because repeated failures may be detrimental to the client's health and well-being.

Health professionals participate in the following preventive activities in a community setting:
1. Parent education regarding (1) feeding of infants and children and (2) appropriate physical activity for the entire family.
2. Early identification of infants and children at risk (i.e., those whose weight/height index is increasing at an undesirably rapid rate, children of obese parents). More intensive efforts should be made to assist these high risk children and their families to increase their activity level and to learn to use food appropriately.
3. Early identification of undesirable weight gain in adolescents and adults.
4. Assistance with selection of a weight control program suited to the needs and income level of the person.
5. Family education regarding danger signals. A marked or persistent unexplained change in food intake may mean that the person needs help in dealing with a medical or personal problem.

Health care providers are frequently called upon to help clients lose weight. In order to perform this function in a responsible manner, they should be knowledgeable about different types of obesity, treatment methods, and limitations of treatment.

Obesity can be subdivided into several categories:
1. Obesity secondary to another condition. Some metabolic disorders (such as hypothyroidism and Praeder-Willi syndrome) lead to obesity. However, obesity arising from serious physical disorders is rare.
2. Recent obesity (adult onset). This type may be due to failure to adjust eating habits with age. It may be quite responsive to treatment.
3. Long term obesity (juvenile onset or developmental obesity). When seen in adults, this type of obesity

tends to be very resistant to treatment. Juvenile onset obesity may often be characterized by an overabundance of fat cells (hyperplastic obesity).

4. Reactive obesity (weight gain following a traumatic emotional experience). This may appear at any time of life. If reactive obesity is detected in an early stage, counseling may help the person find a more constructive means of coping with the problem.

Points to consider before recommending weight reduction

Health professionals should be very cautious about taking the initiative to convince an obese person to reduce and about developing guidelines for a weight loss program. Accurate assessment of the situation is needed. Some pertinent points to consider before recommending weight loss are given here.

Has the person maintained a stable weight for a period of time? There is evidence suggesting that there may be an "equilibrium point" for body weight (a "preferred weight"[9]) and that the body strongly resists weight changes away from that point.[10] Nearly every adult who has been obese for a long time experiences rebound weight gain after a period of weight loss. This might be because his "equilibrium point" is well above usual ideal body weight. No one knows how long a period is required to achieve a new equilibrium state at a lower weight or even if that will occur. It is probably more healthful to maintain a stable elevated weight than to undergo frequent major weight fluctuations. It might be better for the health professional to enlist an obese client's aid in preventing the client's children from becoming obese than to encourage him to lose weight.

Does the person have a history of repeated failure in either achieving or maintaining weight loss? The health care provider should obtain specific data from the client regarding what diets he has followed, weight loss programs in which he has participated, and what caused him to have difficulty in either losing weight or maintaining weight loss.

Are there any appropriate weight reduction methods which truly offer the client a good chance of success? Since many weight loss procedures are expensive, the answer to this question is especially likely to be "no" if the individual is extremely obese and is of low socioeconomic status. Health care workers should try to avoid setting clients up for failure. The poor results associated with most weight loss efforts point up the need for health professionals to take a more active role in prevention of obesity.

Is the client well adjusted to his weight, or is he very strongly motivated to change? If not motivated, chances of success are poor. The most potent motivat-

ing factors appear to be improved appearance (especially in young people) and improved health (primarily in older persons).[11]

Are there health conditions which make weight reduction a high priority item? When a serious health condition is the reason for attempting to reduce, even a moderate weight loss may be adequate to alleviate the current problem. Return to ideal body weight may be an unrealistic goal. However, once improvement in the health condition becomes evident, feedback regarding favorable changes (e.g., reduced blood pressure) may help to motivate the client to continue his efforts.

If change is desired, are expectations realistic? Some clients might believe that weight loss will enable them to get a high paying job or to attract a marital partner. Future problems may be avoided by helping an unrealistic client set more achievable goals.

Will weight loss and weight maintenance be incompatible with maintaining valued social relationships? Some obese persons may have successfully coped with the stigma of obesity by establishing firm bonds of friendship with other obese individuals.[12] Successful weight loss might result in the breaking of these bonds. If weight loss is not a medical necessity, health professional and client should consider whether it is really worthwhile to begin a program that may result in disruption of supportive social relationships.[12]

Client and health professional can choose among a number of approaches to weight loss. Barlow states ". . . almost anything you do with people who overeat is probably going to work for a while."[13] Finding an approach which will result in long term success is more difficult.

Conservative methods of losing weight

BALANCED CALORIE DEFICIT DIETS (REDUCING DIETS)

The traditional means of helping clients lose weight is to prescribe a balanced reducing diet. Usually the caloric level is set at 500 to 1000 kcal. below the estimated maintenance level. The diet is planned to have the qualities listed in Table 18.2, page 198. After following such a diet for awhile, a person may lose less than the expected 0.5 to 1 kg. weekly. (Caloric deprivation causes his basal metabolic rate and, therefore, his energy expenditure to fall.)

Reducing diets are most likely to be effective when relatively little weight (i.e., < 10 kg) needs to be lost or if a person is residing in a health care facility. They work best when accompanied by other conservative weight loss strategies, such as behavior modification and exercise. Broadening the base of a weight loss program may provide a means for helping the client deal with common problem situations and self-defeating behaviors, some of which are listed here.[11]

1. Going off of diet because of undeserved loss or gain of weight or because of reaching a plateau. (Why bother to diet if this weight change occurs anyway?)
2. Rewarding weight loss with a food treat.
3. Going off of diet before goal is reached in response to compliments, to finding that clothes are too large, or to ridicule.
4. Leaving a weight control program because of the belief that success does not require the support of health professionals (or of a group).[14,15] (This may be a problem either before or after the weight loss goal has been reached.)
5. Failing to enlist the assistance of a family member or companion as a means of obtaining regular positive reinforcement.[16]

When a reducing diet is a specific part of treatment, the client is usually given a meal plan which includes a menu pattern, sample menu, and a set of exchange lists (such as "Exchange Lists for Meal Planning," Appendix 5I). The client learns that he won't have to count calories if he uses the number of servings specified in his diet pattern and the serving size indicated in the exchange list. Sometimes the diet counselor provides the client with information about how a small serving of dessert or some other sweet can occasionally be worked into the diet. No specific conservative diet plan has been demonstrated to be superior to other plans.

Many clients benefit from information about calorie labeling of food. A 1979 Food and Drug Administration regulation sets the following rules for calorie labeling:[17]

"A food labeled 'low calorie' may contain no more than 40 calories per serving. Small, calorically dense foods such as candy and potato chips do not qualify even if one piece or one serving provides fewer than 40 kcal.
"A food may be called 'reduced calorie' only if its caloric content is at least ⅓ lower than a similar food for which it can substitute.
"All foods which claim to be reduced in calories must describe the comparison on which the claim is based.
"Foods that are normally low in calories, such as celery, cannot use the term 'low calorie' immediately before the name. . . . However, it may be labeled 'celery, a low calorie food.'
"For a food to be labeled as 'sugar free,' 'sugarless,' or 'no sugar' it must also be labeled as 'low calorie' or 'reduced calorie' . . . or be accompanied by such statements as 'not a reduced calorie food'. . . ."

Unfortunately but understandably, many obese clients find it very difficult to follow a reducing diet long enough to lose a medically significant amount of weight, that is, enough weight loss to result in improved health or decreased risk of certain health problems. When weight loss averages only about 0.5 kg per week, a client easily becomes discouraged with his slow progress. A reducing diet provides little assistance to persons who have a problem with compulsive behavior (i.e., eating binges or snack attacks). Desire to eat may seem to be a "constant companion" during the time a client is on a balanced calorie deficit diet. Because this powerful drive can override even the best intentions, health professionals need to look for supplementary or substitute weight loss and weight maintenance strategies to use for many clients.

A BEHAVIORAL APPROACH TO WEIGHT REDUCTION

Findings of studies which have compared behaviors of obese and normal weight individuals suggest that obese individuals tend to be unusually susceptible to external stimuli, but relatively insensitive to internal stimuli to eat.[18–20] The findings lend support to the validity of using a behavioral approach as a means of achieving weight loss. The approach is suitable for both children and adults.

A behavioral approach to weight loss is distinctly different from traditional diet approaches. Ordinarily emphasis is not on the food a person eats, the reasons why a person eats as he does, or even on the weight loss per se. Rather it is on identifying and *gradually* changing those behaviors which contribute to excessive caloric intake and inadequate energy expenditure. The ultimate goal is the development of a permanent set of appropriate eating and activity habits. These are expected to result in weight loss and weight maintenance. Guidelines regarding food selection and preparation may be introduced into a behavioral program as needed, usually after the program is well underway.

A behavior modification program for weight loss should be directed by someone who is trained by experts in the use of behavior modification techniques for weight control.

When informing clients about a behavioral approach, it is essential to emphasize from the start that a substantial time commitment is required for best results. Length of programs is commonly 14 to 16 weeks.[21] Success with the procedure is strongly dependent upon a systematic, stepwise approach.[22] The health practitioner is firm about the necessity of adhering to guidelines which have been demonstrated to be effective. If a client tries to progress at a faster rate than scheduled, he may experience discouraging setbacks.

A behavioral approach begins with a period of data collection. A form similar to the one shown in Figure 20.2, page 226 may be used. Initially clients are instructed in how to keep the necessary records, but are advised not to try to alter behavior at that time. Early records are used to determine baseline behavior. Just the process of record keeping may result in a reduction in food intake and loss of weight.[23]

Using the records they have kept, clients learn to assess their own eating patterns. They determine when appropriate eating behaviors occur, identify "cues" for undesired behavior, and identify "consequent" events (e.g., pleasure, relief of tension) which help to maintain undesirable habits. If approached with a sense of adventure, this process may "catch the fancy" of children and gain their cooperation.[24]

At first, analysis might be limited to identification of one or two problem behaviors and to identification of the core of appropriate behaviors. (The latter contributes positively to the individual's self-esteem). Therapist and client agree upon techniques to be used for increasing the frequency of existing desirable behaviors and decreasing the inappropriate ones. Cue-avoidance and self-reward for meeting present objectives are integral parts of a behavioral approach. Clients continue to keep records in order to monitor change.

Some of the techniques which might be introduced in behavioral therapy of obesity are listed below.

1. Make eating a "pure activity." Avoid all other activities at mealtime. Concentrate on what you are eating instead.
2. Eat slowly. Leave utensils on plate while chewing. Chew thoroughly. Introduce delays in the meal.
3. Use a distinctive plate (somewhat smaller than the usual dinner plate), bowl, utensils, placemat, and eat only from this place setting.
4. Rid the house of inappropriate food items. Ideally this includes any foods other than salad items which can be eaten without preparation.
5. Shop when not hungry. Take only enough cash with you to cover the items needed.
6. Store food out of sight, in opaque containers.
7. "Program" behaviors which are incompatible with eating but which you enjoy and can easily do. Write a list of these alternate activities and chose one when tempted to eat. (Popular ideas include taking a bath or shower, going for a walk or bicycle ride, pursuing a hobby, calling a friend.)
8. Make a contingency contract with the therapist.
9. Enlist the aid of a companion or spouse to help in reducing exposure to cues for eating, to help increase activity level, and to provide positive reinforcement at appropriate times.
10. Pair activities in new ways. For example, read to the children while waiting for dinner to be prepared; brush the dog while watching TV.

Note: Remember to try to change only one type of behavior at a time to increase your chance of success. Be sure to provide prompt rewards for desirable changes in behavior.

Many of these techniques insert a delay between the stimulus and the response. In other words, barriers to eating are introduced. No food is specifically prohibited. Results of a behavioral approach vary greatly within and among programs. Typical weight loss appears to be about 4 to 9 kg. (9 to 20 lb.) over a period of weeks.

Numerous books have been published so that individuals can learn to practice behavior modification techniques on their own. Little information is available regarding the effectiveness of this approach. Mail correspondence and treatment by telephone have been reported to be successful in promoting weight loss.[25]

Although behavior modification appears to be a useful tool in promoting weight loss, some individuals resist keeping records and fail to follow through with many of the instructions. Adaptations of the usual approach may be needed for people who have trouble reading, writing, or correctly completing forms. Other adaptations may be needed if the family is not supportive of the client's actions.

EXERCISE AND RELAXATION TECHNIQUES

Increased physical activity is a desirable aspect of any weight loss program. Activity should be gradually increased in a healthful manner. It may be advisable for extremely obese persons and middle-aged or older adults to undergo a stress test before engaging in a vigorous activity program. Extremely obese individuals may need close supervision of exercise since even walking may require unusually high energy expenditure.

Obese clients may benefit from learning and practicing relaxation techniques. A brief period of relaxation can be an effective means of coping with stress or dealing with a strong urge to eat.

ASSERTIVENESS TRAINING

Assertiveness training is not usually considered to be a weight control method, but for many people it may be a useful addition to a weight control program. In an assertiveness training program a person learns to state and stand up for his rights even when he knows others disagree with him and will try to block his action. A person learns to handle criticism without resorting to eating. He learns to say "no" when someone pressures him with "Won't you have some of this cake that I made just for you." Some clients may even learn to be assertive with themselves, that is, to stop thoughts that tend to lead to inappropriate eating. Communicating in a clear and open manner is an integral part of assertive behavior.

A GROUP APPROACH TO WEIGHT REDUCTION

Becoming an active participant in a weight reduction group helps many individuals to lose weight. The approval of group members provides a meaningful reward for following a diet or carrying out some other treatment measure. Groups can be used in combination with any conservative approach to weight loss.

All groups include a time for sharing and mutual support. Because there is a chance that group members will become discouraged if one or more members drops out or runs into difficulty, it is sometimes recommended that a group approach be delayed until the weight maintenance period.

The origin of a weight loss group may affect its operation. In some cases health professionals plan and conduct groups to meet an identified need of clients. Sometimes they assist clients in developing their own self-help group. There are nationwide nonprofit self-help weight loss groups, notably Overeaters Anonymous (OA) and TOPS (Take Off Pounds Sensibly). Several of the commercial weight control programs also include a group approach. Table 25.2 summarizes features of some of the nationwide weight loss organizations.

Unfortunately there is limited information regarding the ability of established weight loss groups to promote long term weight loss. Clients should compare costs, services, and success rates before deciding to join a program. (Some programs are very costly and may request a large advance payment.) Since dropout rates are high for many groups (even those which require a sizable deposit), the overall success rate of a group may be much lower than statistics suggest.

If a client is shopping around for a weight control program, he should find out if available programs include practices which might embarrass him and lower his sense of self-esteem. For example, if a client has gained weight (determined in a weigh-in), is this publicly announced? Are group members allowed to make negative comments, to boo, or to provide some

POINTS OF EMPHASIS
Conservative methods of weight loss

* *Reducing diets help clients to know how much and what types of foods to eat in order to achieve a specified weight loss.*
* *Behavior modification helps clients to replace undesirable eating habits with behaviors that promote weight loss and weight maintenance.*
* *Exercise programs, relaxation techniques, and assertiveness training complement weight reduction programs.*
* *A group approach may enhance any type of conservative weight loss program.*

other form of aversive conditioning? An embarassing experience may make some clients feel defeated; instead of being motivated to do better next time they may be motivated to leave the group.

Extreme methods of weight reduction

When obesity is seriously interfering with health and conservative weight loss methods have been unsuccessful, a more vigorous approach is sometimes indicated. Extreme methods, however, are rarely recommended for treating obese children. Health profes-

---

TABLE 25.2 *Features of some of the least costly nationwide weight loss organizations*

COMMERCIAL PROGRAMS	NONPROFIT SELF-HELP GROUPS	
Diet Workshop* and Weight Watchers* Diet plans, menu patterns, and exchange lists are nutritionally sound Separate diet plans are available for men, women, and teens, and for certain conditions but plans are not individualized further	*Overeaters Anonymous (OA)*[26]* A choice is made between two weight reduction diets, or the client uses a plan provided by his physician	*TOPS*[27]* The meetings feature group support, weigh-in
Programs include teaching of behavior modification techniques, directions for preparing reduced calorie foods, exercise (usually geared toward flexibility and toning rather than toward burning up many calories), group support, and assistance with weight maintenance following weight loss	Client follows the 12 Steps of Recovery (patterned after Alcoholics Anonymous) with the help of a sponsor. The program is particularly suitable for compulsive eaters	Educational aspects of program vary widely with the local group
	Program features group support and building of client's self-esteem; there is no teaching regarding diet, food preparation, behavior modification, or other weight loss strategies	Presentations by health professionals are occasionally used.
A confidential weekly weigh-in is a regular feature		Members are encouraged to help each other (i.e., by telephone) between meetings
Payment of a fee for attendance is required (about $3.50/meeting in 1979); advance payment reduces the rate	There is no weigh-in, no fee (Basket is passed for contributions to meet small expenses of local group)	A small charge is made for yearly dues
Details of implementation vary with the organization		

* Physician's approval of participation is recommended.

sionals should be able to inform clients about possible benefits and drawbacks of extreme weight loss methods.

STARVATION

Supervised starvation in a hospital setting has been used as a means of producing rapid weight loss in extremely obese individuals. Starvation ketosis may reduce or eliminate hunger and, because of this, the process is more tolerable than might otherwise be expected. Hospitalization allows close monitoring of the client for physiological and psychological problems which might be precipitated by this drastic procedure. Weight losses have exceeded 43 kg. (100 lb.) in some of the longer fasts.[23]

In addition to cost, one very serious drawback of supervised starvation is that the client loses a large amount of lean body mass. Protein malnutrition is expected and may become clinically evident. Potential side effects and complications of starvation include renal failure, liver disorders, gout, edema, severe hypotension (especially postural hypotension), arrhythmias, polyneuritis, hair loss, incapacitating weakness, and increased susceptibility to infection.

After a starved client resumes a normal diet, repletion of muscle tissue begins and the client gains weight even if caloric intake is not excessive. Many resume inappropriate eating and regain much fat as well. Even so, some clients have reported that they benefited from the temporary weight loss.[28]

PROTEIN SPARING MODIFIED FAST (PSMF) AS A PART OF A PHYSICIAN SUPERVISED COMPREHENSIVE WEIGHT REDUCTION PROGRAM

A protein sparing modified fast is a type of reducing diet which has been recommended as just one part of a physician-supervised comprehensive weight reduction program for individuals who have more than about 22 kg. (50 lb.) to lose. The PSMF by itself would only be a fad diet which could not be expected to result in lasting weight loss; however, the diet may serve a useful purpose when incorporated into a comprehensive program. Features of a comprehensive program are summarized here.[14,15]

1. Complete physical examination
2. Nutrition and diet (in the following sequence over a period of many weeks):
   a. Balanced low calorie deficit diet
   b. Protein sparing modified fast (PSMF)
   c. Weight maintenance diet (following a period of weaning from the PSMF)
3. Behavior modification techniques
4. Problem-solving techniques
5. Assertiveness training
6. Relaxation techniques, visualizations
7. Fitness program
8. Education regarding the above topics

9. Monitoring of all aspects of client's participation: laboratory tests, weight change, fitness level, record keeping (i.e., are diaries consistent with weight and fitness changes?); nutrition knowledge (pencil and paper tests), and completion of assignments

The PSMF diet allows 1.2 to 1.5 gm protein per kg of the client's ideal body weight. Usually this protein is obtained from lean meat, fish, skinless poultry, or shellfish. No carbohydrate is allowed at all, and fat is limited to that present in the high protein foods previously listed. No fat may be added in cooking.

Although a protein sparing modified fast has attractive features, such as weight loss of about 0.2 kg. (⅓ to ½ lb.) or more daily, *this type of dieting holds dangers and should never be attempted by a person on his own.* Blackburn and Bistrian, two leading investigators of this extreme weight loss technique, emphatically state, ". . . the program must be physician-supervised and should be carried out only by people knowledgeable in the metabolism of fasting and its appropriate role in comprehensive weight control therapy."[29] They do not recommend the PSMF when only a small amount of weight must be lost.

A listing of possible side effects of a PSMF points up the need for monitoring and supervision by a physician who is competent in this field:

1. Transient lightheadedness and weakness
2. Gastrointestinal complaints including decreased gut motility and constipation
3. Fluid and electrolyte imbalances. (Sodium, potassium, calcium, magnesium, and phosphate levels require monitoring.) Supplementation is individualized to the client's needs
4. Gout, hyperuricemia. Medication may be required to prevent problems
5. Amenorrhea (missed menstrual periods). Pregnancy testing may be necessary since the diet is contraindicated for pregnant women.
6. Hair loss (temporary).

The physician gives advice regarding changes in medications used for control of chronic diseases. Physiological changes caused by the modified fast nearly always result in a need to decrease antihypertensive drug dosage and diabetic drug dosage. The client must also check with the physician regarding use of over-the-counter medicines.

Those who are familiar with popular carbohydrate-free or low carbohydrate diets (e.g., Dr. Stillman's Quick Weight Loss diet and Dr. Atkin's diet) might note that they are similar to the protein sparing modified fast. They should not be considered safe to use independently. The popular diets may have the additional drawback of raising blood lipid levels.[30,31] Since the popular low calorie reducing diets do not limit calories, they will not necessarily result in loss of adipose tissue.

A comprehensive program of the type described on this page may be an unrealistic option for individuals with limited income. Nevertheless, the program's apparently high long-term success rate for clients who participate fully may help to offset its cost.[14]

SURGICAL TREATMENT

Surgery is occasionally used as a method of treating carefully selected persons whose health is in jeopardy because of extreme obesity. Two types of major surgical procedures are used: jejunoileal bypass and gastric bypass. Jejunoileal bypass decreases the length of functioning small intestine to less than about 84 cm. (25 in.). This change results in both a decrease in food intake (because of gastrointestinal symptoms) and reduced absorption of food. Gastric bypass involves sectioning the stomach to form a small pouch; the greatly reduced stomach size demands marked change in eating habits. Both procedures almost invariably result in medically significant weight loss (about 30 to 60 kg. [66 to 130 lb.] for jejunoileal bypass and an average of 36 kg. [80 lb.] for gastric bypass). Weight is seldom regained.

Relatively few people are good candidates for such drastic means of weight reduction. Among the criteria for jejunoileal bypass are (1) greater than 45 kg. (100 lb.) above normal weight or more than two times normal weight; (2) failure of more conservative weight loss regimens; (3) presence of a disease condition aggravated or caused by obesity; (4) stable adult life pattern; and (5) absence of contraindications to surgery (including ambivalence toward the procedure).[32,33]

Both procedures, especially jejunoileal bypass, pose serious health hazards, including malnutrition. Chronic marked diarrhea almost always results from jejunoileal bypass, but other possible consequences (e.g., liver disease) are more serious. A client who has bypass surgery will require prolonged medical management. Both surgical procedures remain investigational.

STUDY QUESTIONS

1. List several reasons why clients may not keep appointments in clinics and other community agencies. Suggest a way of overcoming each of the problems you identified.
2. Suggest several ways in which a group approach might be useful for promoting improved nutrient intake of outpatients and their families.
3. When using a behavioral approach, why shouldn't rewards be delayed until the therapist can accurately assess the client's progress?
4. Discuss reasons why it is undesirable to advise all obese clients to lose weight.
5. An obese man often rewards himself with food. Suggest strategies that might help him overcome this habit.
6. Identify several reasons why a comprehensive approach to weight loss may be more effective than a reducing diet alone.
7. An extremely obese woman who is a compulsive

eater is in ill health because of her obesity. She has tried many weight loss schemes in the past without lasting success. She says she has heard that bypass surgery is a sure way to lose weight. Discuss points which the health professional might raise in discussing this and other weight loss options with her.

References

*1. Owen, A. Y.: *Community Nutrition in Preventive Health Care Services: A Critical Review of the Literature.* DHEW Publ. No. (HRA) 78-14017. Washington DC: Superintendent of Documents, May 1978.

2. Isaf, J. J., and Alogna, M. T.: Better use of resources equals better health for diabetics. *Am. J. Nurs.* 77:1792, 1977.

3. Ryan, L. K., and Dutton, C. B.: Utilization of a nutrition service in a neighborhood health center. *Am. J. Public Health* 57:565, 1977.

4. Hassell, J., and Medved, E.: Group audiovisual instruction for patients with diabetes: Learning achievements and time economics. *J. Am. Diet. Assoc.* 66:465, 1975.

*5. Strickland, B.: Group dynamics: A point of view. People, interaction, and change. *J. Am. Diet. Assoc.* 69:373, 1976.

*6. Barlow, D. H., and Tillotson, J. L.: Behavioral science and nutrition: A new perspective." *J. Am. Diet. Assoc.* 72:368, 1978.

7. Clark, C. C.: *The Nurse as Group Leader.* New York: Springer Publishing Co., 1977.

8. Mahoney, M. J., and Caggiula, A. W.: Applying behavioral methods to nutritional counseling. *J. Am. Diet. Assoc.* 72:372, 1978.

9. Bruch, H.: *Eating Disorders. Obesity Anorexia Nervosa, and the Person Within.* New York: Basic Books, 1973.

10. Jordan, H. A.: In defense of body weight. *J. Am. Diet. Assoc.* 62:17, 1973.

11. Berman, E. M.: Factors influencing motivations in dieting. *J. Nutr. Educ.* 7:155, 1975.

12. Tobias, A. L.: A word of caution: Don't perpetuate the stigma of obesity. Abstracts, 61st Annual Meeting of The American Dietetic Association, New Orleans, Sept. 1978, p. 70.

*13. Barlow, D. H., and Foreyt, J.: Work session on application of behavior therapy techniques to changing dietary habits. In *Proceedings of the Nutrition-Behavioral Research Conference.* DHEW Publ. No. (NIH) 76-973. Bethesda MD: National Institutes of Health, 1975.

14. Lindner, P. G., and Blackburn, G. L.: Multidisciplinary approach to obesity utilizing fasting modified by protein sparing therapy. *Obesity/Bariatric Med.* 5(6):198, 1975.

15. Blackburn, G. L. (ed.): *Obesity.* Boston: Center for Nutritional Research, 1977.

16. Cormier, A., and Préfontaine, M.: Does behavior modification work for obese young adults? *J. Nutr. Ed.* 9:31, 1977.

17. Calorie labeling. *Cons. Register* 8(21):1, 1978.

18. Schacter, S.: Some extraordinary facts about obese humans and rats. *Am. Psychol.* 26:129, 1971.

19. Drabman, R. S., Hammer, D., and Jarvie, G. J.: Eating rates of elementary school children. *J. Nutr. Ed.* 9:80, 1977.

20. Van Itallie, T. B., and Campbell, R. G.: Multidisciplinary approach to the problem of obesity. *J. Am. Diet. Assoc.* 61:385, 1972.

*21. What's new in weight control? *Dairy Council Digest* 49(2), Mar./Apr., 1978.

22. Levitz, L. S.: Behavior therapy in treating obesity. *J. Am. Diet. Assoc.* 62:22, 1973.

*23. Leon, G. R.: Current directions in the treatment of obesity. *Psychological Bull.* 83:557, 1976.

24. Brownell, K. D., and Stunkard, A. J.: Behavioral treatment of obesity in children. *Am. J. Dis. Child.* 132:403, 1978.

25. Balch, D., and Balch, K.: Establishing a campus-wide behavioral weight reduction program through a university student health service. *J. Am. Coll. Health Assoc.* 25:148, 1976.

26. Lindner, P. G.: Overeaters Anonymous—Report on a self-help group. *Obesity/Bariatric Med.* 3(4):134, 1974.

27. Stunkard, A. J.: The success of TOPS, a self-help group. *Postgrad. Med.* 51(5):143, 1972.

28. Johnson, D., and Drenick, E. J.: Therapeutic fasting in morbid obesity. *Arch. Intern. Med.* 137:1381, 1977.

29. Blackburn, G. L.: The "liquid protein" controversy—A closer look at the facts. *Obesity/Bariatric Med.* 7(1):25, 1978.

30. Rickman, F., et al.: Changes in serum cholesterol during the Stillman diet. *J.A.M.A.* 228:54, 1974.

*31. Council on Foods and Nutrition. A critique of low-carbohydrate ketogenic weight reduction regimens. *J.A.M.A.* 224:1415, 1973.

32. Bray, G. A., and Benfield, J. R.: Intestinal bypass for obesity: A summary and perspective. *Am. J. Clin. Nutr.* 30:121, 1977.

33. Maini, B. S.: Surgical approaches. In Blackburn, G. L. (ed.): *Obesity.* Boston: Center for Nutritional Research, 1977.

* Recommended reading.

26

Nutrition action in the expanded community

". . . most human beings, professional or nonprofessional, provider or consumer, make the easiest choices available to them most of the time, and not necessarily because of what they know is most healthful."[1] Assuming that this statement is true, action to improve the nutritional status of population groups should be directed toward making healthful practices easier and more enjoyable. A health professional does this on a small scale for the clients she serves; however, her actions may have little effect on the community at large. Unless she extends her services through constructive use of available channels of communication and established channels of change, a large proportion of the community may remain ignorant of preventive nutrition measures or unwilling to go to the trouble of changing food-related behavior.

To benefit the people most in need of assistance, it is necessary for any nutrition program to have a well-planned *outreach* component. Outreach refers to publicity about the program—how it works, who is eligible, and what the benefits are. Usually outreach takes the form of notices, brochures, newspaper articles and other printed matter, TV and radio spot announcements, and word of mouth from health care providers and others involved in community agencies. Ideally, all of these will give a hotline number which consumers can call for clarification or for additional information. Verbal messages and hotlines are particularly valuable since many of the people who are most in need of services may be unable to read well, if at all. Bilingual messages are desirable in many communities.

Money to cover outreach expenses is budgeted into some but not all of the federal food programs. Local programs vary widely in funding for and/or knowledge of how to develop effective outreach.

Since many programs do not have extensive outreach, it is incorrect to assume that community members are aware of the resources available to them or of the benefits of participation in a particular program. For instance, low income parents might not know that their children are eligible for free school lunch and breakfast because they cannot read the notices sent by the school.

Some studies have been and are being conducted to find out if frequent use of media can foster desirable change in food behaviors. Results from the Stanford Three Community Study suggest that a media approach can help to lower blood lipid levels in a community but probably not to produce weight loss.[2,3] Studies being sponsored by the National Institutes of Health may indicate what marketing and on-the-spot educational techniques can be used to improve food choices in the marketplace and in eating establishments. It is easier for people to choose what is healthful if they feel it is "the thing to do." Once initiated, behavioral change may be followed by change in attitude.[4] For example, a person may discover that fresh fruit really does make a delightful substitute for rich desserts.

To better reach the community at large, more health professionals are becoming personally involved in initiating and/or implementing wide scale measures to promote nutritional health. They recognize that actions of organizations (government, industry, health care facilities, and others) influence choices that are available to consumers. Therefore, health professionals are beginning to make reliable information available to consumers and are encouraging them to take informed stands on proposed nutrition-related changes. They let consumers know how they can influence nutrition-related policy decisions that are being made by organizations.

STRATEGIES

By making constructive use of available channels, health professionals and other responsible citizens have been able to secure assistance and to initiate and support actions which benefit the nutritional status of large numbers of people. A variety of approaches are briefly described here.

Obtaining information If a consumer has a problem or has questions about any program or agency of the federal government, he can call the nearest Federal Information Center (FIC). This center helps him locate the appropriate agency. Low income families who need help obtaining access to participation in federal, state, or local food programs can be directed to the local Community Action Agency (CAA). The office of the city mayor or of the county commissioner should be able to provide the address and phone number of the local CAA.

Written comments on proposals made by the FDA, USDA, or the FTC When proposals are made, notices are placed in the *Federal Register*, a publication which can be found in large public libraries and in some university libraries. However, since using the *Federal Register* itself may be inconvenient and time consuming, summaries of the food and nutrition-related proposals are prepared and printed in publications such as *FDA Consumer*, the *CNI Weekly Report*, *The Journal of the American Dietetic Association*, and sometimes in daily newspapers. Industry, food industry associations, and organized consumer groups recognize the value of submitting comments and make sure their views are expressed. Comments from health professionals and other individuals, when received, are given serious consideration, especially if they include supportive statements for the stand taken. This avenue of effecting change is seriously underused.

Testimony at public hearings On occasion, announcements appear in newspapers about public hearings to be held around the country by federal agencies or by congressional groups. For example, in the summer and fall of 1978, the FDA, USDA, and FTC jointly held five public hearings to discuss issues related to food labeling. Background information about the topic of the hearing is made available free of charge upon request so that individuals can more adequately prepare their comments. Health care workers can alert consumers to opportunities to make their voices heard.

Affiliation with or support of advocacy or public interest groups Public interest groups are nonprofit organizations which attempt to effect changes in laws and regulations for the benefit of consumers. These groups are generally at least partially dependent upon contributions from people who support the causes they represent. A brief discussion of two of these groups is given below. Others are listed in Appendix 2F.

Action for Children's Television (ACT) started as a small group of concerned parents which grew into a powerful advocacy group. Their persistent effort has resulted in many beneficial changes, including voluntary withdrawal of vitamin commercials from children's television.

Center for Science in the Public Interest (CSPI) is an organization which "seeks to improve the quality of the American diet through research and public education at the national and local levels." They investigate and publicize problems, lobby, and initiate legal action when they feel it is justified. They take very strong stands for a prudent diet and against so-called junk foods and many food additives. CSPI is sometimes criticized for its approach.[5]

Contacting state consumer agencies Consumer agencies at the state level want to learn of consumer complaints, including those related to food, nutrition, and health care. They can advise consumers regarding appropriate channels for seeking corrective action.

Letters or calls to elected officials Many nutrition bills have been before Congress and state legislative bodies in recent years. Health care providers and other concerned citizens should register their opinions with their Representatives and Senators. Many of the bills affect funding of food assistance programs and of government agencies working in the area of food, nutrition, and health. An easy way to keep abreast of nutrition-related bills which are before Congress is to read the weekly newsletter *CNI Weekly Report*.

The impact of public outcry became apparent following FDAs announced ban on saccharin. (No doubt this was reinforced by activity of powerful lobby groups.) A question rises as to how many people who *supported* FDAs action did not bother to write or call to express their views.

Contacting the Better Business Bureau (BBB) When fraudulent practices are discovered or suspected, notification of the BBB may help protect others. The bureau can provide information to consumers only if they have been able to collect reliable information about the business in question.

Letters to food companies and product boycotts Food companies make note of the comments received from their customers. If enough people were to complain about too much sugar in a product and refused to buy that product as well, the company would change the product. The power of organized boycotts became quite evident when consumers boycotted sugar and coffee in response to greatly increased prices. It only took a while before the big drop in sales led to a drop in prices.

Except in the case of organized boycotts, consumers seldom let a company know why they refrain from purchasing a food. If a company makes a change for the better, this might be supported by letters and by increased purchase of the product.

PARTICULAR ISSUES

Children's TV commercials

An example of a nutrition-related area in which consumers, health professionals, and public interest groups have been working to effect change is that of TV advertising directed toward children. In response to petitions from ACT, CSPI, Consumers Union, the Committee on Children's Television, and individuals, the FTC proposed a regulation which would "ban any TV advertising aimed at children too young to understand its selling purpose; ban TV advertising of the sugared food products most likely to cause tooth decay aimed at or seen by older children; and require corrective disclosures in TV advertising of other sugared foods aimed at or seen by older children." It is expected that it will take at least 3 to 5 years before such a rule might become effective, if indeed it does.[6]

The U.S. is not the only nation where concern has been expressed about the effects of advertising directed toward children. The Netherlands took action to control advertising directed toward children some time ago. Sweets cannot be advertised before 8 PM in that country; when candy is advertised, a toothbrush and toothpaste must be pictured at least 10 percent of the time.[7] Similar regulations might be possible in the U.S. if citizens work toward that goal.

Global malnutrition

Global malnutrition is a problem with which America and other prosperous nations have been wrestling and will continue to wrestle for many years. The world has become so small that it is no longer possible to ignore the fact that millions of people living in less affluent nations are chronically malnourished. Most of the world's hungry are concentrated in about 90 developing nations. The Government Accounting Office states that there is evidence that the situation is worsening for these people.[8]

There have been many approaches to solving problems of malnutrition in developing countries, some of which look promising. Both governmental and humanitarian agencies have been involved. The Government Accounting Office states that much of the world relies on the U.S. for expanded food aid and for related development assistance. They suggest that federal programs designed to decrease malnutrition in developing nations should consider the impact on the recipient nation's self-help development, impact on their domestic prices and a number of other points.

The Office of Nutrition within the State Department's Agency for International Development (AID) is an example of a federal agency which has made some big strides on a small budget.[9] One interesting program involves effective use of brief radio messages. For example, one message teaches Nicaraguan mothers that they should feed their children if the children become ill (which is not the usual custom); another suggests a practical means of doing this.

The Food and Agricultural Organization of the United Nations (FAO), the United Nations International Children's Fund (UNICEF), and the World Health Organization (WHO) are among the international groups which have been actively promoting self-help and taking measures to relieve food crises.

Some private citizens who urge eating lower on the food chain do so out of the conviction that this is essential if there is to be adequate food for all the world's population without squandering limited resources. Other approaches to the problem of hunger have involved development of nutritious cereal-based foods for children using indigenous products (Incaparina), teaching improved agricultural methods, developing disease-resistant crops, improving food distribution methods, instituting measures to reduce large-scale food spoilage, and encouraging use of inexpensive, widely available cultural foods which appear to account for the superior nutritional status of some of the inhabitants.[10]

A variety of references on this subject is listed at the end of Part 3.

A national nutrition policy

The United States *needs* a food policy, a nutrition policy, and a health policy which recognize the interrelationships between food, nutrition and health. (P. A. Lachance, 1977)[11]

The objective of a national nutrition policy is to develop a workable, coordinated plan for actions that will result in improved nutritional status for the population. (J. Dwyer, 1977)[12]

To date the U.S. has no formulated national nutrition policy. From time to time general policy statements have been made by government agencies or officials, as illustrated by the following:

All citizens shall have access to an adequate and safe supply of food and ability to identify, select, and prepare an optimal diet, irrespective of social or economic status. (A statement of nutrition policy for the Department of Health, Education and Welfare [Draft])[13]

Numerous governmental agencies and offices are involved in activities which can affect the nutritional status of the population either directly or indirectly, but these efforts are by no means coordinated. In actuality, sometimes the efforts of one agency work at cross purposes to those of another. For example, efforts by DHEW to try to persuade people to limit their intake of high fat meat are hampered by USDAs giving top grade (and therefore high appeal) to beef which is heavily marbled with fat. Even nutrition education efforts have been conducted in a haphazard fashion. In 1977 more than 30 nutrition education programs were administered by 2 federal departments and 11 agencies.

The National Nutrition Consortium, an organization composed of representatives of all the major professional societies in food, nutrition, and dietetics, has recommended the following five basic goals for a national nutrition policy:

(a) Assure an adequate wholesome food supply, at reasonable cost, to meet the needs of all segments of the population—this supply to be available at a level consistent with the affordable lifestyle of the era;
(b) Maintain food resources sufficient to meet emergency needs and to fulfill a responsible role as a nation in meeting world food needs;
(c) Develop a level of sound public knowledge and responsible understanding of nutrition and foods that will promote maximal nutritional health;
(d) Maintain a system of quality and safety control that justifies public confidence in its food supply;
(e) Support research and education in foods and nutrition with adequate resources and reasoned priorities to solve important current problems and to permit exploratory basic research.[14]

This statement was not well publicized and received relatively little attention; many health professionals and other consumers were largely unaware of a need for a national nutrition policy. The picture changed dramatically in 1977 when the Senate Select Committee on Nutrition and Human Needs published *Dietary Goals*. Media coverage and the goals themselves sparked considerable debate and stimulated increased interest in a national nutrition policy.

A national nutrition policy could influence agricultural production and practices of the food industry as well as consumer choices and the thrust of nutrition education efforts. There is concern about making major policy decisions without sufficient scientific findings to justify them. There is fear by some that basic rights will be infringed by hastily formulated policies. These are, of course, possibilities and are good reasons for consumers and health professionals alike to become involved in the decision-making process. Freedom need not be incompatible with measures to promote health, but achievement of a good combination of the two requires citizens to assume some responsibility for influencing formulation of policy. The process will take time, but consumer interest will expedite it.

In North Karelia, Finland, citizens were so concerned about their risk of cardiovascular disease (by far the highest in the world) that they demanded and received governmental assistance with dealing with the problem.[15,16] This suggests that a grass roots effort might become the stimulus for initiation of national policies.

Norway is one country which has developed a national nutrition and food policy.[17] The policy aims to encourage healthy dietary habits; its stated goals are similar to those listed in *Dietary Goals of the United States*. (Norway has similar health problems, namely diseases of overabundance.) Norway has taken a big step by formulating proposals for implementing an overall nutrition policy. These include agricultural

and fisheries policies; price policies; changes in industrial processing, imports, and marketing; and ongoing research and education. New administrative arrangements and selective use of subsidies are designed to encourage the desired changes. The Norwegian Ministry of Agriculture clearly states its stand: "In deciding on consumer subsidies, in the government's opinion, it is important to aim at influencing the consumption of food in the desired direction, with regard to nutrition and health."[17] The Norwegian position might be compared to the position of the U.S. Public Health Service:

The government's function is to enable people to make sound decisions about their health, to equip them with information and skills and other resources to translate these decisions into action, and to aid in the removal of legal, economic, physical or other barriers that might prevent them from acting accordingly . . .
. . . the proposals are intended solely to provide opportunities and incentives for people to assume full responsibility for their own health.[18]

A nutrition policy suitable for the U.S. would of necessity be far more complex than the Norwegian policy for many reasons, including the much larger size of the nation, greater heterogeneity of the population, and independent governmental powers of each of the 50 states, Puerto Rico, and U.S. territories.

Consumers have a stake in the outcome whether or not the government adopts a coordinated plan of action with clearly defined goals. Right now government policies influence what Americans eat and the kinds of nutrition services that are available to them. No action is a form of action. Progress depends on "broad and vigorous involvement by consumers and by health professionals in the further development of public policy."[19] Suggested readings are listed at the end of Part 3.

STUDY QUESTIONS

1. A parent is upset about the effect that television commercials are having on her children's attitudes toward food. Discuss several constructive means of trying to deal with the source of the problem (while allowing the child to watch a "reasonable amount" of TV).
2. Identify a food product you are dissatisfied with for nutrition-related reasons. Draft a letter to the manufacturer stating your concerns about their food product.
3. Identify some of the larger developing nations where malnutrition is a serious problem. List several reasons for the existence of malnutrition in one of those nations.
4. Describe some of the approaches which have been used to decrease malnutrition in developing nations.
5. List at least five reasons supporting the desirability of establishing a national nutrition policy.

References

*1. Milio, N.: A framework for prevention: Changing health-damaging to health-generating life patterns. *Am. J. Public Health* 66:435, 1976.

2. Farquhar, J. W., et al.: Community education for cardiovascular health. *Lancet* 1:1192, 1977.

3. Stern, M. P., and Taylor, C. B.: Response of dietary patterns to a two-year cardiovascular health education campaign: The Stanford Three Community Study. In *Proceedings of the Nutrition-Behavioral Research Conference.* DHEW Publ. No. (NIH) 76-978. Bethesda MD: National Institutes of Health, 1975.

*4. Evans, R. I., and Hall, Y.: Social-psychologic perspective in motivating changes in eating behavior. *J. Am. Diet. Assoc.* 72:378, 1978.

5. Food Day at the White House. A Staff Report. *Nutr. Today* 12(6):16, 1977.

6. TV ads directed at children. *Consumer Register* 8(10): May 15, 1978.

7. Slattery, J.: Dental health in children. *Am. J. Nurs.* 76:1159, 1976.

8. *Food and Agriculture Issues for Planning.* General Accounting Office. Washington DC: USGAO CED-77-61. April 22, 1977.

9. ———. AID's nutrition office has wide-spread impact. *CNI Weekly Report* 7(28):4, 1977.

*10. Wishik, S. M., and Van der Vynckt, S.: The use of nutritional "positive deviants" to identify approaches for modification of dietary practices. *Am. J. Public Health* 68:36, 1976.

11. LaChance, P. A.: National nutrition programs—perspective and policy. *J. Am. Diet. Assoc.* 71:489, 1977.

12. Dwyer, J.: Challenge of change—nutrition and policy. *J. Nutr. Ed.* 9:54, 1977.

13. A statement of nutrition policy for the Department of Health, Education, and Welfare. (Draft) Nutrition and Health Select Committee on Nutrition and Human Needs, U.S. Senate Dec. 1975, Appendix W, p. 238.

14. Guidelines for a National Nutrition Policy. National Nutrition Consortium. Prepared for Senate Select Committee on Nutrition and Human Needs, Washington, DC: U.S. Government Printing Office, 1974.

15. Puska, P., et al.: The North Karelia Project: A programme for community control of cardiovascular diseases. *Scand. J. Soc. Med.* 4:57, 1976.

*16. Puska, P.: High-risk hearts. *World Health.* Oct. 1976, p. 12.

17. *On Norwegian Nutrition and Food Policy, Report No. 32 to the Storting (1975–76),* Royal Norwegian Ministry of Agriculture, Nov. 7, 1975.

18. *Forward Plan for Health.* FY 1978–82. DHEW. Washington DC: U.S. Govt. Printing Office, 1976.

19. Lee, P. R.: Nutrition policy—from neglect and uncertainty to debate and action. *J. Am. Diet. Assoc.* 72:588, 1978.

* Recommended reading.

Part 3

Bibliography and Additional Recommended Readings

Aspinall, M. J.: Use of a decision tree to improve accuracy of diagnosis. *Nurs. Res.* 28:182, 1979.

Austin, J. E.: What comes first in feeding the hungry? *Nutr. Today* 13(6):21, 1978.

Bayer, M., and Brandner, P.: Nurse/patient peer practice. *Am. J. Nurs.* 77:86, 1977.

Bistrian, B., et al.: The better gauge to protein depletion. *RN* 39:ICU1, July 1976.

Borgstrom, G.: *The Food and People Dilemma.* Belmont CA: Wadsworth Publishing Co., 1973.

Burkitt, D., and Meisner, P.: How to manage constipation with a high-fiber diet. *Geriatrics* 34(2):33, 1979.

Byrne, J.: Lab report—tests that measure protein metabolism. *Nursing 77.* 7(10):13, 1977.

El-Beheri, B.: Dietetic audit—a giant step for nutritional care. *J. Am. Diet. Assoc.* 74:321, 1979.

Gifft, H. H., Washbon, M. B., and Harrison, G. G.: *Nutrition, Behavior and Change.* Englewood Cliffs NJ: Prentice-Hall, 1972.

Goodwin, M. T., and Pollen, G.: *Creative Food Experiences for Children.* Washington DC: Center for Science in the Public Interest, 1974.

Granz, K.: Strategies for nutritional counseling. *J. Am. Diet. Assoc.* 74:431, 1979.

Hegsted, D. M.: Food and nutrition policy: Probability and practicality. *J. Am. Diet. Assoc.* 74:534, 1979.

Ikeda, J.: *For Teenagers Only: Change Your Habits to Change Your Shape.* Palo Alto: Bull Publishing Co., 1979.

Jordan, H. A., Levitz, L. S., and Kimbrell, G. M.: *Eating Is Okay. A Radical Approach to Successful Weight Loss.* New York: Rawson Associates, 1976.

Katz, D., and Goodwin, M. T.: *Food: When Nutrition, Politics, and Culture Meet, An Activities Guide for Teachers.* Washington DC: Center for Science in the Public Interest, 1976.

Keithley, J.: Proper nutritional assessment can prevent hospital malnutrition. *Nursing 79.* 9(2):68, 1979.

Lewis, C. W.: Body image and obesity. *J. Psychiatr. Nurs.* 16(1):22, 1978.

Nash, J. D., and Long, L. O.: *Taking Charge of Your Weight and Well-Being.* Palo Alto: Bull Publishing Co., 1978.

Patient Teaching. *Nurs. Digest* 6(1) Spring 1978.

Schneggenberger, C.: History-taking skills, How do you rate? *Nursing 79.* 9(3):97, 1979.

Sims, L.: The community nutritionist as change agent. *Family and Community Health* 1(4):83, 1979.

Stuart, R. B., and Davis, B.: *Slim Chance in a Fat World* (Condensed ed, rev). Champaign IL: Research Press Co., 1978.

Wortman, S., and Cummings, R. W., Jr.: *To Feed This World: The Challenge and the Strategy.* Baltimore: Johns Hopkins University Press, 1978.

Diet Changes for Meeting Special Needs

27

Diet changes and stress

The type and degree of dietary change required for an individual should be based on the health professionals' assessment of how stressors have affected an individual's intake, absorption, utilization, and/or excretion of nutrients. The stressors which sometimes make diet modification necessary may be of the following types: (1) stressors related to disease, injury (trauma), or surgery; (2) stressors related to hospitalization or other forms of restriction of activities of daily living; or (3) stressors related to medications, radiation therapy, and other forms of treatment.

Some physiological responses produced by a stressor are localized and specific. Other physiological responses to any stressor are generalized and nonspecific. (They affect the body as a whole.) The *general adaptation syndrome* is a term used to refer to the nonspecific responses.[1]

EFFECTS OF STRESS ON GASTROINTESTINAL FUNCTION

Stressors such as isolation, injury (including surgery), and disease can influence the nutritional status of an individual via stimulation of the sympathetic nervous system. Different stressors may produce generalized physiological responses which are the same in type but not necessarily in degree. During stress the body gives priority to supplying the heart and striated muscle with blood to prepare for "fight or flight." In support of this, messages from the sympathetic nervous system cause constriction of blood vessels to the gastrointestinal tract. Catecholamines, which are

hormones released during stress, cause decrease in muscular activity of the tract. Decreased motility may cause development of anorexia, abdominal distention, gas pains, and constipation, all of which contribute to reduced food intake.

If stress is intensified, the parasympathetic nervous system may be stimulated. This occasionally results in hunger, but often causes nausea, vomiting, and diarrhea.

Progressive (transitional) diets

Modification of diet often enables an individual to tolerate food better when experiencing physiological or psychological stress. Progressive (transitional) diets are often used when any one of a number of conditions results in gastrointestinal manifestations of the stressed state, such as nausea and vomiting. These progressive diets are not reserved for use within health agencies.

The diets included in the progressive series are clear or surgical liquid, full liquid, soft, light, and house (regular). Sometimes the term light diet is used in place of soft diet. Many health agencies omit the light diet from the series because it hardly differs from the soft diet. Appendix 5A gives a listing of foods commonly included in the first three progressive diets. These diets are altered in texture, fiber, and flavor.

In a hospital setting the diet order is often written "Clear liquid → house, as tolerated." The nurse or dietition is then expected to use judgment in progressing an individual from one diet to the next. Similar judgment may be required of the client at home. Judgment should be based on understanding of the purposes and characteristics of each diet.

CLEAR (SURGICAL) LIQUID DIET

A clear liquid diet is planned to require a minimum of digestion and may, therefore, be appropriate when the stressed state is acute. Its major contributions are toward maintenance of fluid and electrolyte balance, along with stimulation of gastrointestinal function. Since the liquids given provide no fiber, the size and number of stools is expected to be less than normal for the individual. Unless special formulas are used, the only nutrients provided in significant amounts are water, sugar, small quantities of water-soluble vitamins (from clear fruit juices) and variable quantities of sodium and potassium (primarily from clear broth).

The volume of liquid served at each feeding is small, often beginning with frequent sips and progressing to about 180 cc. every hour or two during the day. If there is no contraindication, the liquid served may be frozen (ice chips, popsicles) or gelled (flavored gelatin dessert). Hard candies are usually allowed if the client is able to manage them safely and comfortably. Allowed changes in flavor, texture, and temperature help reduce the feeling of sensory deprivation experienced by many individuals on liquid diets. The diet should be used for the shortest possible time (usually only one to two days) unless nutritionally complete clear liquid formulas are used.

FULL LIQUID DIET

As the stressed individual's gastrointestinal function improves, a clear liquid diet is progressed to full liquids. This is achieved by adding a variety of more nourishing fluids. A full liquid diet makes nutritional adequacy possible, while minimizing "work" associated with the ingestion of food. Because no chewing is necessary, little energy is required to consume the diet. Under most circumstances, the possibility of gagging is minimized by liquid feedings. Food particles are so small that they are very susceptible to enzyme activity; therefore, digestion is promoted.

All foods which are liquid at body temperature are allowed, including ice cream if it is free of nuts, fruit pieces, and other particles. Ice cream and other high fat fluids may need to be restricted, however, if they cause distress related to slow emptying of gastric contents into the duodenum. Milk or milk-based formulas usually provide the basis for the diet. Many alternatives are available for use by individuals who are intolerant of milk because of lactose intolerance or allergy. A variety of strained foods may be used on a full liquid diet if they are diluted with juices, broth, milk, or other fluids.

The maximum volume of the feeding varies with the client and his tolerance of the diet. Frequent feedings, every 2 to 3 hours during the day, are suggested to provide recommended levels of nutrients without undue abdominal distention. Assessment of nutritional adequacy should be an ongoing process. Achiev-

ing nutritional adequacy on a full liquid diet is often difficult because liquids give a temporary feeling of fullness even if energy nutrient intake is low and because monotony tends to dull the appetite.

If possible, therefore, the client is normally progressed to the soft diet when full liquids are well tolerated. In some cases this will occur in a matter of hours; in others it will be a matter of days or weeks.

SOFT DIET

The soft diet is often ambiguously described as "easy to digest." It is hoped that the diet will provide foods which will be well tolerated even though the individual's gastrointestinal function has not completely returned to normal. The rationale for the restriction of certain groups of foods is based more on empirical observation than on results of scientific investigation. Foods which are included tend to be low in fiber, soft or tender in texture, and rather bland in flavor, as listed in Appendix 5A.

There is a movement toward liberalizing a soft diet if the client requests restricted foods and normally tolerates them. If a client requests one of these foods, the health professional should check on the policy within the agency.

Limiting the fat content of the diet is desirable in certain circumstances. Decreasing fat intake reduces the time food remains in the stomach, an advantage to a stressed individual who has symptoms related to slowing of the digestive process. Keeping meals small in size and offering nutritious snacks is helpful in promoting both comfort and adequate nutrition for the client.

POINTS OF EMPHASIS
Progressive diets (clear liquid → regular)

- *Offer a variety of flavors, textures, and temperatures within diet restrictions.*
- *Offer small, frequent feedings.*
- *Avoid continued feeding of nutritionally incomplete diets (clear liquid in particular).*
- *When fat is added to the diet, assess how well it is tolerated.*
- *Advance the client to a normal diet as soon as possible.*

EFFECTS OF STRESS ON METABOLISM OF ENERGY NUTRIENTS

Prolonged or acute stress can cause protein-energy malnutrition. This is only partially due to impairment of gastrointestinal function. The stress process affects nutrition in many ways. Stimulation of the sympathetic nervous system during stress causes chemical and hormonal responses which in turn affect the metabolism of energy nutrients. The major metabolic changes which occur as a result of stress are summarized in Table 27.1.

It should be noted that all but one of the changes in Table 27.1 are catabolic and can lead to reduction of both adipose tissue and lean body mass (muscle tissue). In many cases the overall metabolic rate is increased and the client is described as being in a *hypermetabolic* state. The hormone insulin does not significantly counteract catabolic effects during severe stress for two reasons: (1) release of insulin is inhibited by catecholamines (norepinephrine and epinephrine)[3] and (2) insulin resistance in muscle and adipose tissue is stimulated by glucocorticoids.[4]

Catabolic processes increase the level of circulating fuels (glucose and fatty acids), making energy readily available as for "fight or flight." The catabolism of muscle tissue results in increased levels of circulating amino acids. These amino acids are then available for maintenance of organs and for synthesis of essential blood proteins and enzymes. *Visceral protein* is a term which is sometimes used to refer to all of these vital proteins. Visceral proteins are maintained at the expense of muscle tissue. Rapid weight loss is an early indication of extensive protein catabolism.

The general diet order "High protein, high calorie (house or soft)" is sometimes written for clients whose nutritional needs are increased by stress. Health team members may need to interpret this order to the client and guide him in making appropriate food choices. In most circumstances, 1.5 to 2 gm. protein per kg. of body weight provides an adult with ample protein for repairing body tissue and/or meeting other moderately increased needs. This amount of protein is comparable to normal intake for most American adults and, thus, can be achieved by eating average portions of food

TABLE 27.1 *Metabolic changes associated with the stress process*[2]

METABOLIC EFFECT	CAUSATIVE AGENTS		RESULTS OF ACUTE OR PROLONGED STRESS
	Regulatory Substance	Stimulus for its Production or Release	
Lipolysis (release of fatty acids from fat cells) which *increases the free fatty acid levels of the blood*	Norepinephrine (a catecholamine), the chemical transmitter at the sympathetic nerve endings	Activation of sympathetic nerves initiated by stressor	Loss of adipose tissue
	Adrenocorticotropin (ACTH secreted by the anterior pituitary)	Excitement by hypothalamus (initiated by stressor) stimulates pituitary	
	Cortisol (a glucocorticoid secreted by the adrenal medula)	ACTH	
	Epinephrine (a catecholamine secreted by the adrenal medulla)	Nervous stimuli	
	Glucagon (secreted by the alpha cells of the islets of Langerhans)	High levels of plasma amino acids	
Gluconeogenesis (formation of glucose from amino acids) *which increases the blood glucose level*	Cortisol Glucagon High blood levels of free fatty acids	See above	Decrease in lean body mass
Glycogenolysis (hydrolysis of glycogen to form glucose) *which increases the blood glucose level*	Epinephrine Glucagon	See above	Decrease of liver glycogen stores
Protein catabolism (release of amino acids from body tissue) *which increases the level of circulating amino acids*	Cortisol	See above	Decrease in lean body mass
Protein anabolism	Growth hormone		Repair of injured tissue, synthesis of visceral proteins

from the meat, milk, and grain groups. If the appetite for meat is small, cereal with milk, custard, a milk-based beverage, or other significant protein sources might be offered between meals. If meat is avoided because the client finds it dry or tiring to chew, the health care worker might suggest a change in consistency or substitution of some protein sources which the client might enjoy more—perhaps an egg dish, a tuna sandwich, or a cup of chowder. Taking measures to increase caloric intake will usually result in increased protein intake as well.

POINTS OF EMPHASIS
Acute stress

• *Frequently assess the nutritional status of clients who are experiencing prolonged or acute stress. Be especially alert for signs of protein-energy malnutrition.*

• *Implement a nutritional care plan which will promote recovery and minimize the possibility of complications.*

INFECTION

Infection can pose a severe nutritional threat, especially in persons whose nutritional status is initially borderline.

Infection may result in decreased intake and absorption of nutrients, altered metabolism, and increased urinary losses of some nutrients. Negative nitrogen balance appears to be the most general nutritional consequence of an infectious disease. At the onset of a febrile response, urinary losses of nitrogen rise sharply, reflecting marked tissue catabolism. Negative nitrogen balance may be most marked in sepsis (infection characterized by the presence of microorganisms or their toxic products in the bloodstream). Occasionally, negative nitrogen balance develops in subclinical infections, even though the affected person has neither anorexia nor appreciable fever.[5] Appropriate feeding of protein and calories usually can lessen the amount of nitrogen lost during infection.

At present there are no specific instructions regarding micronutrient requirements during infection.[6] It is not clear, for example, if administering vitamins will benefit a well-nourished person when he develops an infection.[7] Supplementation appears to be indicated in long term infection; it is strongly advised in persons who were at nutritional risk before they became infected.

SURGERY

Preoperative nutrition

Surgery is an example of a stressor which intiates the stressed state and, thus, alters the process of nutrition. When surgery is elective, the health team should assess if and how nutritional status is to be improved preoperatively. In making the assessment, health care providers should give special attention to the following:

1. Fluid and electrolyte balance. If the client is not in balance, additional stress caused by surgery may precipitate a life-threatening crisis.
2. Prothrombin time. If abnormally long, vitamin K may be needed to allow normal blood clotting.
3. Adequacy of vitamin C and zinc intake (determined from diet recall or from laboratory tests). These nutrients are vital to wound healing.
4. Signs of protein-energy malnutrition. If reserves are low or absent, a client is at greater risk of complications during and after the surgical procedure.

In setting goals involving diet change, health care workers give recognition to relationships between surgery and nutritional status:

1. Good nutritional status prior to surgery improves the prognosis of the outcome of surgery. It decreases the risk of complications both during and after surgery. A well-nourished individual has better reserves for coping with the stresses of surgery and with the reduced nutrient intake which usually accompanies an operation.
2. Good preoperative nutritional status is of special benefit to infants, children, and the elderly, all of whom may have more limited capacity to tolerate stress than does the normal adult.
3. Extreme obesity is a special type of nutritional problem which increases risks during and after surgery. The miles of extra blood vessels needed for nourishing excess adipose tissue increase the work of the heart. Adipose tissue is more susceptible to wound dehiscence and to infection than is muscle tissue. The risk of pulmonary complications is increased since obese individuals breathe poorly when lying on their side.[8] Risks will be reduced if an obese client loses adipose tissue prior to surgery but maintains other nutrient stores. Fat reduction may also alleviate hypertension and improve the management of diabetes mellitus in affected individuals, thereby increasing their ability to adapt to the stress of surgery.
4. Vitamin and mineral (electrolyte) replacement can usually be achieved quickly. Protein replacement proceeds slowly, often requiring weeks. In severe protein deficiency, fluid balance is dependent on protein replacement. Correction of obesity may require months.

If it is determined that surgery is to be postponed until nutritional deficits or excesses are corrected, health team members should work with the client and his family in developing a realistic diet plan for achieving specified goals.

Prior to gastrointestinal surgery a modified diet (low residue or clear liquid diet) may be ordered to minimize gastrointestinal contents and flatus. Clients whose nutritional status is poor or borderline should be given a nutritionally complete modified diet even though the modification is required for only a short time, (perhaps for two to three days). Malnourished clients can ill afford even brief periods of inadequate nutrition.

Postoperative nutrition

Surgery initiates gastrointestinal and metabolic changes associated with stress. How long these responses continue depends on the nature of the surgery, other stressors present (such as infection), the ability of the individual to adapt, and the medical interventions employed.

Suitable diet modification is affected by each of these variables. Postoperatively a client must depend upon health professionals for an adequate supply of essential nutrients in a form which can be tolerated.

Postoperative nutritional care must be tailored to the client's needs. Often the first feedings are parenteral feedings; these may soon be followed by the progressive series of diets. If the stress is severe, specialized parenteral feedings may be necessary to promote adequate nutrition. If use of the gastrointestinal tract is safe, as is the case following many minor operations, parenteral feedings may be omitted and clear liquids are given as the first nourishment. It is preferable to introduce nutrients by mouth when there are no contraindications. Specialized oral feedings are available for clients who cannot tolerate the usual dietary progression.

It is important for health care providers to meet the client's increased nutritional needs to prevent loss of lean body mass and to decrease the likelihood of infection and other complications.

EFFECTS OF PHARMACOLOGICAL AND RADIATION THERAPY AND OTHER TREATMENTS ON NUTRITIONAL STATUS

Drug and radiation therapy are two other types of stressors which have both generalized and specific effects in relation to nutritional status of a client. These stressors therefore may lead to a need for diet change. In recent years there has been increased awareness of interrelationships between these stressors and nutritional status. Frequently the nutritional status of an individual affects the amount of drug or radiation therapy which can be tolerated. On the other hand, a treatment may adversely affect a person's nutritional status.[9]

The health worker should distinguish between purposes of drugs and their side effects as related to nutrition. Some drugs are given because they interfere with the absorption or metabolism of a specific nutrient. If drug-nutrient interaction is part of the mechanism of the therapeutic action of a drug, careful monitoring is required to balance the benefits against the associated nutritional risks. Using the drug methotrexate in the treatment of cancer is an example of this. (Methotrexate interferes with utilization of folic acid, and this is partly responsible for its chemotherapeutic effect.)

More often it is the side effects of drugs, radiation therapy, and other treatments which seriously interfere with nutritional status. Sometimes these stressors greatly increase nutrient losses via the gastrointestinal tract or urine. Side effects of some medications include decreased absorption or altered metabolism of specific nutrients. Direct or indirect exposure of the gastrointestinal tract to radiation frequently results in damage to the mucosal cells and serious interference with digestive processes. The most common side effects of pharmacological and radiation therapy result in reduced intake of food.

One or more of the following symptoms is produced by a wide variety of drugs, radiation therapy, and other stressful treatments: dry mouth, unpleasant metallic taste, anorexia, nausea, vomiting, heartburn, abdominal distress, gastric irritation, diarrhea, and constipation. When some of these symptoms are present, the client tends to lose interest in food. Nutrient intake drops and nutrient reserves may be depleted. Health professionals need to intervene with measures to increase food intake.

Side effects of any drug are most likely to be a source of problems when high dosages are used over a period of time or when individuals are at nutritional risk because of age (children and elderly), chronic illness, or a history of poor to marginally good food intake.

Antineoplastic drugs and cytotoxic agents (drugs used in the treatment of cancer) invariably have some nutrition-related side effects, some of which are summarized in Table 27.2. Antimicrobial agents (e.g., penicillin, isoniazid, sulfonamides) are also commonly involved in drug-nutrient interactions which can have a significant effect on a person's health. For example, when given orally or by suppository or enema, many antimicrobial agents interfere with normal bacterial production of vitamin K. There are so many antimicrobials in use that the health professional should be sure to check current literature concerning possible drug-nutrient interactions. Some other types of drug-nutrient interactions are identified in relation to client care in the remaining chapters of the text.

The route of administration of drugs is in some cases related to the occurrence of gastrointestinal side effects. For example, drugs taken by mouth may pro-

TABLE 27.2 Cancer chemotherapeutic agents that can adversely affect nutritional status

EFFECTS

DRUG	Stomatitis	Nausea	Vomiting	Diarrhea	Oral ulcerations	Constipation	Ulceration of buccal mucosa	Gingivitis	Metallic taste	Prolonged anorexia	Abdominal pain	Glossitis
actinomycin D	X	X	X	X	X							
bleomycin	X	X	X									
cyclophosphamide		X	X									
cylarabine		X	X	X	X							
doxorubicin	X	X	X	X								
5-fluorouracil	X	X	X	X	X							
hydroxyuria	X	X	X	X		X	X					
melphalan		X	X									
6-mercaptopurine	X	X	X									
methotrexate	X	X	X	X	X			X				
nitrogen mustard		X	X	X					X			
nitrosoureas		X	X								X	
vinblastine	X	X	X	X		X					X	X
vincristine		X	X			X					X	

From Visconti, J. A.: Drug-food interaction. *Nutrition in Disease.* Columbus, OH: Ross Laboratories, May 1977, p. 18. Used with permission.

duce nausea and vomiting as a result of their presence in the gastrointestinal tract. If these drugs are given by injection or intravenously, the gastrointestinal side effects will be less marked unless the drug acts directly on the vomiting center of the brain. Taking food with drugs which topically irritate the digestive tract may reduce the occurrence of gastrointestinal side effects because of the mixing and dilution which occur. However, some drugs must be administered when the stomach is empty in order to promote their maximum absorption. Some drugs result in damage to the intestinal tract even when given parenterally.

quency of feeding, or timing of feeding may alleviate gastrointestinal symptoms, increasing the comfort of a person who is being treated with irritating drugs or radiation of the gastrointestinal tract. Diet modification can reduce the fluid retention which is a side effect of steroids.

Diet changes or nutrient supplements are in order if a drug causes excessive excretion of one or more essential nutrients. If adequate nutritional status can be attained and maintained during therapy, it may be possible for the client to tolerate high dosages, thus increasing the potential for therapeutic effectiveness.[9]

> **POINTS OF EMPHASIS**
> *Drug and radiation therapy*
>
> • *Drugs and radiation therapy cause many types of side effects which can interfere with normal nutrition.*
> • *Drugs taken by mouth are often topically irritating to the gastrointestinal tract.*
> • *Some drugs irritate the gastrointestinal tract even if given parenterally.*

MODIFIED DIETS AS RELATED TO SIDE EFFECTS OF TREATMENTS

There are numerous examples of cases in which diet modification is used because of certain side effects of therapy. Diets modified in texture, fiber, flavor, fre-

STUDY QUESTIONS

1. Keep a 24-hr. food intake record for a patient on a clear liquid diet. (Include parenteral feedings, if any.) Determine the patient's caloric and nutrient intake. Compare intake with the RDA. Explain why the patient should be quickly progressed to a more adequate diet.
2. Use Table 27.1 to answer the following questions:
   a. Why may the blood glucose level be high normal during stress even though no food has been eaten recently?
   b. What hormones result in increased blood levels of free fatty acids?
   c. During stress the level of circulating amino acids is increased. What is the source of these amino acids?
   d. Name three ways in which cortisol affects the

fuels circulating in the bloodstream during stress.

3. Individuals undergoing radiation therapy should be assisted to meet nutrient requirements by diet modification and supportive medication if necessary. This results in the normal benefits of good nutrition. What additional benefits does the individual gain?

4. Look up side effects of medications used to reduce gastrointestinal discomfort. Determine if any of these may affect nutritional status. Suggested medications:

Aluminum hydroxide

Sodium bicarbonate

Phenothiazides such as prochlorperazine

References

*1. Selye, H.: The evolution of the stress concept. *Amer. Scientist* 61:692, 1973.

2. Montgomery, R., et al.: *Biochemistry: A Case Oriented Approach,* ed. 2. St. Louis: C. V. Mosby Co., 1977.

3. Porte, D., Jr., and Robertson, R. P.: Control of insulin secretion by catecholamines, stress and the sympathetic nervous system. *Fed. Proc.* 32:1792, 1973.

4. Burns, T. W., et al.: Studies on the interdependent effects of stress and the adrenal cortex on carbohydrate metabolism in Man. *J. Clin. Invest.* 32:781, 1953.

5. Beisel, W. R.: Magnitude of the host nutritional responses to infection. *Am. J. Clin. Nutr.* 30:1236, 1977.

6. Scrimshaw, N. S.: Effect of infection on nutrient requirements. *Am. J. Clin. Nutr.* 30:1536, 1977.

7. Vitale, J. J.: The impact of infection on vitamin metabolism: An unexplored area. *Am. J. Clin. Nutr.* 30:1473, 1977.

8. Shafer, K. N., et al.: *Medical-Surgical Nursing,* ed. 6. St. Louis: C. V. Mosby Co., 1975.

*9. March, D. C.: *Handbook: Interactions of Selected Drugs with Nutritional Status in Man,* ed. 2. Chicago: The American Dietetic Association, 1978.

* Recommended reading

28

Alterations in fluid and electrolyte balance

CAUSES OF FLUID AND ELECTROLYTE IMBALANCES

A health professional who can detect changes in intake or output of fluid and electrolytes can often take remedial action to prevent or retard the development of serious problems. Those who know the principles and characteristics of diets modified in fluid or electrolytes can assist the client to cooperate with his plan of care in order to stabilize or improve his condition.

Alterations in fluid and electrolyte balance commonly develop in a variety of diseases and injuries (including surgery). Fluid and electrolyte imbalances also arise as a result of such stresses as strenuous physical exercise, exposure to extreme heat, use of some pharmacological agents, radiation therapy, and fasting. Any of these stresses may result in altered input, output, distribution, or metabolism of water and/or nutrient electrolytes (sodium, potassium, calcium, magnesium, chloride, and phosphate). Hydrogen and bicarbonate ion concentration may also be altered by stress, resulting in acid-base imbalances.

Fluid and electrolyte imbalances develop much more quickly in the very young and in the elderly than they do in other age groups. In infants the rate of turnover of fluid is seven times as great as that occurring in adults. In addition, there is greater potential for loss of fluid by infants and young children than by older individuals because of the child's large body surface in proportion to body weight. The higher metabolic rate of infants and young children causes a proportionately higher acid production, increasing their susceptibility to imbalances in hydrogen ion and other electrolytes. Immaturity of body systems, such as the renal and endocrine systems, predisposes infants toward rapid shifts in fluid and electrolyte balance.

When older adults are compared to younger ones, they are more susceptible to rapid and serious changes in fluid and electrolyte balance. This is a result of the older person's lower water content.

To determine if a fluid and electrolyte problem is likely to develop, stabilize, or resolve, health professionals assess intake and output of substances involved. Table 28.1 identifies factors which may alter input or output of water and/or electrolytes and the type of imbalance to anticipate in each case. Diet modification is often one of the principal means of preventing these imbalances and of restoring balance, as explained in the following sections of this chapter.

Altered distribution of fluid and electrolytes within the body may take many forms. Examples include the development of swollen ankles in a person who sits most of the day, a shift of potassium from intracellular to extracellular fluid as a result of thermal injury, and increased demineralization of bone associated with immobility. Relations between diet and altered distribution of fluid and electrolytes are discussed in conjunction with the particular electrolytes.

TABLE 28.1 Factors related to specific alterations in fluid and electrolyte balance

FACTORS INFLUENCING FLUID AND ELECTROLYTE BALANCE	TYPE OF ALTERATION WHICH MAY DEVELOP
ALTERED INPUT OF WATER AND/OR ELECTROLYTES	
Decreased	
Partial or complete abstinence from food and/or fluid; allowing the client nothing by mouth	Dehydration if fluid intake is low / Potassium deficit if food intake is very low
Concentrated tube feedings without supplemental water	Dehydration
Malabsorption	Deficits of water and electrolytes
Depressed ability to absorb calcium in chronic renal failure	Calcium deficit (hypocalcemia)
Increased	
Bizarre eating or drinking behavior associated with contests or psychiatric disorders	Fluid overload with dilutional hyponatremia is most common
Excessive intake of milk with antacids as in home treatment of peptic ulcers	Calcium excess
Excessive calcium absorption in idiopathic urolithiasis	Calcium excess in urine (hypercalcuria)
Too rapid intravenous infusions	Fluid overload / Deficits or excesses of electrolytes depending on nature of the IV solution and the rate at which it is infused
ALTERED OUTPUT OF FLUID AND/OR ELECTROLYTES	
Altered renal losses	
Increased urine production (polyuria) as in:	Dehydration / Variations in hormones and renal integrity cause different types of electrolyte imbalances
Uncontrolled diabetes mellitus	
Diabetes insipidus (deficiency of antidiuretic hormone)	
Some types of renal disease during the stages of diuresis	Sodium and potassium deficit
Diuretic therapy	Depletion of sodium and water could result from excessive use of any diuretic / Potassium, magnesium, and/or zinc depletion may occur with furosemide, thiazides, and ethacrynic acid
Decreased or absent urine production (oliguria and anuria respectively) as in:	Retention of water and electrolytes
Chronic or acute renal failure	
Congestive heart failure, shock	
Excessive production of antidiuretic hormone	
Altered aldosterone levels:	
Increased aldosterone production	Sodium retention, potassium loss
Decreased aldosterone production as in Addison's disease or adrenalectomy	Potassium retention, sodium loss
Other types of drug therapy:	
Mineralocorticoids	Retention of sodium and water
Glucocorticoids	
Androgens	
Estrogens	
Altered extrarenal losses	
Diaphoresis (excessive perspiration) as in fevers, myocardial infarction	Dehydration and sodium deficit (As much as 1L. of fluid may be lost during each episode of acute diaphoresis requiring linen change[1])
Increased insensible perspiration associated with hot, dry environmental conditions	Dehydration and sodium and potassium deficit
Increased perspiration associated with vigorous physical activity, especially in hot weather	
Increased sodium concentration in perspiration (cystic fibrosis)	Sodium deficit
Vomiting	
Of gastric contents (repeated)	Dehydration, chloride deficit (alkalosis)
Deep vomiting of bilious contents	Dehydration, sodium deficit (acidosis)
Increased respiratory rate	Dehydration
Decreased respiratory loss due to high humidity	Fluid overload in individuals with impaired renal function (ultrasonic nebulization may actually result in absorption of up to 1000 cc. water in 24-hr[1])
Diarrhea	Extra secretion of potassium, sodium, and water compounds effects of decreased absorption
Fistula drainage, drainage tubes	The type of electrolyte deficit which may develop depends on the composition of the interestinal secretion in the part of the tract the fistula drains
Exudates due to loss of skin as in trauma, burns, infection, ulceration, certain inflammatory diseases	Dehydration and sodium depletion

RETENTION OF SODIUM AND WATER

Effects

Sodium retention is one of the most common electrolyte imbalances. Water is usually retained whenever sodium retention occurs, as in congestive heart failure and chronic renal failure. Retention of 20 mEq. (460 mg.) Na* per day results in accumulation of about 1 L. of extracellular fluid per week.[2] This would show up as a gain of 1 kg. (2.2 lb.) on the scale.

Most of the excess sodium and water moves from the blood to the interstitial fluid, allowing maintenance of a relatively normal blood volume. When fluid retention is observable, the condition is called edema. Edema often takes the form of puffiness in the fingers and ankles or sometimes *anasarca* (edema of the entire body).

Retention of sodium and water can seriously impair health and cause extreme discomfort. A significant increase in workload of the heart results from retention of these nutrients. The overworked heart may fail. Congestion in the lungs (pulmonary edema) may lead to severe, sometimes fatal, respiratory distress. Excessive fluid in the extremities may interfere with mobility and activities of daily living.

* When referring to intake of sodium and potassium, some health care agencies use the unit *milliequivalents* (mEq.) while others use the unit *milligrams*. The method for converting from one unit to another is shown in the Conversion Table on page 301.

Reducing Na intake, sometimes in conjunction with diuretic therapy, increases net Na excretion. This may have the following beneficial effects: (1) decrease in workload of the heart, both at rest and during exercise; (2) prevention or control of hypertension (due to reduction in fluid volume and perhaps to specific effects of decreased sodium)[3]; (3) relief from discomfort and potentially dangerous side effects of edema; (4) improved mobility; or (5) prevention of development of edema.

Some types of edema which are due to fluid distribution problems (Table 28.2) cannot be relieved by a sodium restricted diet. Health professionals should be able to distinguish between types of edema which usually benefit from sodium restriction and those which do not.

POINTS OF EMPHASIS
Fluid and electrolyte imbalances

• *Injury, disease, medications, extremes of diet, or other stresses may lead to fluid and electrolyte imbalances, especially in the very young and in the elderly.*

• *The type of fluid and electrolyte imbalance which may develop can be predicted from knowledge of composition of fluids lost, effects of medications and treatments, and alterations in normal intake.*

• *Observable retention of sodium and water (edema) is often, but not invariably, alleviated by sodium restriction and/or prescribed diuretics.*

TABLE 28.2 *Factors which may interfere with normal movement of fluid and lead to its accumulation in the interstitial space*

FACTOR	COMMENT
Decreased blood oncotic pressure	Less fluid moves back into the capillary when blood oncotic pressure is low. Low serum albumin level causes decreased blood oncotic pressure. This may occur in protein deficiency (especially in kwashiorkor and advanced anorexia nervosa), nephrosis, cirrhosis of the liver, and burns. Recommended sodium intake varies with the type and stage of the disease. Diet modification to restore oncotic pressure usually takes precedence over sodium restriction, except in cirrhosis.
Increased blood hydrostatic pressure at the venous end of the capillary	Less fluid moves back into the capillary when there is this increased force opposing movement of fluid back into the capillary. This occurs in congestive heart failure, cirrhosis of the liver, and edema associated with body position and lack of activity (dependent edema). Dependent edema is not responsive to sodium restriction; other types are. In cirrhosis, increased venous pressure occurs primarily in the portal vein, so that fluid accumulates in the peritoneal cavity. This type of edema, which is characterized by greatly increased abdominal girth, is called ascites.
Increase in capillary permeability associated with the inflammatory process	The resulting fluid accumulation is localized, such as that occurring in tissue injury. Sodium restriction is not beneficial.
Decrease in movement of interstitial fluid into lymphatic circulation due to lymphatic block	The area in which edema develops is that which is normally drained by the affected lymphatics. Sodium restriction is generally not necessary

Sodium restricted diets

There are several levels of sodium restricted diets which are commonly used for the prevention, control, or amelioration of fluid retention and hypertension. The most widely used of these are the levels established by the American Heart Association (AHA),[4-6] namely:

Strict—500 mg. (22 mEq.) sodium—Used to reduce edema. Occasionally used as a maintenance diet when sodium output is very low.

Moderate—1000 mg. (43 mEq.) sodium—May be used to relieve mild edema, or as a maintenance diet for prevention of edema or control of hypertension.

Mild—3-5 gm. (130-215 mEq.) sodium—Frequently used as a maintenance diet to prevent the development of edema, as for individuals on steroid therapy, or to control blood pressure. The term "No Added Salt Diet" is used for this diet in some health agencies, but the practice is to be avoided because it is vague and may be misleading to clients.

A severe sodium restricted diet (250 mg. or 12 mEq. Na) is occasionally prescribed for short periods of time when drastic reduction in sodium intake is indicated, as in severe congestive heart failure. Other levels of sodium intake may be prescribed according to the client's need. A 2000 mg. (86 mEq.) sodium diet, although not one of the levels set by the AHA, is a commonly prescribed level of sodium restriction used primarily as a maintenance diet.

In setting the level of sodium restriction, the physician and other health team members should consider what is most realistic and beneficial for the client in terms of both diet and diuretic therapy. The client who habitually refuses to take a diuretic because of its side effects may be able to avoid edema or control hypertension by reducing sodium intake. Conversely, a client who eats all his meals at a cafeteria and, therefore, finds it impossible to follow a moderate sodium restricted diet can perhaps be maintained on a mild sodium restriction with an increased dosage of diuretic.

There is no one level of sodium restriction which is

Conversion Table for Milliequivalents and Milligrams

MINERAL	EQUIVALENT WEIGHT
Sodium	23
Potassium	39

A. To convert mEq to mg, multiply the number of mEq of the electrolyte by the equivalent weight of that electrolyte.

Example: 22 mEq Na = ? mg Na
$$22 \times 23 = 506 \text{ mg Na}$$

B. To convert mg. to mEq, divide the number of mg of the electrolyte by the equivalent weight of that electrolyte.

Example: 200 mg K = ? mEq K
$$\frac{200}{39} = 5.1 \text{ mEq K}$$

C. To convert weight of salt to weight of sodium, multiply weight of salt times 0.4. (Salt = about 40% sodium by weight)

Example: 5 gm salt contains how much sodium?
$$5 \times 0.4 = 2.0 \text{ gm (2000 mg) Na}$$

correct for every person with the same disease. The nurse or dietitian may wish to initiate a health team conference if the diet and/or drug order(s) appear to be unrealistic for the client.

SOURCES OF SODIUM

Distinguishing between the characteristics of various sodium restricted diets requires familiarity with sources of Na and their significance. Sources include food and seasonings, water, and medications.

Food and seasonings are the largest contributors to sodium intake. Foods differ in Na content depending on (1) the amount inherently present in the food (naturally occurring Na) and (2) the amount of Na added in processing (Table 28.3). Foods naturally containing significant amount of Na include milk and

TABLE 28.3 *A comparison of some foods which are* naturally *high in sodium with foods which contain* added *sodium.*

NATURALLY HIGH IN SODIUM		CONTAIN ADDED SODIUM	
Food	Amt. of Na (mg)	Food	Amt. of Na (mg)*
240 ml (1 c) skim milk	125	240 ml (1 c) buttermilk	315
85 gm (3 oz) portions of foods from meat group:		85 gm (3 oz) portions of foods from the meat group:	
Fresh roast pork	61	Cured baked ham	637
Beef liver	156	Sausage	630
Lobster	120	Imitation sausage (meat analog)	850
Shrimp	160	Bologna	1100
		Sardines, canned, drained	700
120 ml (½ c) cooked spinach	45	120 ml (½ c) canned spinach	242
120 ml (½ c) cooked celery	66		

* Subject to considerable variation among different brands.

milk products (excluding butterfat), eggs, meat, fish, poultry, and a few vegetables such as celery, greens, carrots, beets, and turnips. One serving of a food which is "naturally high in sodium" contributes Na in the range of about 30 to 160 mg. (as in 120 ml. [½ c.] cooked carrots and 85 gm. [3 oz.] cooked shrimp). Animal fats and plant foods other than those previously mentioned are very low in Na unless it has been added in processing.

Salt is the additive most commonly responsible for the high sodium content of many processed foods. Salt is approximately 40 percent Na by weight. One teaspoon of salt (5 gm.) provides about 2 gm. of sodium. It is not unusual for one serving of a commercially prepared food such as seasoned rice or soup to contain 500 mg. to 1 gm. Na. Foods which have been prepared with or stored in brine contain added salt. (Brine is a concentrated solution of salt dissolved in water.) A large dill pickle, for example, contains about 2 gm. Na absorbed from the brine used in its preparation.

Moderately large increases in sodium content of foods result from use of additives such as monosodium glutamate (a flavor enhancer which contains 735 mg. Na per tsp.), bicarbonate of soda (commonly called baking soda—1335 mg. per tsp.), and baking powder (390 mg. Na per tsp.).

Smaller amounts of Na are contributed by miscellaneous sodium containing compounds such as sodium nitrite, benzoate of soda, sodium saccharin, sodium propionate, and others. Sometimes the amount of Na contributed by one of these additives is so small that it can easily be incorporated in a sodium restricted diet.

The sodium content of water in different parts of the country ranges between practically 0 to 120 mg. Na or more per L. The amount in the local water supply can be determined by calling the local health department or the local branch of the American Heart Association. In hard water areas it may be advisable for a health professional to ask the client if there is a water softener operating in his home. Water softeners remove the minerals which cause water to be hard and replace them with Na. Hartshorn gives suggestions for dealing with this situation.[8]

A wide variety of medications, including nonprescription drugs, contain Na. Cautions against use of sodium-containing proprietary medications become important with increasing severity of the sodium restriction.

A given level of sodium intake can be achieved by innumerable combinations of sodium sources. The greater the amount of Na allowed, the greater the choice of foods.

DIET DESCRIPTIONS

For any given level of sodium restriction, the emphasis should be on achieving a diet which is tailored to meet the individual's various needs without exceeding the sodium intake allowed. Sample plans for sodium restricted diets are given in Appendix 5D. It is to a client's benefit to distinguish between significant and insignificant sources of Na for his level of restriction. This is done in the following diet descriptions.

500 mg. (22 mEq.) sodium diet The Na which occurs naturally in food usually contributes *all* of the Na allowed on a 500 mg. Na diet. *No* foods are used which have been processed with sodium-containing additives, unless the amount of Na involved is exceedingly small. In fact, this diet is so low in Na that there are restrictions imposed on use of foods previously identified as naturally containing significant amounts of Na. If water contains more than 20 mg. Na per L., use of distilled water for beverages and cooking is recommended.

A plan for a 500 mg. sodium diet might include the following foods for one day:

	Na (mg)
490 cc (2 c) milk (120 mg. Na/c)	240
1 large egg	60
120 gm (4 oz) fresh meat, fish, poultry	100
Any of the vegetables which are naturally *low* in sodium *and*	
Other foods, either fresh or processed without added sodium, as desired to round out the menu and meet nutritional needs	100
Total	500

Unless the appetite is very large, the intake of allowed fruits, vegetables, and cereals is unlikely to contribute more than 50 mg. Na per day. Thus it may be possible to incorporate an extra 60 gm. of meat or some other sodium source into a 500 mg. Na diet. Variations in use of foods which are naturally high in Na are also possible. A dietitian or nutritionist can adapt plans to meet an individual's nutritional needs.

A sample menu for a 500 mg. Na diet is given in Table 28.4. Amounts of food are specified only for those foods which *must be limited* because of their natural sodium content. Many other variations are possible. Distribution of food into meals can be changed as needed to fit in with the client's lifestyle.

250 mg. (11 mEq.) sodium diet This low level of sodium intake can be achieved by following the 500 mg. Na plan (given prior to this diet) with the substitution of specially processed low sodium milk for ordinary milk. Although low sodium milk is lower in certain nutrients than is milk, it makes an important nutritional contribution which cannot be equalled by any other food which is low in Na. Low sodium milk is somewhat unpalatable. It is most apt to be accepted if served icy cold, perhaps with a low sodium flavoring added. It is quite acceptable when used in low sodium milk-based puddings, cream soups, cream sauces, and bakery products. Low sodium milk is more expensive than is ordinary milk and may be hard to obtain. Its use is seldom justified on diets which allow more than 250 mg. Na.

TABLE 28.4 *Sample 500 mg. (22 mEq) sodium diet*

BREAKFAST
Frozen orange juice
1 soft cooked egg
Low sodium toast with
Low sodium margarine or butter and regular jelly
Coffee with 30 ml (2 tbsp) milk

LUNCH
Sandwich made with low sodium bread, 60 gm (2 oz) unsalted sliced roast beef, lettuce, tomato, onion, and low sodium mayonnaise
Fresh fruit (any type)
240 ml (1 c) skim milk
Homemade low sodium spice cookies

SNACK
Salt-free crackers with low sodium peanut butter
Lemonade

DINNER
85 gm (3 oz) (edible portion) broiled chicken, cranberry sauce
Baked potato with 30 ml (2 tbsp) sour cream and chives
Cooked fresh or frozen broccoli with low sodium margarine or butter and lemon if desired
180 ml (¾ c) skim milk
Homemade low sodium whole wheat rolls
Tossed salad with homemade low sodium salad dressing
Tea with lemon

± 1900 kcal*

* A considerable range of calories is possible depending on portion sizes and recipes used.

1 gm. (43 mEq.) sodium diet If the amount of sodium allowed exceeds 500 mg. daily, it is possible to increase the intake of foods which naturally contain significant amounts of sodium. Alternatively, it is possible to include some foods or flavorings which contain salt or other sodium additives.

Allowing a client to participate in deciding how the extra Na is to be added may maximize the possibility that he will comply with the diet. The American Heart Association plan for a 1 gm. sodium diet has a section entitled "The other 500 mg. sodium." This section groups some commonly liked salted foods according to their sodium content. The client may use the lists to determine the serving size of a food which would provide a given amount of Na (i.e., 200 mg. or 500 mg.). By referring to a table of food composition or to nutritional labels, the health professional could expand the lists to include foods the client would particularly like to use occasionally. Table 28.5 is an example of an individualized list which the dietitian might provide for a client. No food is definitely contraindicated because of its sodium content, as long as the client is willing and able to limit portion size to that which fits in with his diet. In fact the AHA plan indicates that a *scant* ¼ tsp. of salt may be used as a means of adding 500 mg. Na to the diet. If this method is chosen, the client should have his own salt shaker. The allowed amount of salt is added to an empty shaker each morning. Any salt remaining at the end of the day is emptied from the shaker, not added to the next day's allowance.

Some health agencies have diet forms which group foods according to sodium content, either by mg. of Na or by "points." (One point usually equals 1 mEq. Na.) The client knows the sodium allotment for the day and is shown how to exchange foods of equal sodium content. This allows for maximum variety within the restriction.

Many clients feel most comfortable following a regular pattern rather than choosing different sources of Na each day. One of many possible designs for a 1 gm. sodium diet includes the 500 mg. sodium foundation diet with the incorporation of:

	Na (mg)
2 slices thinly sliced regular bread (120 mg Na/slice)	240
20 gm (4 tsp) regular butter or margarine	200
1 serving vegetable naturally rich in Na	60
Total	500

Many clients find that they prefer to distribute their salt-containing food. Regular butter or margarine

TABLE 28.5 *Individualized list of sodium-containing foods*

A. Foods providing about 50 mg sodium:
   5gm (1 tsp) margarine
   10gm (2 tsp) regular peanut butter
   4 ml (scant teaspoon) prepared mustard

B. Foods providing about 100 mg sodium:
   5ml (1 tsp) Worcestershire sauce
   180 ml (6 oz) Shasta Club soda

C. Foods providing about 150 mg sodium:
   30 gm (2 Tbsp) regular peanut butter
   15 ml (1 Tbsp) regular catsup

D. Foods providing about 200 mg sodium:
   30 gm (1 oz) cheddar cheese
   60 gm (2 oz) cottage cheese
   30gm (¼ c) canned drained tuna
   15 ml (1 Tbsp) regular French dressing

E. Foods providing about 500 mg sodium:
   ½ bouillon cube
   75 gm (2½ oz) canned corned beef

Directions: Each day you may use an extra 500 mg sodium in your diet plan. Many combinations are possible, for example:

   2 foods from group C + 1 food from group D
   2 A's + 2 B's + or 1 D
   or
   Only 1 E

Be sure to measure carefully!

Follow your diet plan carefully to be sure you get enough nutrients without getting too much sodium. Call me if you have any questions.

Anne Morgan, R.D.   289-2468
Dietitian   Phone number

might be used to flavor potatoes, other vegetables, rice, pasta, fried egg, broiled fish, low sodium toast, or sandwiches. Regular bread used in a sandwich compliments unsalted meat.

2 gm. (87 mEq.) sodium diet The design of a 2 gm. sodium diet may vary considerably, particularly in relation to an individual's caloric requirements. A client who has a small food intake requires relatively few restrictions to stay within the 2 gm. of Na allowed. For example, a diet low in calories could be planned to include several salt-containing foods on a regular basis, such as bread, ready-to-eat cereal, natural cheddar cheese, and peanut butter. A client who is very active would quickly exceed the Na allowance if larger amounts of these same salt-containing foods were used.

A Chinese-American or Japanese-American client would probably want the plan to allow for the use of some soy sauce. An Orthodox Jew would want to have a plan that would allow for the use of kosher meat.* Health workers should find out if a Mormon has large stores of canned salted food on hand so that it can be incorporated into the diet if possible.

3 to 5 gm. (130–215 mEq.) sodium diet Plans developed by different health agencies for diets which are mildly restricted in Na vary somewhat, reflecting the fact that there is more than one way to achieve the same result. The American Heart Association plan allows half the usual amount of salt and monosodium glutamate in cooking and at the table, but prohibits use of all other salty seasonings and highly salted foods. Many plans such as the one shown in Appendix 5D aim for the lower level of Na. These stricter plans usually specify that minimal amounts of salt may be used in cooking, but instruct the client to *avoid* (1) addition of salt at the table, (2) use of salty seasonings (including monosodium glutamate) at any time, and (3) use of highly salted processed foods. Again, the diet counselor may adapt the plan to promote greater acceptance and compliance by the client.

A distinction is made in the types of cheese allowed on the 3 to 5 gm. sodium diet. Processed cheeses are to be avoided. Processed cheeses include American cheese, cheese food, and cheese spread, all of which are much higher in Na than the natural cheeses from which they are made. Bleu, Roquefort, feta, camembert, gorgonzola, and any other highly salted natural cheese should also be avoided on the 3 to 5 gm. sodium diet.

Although 2 gm. and 3 to 5 gm. sodium diets are commonly called mild sodium restrictions, many clients do not share this view. If asked to eliminate some of their favorite foods which happen to be high in Na content, clients are apt to view their Na restriction

as severe. Health professionals should take care to identify and acknowledge the client's attitudes rather than point out the "mildness" of a restriction.

POINTS OF EMPHASIS
Sodium restricted diets

• *The degree of Na restriction is based on client's immediate health condition and on his ability to comply with restrictions.*
• *The type of processing a food has undergone often has a marked effect on its Na content and therefore its suitability for a particular level of Na restriction.*
• *Salt, salty seasonings, and foods processed with large amounts of Na are avoided unless careful plans are made by the diet counselor for their occasional controlled use.*
• *Strict Na controlled diets (500 mg. Na or less) are usually free of foods which contain added Na.*
• *Some foods containing added Na can be worked into diets which allow more than 500 mg. Na.*
• *Foods which are "naturally high in sodium" are carefully controlled when the allowed daily Na intake is less than 2 gm.*

Promoting compliance

Many clients are initially unaware of what the words *sodium restriction* mean. If clients are told that they are on a 2 gm. sodium diet, some become afraid that they will have to learn the metric system or calculate their diets each day. On the other hand, if clients are told that they are on a "no added salt" diet or a "mild salt restricted diet" some will jump to the conclusion that they can eat just as they did previously as long as they don't salt their food—not realizing that many of the foods they ordinarily eat are excessively salty. Health care workers can sometimes prevent difficulties in teaching if they clarify the meaning of the diet order when the client is first exposed to it and then get feedback from the client regarding his understanding.

A sodium restricted diet is almost always used for a long period of time—often for the remainder of the client's life.

Much effort may need to be expended by health professionals to help any client on a sodium restricted diet to accept the discipline of a long term commitment and to motivate him to learn how to follow his diet. It might be helpful to use one or more of the following approaches, if applicable to the situation:
1. Show the client how his blood pressure has decreased with treatment, and link this desired result to both diet and medication.

---

* Often instructions are given for reducing the salt content of kosher meat by soaking cut up pieces in water.[9]

2. Point out how pedal edema, abdominal girth (in the case of ascites) or body weight has decreased with treatment. Encourage the client to participate in taking measurements and/or recording data.
3. Show the client how his urinary excretion of Na has decreased as a result of following the diet. (Use data obtained from 24-hr urine samples.)
4. In all cases find out if the client understands why decreased fluid retention and/or blood pressure are beneficial *to him*. Help him to value and work toward achieving or maintaining these decreases.
5. Encourage the client to try to detect natural flavors of foods which may previously have been masked by heavy salting.
6. Assist the client to develop the skills he will need to make implementation of the diet practical and, if possible, enjoyable.

COOKING AND FAMILY INVOLVEMENT

There are numerous ways to improve the palatability of a sodium restricted diet. Some of these have been incorporated in the menu in Table 28.4. Close attention to texture, temperature, and flavor contrasts, freshness, and eye appeal work wonders. Meat, fish, and poultry are very flavorful if charcoal broiled or cooked in a smoker. Foods may be seasoned with herbs, spices, and seeds, all of which are low in Na unless mixed with salt. Dried vegetable flakes and powders, with the exception of celery flakes and powder, are also low in Na. Lemon, vinegar, table wine, fruit, and vegtables may be used to create interesting low sodium flavor combinations. Although lists of allowed seasonings may be helpful to a client, some individuals are at a loss to know what flavorings complement a particular meat, vegetable, or cereal product. Many health agencies have publications providing suggestions for flavoring, cooking, and garnishing low sodium foods to improve their taste and appearance. If one of these publications is not available, the client might appreciate being given the names of some reliable references, such as those listed at the end of Part 4. Individuals who can be motivated to develop a spirit of adventuresomeness may discover interesting new flavors and food combinations which make food more enjoyable. For individuals who find change more difficult, a sodium restricted diet may be tolerable at best.

Many clients are unaware that some of the seasonings they are accustomed to using are high in Na. Health professionals should not assume that clients can taste the salt. Some disease conditions which require Na restriction may interfere with ability to detect saltiness.[10] Commonly used high sodium seasonings and condiments are listed in Appendix 5D. Even though substitutes are avaliable for many of them, such as fresh cloves of garlic or garlic powder in place of garlic salt, the resulting taste is different. Therefore, a person accustomed to using salty seasonings may need much support while he is adjusting to the changes. Extra support may also be needed by those accustomed to using many presalted convenience foods as the basis of their meals, such as TV dinners, canned main dishes, or mixes for the preparation of casseroles. Not only will the person need to adjust to the taste of unsalted food, but he may have to spend considerably more time preparing food if a varied diet is to be eaten.

Suggesting ways to fit the modified diet to the usual eating pattern may be helpful. Several options are possible. The cook may season the family's food with sodium-containing ingredients after the client's portion has been removed. Some families would rather allow each person to season food to taste at the table. (Some clients will be bothered by observing others making liberal use of the salt shaker. Placing shakers of herbs, spices, or salt substitute, if allowed, on the table may give the client a psychological lift.) Other families decide that it would be a good idea for everyone to decrease use of added salt. Everyone adapts to the change together. (Occasionally a client objects strongly to this option if he feels he is depriving others of one of the pleasures of life.) The most satisfactory manner of dealing with the sodium restricted diet is an area of concern which the health professional should encourage the family to discuss.

LABEL READING

It is not always necessary or appropriate for clients on mild sodium restricted diets to learn to read labels. A client who has a stable eating pattern can usually rely on his individualized diet form as a simple and safe guide for choosing foods. However, sometimes a client on a low level of sodium restriction (or the person assisting him) may need to develop label reading skills in order to comply with the diet. If this is the case, guided practice should be provided. Simply directing a client to read labels is not enough. The dietitian is well equipped to determine just how much a client needs to learn about label reading and to provide related learning experiences. Prior to discharge she may want to make sure the client can use sample labels and his diet form to determine (1) if specified foods are allowed on his diet and (2) if the amount of a specified food must be controlled.

Health professionals should be aware of some of the potential problems and misconceptions associated with label information and sodium restricted diets:

1. Many clients get confused about the difference between sodium and salt. They may accidentally miss the word "salt" in the list of ingredients (easy to do with fine print) and they may not realize that the listed Na content (e.g., 590 mg. Na per serving) indicates that the product is not suitable for their diet. Conversely, an individual may avoid buying salt-free crackers because he notices that the

sodium content is 10 mg. per 100 gm. He may do without crackers altogether or select a brand that does not include information about Na content. Such mistakes might be avoided by using the diet form rather than labeling information.

2. Ingredient listing can be easily misinterpreted. For example, those who know that ingredients are listed in descending order by weight may think that canned soup is much lower in Na than is soup prepared from a dry mix. The two types of soups are actually comparable in Na content when diluted according to directions. Diet forms clearly indicate that all types of commercial soups are to be avoided unless they are marked *low sodium*.

3. Referring to ingredient listings may also give rise to the impression that two foods are very similar in Na content, although they are actually very different.

Clearly, if label reading is a skill which the client needs, the dietitian will need adequate time for teaching. She should be notified of the discharge diet order well in advance of discharge.

SALT SUBSTITUTES AND LOW SODIUM PRODUCTS

A client on a sodium restricted diet should be warned not to use salt substitute without a doctor's permission, even if the product is available without a prescription in the state in which he lives. Salt substitutes contain potassium instead of sodium chloride. Since some individuals who are restricted in sodium should also restrict potassium intake (because of impaired renal function), salt substitute is not safe for everyone.

A mixture of sodium chloride and potassium chloride is commercially available (e.g., Lite Salt). Since some clients confuse this product with sodium-free salt substitute, they should be warned against its use unless it has been planned into the diet.

Clients often have unrealistic expectations for a salt substitute. They should be advised that although it looks like salt, it does not taste like salt. When first trying it, caution is advised. Some clients find its taste very objectionable. Some find it to be more acceptable with some food than with others. A light sprinkling on a small portion of food is a good practice when using salt substitute for the first time.

Low sodium dietetic products are available in most supermarkets. These foods contain no added Na, but do contain as much Na as is found in comparable fresh products or in the original ingredients. Foods naturally containing significant amounts of Na, such as tuna and spinach, cannot be freely used on the lower levels of Na restriction even if they are marked "Low sodium dietetic." Other low sodium dietetic products, such as low sodium crackers, are so low in Na that their use does not need to be controlled.

Low sodium dietetic products are more expensive than their salt-containing counterparts and should not be recommended unnecessarily.

There are several popular ready-to-eat cereals which are free of added Na as usually purchased. They include shredded wheat, puffed wheat and rice, wheat germ, and some brands of granola. They are likely to be better buys than are low sodium dietetic ready-to-eat cereals.

Special products which are most apt to be useful, at least for the stricter diets, include low sodium canned peas and tomatoes (fresh ones are often unavailable, very expensive, of poor quality, or impractical); other low sodium canned vegetables if fresh or frozen ones cannot be used; low sodium canned tomato and vegetable juices; low sodium peanut butter (freshly ground peanut butter with no added salt is available at some stores and may cost much less than the brand name dietetic product); low sodium soups; low sodium tuna and salmon; low sodium mayonnaise; low sodium cheese and cottage cheese (these taste *very* different from the usual product and are often poorly accepted).

Some low sodium dietetic products which are available contain added potassium. Low sodium bouillon cubes, catsup, mustard, and relish are some of the items in this category. This is of no concern unless potassium intake needs to be restricted; however, foods and condiments containing potassium chloride taste very different from the usual product.

EATING OUT

Most clients on sodium restricted diets want to eat away from home at least occasionally. They will probably be able to do so without exceeding their sodium allowance if they learn about appropriate foods to order and ways to avoid offending a hostess. The ease with which meals can be eaten away from home depends on the level of sodium restriction, the frequency of eating out, and the types of places where food is eaten. Choices will usually be *very* limited for 500 to 1000 mg. sodium diets. It is not realistic to expect a person to regularly eat well-balanced, varied meals in a cafeteria or restaurant unless 3 to 5 gm. sodium daily is allowed.

A consumer can expect the following items to be free of *added* sodium in restaurants: baked potato (without added butter—unsalted butter is occasionally available upon request and unseasoned sour cream is quite low in sodium); salads prepared from raw vegetables, with oil and vinegar or lemon juice used as a dressing; fresh or canned fruits or fruit juices; milk, tea, or coffee (excluding specialty coffees, e.g., cafe au lait, mocha); boiled eggs; puffed wheat and rice, shredded wheat.

It is usually possible to request that broiled steak, chops, chicken, or fish be prepared without added salt or sauces. Inside slices of roasts or turkey are relatively free of added salt as long as gravy or drippings are not served on the meat.

The consumer should expect bread products, cooked vegetables, combination dishes, and desserts other than fruit to contain added sodium. The dietitian can tell the client who is on a mild sodium restricted diet the number of servings of bread products and plain cooked vegetables which may be included in a restaurant meal.

No matter what the level of sodium restriction, the client should be advised to avoid eating soups, gravy, sauces, stuffing, pizza, and other mixed dishes since they are all likely to be highly salted. Plain foods are more appropriate choices when eating out.

Sometimes clients on sodium restricted diets feel reluctant to accept an invitation to dine at the home of a friend. Friends are usually glad to adapt a meal to make it low in Na as long as they are given some guidelines in advance. They usually are willing to omit salt during cooking (allowing guests to salt food to taste) and to serve salty sauces separately from meat or vegetables.

If an individual wants to attend a party where most of the food is expected to contain too much added Na, eating in advance may be advisable. The client may want to check with the hostess to find out if she would mind if he brought his own food. Hunger is a powerful drive and can ruin the best intentions when low sodium foods are unavailable.

POINTS OF EMPHASIS

Promoting compliance with a sodium restricted diet

• *Provide the client with specific feedback regarding how the diet is actually benefiting his health.*

• *Remember that some clients who require Na restriction may have impaired ability to taste salt.*

• *Avoid confusing the client regarding the need to read labels. For some clients the diet plan is a much better guide.*

• *Recommend plain foods when dining out. Most sauces and combination dishes contain more Na than is allowed on any sodium restricted diet. The client should use his diet plan as a guide.*

• *Do not recommend use of potassium-containing salt substitutes without a physician's approval.*

• *Inform client regarding the suitability of low sodium dietetic foods for his diet.*

NURSING PROGRESS NOTE

The following **SOAP** note written by a registered nurse reflects a common situation involving fluid retention and sodium restricted diets. The plan would obviously vary with the ability of the client to learn, the availability of a dietitian in the particular agency, and agency policies.

Nursing Progress Note 1/7/80
Problem #1 Fluid Retention

S. Client stated, "Wedding ring is uncomfortably tight. I get short of breath if I walk around the house. I haven't been able to lose weight even though I've cut way down on the amount I eat. I'm too tired to cook so I use convenience foods like canned soup a lot. I take my "water pill" every day. I posted my low salt diet sheet in the kitchen."
O. Weight has increased 5 kg. since last clinic visit 2 mo. ago.
A. Frequent use of convenience foods has resulted in excessive sodium intake. Client unable to distinguish between fluid retention and "getting fat." May need assistance with meal preparation.
P. Have client participate in obtaining and recording daily weight. Relate significant weight changes to medication and diet. Assess need for assistance with cooking and other household duties. Contact the dietitian about visiting client. Request order for diet instruction.

Fluid restriction

RATIONALE FOR RESTRICTION OF WATER

Although a sodium restricted diet is very helpful in ridding the body of excess fluid or preventing fluid accumulation, it is sometimes essential to restrict water as well as Na intake. This modification is usually termed a fluid restriction. In congestive heart failure or other diseases in which cardiac output is low, fluid restriction must often be employed to promote diuresis or to prevent life-threatening hyponatremeia. A person who is anuric (produces no urine) or oliguric (produces a decreased amount of urine) must limit intake of water-containing fluids even if he is treated by dialysis (a method of removing wastes from the blood). By avoiding excess fluid accumulation, persons with reduced renal output help control their blood pressure and reduce the chance of pulmonary congestion.

When proper fluid balance requires control of fluid intake, the amount of fluid allowed is based on the client's estimated *total* water loss. Average ranges are indicated in Table 15.1 page 161. These values differ depending on the environmental temperature, humidity, and the body surface area and activity of the individual. They also vary with certain disease conditions, as covered in Table 28.1.

A fluid restriction usually allows an adult about 600 to 800 cc. (ml.) to cover insensible fluid losses. Any fluid allotment below 2000 cc. daily is considered to be a restriction. Health team members need to recognize when change in environment or health status might require an adjustment in the amount of fluid allowed.

If a client with decreased renal output carefully follows a sodium restricted diet, his decreased thirst may make it unnecessary to teach him how to restrict fluids. Preliminary studies have found that a simplified diet instruction (sodium restriction only) was associated with improved adherence to the diet as measured by weight gain and blood pressure.[11]

RESTRICTED ITEMS

When a fluid restriction is ordered, limits are placed on intake of all aqueous liquids. Thus the client limits intake of juices (including syrup in which fruit is packed), milk, soups, coffee, beer, soft drinks, and so forth. Foods which liquefy at body temperature, such as gelatin desserts, ice cream, sherbet, popsicles, and ice chips, are also restricted. Puddings and cooked cereal are counted as fluids in some health agencies. Other foods have a high water content but are not usually counted. However, if an individual greatly increases use of fruits and/or vegetables when a fluid restriction is imposed, he defeats the purpose of the restriction.

FLUID RESTRICTION PLAN

When a hospitalized client is placed on a fluid restriction, a fluid restriction plan should be developed by the nurse in cooperation with the dietitian and, if possible, the client. In developing the plan the nurse may need to clarify the order with the physician. For example:

1. Are medications in aqueous solution to be included in the restriction? (30 cc. Mylanta q. 2° contributes a large amount of water.)
2. Is an IV to be included?
3. Is the allowable amount of oral fluid adequate for meals and for fluid needed between meals? (Doctors are usually willing to change the form in which a medication is given, if possible, or the amount of the fluid restriction if there is a good reason to do so.)

The nurse and dietitian also need to consider the amount of fluid the client appears to need between meals:

1. How much fluid is needed to administer medications by mouth? Does the client require a relatively large amount of fluid because of difficulty swallowing tablets and capsules or because the medication needs to be diluted to reduce gastric irritation?
2. Does the client request ice chips or other fluid between meals because of an unpleasant taste in the mouth or for some other legitimate reason?

The client's preferences at mealtime should also be considered. He may need to choose between coffee or milk in the morning or he may want to settle for very small servings of each. If a plan is worked out *with* the client, he is more apt to cooperate with it. Such cooperation is essential since the client ordinarily has free access to water unless immobilized.

Some clients who are being discharged on a fluid restriction like to follow a set plan which specifies the amount of fluid they may have at specified times and meals. Other clients prefer to keep a running total of fluid intake to allow for more variety. Those who take all of their fluid at home may want to use the following method of keeping track of fluid intake.

In the morning a pitcher or other container is filled with water in the amount of the day's fluid restriction (e.g., 1000 cc.). This pitcher is usually stored in the refrigerator. When the client wants some juice (or any other fluid), he pours out of the water pitcher an amount of water equal to the amount of juice he will consume. If he wants water, he takes it from the pitcher. If the pitcher is clear, the client can easily see if the fluid level is dropping too quickly to last the whole day. As long as he remembers to pour the correct amount of water out of the pitcher, he won't have to do any arithmetic to make sure he is getting the correct amount of fluid.

> **POINTS OF EMPHASIS**
> *Restricting fluid intake*
>
> • *All beverages and foods which are liquid at body temperature are included in the fluid restriction. Some liquid medications may also be included.*
> • *Planning fluid distribution needs to consider acceptability of meals, client's special fluid needs, and client's preferences.*
> • *Restricting Na intake helps reduce thirst and, thus, makes control of fluid easier.*

Encouraging fluids

RATIONALE FOR ENCOURAGING FLUIDS

Adequate hydration is vital to all body processes. Thirst is not always a reliable guide for fluid consumption, particularly when illness, injury, or other stresses are present. Intracranial lesions which produce loss of motor function, difficulty in swallowing, and a decreased level of consciousness may interfere with thirst. Individuals who are losing extra fluid because of illness will seldom increase their fluid intake on their own. If not encouraged to take liquids, dehydration may quickly ensue. This is particularly true of the very young and the elderly.

Individuals with diabetes insipidus are unable to concentrate their urine owing to lack of (or resistance to) antidiuretic hormone. These persons must drink large volumes of water daily unless their condition is satisfactorily controlled by treatment with the drug vasopressin (antidiuretic hormone). If they are vasopressin resistant, their fluid requirement (and polyuria) can be decreased by decreasing dietary intake of sodium and of protein.[12]

Even if the state of hydration is normal, it is sometimes desirable to maintain a high fluid intake to increase urine flow and keep the urine concentration dilute. Maintaining a large volume of dilute urine is helpful in treating and preventing the recurrence of urinary tract infection or renal calculi (kidney stone) formation.

METHODS OF ENCOURAGING FLUIDS

When a high oral fluid intake is desirable, this might be noted by the terms "encourage fluids," "push fluids," or "force fluids." The latter term should never be interpreted to mean that force should be employed. If adequate hydration cannot be achieved by the oral route with the client's cooperation, the physician will write an order for intravenous fluids. Sometimes an order is written to "push fluids" so that intravenous fluids may be safely discontinued.

It is often unrealistic to expect clients to take more fluid just because they are advised to do so. Intravenous fluids reduce thirst making it difficult for the client to increase intake. Fever and dehydration may temporarily impair mental functioning enough to cause even the most intelligent individual to ignore good advice. Rather than asking if the client wants a drink, a beverage should be offered frequently. Well-liked juices, carbonated beverages, and broth are good choices, as are gelatin desserts, popsicles (or the variation on the popsicle which comes in a plastic envelope), fruit ice, and sherbet. When dehydration is the threat, fluid intake must temporarily be given priority over a well-balanced diet. Frequently offering different liquids in *small* cups, glasses, and bowls generally produces better results than giving larger portions less often.

SODIUM DEFICIT

Conditions leading to a net loss of sodium are no less serious than those causing retention of sodium and water. A person with cystic fibrosis can quickly become dangerously salt-depleted in hot weather because of unusually high loss of salt in perspiration. Likewise, a renal patient who experiences wasting of sodium may develop signs and symptoms of sodium deficit.

When the problem is sodium deficit, diet modification is usually made without a specific diet order. For example, a person with cystic fibrosis is encouraged to salt his food and to eat salty foods which are compatible with other aspects of his diet. Rather than keeping track of exactly how much sodium is used, the individual and his family are taught to recognize signs and symptoms indicating the need for more salt.

For the client who is experiencing sodium wasting because of renal disease, the need for controlled intake is more important. It may be necessary to walk a tightrope between inadequate and excessive intake. A specific amount of added salt may be provided in the form of a salt packet on the client's tray. This means that a salt packet appearing on the tray of a patient on a 3 gm. sodium diet may not be a mistake. Dietary departments have a definite procedure for clearly identifying whether salt packets should or should not be on the client's tray. Since the procedure is not necessarily the same in every health agency, the health professional needs to check her agency's policy.

ALTERATIONS IN POTASSIUM BALANCE

HYPOKALEMIA

Hypokalemia may be defined as any serum potassium level below 3.5 mEq. per L. During hypokalemia the heartbeat is more rapid than usual (tachycardia). The client may experience nonspecific symptoms such as anorexia, malaise, or muscle weakness. If the potassium level is sufficiently depressed, cardiac arrest may ensue.

HYPERKALEMIA

Hyperkalemia may be characterized by serum potassium levels above 5.5 mEq. per L. and a slow heart rate (bradycardia). Symptoms, again, are relatively nonspecific. In fact, some of them, such as muscle weakness, are similar to symptoms of hypokalemia. Mental confusion; numbness or tingling of the hands, feet, and/or scalp; and difficulty breathing and speaking are likely to develop. If the potassium level is sufficiently elevated, cardiac arrhythmias may develop, followed by cardiac arrest. If the kidneys are not functioning normally it is difficult to remove excessive potassium from the blood quickly and safely.

Clearly it is desirable to assist the client to maintain potassium within normal limits. Often this can be done by balancing intake against output. Thus, a client who retains excess potassium owing to decreased urine formation or decreased production of aldosterone (in adrenal gland insufficiency) is placed on a potassium restricted diet. Conversely, a person who is potassium depleted, for reasons such as starvation or chronic use of thiazide diuretics, is encouraged to increase potassium intake.

SERUM POTASSIUM AS AN INDICATOR OF TOTAL BODY POTASSIUM

The state of potassium balance can be difficult to determine since most of the potassium is within body cells. Accurate direct measurement of intracellular potassium is not feasible. Unfortunately, the small fraction of potassium circulating in the blood sometimes does not accurately reflect the cellular level. The body may be severely depleted of potassium (low intracellular potassium) while the serum potassium level is normal or elevated. Shifts in potassium distribution from one fluid compartment to another are responsible.

Diets modified in potassium content

Whether the diet is to be high or low in potassium content, a few facts about the distribution of potassium in foods can be useful in determining which forms of foods and cooking methods are most compatible with the diet (Table 28.6).

Potassium is an essential component of all living cells, both plant and animal. It is present in all foods except purified separated food components such as sugar, cornstarch, and vegetable oil. Since potassium is associated with protein in the cell, high protein foods, whether of animal or plant origin, tend to be high in potassium unless they have been refined or purified.

Potassium is highly soluble in water. Food preparation methods involving soaking or cooking cut-up pieces of food cause potassium to diffuse out of the food into the water. Canned fruit is lower in potassium than is fresh fruit if the syrup is not consumed. The water-soluble portion of meat drippings is high in potassium while the fat from meat is nearly potassium-free.

Canned, fresh, and frozen fruit juices are similar in potassium content. Foods retain their original potassium content if baked or fried. Dried foods are much higher in potassium content than their fresh counterparts when equal weights are compared. Although there would be no difference in potassium intake if the same number of pieces of fruit were eaten, the small size of dried fruit invites larger consumption. (For example, about 43 dried grapes are packed into a tiny 15 gm. box of raisins.)

Dilution obviously decreases potassium content. Fruit drinks, fruit nectars, and cranberry juice cocktail are diluted fruit juices and are correspondingly decreased in potassium content. Instant coffee has only about half as much potassium as does brewed coffee.

The potassium in grains is found primarily in the germ and bran; refined grain products are lower in potassium than is whole grain. Thus, when it is important to alter potassium intake, adjusting cooking methods and forms of food used may be very helpful.

HIGH POTASSIUM DIETS

Rationale Diets modified to be high in potassium content can be extremely beneficial for thousands of individuals who lose excessive amounts of this mineral in the urine. The most common cause of urinary potassium wasting is the use of diuretics, particularly the furosemides (Lasix) and thiazides (Diuril). Combination medications used in the treatment of hypertension frequently contain a diuretic; therefore, the composition of antihypertensives should be ascertained to determine whether potassium requirement is likely to be increased.

In a society like ours, which tends to rely on pharmaceutical agents, potassium salts are often prescribed to assure adequate potassium intake. For many clients a high potassium diet would be more appropriate. Despite attempts by drug companies to mask the bitter taste of potassium supplements, most clients find them unpleasant at best. "Vile" and "nauseating" are common descriptors. Potassium supplements are irritating to the wall of the stomach and intestine and have the potential for causing ulceration. Clients who could meet potassium requirements by dietary means are exposed to unnecessary risks, unpleasant taste, and extra expense when potassium supplements are prescribed instead. Their food intake may fall below optimal, especially if good mouth care is not practiced.

The taste and side effects of potassium supplements probably contribute to a significant amount of noncompliance. This can be particularly dangerous to those individuals using digitalis preparations since hypokalemia potentiates the action of digitalis on the heart.

Increasing potassium intake by 50 mEq. per day Diet modifications can usually be made which will increase potassium intake by up to 2000 mg. (50 mEq.) daily without significantly increasing intake of sodium or calories.[13] The individual chooses from a variety of potassium-rich foods, and may wish to use a salt substitute as well. Table 28.7 shows how a day's menu might be changed to increase potassium intake by about 50 mEq. Usually fewer changes are needed since the maintenance dose for potassium is often about 20 mEq. per day. The extra banana and orange juice which are commonly suggested can easily add 20 mEq. of potassium. Many other high potassium foods could be used instead of bananas and oranges. A list of possible substitutes is in Appendix 5E.

TABLE 28.6 *Relation of potassium content to the form of different types of foods*

TYPE OF FOOD	FORMS HIGHEST IN POTASSIUM	FORMS MODERATE IN POTASSIUM	FORMS LOWEST IN POTASSIUM
Grains	Bran, germ	Whole grain	Refined
Fruits*	Dried, raw, frozen whole	Canned (drained)	Fruit *drinks*
Vegetables*	Dried, raw, baked, fried	Frozen (steamed or cooked in very little water)	Soaked and cooked in large volume of water; canned (drained)
Candies	Chocolate, nut, raisin coconut		Hard candy
Coffee (including decaffeinated)	Brewed, strong		Instant, weak
Other	High protein foods		Highly refined foods

* Different types vary widely in potassium content

ORIGINAL FOOD SELECTION	MODIFIED FOOD SELECTION	CHANGE IN POTASSIUM CONTENT	CHANGE IN KCAL
4 slices white enriched bread	Substitute 4 slices whole wheat bread	+290	—
120 ml (½ c) rice or pasta	Substitute 1 potato boiled in skin	+500	—
120 ml (½ c) gelatin	Substitute 1 medium banana	+440	+30
No vegetable at lunch	Add 120 ml (½ c) cooked frozen spinach	+340	+23
No salad at dinner	Add 1 sliced tomato (medium)	+300	+27
240 ml (1 c) farina at breakfast	Substitute 240 ml (1 c) oatmeal	+120	+20
	Omit 15 gm (1 Tbsp) margarine or butter or 100 kcal worth of other food which is primarily a source of empty calories	—	−100
	Total	1990	0

POTASSIUM RESTRICTED DIETS

Rationale Diets are modified to be reduced in potassium content when there is interference with urinary excretion of potassium, as in acute or chronic renal failure. The smaller the amount of potassium excreted the stricter the potassium restriction must be. In acute hyperkalemia, potassium intake may be entirely prohibited. Analysis of 24-hr urine specimens can provide good estimates of potassium excretion.

Potassium free diet A variety of dietary restrictions are imposed on clients who are anuric and who have seriously elevated levels of potassium and other potentially toxic substances. The potassium restriction is probably the most critical. Some foods containing negligible amounts of potassium are identified in Appendix 5G. This table also identifies commercial supplements which are high in calories but low in potassium. Some of these foods and supplements might be offered to a client with acute hyperkalemia if he is able to tolerate foods by mouth. Food selection is, of necessity, very limited. A diet comprised only of these foods would be nutritionally inadequate and would only be used as a temporary measure.

1.5 to 3.0 gm. (58 to 117 mEq.) potassium diets Chronic renal failure from any cause is the condition most frequently necessitating a potassium restricted diet. The amount of potassium allowed is usually between 1.5 gm. (58 mEq.) and 3.0 gm. (117 mEq.) daily, depending on potassium output. Output includes potassium lost in the urine and during dialysis, if used. If vomiting and/or diarrhea are present, an additional amount of potassium is allowed to cover these extra losses.

A potassium restriction is seldom the only diet restriction recommended for a client with chronic renal failure. Sodium, fluid, protein, and phosphorus intake are likely to be controlled as well (Appendix 5G); however, consideration of potassium as a single entity is useful. Adherence to the potassium restriction on a daily basis may make the difference between life and death. Potassium is so widely distributed in food that relatively small contributions from single foods quickly add up to substantial amounts of the mineral.

NURSING PROGRESS NOTE

During the course of a client's hospital stay, events such as the one reported in the following nursing progress note may reveal the need for teaching to prevent or alleviate hyperkalemia.

Nursing Progress Note 8/11/79
Problem #2. Hyperkalemia

S. "I thought fruit was allowed since it is served to me at mealtime. I'm really tired of the hospital food, it's pretty tasteless without salt. Besides, Jim spent a lot of money on that fruit basket and would have been disappointed if I hadn't eaten any."

O. I. 500 cc. O. 300 cc.   Se K 9/16: 5.3 mEq./L
Ate undetermined amount of fruit from fruit basket brought in by friend. Consumed all food served on 2 gm. K, 2 gm. Na diet. Nurse had told client not to eat any fruit from basket because of its high potassium content—unless a plan could be worked out with the dietitian.

A. Client appears not to understand the importance of limiting potassium intake and wants more variety in diet. May not know how to tactfully handle gifts of food.

P. 1. Explain purpose of potassium restriction and obtain feedback. Request reinforcement by physician.
2. Monitor heart rate for arrhythmias.
3. Role play ways of dealing with gifts of food such as chocolate candy.
4. Ask dietitian to discuss ways of increasing palatability of diet with client and to inform client of procedure to follow to see if foods brought in by family and friends can be worked into the diet.

Additional measures for maintaining potassium balance

An individual who requires a potassium restricted diet may be vulnerable to increases in serum potassium levels even if he does not exceed the allowed amount of potassium in a day. Additional measures can be taken by the client to help avoid this potentially dangerous situation.

1. Maintain nitrogen balance by consuming an adequate amount of protein and calories. Inadequate intake results in cellular breakdown which tends

to release intracellular potassium into the extracellular fluid and causes increased serum potassium level.

2. Include at least moderate amounts of carbohydrate (about 40 percent of calories) in the diet. When carbohydrate moves into the cells, potassium from the extracellular fluid is carried into the cell with it.

3. Exercise within the limits set by the physician. If on bedrest, regularly perform allowed range of motion exercises. Exercise helps prevent breakdown of muscle tissue and increases movement of glucose into the cell.

4. Avoid saving high potassium foods for use in one meal or for another day. Potassium is rapidly absorbed from the gut. A potassium load could cause a temporary but dangerously sharp increase in serum potassium level.

5. Find out in advance from the physician what changes in urine output and other indicators of health status are serious enough to warrant a call to the physician.

POINTS OF EMPHASIS
Maintaining potassium balance

• *Practically every food contains potassium. Content varies widely even within food groups and with type of processing of a single food.*

• *High potassium diets can be planned for clients taking diuretics which cause potassium loss. This reduces or eliminates the need for potassium supplements.*

• *If a condition leads to hyperkalemia, dietary potassium restriction reduces the chance of serious complications. Intake of nearly every food must be controlled to promote desired low potassium intake.*

• *Intake of protein, calories, and carbohydrate can influence distribution and serum level of potassium.*

ALTERATIONS IN CALCIUM AND PHOSPHORUS BALANCE

Controls of calcium and phosphorus balance

Alterations in calcium and phosphorus balance are most likely to be noticed because of bone changes or because calcium salts are deposited in inappropriate places, rather than because of changes in serum calcium and phosphorus levels. The reason is that compensatory mechanisms are geared toward keeping serum calcium levels within normal limits, which is necessary for the preservation of life itself. A serum calcium within the narrow range of 9.2 to 10.4 mg.

per 100 ml. is required for normal cell permeability and neuromuscular irritability. Hypercalcemia may cause respiratory failure or cardiac arrest, while hypocalcemia may cause tetany. Serum phosphorus levels can vary rather widely without causing immediate drastic effects.

Compensatory effects mediated by parathyroid hormone (PTH) are reduced if stores of calcium in the bone are already seriously depleted, renal excretory function is impaired, vitamin D deficiency exists, production of vitamin D hormone is impaired, or calcium intake is very low. When there is malfunctioning of the parathyroids, serum calcium level changes rapidly.

Disease conditions associated with calcium and phosphorus imbalance

RICKETS AND OSTEOMALACIA

Rickets is a calcium-phosphorus imbalance characterized by slightly lowered serum calcium level, seriously depressed serum phosphate level, progressive weakening of the bones, and a variety of other symptoms. Rickets is most apt to occur during periods of rapid growth. Ingestion of vitamin D or irradiation of the skin with ultraviolet light promptly cures rickets; however, bone malformations tend to persist. Either sunlight or vitamin D can prevent the development of rickets. One case of rickets owing to calcium deficiency has been reported.[14]

Osteomalacia is the adult version of rickets. In the U.S. it is most commonly seen in individuals with renal failure, liver disease, or prolonged malabsorption states. Women who bear and breast feed several children without obtaining an adequate supply of vitamin D and calcium are likewise susceptible to this bone disease.

CHRONIC RENAL FAILURE

In chronic renal failure, a series of events involving calcium-phosphorus imbalance may result in bone disease unless medical and dietary measures are used to control the situation. The physiological changes are summarized as follows[15]:

1. Decreased glomerular filtration rate (GFR) produces a transient rise in serum phosphate.

2. Increased serum phosphate depresses serum calcium. This stimulates the parathyroids to secrete more parathyroid hormone (PTH).

3. PTH acts to normalize serum levels of calcium and phosphate. In normalizing serum calcium and phosphate levels, the bone loses calcium.

4. Production of vitamin D hormone is impaired in chronic renal failure. Lack of active vitamin D greatly reduces absorption of calcium from the in-

testinal tract and interferes with normal bone calcification.

5. PTH levels become progressively higher with continuing decreases in the GFR. Secondary hyperparathyroidism and accompanying bone disease gradually develop.

6. When the GFR falls below 25 ml. per minute (normal 125 ml. per min.), phosphate excretion is severely limited (despite high PTH levels) and serum phosphate level remains elevated.

Thus, when renal function is seriously impaired, physiological adaptations to normalize serum calcium and phosphorus levels result in secondary hyperparathyroidism and bone disease. Adaptive ability decreases along with decreasing renal function.

Reducing phosphorus input   In experimental animals, reducing "input" of phosphorus retards the preceding undesirable course of events which accompanies chronic renal failure[16]; the effect of reduced phosphorus intake on humans is under study. Use of a 600 to 700 mg. phosphorus restriction along with a controlled protein intake of 0.6 gm. per kg. is reported to reduce incidence of bone disease in chronic renal failure if begun when serum creatinine is about 3 mg. per 100 ml. Severe restriction is difficult since phosphorus is very widely distributed in nutritious foods. A very low phosphorus diet using normal foods would be deficient in content of other essential nutrients.

Fortunately, aluminum hydroxide compounds (commonly used antacids such as Amphojel, Basaljel and Alu-Caps) can bind dietary phosphorus and, therefore, are helpful in the treatment of chronic renal failure. *If taken with a meal,* aluminum hydroxide ties up phosphorus in an insoluble compound which is not well absorbed. Instead the phosphorus is excreted in the stool. Thus, aluminum hydroxide compounds are sometimes called phosphate binders. The larger the dose of aluminum hydroxide preparation taken, the greater the amount of phosphorus which is bound and the smaller the amount of phosphorus absorbed into the bloodstream. Theoretically, increasing the dose of aluminum hydroxide should make dietary phosphorus restriction unnecessary. In practice, most clients cannot tolerate large doses of the antacid because it is unpalatable and produces side effects such as constipation and nausea. Ingenious means of transforming Amphojel into a more acceptable form have been developed, such as using it as an ingredient in cookies.[18]

The safety of prolonged use of high doses of aluminum hydroxide preparations by clients who are undergoing dialysis is uncertain. Small amounts of aluminum may be absorbed, accumulate, and contribute to dialysis encephalopathy[19,20] and osteodystrophy.[19] Since dialysis cannot effectively reduce the serum phosphorus level, even those clients who are being dialysed regularly need to take measures to reduce phosphorus intake and absorption. Dietary phosphorus restriction, if ordered, is usually 0.8 to 1.2 gm. phosphorus per day (compared to an RDA of 0.8 gm.). Many foods contain *extra* phosphorus because phos-

phorus-containing compounds have been added in processing.* Examples are listed here. Most of these foods are high in added sodium as well.

Carbonated beverages: cola and others made with phosphoric rather than citric acid

Cheese: American, cheese food, cheese spread, other *processed* cheeses

Fabricated potato chips (e.g., Pringles)

Instant pudding

Processed meats: bologna, hot dogs, ham, Canadian bacon, and others

Refrigerator bakery products

Salad dressings of many types

Increasing calcium input   A high calcium diet cannot usually be employed in chronic renal failure since it is incompatible with other necessary dietary restrictions; therefore, calcium supplements are given in an attempt to increase calcium absorption. These may be of little effect without vitamin D hormone to promote their absorption.

Neither irradiation of the skin with ultraviolet light nor administration of vitamin D (ergocalciferol or cholecalciferol) solves the problem of an inadequate supply of vitamin D hormone in chronic renal failure. Analogs of active vitamin D (such as Hytakerol) can reverse bone changes in many patients with chronic renal failure[21,22] and may promote growth of children.[23] They are given after serum phosphorus levels have been brought down to normal levels. These vitamin-D-like substances must be administered cautiously since they may be toxic at low dosage. Unfortunately, the expense of compounds with vitamin D hormone activity is prohibitive for many clients.

CALCIUM-CONTAINING RENAL CALCULI

The changes leading to formation of calcium-containing kidney stones are not all well identified. Such stones are most apt to occur in individuals predisposed by heredity, geographical location, immobilization, chronic urinary infections, or hyperparathyroidism. Although diet is not effective in dissolving stones and is not thought to be a principal cause of stone formation in well-nourished individuals, dietary changes may be recommended to reduce the chance of recurrence of stone formation.

It is helpful to keep certain facts and principles in mind when considering the relationship of diet to stone formation:

1. Renal calculi are salts which have precipitated out of the urine. There are a number of different types of salts involved, but one person will ordinarily be susceptible to just one kind of stone. The composition of the stone can be determined only if a stone is available for analysis. Calcium is the cation most commonly found in renal calculi.

* Look at the ingredient listing on the label for the words *phosphate* (any type) or *phosphoric acid.*

2. The higher the concentration of the involved cation, anion, or both, the greater the chance that the salt will precipitate out of the urine.
3. The solubility of salts is influenced by pH. The effect of pH differs for different salts. The solubility of calcium phosphate salts increases with increased acidity of the urine.

Diet modifications sometimes recommended Using the preceding information, the following adjustments in diet may be ordered:

1. If the composition of the stone is not known, the only justified dietary measure is to increase fluid intake to more than 2.5 L. (2½ qts.) per day. Diluting the urine decreases the concentration of both the involved anion and cation and maintains high urine flow. The diet order may be written as "encourage fluids to >2500 cc q d," or just "encourage fluids." The client should be encouraged to take 250 to 300 cc. each hour while awake and when he voids at night. A large fraction of the fluid should be in the form of water.[24]
2. If the composition of the stone is known, mild restriction of dietary intake of one or both of the involved ions, or foods leading to the formation of those ions, may be recommended. Calcium is the substance most likely to be restricted. When calcium oxalate stones are identified, reduction in use of foods high in oxalates may be suggested to coincide with the calcium restriction. Guidelines for calcium restricted diets with modifications for oxalate restriction are found in Appendix 5F.
3. If the composition of the stone is known, food may be used in conjunction with pharmaceutical agents to control the pH of the urine. The purpose is to maximize the solubility of the offending salt. An *acid ash* diet might be recommended when an individual has been diagnosed to have calcium phosphate stones. An acid ash diet includes a high proportion of foods which tend to produce an acidic urine and a low proportion of foods which tend to make the urine alkaline. Staple foods which produce an alkaline urine are not prohibited since the diet would then be nutritionally inadequate. Guidelines for an acid ash diet are included in Appendix 5F.

STUDY QUESTIONS

1. Are foods which are naturally high in sodium usually eliminated from sodium restricted diets? Explain.
2. If a doctor writes an order for a 500 mg. NaCl diet, what level of sodium restriction would this be? Would any double checking with the doctor be advisable? Explain.
3. A food product states on the label that it contains 350 mg. of sodium. How many mEq. of sodium would this be?

4. If a person tolerates potassium supplements poorly, how could he adjust his diet to include an extra 20 mEq. of potassium daily?
5. What method of cooking is most effective for decreasing the potassium content of foods? What disadvantage does this cooking method have?
6. When a fluid intake of 3 L. daily is advised, list several suggestions to help a client achieve this goal when he is at home.
7. If a person on a fluid restriction repeatedly gains an excessive amount of weight, what kind of information should health care workers obtain from the client in order to improve the plan of care?

References

1. Secor, J.: *Patient Care in Respiratory Problems.* (Monographs in Clinical Nursing, Vol. 1.) Philadelphia: W. B. Saunders Co., 1969.
2. Meneely, G. R., and Battarbee, R. D.: Sodium and potassium *Nutr. Rev.* 34:225, 1976.
3. Morgan, T., et al.: Hypertension treated by salt restriction. *Lancet* 1:227, 1978.
*4. *Your Sodium Restricted Diet: 500 Mg.* Dallas: American Heart Association, 1958.
*5. *Your Sodium Restricted Diet: 1000 Mg.* Dallas: American Heart Association, 1958.
*6. *Your Sodium Restricted Diet:* Mild Restriction. Dallas: American Heart Association, 1958.
7. Weickart, R.: *Sodium in Food, Medicine and Water.* Lombard IL: Water Quality Assoc., C.I. 2–76.
*8. Hartshorn, E. A.: Food and drug interactions. *J. Am. Diet. Assoc.* 70:15, 1977.
9. Kaufman, M.: Adapting therapeutic diets to Jewish food customs. *Am. J. Clin. Nutr.* 5:676, 1957.
10. Contreras, R. J.: Salt taste and disease. *Am. J. Clin. Nutr.* 31:1088, 1978.
11. Rupp, J. W., Stone, R. A., and Gunning, B. E.: Sodium versus sodium-fluid restriction in hemodialysis: Control of weight gains and blood pressures. *Am. J. Clin. Nutr.* 31:1952, 1978.
12. Blalock, T., et al.: Role of diet in the management of vasopressin-responsive and -resistant diabetes insipidus. *Am. J. Clin. Nutr.* 30:1070, 1977.
13. *When you need extra potassium.* Boston: Nutrition Education Committee, Greater Boston Chapter, Massachusetts Heart Association, 1973.
14. Kooh, S. W., et al.: Rickets due to calcium deficiency. *N. Engl. J. Med.* 297:1264, 1977.
*15. Schoolwerth, A. C., and Engle, J. B.: Calcium and phosphorus in diet therapy of uremia." *J. Am. Diet. Assoc.* 66:460, 1975.
16. Ibels, L. S., et al.: Preservation of function in experimental renal disease by dietary restriction of phosphate. *N. Engl. J. Med.* 298:122, 1978.
17. Fiaschi, E., Maschio, G., and D'Angelo, A.: Low-protein diets and bone disease in chronic renal failure. *Kidney Int.* 13(Suppl 8): s-79, 1978.
18. Margie, J. D., et al.: *The Mayo Clinic Renal Diet Cookbook.* New York: Golden Press, 1974. (Available from National Kidney Foundation)
19. Ward, M. K., et al.: Osteomalacic dialysis osteodystrophy: Evidence for a waterborne oetiological agent, probably aluminum. *Lancet* 1:841, 1978.
20. Kaehny, W. D., Hegg, A. P., and Alfrey, A. C.: Gastrointestinal absorption of aluminum from aluminum-containing antacids. *N. Engl. J. Med.* 296:1389, 1977.
21. Coburn, J. W., Hartenbower, D., and Brickman, A. S.: Advances in vitamin D metabolism as they per-

tain to chronic renal disease. *Am. J. Clin. Nutr.* 29:1283, 1976.

22. Coburn, J. W.: Vitamin D and calcium in patients with renal disease. Presentation at the 60th Annual Meeting of The American Dietetic Association, Los Angeles, Oct. 14, 1977.

23. Chesney, R. W., et al.: Increased growth after long-term 1 α 25-vitamin D_3 in childhood renal osteo-dystrophy. *N. Engl. J. Med.* 298:238, 1978.

24. Smith, L. H., Van den Berg, C. J., and Wilson, D. M.: Nutrition and urolithiasis. *N. Engl. J. Med.* 298:87, 1978.

* Recommended reading.

29

Alterations in levels of nitrogenous compounds

A dramatic or insidious change in blood level of one or more nitrogenous compounds poses a threat to a client's well-being. The nitrogenous substances discussed in this chapter are compounds which are influenced by *both* illness and diet. They include the waste products urea, ammonia, and uric acid and the essential blood constituents albumin and amino acids. Creatinine is not covered in detail because diet has little effect on blood creatinine level.

Health professionals assist clients to avoid problems associated with altered levels of nitrogenous substances by being alert for conditions which tend to precipitate problems, detecting early changes, and tailoring care of the client to attain or maintain normal levels. This requires some familiarity with factors governing the presence of these compounds in the blood.

Ammonia (NH_3) is a nitrogenous substance produced endogenously when the amino group ($-NH_2$) is removed from an amino acid in the process called deamination. Ammonia is also produced during digestion when intestinal bacteria act on protein breakdown products. Ammonia can be rapidly absorbed from the gut. It does not ordinarily accumulate in the blood because it is rapidly incorporated into urea, primarily in the liver. Urea circulates in the bloodstream until it is excreted by the kidneys. Small amounts of ammonia are also excreted via the kidneys.

A high dietary intake of protein results in increased endogenous production of both ammonia and urea. Catabolic conditions also increase production of these nitrogenous waste products.

RELATION OF DISEASE STATES TO ALTERATIONS IN NITROGENOUS COMPOUNDS

Impaired renal function Impaired renal function (of many types) is the most common cause for accumulation of urea. *Uremia* means an elevated blood urea level, but the term is more commonly used to refer to the uremic syndrome, that is, all of the signs and symptoms of renal failure. *Azotemia* refers to elevated levels of many types of nitrogenous waste products in the blood.

An elevated blood urea nitrogen (BUN) appears to contribute to development of anorexia, nausea, vomiting, lethargy, appearance of crystals of urea on the skin (uremic frost), and a uriniferous breath odor. "Middle molecules" (nitrogenous compounds which are so named because their size is intermediate between that of urea and of protein) are poorly defined compounds which also accumulate in uremic individuals and are thought to be toxic.[1]

If renal disease (e.g., nephrosis) increases the permeability of the renal tubules, large amounts of albumin may be lost in the urine (albuminuria). This may cause a serious *decrease* in serum albumin level. Dietary intake of protein may need to be increased to cover urinary protein loss.

Liver disease Diseases of the liver such as cirrhosis and hepatic failure are apt to interfere with conversion of ammonia to urea, causing elevated blood ammonia levels. High levels of ammonia in the blood are linked with hepatic encephalopathy and death. Hepatic encephalopathy is a syndrome of neurological changes. Early signs and symptoms include decreased regard for personal appearance, day-night reversal of sleep patterns, restlessness, euphoria, and mild confusion. Late signs include psychotic behavior, stupor, and asterixis (flapping tremor of the hand).

Liver disease may also lead to *imbalances* of amino acids in the blood. These imbalances have been implicated in the development of hepatic encephalopathy. Amino acid imbalances which occur in liver disease appear to alter the production of neurotransmitters (chemical compounds released from nerves which cause biological responses in adjoining cells). False neurotransmitters may be produced. Since neurotransmitters influence behavior and state of consciousness, an imbalance among them appears to help explain why serious neurological changes sometimes develop in hepatic failure.[2]

Another potentially serious problem in liver disease is a marked decrease in serum albumin level. This may result from pooling of albumin-rich fluid in the peritoneal cavity (ascites). A marked increase in abdominal girth is characteristic of ascites. Albumin retained in ascites fluid is not available for serving its usual functions. The liver increases albumin production in an attempt to normalize serum albumin level, but adequate compensation is generally impossible. If liver disease is severe or if intake of protein is inadequate, albumin *synthesis* may be impaired, further aggravating the problem.

Aminoacidurias Genetic defects which cause lack of any enzyme involved in amino acid metabolism can result in accumulation of specific amino acid(s) and of byproducts of the amino acid(s) in the blood and urine. Phenylketonuria (PKU) is an example of this type of genetic defect. If untreated, this condition causes severe mental retardation.

Hyperuricemia If ketones or other acidic substances successfully compete with uric acid for excretion by the renal tubules or if there is excessive production of uric acid due to gout, blood uric acid level rises. When blood uric acid level is sufficiently high, uric acid crystals may be deposited in joints or uric acid kidney stones may form.

MEANS OF PHYSICALLY OR PHARMACOLOGICALLY REDUCING BLOOD LEVELS OF NITROGENOUS COMPOUNDS

An understanding of the role of diet modification in the control of blood levels of nitrogenous compounds requires familiarity with artificial methods of ridding the body of these substances. To date technology is *not* sufficiently advanced to provide a practical means for continuous and selective removal of each toxic nitrogenous compound from the blood. Although there are reasonably good means of removing certain wastes from blood, the amount which can be safely removed in a period of a few hours is limited, if it is possible to remove the waste at all. Individuals with genetic defects such as phenylketonuria cannot take medication or undergo a special treatment in order to keep certain blood amino acids and their byproducts from accumulating.

DIALYSIS TREATMENTS

Principles A somewhat nonselective cleansing of the blood can be achieved on an intermittent basis by making use of dialysis treatments. Dialysis is primarily used with clients who have renal failure. Dialysis treatments involve bringing body fluid into indirect contact with another fluid (dialysate), the two being separated by a semipermeable membrane. Certain nitrogenous wastes—urea and creatinine in particular—can be removed from the blood by dialysis. Excess water and electrolytes can also be removed at the same time. Dialysis inadvertently causes losses of nutrients circulating in the blood unless those nutrients are bound to protein. Certain nutrients may also be *supplied* to the individual via dialysis.

Diet control is a valuable adjunct to dialysis. By limiting the accumulation of urea, fluid, and electrolytes, diet control facilitates safe removal of wastes in a reasonable period of time. If diet is controlled the client is likely to have a smoother course of dialysis treatments.

Types Two types of dialysis are commonly used for removing waste products from the body: peritoneal dialysis and hemodialysis. Both types make use of diffusion, osmosis, and filtration, but they differ in the method used for bringing extracellular fluid in contact with dialysate.

Differences in type of dialysis produce some differences in results which are of nutritional significance. These are summarized in Table 29.1. When comparing the rate of removal of waste products, health professionals should remember that a faster rate is not necessarily better.[3]

PHARMACOLOGICAL AGENTS AND TREATMENTS

A number of pharmacological agents (e.g., mannitol salt solution, bacterial enzymes, and charcoal) are being tested for use in removing wastes in the treatment of chronic renal failure.[6] If they are used, health care workers should be alert to drug-nutrient interactions.

Lactulose (Cephulac) and neomycin sulfate are

TABLE 29.1 *Features of hemodialysis and peritoneal dialysis which may be related to diet management*

	HEMODIALYSIS	*PERITONEAL DIALYSIS*
Rate of removal of nitrogenous wastes	Relatively rapid. If the BUN is very high and falls rapidly, adverse reactions such as cerebral edema are possible. Controlled protein intake reduces this problem	Slow
Rate of removal of potassium	Dependent on concentration of potassium in dialysate vs its concentration in the blood. The rate of removal of potassium is highest at the start of the treatment and tapers off owing to equalization of the concentration of potassium in dialysate and blood. If the blood concentration of potassium is unduly high, removal of the extra potassium is possible, but only at considerable risk to the client. Dietary restriction of potassium helps prevent this problem	Dependent on concentration of potassium in dialysate Repeated exchanges allow gradual removal of potassium
Removal of sodium	Related to removal of water as well as to the amount of sodium in the dialysate Serum sodium levels are usually within normal limits when dialysis begins, but total body sodium and water must be reduced. Rate of removal can be varied, but rapid removal is hazardous. Dietary restriction of sodium and fluid helps prevent this problem	Same as for hemodialysis but rate of removal is generally slower, allowing more to be safely removed There is some disagreement regarding the optimum amount of sodium and fluid restriction
Removal of phosphate	Low Control of dietary intake of phosphorus is recommended	Low
Loss of intact protein (primarily albumin)	Negligible—too large to pass through cellophane membrane	About 3–33 gm albumin per treatment[5]
Loss of amino acids	16–20 gm per 6 hour treatment[4]	Variable
Loss of vitamins	Ascorbic acid B complex vitamins, except riboflavin (B_2) and cyanocobalamin (B_{12}) Supplementation recommended	Supplementation recommended
Damage to RBCs	Some mechanical injury occurs Injury and blood loss increase need for nutrients for hematopoesis	Negligible
Net diffusion of glucose from dialysate to ECF	Usually has minor effect on blood sugar level	May cause significant rise in blood sugar level, sometimes resulting in hyperglycemia. A small source of calories
Usual duration of treatment during *maintenance* dialysis	4–6 hr; partially dependent on diet	8–12 hr; partially dependent on diet
Usual number of treatments weekly during maintenance dialysis	2–3; partially dependent on diet	3–5; partially dependent on diet
Relationship between meals and treatment	Meals may be taken during hemodialysis Some facilities allow liberal intake when the client is undergoing hemodialysis while other facilities feel it is more educationally sound to provide the client with his customary fare	Abdominal discomfort may produce anorexia Food is tolerated best if the meal is small and the client starts eating at the end of the "dwell time." This problem is avoided by giving peritoneal dialysis treatments at night

among drugs which might be used to reduce the serum ammonia level, as in clients who have certain liver diseases. These drugs do not eliminate the need for a modified diet. Neomycin may contribute to deficiencies of several nutrients if therapy is prolonged.

Uricosuric agents such as probenecid and sulfinpyrazone increase urinary excretion of uric acid, reducing serum uric acid levels. Allopurinol (Zyloprim) is a different type of drug which reduces biosynthesis of uric acid and thereby reduces blood uric acid level. Drug therapy is generally more effective than use of modified diets in controlling blood uric acid level.

DIET MODIFICATION

Principles to help normalize levels of nitrogenous compounds A diet modified in protein and/or specific amino acids is a useful adjunct in treatment of conditions characterized by altered levels of nitrogenous compounds. When determining the extent to which protein and/or amino acid intake should be modified in any disease condition, the health team considers and balances a number of factors:

1. How much protein/essential amino acid does the individual require for growth and/or maintenance of body tissue?
2. What nondietary means are or should be used to decrease blood levels of toxic nitrogenous substances?
3. What level of intake of protein and/or specific amino acids will result in dangerous increases in nitrogenous compounds?
4. What modifications are compatible with the individual's willingness and ability to comply with diet control?

The health team also directs attention toward promoting maximal protein sparing so that amino acids will be used for anabolic purposes.

Safely meeting the nitrogen requirement

When abnormal accumulation of nitrogenous compounds or amino acid imbalance is present, it may be necessary to walk a tightrope with regard to dietary intake of protein or particular amino acids. To achieve the desired state of nitrogen balance, the diet must include adequate amounts of all essential amino acids, total protein, and other nutrients. Otherwise balance between anabolism and catabolism of protein will be upset in favor of net breakdown. This would result in muscle wasting which would, in turn, release the very substances to be avoided. Muscle tissue is, after all, a source of amino acids.

Use of protein of high biological value is usually favored when protein intake must be restricted. Complete protein provides adequate amounts of essential amino acids without an unnecessarily large surplus of nonessential amino acids. In some cases use of a complete mixture of essential amino acids may be preferable to feeding intact protein.[1]

Variability in human requirements for protein and for essential amino acids is so great that careful monitoring of the individual's status is essential. Too high an intake of protein or specific amino acids accelerates dangerous accumulations of nitrogenous compounds. Inadequate intake prevents growth of children, prevents repletion of body tissue of malnourished individuals, and causes the development of protein-energy malnutrition. Guidelines based on age (for children), ideal body weight, urinary protein loss (if any), and current nutritional status can provide a reasonable starting point for determining protein needs. Sub-sequent monitoring of anthropometric, laboratory, and food intake data often reveals the need for diet adjustments.

Providing for maximal protein sparing and utilization of amino acids for anabolic purposes

Whenever there is a condition causing alteration in levels of nitrogenous compounds in the blood, the plan of care should include measures to promote use of dietary protein for anabolic purposes rather than for energy. Providing enough calories to cover metabolic demands for maintenance, activity, and growth or repletion (if applicable) permits utilization of protein for its many nonfuel functions. It is easy to forget that fuel is the body's first priority and that protein catabolism will increase if the fuel supply is inadequate.

Distributing the protein allowance into at least three feedings is generally recommended. (Avoiding a high intake at any one time reduces hepatic deamination of amino acids.)

Exercising the body promotes normal balance between anabolism and catabolism and thus helps to control the production of nitrogenous wastes. Health care workers should encourage or assist the client to exercise to whatever extent is allowed.

Necrosis of body tissue and fever are both associated with increased protein catabolism. Nursing measures can be implemented to prevent, identify, or reduce these problems. Examples include frequent turning and other measures to prevent development of pressure areas, protecting the client from infection, frequent checks of vital signs, and fever control measures.

POINTS OF EMPHASIS
Increasing the effectiveness of dietary protein

• *Encourage and facilitate intake of enough calories to maintain body weight.*
• *Promote physical exercise within prescribed limits.*
• *Distribute protein throughout the day.*
• *If protein intake is restricted, emphasize use of protein of high biological value.*
• *Take measures to prevent infection, necrosis, or other causes of increased catabolism.*

Safely promoting dietary compliance

The more normal the diet, the greater the likelihood that the client will feel able to adhere to a diet prescription. Since Americans are accustomed to an unnecessarily high protein intake, any degree of control of protein is usually considered to be restrictive, even if it allows a protein intake which meets Recommended Dietary Allowances. Compliance with a protein restricted diet usually requires limiting intake of most normal foods.

Since protein is an integral part of every type of cell, the only foods which are protein free are "separated" ingredients such as vegetable oil, cornstarch, and sugar.

When dietary intake of protein and/or specific amino acids must be restricted, the use of an exchange system simplifies the process of planning a varied diet. The exchange system used depends on which nutrients need to be restricted. Appendix 5G gives examples of exchange lists used for clients with renal disease who require a diet which is modified in protein, potassium, and sodium. A simpler set of exchange lists may be used for clients with liver disease since they do not usually need to restrict potassium intake. Food lists used in planning meals for children with phenylketonuria can be found in references listed at the end of Part 4.

SPECIAL CONSIDERATIONS IN DIETARY TREATMENT OF SPECIFIC DISEASE CONDITIONS

Acute renal failure

In acute renal failure the kidneys "shut down" suddenly in response to a severe stress such as hemorrhage, major surgery, or nephrotoxic agents (chemicals or drugs toxic to the kidneys). Nutritional demands are often greatly elevated, but appetite is lacking. Total parenteral nutrition and dialysis treatments may be necessary for the survival of the affected person. In acute renal failure from any cause, enteral feedings are severely restricted, if allowed at all. Enteral intake may be limited to "free" foods listed in Appendix 5G. These foods will not provide adequate nourishment and serve mainly to spare some protein.

Chronic renal failure

Although cure of chronic renal failure is seldom possible, treatment can greatly improve the client's feeling of well-being and can sometimes prolong his life for many years. One of the principal aspects of treatment is dietary control.

CONSERVATIVE MANAGEMENT

Conservative management of chronic renal failure involves diet and medication but not dialysis treatments. Conservative management is of value if the

glomerular filtration rate (GFR), measured by creatinine clearance, is above 4 ml. per minute. Conservative management is less effective than maintenance dialysis, but it is useful for clients who are unwilling or temporarily unable to undergo dialysis treatment.

Diet management includes control of protein, phosphate, sodium, potassium, and fluid and maintenance of adequate caloric intake. Restricting protein while maintaining caloric balance reduces urea production. When the BUN is elevated and dietary intake of protein is restricted, some of the accumulated urea in the blood may be used as a source of nitrogen for the formation of nonessential amino acids. Simplified, this reaction might be viewed as the opposite of deamination:

$$urea + keto\ acid \rightarrow amino\ acid$$

To favor this reaction, some physicians have severely curtailed clients' protein intake to about 18 to 22 gm. of high quality protein per day—as in the Giordano-Giovanetti diet.[8] Adherence to such a restricted diet has generally been poor and the value of this type of diet has been questioned.[9] It is uncertain whether diets providing less than 0.6 gm. protein per kg. body weight per day are nutritionally adequate and capable of preventing wasting of muscle tissue.[10] If the GFR is above 4 ml. per min., clients who are allowed 0.6 gm. protein per kg. per day appear to have as much symptomatic relief as do persons who are allowed only 0.3 gm. per kg. per day, and the higher intake is reported to increase clients' sense of well-being.[11]

KETOACID AND HYDROXYACID ANALOGUES OF AMINO ACIDS

Synthetic compounds called ketoacids and hydroxyacids have been used as protein substitutes on an experimental basis.[12] These compounds have the carbon skeletons of essential amino acids but differ in that they lack the amino group. In the body these ketoacids or hydroxyacids can pick up an amino group from urea, thus forming essential amino acids and reducing the BUN. The beneficial effect of ketoacids on protein metabolism may be greater than can be accounted for by this transamination reaction.[13] Unfortunately these synthetic compounds have several drawbacks. Since ketoacids or hydroxyacids are primarily effective when protein intake is restricted, their use does not result in a normal diet. Both ketoacids and hydroxyacids are expensive, and the ketoacids have a particularly unpleasant taste. Thus, although incorporating these compounds into the diet may promote maintenance of body tissue and control of the BUN, clients may not feel that the benefits outweigh the disadvantages. These compounds may become useful in tube feeding or parenteral feeding of persons who must be protein restricted.

TABLE 29.2 *Sample dinner menu pattern and sample menu for a diet providing 40 gm protein, 1 gm sodium 2 gm potassium*

Food list	MENU PATTERN No. of servings	SAMPLE MENU*†
Unsalted meat list	1	Casserole made with 30 gm (1 oz) cooked beef
#2 vegetable list	1	60 ml (¼ c) mushrooms and ½ green pepper
Low protein products	1	120 ml (½ c) imitation pasta
#1 fruit list	1	120 ml (½ c) canned applesauce
Dairy list	1	120 ml (½ c) whole milk
Fats	15 gm (1 Tbsp) salted margarine	15 gm salted margarine
Miscellaneous		
Dessert		3 low protein cookies
Herbs and spices		As desired, with casserole and applesauce

* This menu provides about 700 kcal
† See Appendix 5G for other choices

An average daily allowance of about 35 to 40 gm. protein (about 0.67 gm. protein per kg. of ideal body weight) is usually allowed in the conservative management of adults with chronic renal failure. Children are allowed more protein per kg. of ideal body weight, but their total intake is usually less than 40 gm. protein because of their smaller size. Conservative management of children with chronic renal failure is accompanied by failure to grow and is seldom used except, perhaps, on a temporary basis.

Numerous combinations of foods can be used to achieve a 40 gm. protein intake, using choices from the exchange groups in Appendix 5G. A dinner menu pattern and sample menu for a 40 gm. protein, 1 gm. sodium, 2 gm. potassium diet are shown in Table 29.2. A multiple restriction of this type is generally required in the treatment of chronic renal failure. The specific allowance of each of the restricted nutrients would be determined on an individual basis. The effectiveness of the protein restriction can be monitored by use of several types of data as suggested in Table 29.3.

A 40 gm. protein diet is not simple to follow. Exact portion sizes are specified and foods are carefully described in Table 29.2 because this much attention to detail is essential to compliance with the diet order and to keeping the disease under control.

Portion sizes of high protein foods are so small that it takes an imaginative cook to prepare appealing meals which stay within the protein allowance. Some

clients like to "stretch" their protein occasionally by using it in combination with other ingredients. For example, a small measured amount of egg and milk may be used in preparing french toast; cooked meat, egg, fish, and poultry all combine well with mayonnaise and finely diced raw vegetables to make sandwich spreads. Cookbooks such as *The Mayo Clinic Renal Diet Cookbook* present enticing recipes as well as practical suggestions for learning to plan, prepare, and enjoy a "renal" diet.[16]

Fluid and electrolyte restrictions complicate diet planning. The need for an adequate caloric intake compounds the problem even more. Suggested amounts of sweets and fats are indicated on the menu pattern to encourage the client to meet his caloric requirements. Since sweets and fats become objectionable when eaten in quantity, special low protein products are often recommended to help increase caloric intake.

Wheat starch and low protein pasta are examples of products which have been specially developed for use in low protein diets. A fairly complete list of special low protein products is included in Appendix 5G. Wheat starch is substituted for flour in preparing low protein bread, cookies, cake, muffins, and other baked goods using special recipes. Ready-made low protein baked goods are also available. Low protein baked goods generally have a heavier, more open texture and flatter taste than do their normal counterparts. Low

TABLE 29.3 *Data useful for assessing effectiveness of protein restricted diet in chronic renal failure*

TYPE OF DATA	INDICATORS OF EFFECTIVENESS
Laboratory tests:	
BUN or SUN	Significant decrease
Serum urea nitrogen:	
Serum creatinine (ratio)	Significant decrease (the ratio adjusts for changes in renal function), a ratio of ≤10:1 indicates compliance with diet[4]
Anthropometric measures	Stable measurements or gradual increase*
Behavioral	Increased appetite and tolerance for food
Food diary	Improved sense of well being Food intake fits diet plan

* If measurements indicate loss of lean body mass, dietary treatment is not necessarily responsible[15]

protein bread tends to be rubbery; some clients find it to be practically inedible.[17] Since special low protein products are not available in supermarkets and are expensive, health care workers should tell clients how they can be obtained and used to best advantage.

Vitamin supplementation is recommended as a part of conservative management of chronic renal failure because the diet is low in water-soluble vitamins. Table 29.4 summarizes recommended nutrient intakes for uremic clients.

MAINTENANCE DIALYTIC THERAPY

Dialysis, used in conjunction with diet and drug therapy, has enabled many individuals to lead changed but meaningful and productive lives. With adequate motivation, teaching, and supportive services, persons maintained by dialysis have the prospect of continuing their formal education, working to support themselves and their families, and/or managing a comfortable, happy home.

Fortunately, regular use of dialysis treatments for maintenance of the individual with chronic renal failure allows considerable liberalization of the diet. There are several reasons why this occurs: (1) dialysis removes small nonprotein nitrogenous waste products so that these toxins should not accumulate to dangerously high levels; (2) dialysis increases the protein requirement (see Table 29.1); and (3) dialysis removes excess fluid and electrolytes so that balance can be achieved with a higher level of intake.

An adult who is being maintained by dialysis is usually allowed *at least* 1 gm. protein per kg. of body weight. The allowance is higher for children when based on body weight, ranging up to 3 to 4 gm. of protein per kg. of body weight. It is common for an adult to be allowed 60 to 80 gm. protein; more than half of the protein should be of high biological value.[14] This level of protein intake has been reported to be associated with (1) adequate control of the BUN, (2) nitrogen balance or positive nitrogen balance, and (3) satisfactory feeling of well-being. Most new dialysis patients require a relatively generous intake of protein and calories to restore serum albumin levels and to

TABLE 29.4 *Recommended dietary intakes for uremic patients undergoing and not undergoing maintenance dialysis*

COMPONENT	NO DIALYSIS*	HEMODIALYSIS (HD) OR PERITONEAL DIALYSIS (PD)
Protein	Men: ≥40 gm/day (0.55–0.60 gm/kg/day) (28 gm of high biologic value) Women, small men: ≥35 gm/day (23–25 gm of high biologic value)	HD: 1.0 gm/kg/day PD: 1.2–1.5 gm/kg/day (>50% of high biologic value)
Calories	≥35 kcal/kg/day unless patient is obese	
Vitamins	(Quantities to be supplemented)	
Thiamine (mg/day)	1.5	1.5
Riboflavin (mg/day)	1.8	1.8
Pantothenic acid (mg/day)	5	5
Niacin (mg/day)	20	20
Pyridoxine hydrochloride (mg/day)	5	10
Vitamin B_{12} (μg/day)	3	3
Vitamin C (mg/day)	70–100	100
Folic acid (mg/day)	1	1
Vitamin A	None	None
Vitamin D	Not established	Not established
Vitamin E (IU/day)	15	15
Vitamin K	None†	None†
Minerals	(Range of total intake)	
Sodium (mg/day)	1000–3000	750–1000
Potassium (mEq/day)	40–70	40–70
Phosphorus (mg/day)‡	600–1200	600–1200
Calcium (mg/day)	1000–2000§	1000–1500§
Magnesium (mg/day)	200–300	200–300
Trace elements	Unknown	Unknown
Water	Up to 3000 ml/day as tolerated	Usually 750–1500 ml/day

From Kopple, J. D.: Nutritional management of chronic renal failure. *Postgrad. Med.* 64:135, Nov 1978, p. 137. © Copyright McGraw-Hill, Inc. With permission.
* Glomerular filtration rate >4–5 ml/min but <15–25 ml/min
† May be needed in patients receiving antibiotics
‡ Phosphate binders (aluminum carbonate, aluminum hydroxide) usually needed as well
§ Dietary intake usually must be supplemented to provide these levels

replete wasted muscle. However, taking more protein than allowed is generally associated with an unnecessarily high BUN/creatinine ratio, excessive prosphorus intake, and excessive potassium intake. (Many foods which are high in protein are also high in these two minerals.)

A typical diet order for an anuric, 70 kg. male who is maintained by 5-hr. hemodialysis treatments three times per week might be 80 gm. protein, 2 gm. sodium, 2 gm. potassium, 1 gm. phosphorus, and 800 to 1000 cc. fluid per day. These amounts vary with an individual's size, nutritional status, and renal function and with frequency and duration of hemodialysis treatments. The fluid allowance, for example, would be increased by 400 cc. daily if the individual excreted that much urine each day.

Competent health care workers make a concerted effort to help children who are treated with hemodialysis to eat as much as they are allowed.[18] Children on hemodialysis usually grow but seldom exhibit desirable rates of growth. Inadequate food intake may be a contributing factor in some circumstances.[19]

Some physicians recommend use of polyunsaturated rather than saturated fats in the diets of dialysis patients in the hope that this will reduce the risk of atherosclerosis.[5] Limiting carbohydrate intake to about 30 to 35 percent of the calories may also be helpful in controlling blood lipid levels.[20]

Cardiovascular disease is the leading cause of death among dialysis patients. Minor dietary indiscretions may be somewhat less serious for individuals who are dialysed than for conservatively managed clients, but compliance is associated with better health and reduced risk of complications. Possible nutrition-related complications are summarized in Table 29.5.

Diet for a client being maintained by peritoneal dialysis usually includes more than 1.2 gm. protein per kg. body weight per day (Table 29.4). In fact, protein intake may need to be encouraged to be sure that protein lost during peritoneal dialysis is replaced and nitrogen balance achieved. For previously malnourished adults, an intake of 1½ gm. protein per kg. of body weight has been accompanied by a desirable state of positive nitrogen balance.[5] Careful monitoring and assessment of the client make it possible to develop a satisfactory individualized diet plan. Nutrient intakes recommended for clients treated by dialysis are summarized in Table 29.4.

Health care workers need to inform a client who is being maintained by dialysis about whether or not he is staying within the limits set for interdialytic weight gain (amount of weight gained between dialysis treatments), serum electrolyte levels, blood urea/creatinine ratio, and blood urea nitrogen level. If dietary indiscretions are suspected, the health professional may want to guide the client in determining for himself what mistakes he made and how to correct them. The health care worker identifies whether lack of knowledge, lack of motivation, or depression or some other stress was involved; then she adapts follow-up care accordingly.

Health professionals who deal with clients on maintenance dialysis will find a high incidence of noncompliance. They should be prepared to deal with it nonjudgmentally, empathetically, and constructively. Noncompliance with one or more aspects of treatment is alarmingly high. One report cities that 3.4 percent of the hemodialysis clients studied *died* as a consequence of noncompliance with treatment, particularly with regard to dietary aspects.[21] For some clients eating is one of the few possible sources of satisfaction.

Because eating behavior is closely tied to the emotions, food intake often serves as a barometer of the client's success in coping with other stresses. A period of increased hope and confidence (associated with increased physical well-being), characteristic of the first

TABLE 29.5 *Possible nutrition-related complications in dialysis patients*

PROBLEM WITH COMPLIANCE	COMPLICATIONS THAT MAY RESULT
Excessive protein intake	Increased risk of problems during dialysis
Excessive sodium and fluid intake	Severe hypertension, congestive heart failure, pulmonary edema
Excessive intake of fluid alone	Same as above. Nausea, vomiting, muscle cramps and other vague symptoms may also develop
Excessive potassium intake	Muscle weakness, cardiac arrhythmia, cardiac arrest
High phosphorus intake	Bone disease
Failure to take prescribed medication:	
Phosphorus-binding agents	Bone disease
Calcium salts	Bone disease
Source of vitamin D	Bone disease
Multivitamins (water soluble)	Symptoms of vitamin deficiency
Folic acid and iron	More severe anemia (see below)

FACTORS NOT USUALLY RELATED TO DIET COMPLIANCE	
Change in glucose tolerance	Impaired glucose tolerance in previously normal persons; in contrast, diabetics may require less insulin
Elevated blood lipid levels	Atherosclerosis, myocardial infarction
Lack of erythropoietin	Severe anemia

few weeks of dialysis treatment, is usually followed by a longer period of discouragement. Clients may fail to eat when they are depressed or they may eat too much as a means of dealing with anxiety. Some clients *choose* to eat and drink whatever they want with full knowledge of the probable consequences. They may prefer to "live it up" temporarily and then assume a "sick role" rather than to remain in the confusing role of a "marginal man" who is neither sick nor well.[22] If a client makes this choice, he needs acceptance, not condemnation, from health team members. Other clients on maintenance dialysis adapt quite well to their new life situation, accept their disease and limitations, and work around them.

One study[23] indicates that incidence of noncompliance among dialysis clients appears to be unrelated

---

POINTS OF EMPHASIS
Dietary treatment of chronic renal failure

• *Conservative management (treatment by diet and drugs only) requires a glomerular filtration rate of at least 4 ml/minute.*

• *Conservative management includes strict control of intake of protein (about 0.6 gm. protein/kg. of body weight per day for adults, more per kg. for children). Lower protein intakes are sometimes indicated. Intake of potassium, sodium, fluid, and sometimes phosphorus must also be controlled.*

• *The purpose of diet modification is to achieve a balance between intake and output, alleviate symptoms, and maintain satisfactory nutritional status.*

• *Dialysis treatments allow some liberalization of the diet.*

• *Protein is so widely distributed in foods that portion sizes of most foods must be strictly controlled to stay within diet guidelines.*

• *Use of special low protein products may be necessary to achieve adequate caloric intake. High priority should be given to meeting caloric needs.*

• *Appropriate vitamin-mineral supplementation is recommended to offset inadequacies of restricted diets and, if applicable, losses during dialysis treatments. An active form of vitamin D is often needed.*

• *Detailed monitoring is needed to provide information about the effectiveness of diet, medications, and dialysis treatments. Assessment should give close attention to the client's nutritional status.*

• *Noncompliance with treatment measures is common and is a potential source of serious complications. Health professionals need to show acceptance and understanding and to develop new approaches to help clients meet their varied needs.*

---

to mastery of facts pertinent to diet control or to the degree of dietary restriction. Noncompliance tended to *increase* the longer a person had been a dialysis client. Apparently health professionals need to (1) more fully understand the needs and desires of clients with chronic renal failure,[17] (2) find better ways to motivate individuals to follow prescribed regimens, and (3) assist individuals in learning to cope with the many extra stresses associated with dialysis. A team effort is needed to help the client develop viable solutions to a variety of problems.

The teaching schedule for a client who is new to maintenance dialysis should be carefully planned since there is a great deal which must be learned before discharge. Long term follow-up meetings with the dietitian will no doubt be desirable after discharge. Putting a diet into practice in a family setting, boarding house, or restaurant is not as easy as learning how to use a diet form.

Supportive groups may be found in communities across the U.S. Many clients benefit from informal social and educational group meetings with other individuals who require maintenance dialysis. Information about such groups and other community resources can be obtained from the National Kidney Foundation.

Liver diseases

A diet modified in protein content is often of value in the treatment of diseases of the liver, such as chronic cirrhosis and acute viral hepatitis. Two opposing factors must be kept in mind: (1) a person with a diseased liver requires an increased supply of amino acids to allow regeneration of liver tissue, replenishment of serum proteins, and correction of protein-energy malnutrition and (2) when hepatic function is severely diminished, the serum level of ammonia and perhaps other protein metabolites may rise dangerously unless protein intake is very low.

Nitrogenous compounds accumulate in severe hepatic failure because less blood actually reaches the liver, the principal site for detoxification and amino acid catabolism. Congestion in the liver stimulates formation of collateral blood vessels which shunt a part of the blood around, rather than to, the liver. A surgically constructed shunt (such as a portocaval shunt) also reroutes much of the blood away from the liver. Natural and surgical shunting increase the likelihood of development of hepatic encephalopathy, but a surgical shunt definitely is associated with greater risk of this complication.

Whether the diet for a client with liver disease is to be high, intermediate, or low in protein varies with the individual's immediate clinical status. In uncomplicated viral hepatitis, modified diets have not been found to improve the course of the disease.[24]

A person with relatively mild to moderate liver disease may be placed on a moderately high protein diet (e.g., up to 70 to 80 gm. daily) if he is alert, oriented, and free of signs of hepatic encephalopathy. Spindly arms and legs of a person with cirrhosis (in sharp contrast to a belly which protrudes due to ascites) signal the need for a somewhat generous protein intake if it can be tolerated. A vegan diet may help to avoid excessive protein intake and may have a more favorable amino acid pattern for certain clients with liver disease.[24a]

It may be desirable for the client to avoid foods which contain much ammonia.[25] Among foods which have been found to contain enough ammonia to significantly increase serum ammonia levels of cirrhotic persons are salami, blue cheese, cheddar cheese, and gelatin. (The first three of these would probably be in the "Foods to Avoid" column of the diet plan anyway, because of their high sodium content. Abstinence from alcohol is essential to prevent further liver damage.

In severe hepatic cirrhosis, protein intake is usually restricted to 60, 40, or 20 gm. protein; it may be completely eliminated from the diet for a brief period. One meal from a 20 gm. protein diet for possible use in hepatic disease is described in Table 29.6. The menu shown is low in sodium as well as in protein. More severe sodium restriction (down to about 250 mg. or 11 mEq. sodium daily) is sometimes beneficial for persons with hepatic insufficiency because they have increased levels of circulating aldosterone and, therefore, tend to retain sodium avidly. It is often unrealistic to expect a person with severe liver disease to eat what is served. Belligerency or unresponsiveness associated with impending hepatic encephalopathy make obtaining a client's cooperation quite difficult. Intensive nutritional support may be necessary to help the client achieve desirable intake.

Providing the client with carbohydrate is emphasized in liver disease. Carbohydrate decreases protein catabolism, provides needed energy, helps maintain or replete glycogen stores in the liver and helps maintain a normal blood glucose level. Glycogenolysis in the liver may be seriously impaired by liver damage, causing a tendency toward a low blood sugar level.

Generally a moderate fat intake is tolerated unless liver function is severely altered or the bile duct is occluded. Including some fat in the diet increases palatability—an important consideration since anorexia is a common complaint in any type of liver disease.

When encephalopathy is moderate or marked, enteral protein intake is completely eliminated. In this case, small frequent feedings of carbohydrate by mouth

TABLE 29.6 *One meal from a 20 gm protein, 500 mg sodium diet*

BREAKFAST
120 ml (½ c) orange juice
  1 soft cooked egg (medium)
120 ml low protein cereal with 5 gm (2 tsp) regular margarine and sugar
  1 slice low protein toast with
  5 gm (2 tsp) unsalted margarine and
 15 gm (1 Tbsp) jelly

(e.g., fruit juices, carbonated beverages, hard candy), if possible, or continuous intravenous administration of dextrose in water are recommended to help maintain normal blood glucose levels. Health care workers must take care to follow orders closely when giving fluids. Both fluid overload and dehydration are especially threatening to persons with severe liver disease. When oral feedings are used, extra carbohydrate is sometimes added to fruit juice or other allowed beverages in the form of corn syrup or special supplements such as Polycose (Appendix 5G). These beverages are served thoroughly chilled or as a frozen slush to avoid an objectionably sweet taste.

Unfortunately, there is seldom a clear dividing line regarding optimal protein intake in liver disease. It may be critical for the nurse and other health professionals to closely assess for signs of impending hepatic encephalopathy, as suggested in Table 29.7. Such assessment may indicate that the liver is unable to adequately handle the protein being given. If danger signs appear, the nurse should avoid giving protein, pending a change in diet order, and should notify the physician. When a person with serious liver disease is discharged or treated on an outpatient basis, a health professional should teach family members or significant others to identify signs that warn of the need for medical care.

If encephalopathy is developing, it is likely that medical treatment will initially restrict enteral feeding of protein or amino acids to no more than 20 gm. per day. This reduces the amount of substrate which intestinal bacteria can convert to ammonia and also reduces ammonia production within the body. Lactulose or neomycin may be given to decrease ammonia absorption. When improvement of the patient's condition becomes evident, enteral protein intake is increased gradually (increments of 10 gm. protein every 3 to 5 days, if tolerated) to about 40 to 50 gm. daily.

To help prevent the development of encephalopathy, health care workers should take measures to assist the client to (1) maintain fluid balance, (2) maintain a normal serum potassium level, and (3) have a daily or more frequent bowel movement. Often the client can be motivated to assume these responsibilities himself at home. Consuming fruits and juices high in potassium (Appendix 5E) may help prevent serum potassium levels from falling; they also help promote fluid balance and regular bowel movements. Soft high fiber foods are recommended to help prevent constipation. Use of lactulose promotes passage of several soft stools daily. Uncooked or gas-forming vegetables are usually avoided since they may be overly filling or cause discomfort. If the person has developed esophageal varices as a result of portal hypertension, a soft diet may be ordered to reduce the risk of rupturing a varix.

Research with animals and humans suggests that specially formulated intravenous feedings of amino acids may be helpful in treatment and perhaps prevention of hepatic encephalopathy.[28] The value of intravenous or enteral feeding of α-ketoacids in liver disease is also being investigated.[2]

TABLE 29.7 *Hints to aid assessment of developing hepatic encephalopathy*[26]

ACTION	EXAMPLE
Clearly document mental status in medical record so that *change* can be easily identified	11/8/79 3 PM S. At lunch time patient stated, "I feel fine. I can manage by myself; just leave me alone." O. Oriented to time, place and person, does not maintain eye contact, frequently stares at wall. Was clumsy and messy when feeding self. Constantly picks at clothes. 11/9/79 10AM O. Difficult to arouse. Mumbling. Responds to name but is not oriented to time or place.
Administer timed number connection tests[27] Maintain handwriting chart (dated samples of the client's handwriting) for early identification of subtle changes	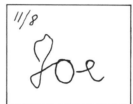 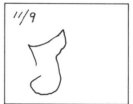
Keep accurate record of daily weights	
Keep accurate I & O records	
Routinely search for precipitating factors	Increased arterial NH_3 level? Hypokalemia? Constipation? Infection? Dehydration?

POINTS OF EMPHASIS

Diet in hepatic disease

• *Ongoing monitoring of response to diet may save a life.*
• *Moderately high intake of protein helps promote regeneration of liver and muscle tissue and of serum proteins but is contraindicated in impending or existing hepatic encephalopathy.*
• *High caloric intake compensates for increased metabolism, spares protein, and/or promotes anabolism. Moderate amounts of fat can usually be tolerated. Large amounts of carbohydrate are encouraged to maintain normal blood glucose levels.*
• *Alcohol should not be consumed.*
• *The need for vitamin and mineral supplementation should be assessed since malnutrition commonly accompanies liver disease.*
• *Intensive nutritional support may be needed to counteract anorexia or inability to eat.*

Phenylketonuria (PKU)

People who have the inborn error of metabolism called phenylketonuria (PKU) lack the enzyme phenylalanine hydroxylase. This enzyme is required for the synthesis of tyrosine (a semiessential amino acid) from phenylalanine (an essential amino acid). Figure 29.1 illustrates how lack of this enzyme affects a number of metabolic reactions. If the affected person is not treated, phenylalanine and phenylpyruvic acid accumulate in the blood.

If elevated blood levels of phenylalanine persist, serious damage to the central nervous system is inevitable. Early detection and treatment are crucial to the prevention of mental retardation. Lack of treatment results in *irreversible* brain damage.

Nearly every state has a law mandating testing of the newborn for PKU prior to discharge of the infant from the hospital. A simple blood test (most commonly the Guthrie test) on about the fourth or fifth day of life is used to screen for PKU. Positive results require further testing to establish a definite diagnosis. In older infants a diaper test may be used as an even simpler (but less reliable) screening method.

MEASURES USED TO REGULATE BLOOD PHENYLALANINE LEVELS

Diet modification makes it possible for a child with PKU to grow to normal size and develop normal intellectual capacity. Dietary control appears to be of greatest importance during the first 6 years of life, the period when brain growth is rapid. Most physicians now feel that a liberalized diet can be safely tried for older children and adults with PKU. In females, however, dietary control is important prior to and during pregnancy. The level of phenylalanine in fetal blood becomes dangerously elevated if maternal levels are high. Dietary control of pregnant women with PKU may help reduce incidence of fetal mortality, mental retardation, and other birth defects. If a female with PKU is planning to become pregnant in the near future, it is advisable for her to consult her physician and nutritionist about altering her diet *in preparation* for pregnancy.

Diet is used to maintain serum phenylalanine level within an established range. At the time of writing, a national study is under way to determine whether a range of 1 to 5.4 mg. per 100 ml. or 5.5 to 10 mg. phenylalanine per 100 ml. is most satisfactory.[29]

Once serum phenylalanine levels are regulated, the diet must include enough phenylalanine, total protein, and calories to support normal growth and maintenance of body tissues. These amounts vary with body size, rate of growth, and, in the case of calories, metabolic rate and activity. Regular monitoring of blood level of phenylalanine is necessary to determine if any changes should be made in the diet prescription.

Diet for an individual with PKU requires the use of one or more specially formulated products. If normal foods were used to meet even the bare minimum need for protein, phenylalanine intake would be much too high. The phenylalanine content of protein averages

about 5 percent; therefore, use of all protein-containing foods must be strictly controlled.

Several products are available to provide the individual with a majority of his daily protein intake: Lofenalac, Mead Johnson Product 3229, Aminogran, Albumaid XP, Cymogran, and Minafen. These products are similar in that they contain fat, carbohydrate, vitamins, minerals, and amino acids. Lofenalac, Cymogran, and Minafen contain a small amount of phenylalanine (although much less than does milk). M.J. #3229 and Albumaid XP are essentially free of phenylalanine. Since the phenylalanine content of all of these formulas is below minimum requirements, other foods can and must be used to provide the correct amount of phenylalanine for the individual.

Lofenalac is the formula traditionally used in the U.S. as the foundation of the diet for infants and children with PKU. During infancy a prescribed small amount of milk is added to the Lofenalac to provide needed phenylalanine. The two are mixed together to make sure that all essential amino acids are present at the same time and to minimize the chance that Lofenalac will be refused because of its taste. (Infants like milk better.) Products free of phenylalanine are advantageous if it is desirable to allow more liberal use of phenylalanine-containing foods.[30]

The nurse who has contact with parents at the time their infant is diagnosed to have PKU may play a vital role in interpreting the meaning of the diagnosis. She may discuss the many ways in which health team members can be of assistance in promoting normal growth and development of their child. Doctor, nurse, nutritionist, social worker, psychologist, and technicians all provide needed services. In many states the cost of special formula is assumed by the state.

Successful control of PKU requires a team effort in which the family plays a leading role. Family members must learn how to (1) plan the baby's diet, (2) monitor food intake, (3) take blood samples, (4) keep accurate

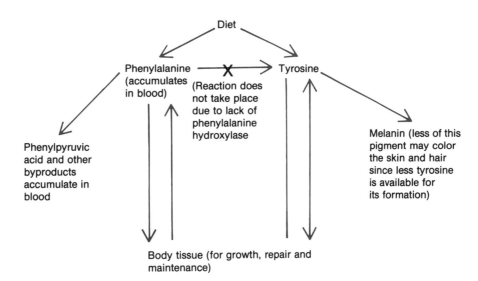

FIGURE 29.1. Alterations in metabolism in phenylketonuria (PKU).

records of the child's food intake and state of health, (5) cope with the child's normal developmental stages without major digressions from the diet, and (6) help the child to develop normally. Besides helping parents master necessary skills, the health team may be able to help them voice their fears, concerns, and feelings of guilt and frustration and to help them develop a healthy outlook.[31]

Gout and hyperuricemia

Dietary modifications to decrease or control blood uric acid levels can be helpful adjuncts to the use of pharmacological agents. The most useful dietary measures are directed toward facilitating excretion of uric acid.

Normal intake of carbohydrate prevents formation of excess ketones. This is desirable since ketones, if present in increased amounts, reduce the amount of uric acid which can be excreted. Retention of extra uric acid may exacerbate symptoms of gout. Low carbohydrate diets and very low calorie diets should be avoided by individuals with gout, especially during an acute attack. This does not imply that the obese individual with gout should not lose weight, but that weight should be lost gradually by means of a well-balanced diet when the gout is under control.

An increased serum level of lactic acid associated with alcohol intake also interferes with uric acid excretion; therefore, individuals who have gout are encouraged to omit alcoholic beverages altogether or to at least limit alcohol consumption.

Although uric acid is produced when purines are broken down in the body, limiting dietary intake of purines is thought to be relatively ineffective in reducing uric acid levels. The *endogenous* supply of purines is large, especially in individuals with gout. Nonetheless, purine restricted diets are still sometimes ordered by the physician.

A mild purine restricted diet doesn't pose much of a hardship for most clients because the principal foods eliminated are organ meats, anchovies, sardines, caviar and other fish roe, meat-based gravy, broth, and beer and wine. Avoidance of these foods may be helpful for some clients when the uric acid level is first being brought under control by drugs.[32] More severe purine restriction can pose a nutritional threat since it limits most foods from the meat group and certain other valuable sources of nutrients.

To help avoid development of uric acid kidney stones when hyperuricemia is present, the most effective dietary measure is to encourage high fluid intake. Maintaining a somewhat alkaline urine may also be helpful.

STUDY QUESTIONS

1. Ms. T. is following a 60 gm. protein, 2 gm. sodium, 2 gm. potassium diet with a 1000 cc. fluid restriction. If she is still hungry after finishing all of her allowed protein-containing foods, what might you suggest that would increase her caloric intake while fitting in with her restrictions?
2. Identify two reasons why more protein is allowed for a person who is being dialysed than for a person who is being conservatively managed for chronic renal failure.
3. Mr. S. has chronic renal failure. His GFR is about 8 ml. per minute. At the present time he is unwilling to undergo dialysis treatments but wants to get better. What type of diet will probably be prescribed? In what ways can a modified diet benefit him?
4. Ms. J. is hospitalized with cirrhosis of the liver. She has been placed on a 40 gm. protein diet. In the late afternoon she has a flapping tremor of the hand and she throws objects and exhibits other signs of abnormal behavior. At this time her tray is delivered. What should be done about feeding her? Why?
5. What problem would arise if parents consistently forgot to give their young infant (who has PKU) the prescribed amount of milk in addition to Lofenalac? Why?
6. If a person has gout, why is it helpful for him to avoid following low carbohydrate reducing diets or drinking alcohol?

References

1. Smith, L. J.: Large surface area dialysis. Innovations and patient management. *Nurs. Clin. North Am.* 10(3):481, 1975.
2. Aguirre, A.: Parenteral nutrition in hepatic failure. In J. E. Fischer (ed.): *Total Parenteral Nutrition.* Boston: Little, Brown & Co., 1976.
3. Shinaberger, J. H., and Blumenkrantz, M. J.: Dialysis therapy and transplantation in uremia: Which to use when. *Postgrad. Med.* 64(5):169, 1978.
4. David, D. S., et al.: Dietary management in renal failure. *Lancet* 2:34, 1972.
*5. Blumenkrantz, M. J., et al.: Nutritional management of the adult patient undergoing peritoneal dialysis. *J. Am. Diet. Assoc.* 73:251, 1978.
6. Friedman, E. A., Delano, B. G., and Butt, K. M.: Pragmatic realities in uremia therapy. *N. Engl. J. Med.* 298:368, 1978.
7. Giordano, C., DeSanto, N. G., and Senatore, R.: Effects of catabolic stress in acute and chronic renal failure. *Am. J. Clin. Nutr.* 31:1561, 1978.
8. Giovannetti, S. and Maggiore, Q.: A low nitrogen diet with protein of high biological value for severe chronic uremia. *Lancet* 1:1000, 1964.
9. Varcoe, A. R., et al.: Anabolic role of urea in renal failure. *Am. J. Clin. Nutr.* 31:1601, 1978.
10. Ritz, E., et al.: Protein restriction in the conservative management of uremia. *Am. J. Clin. Nutr.* 31:1703, 1978.
11. Kopple, J. D., and Coburn, J. W.: Metabolic studies of low protein diets in uremia. *Medicine* 52:583, 1973.
12. Walser, M.: Keto-analogues of essential amino acids in the treatment of chronic renal failure. *Kidney Int.* 13 (Suppl. 8): S-180, 1978.
13. Wrong, O.: Nitrogen metabolism in the gut. *Am. J. Clin. Nutr.* 31:1587, 1978.
*14. Kopple, J. D.: Nutritional management of chronic renal failure. *Postgrad. Med.* 64(5):135, 1978.
15. Bianchi, R., et al.: The metabolism of human

serum albumin in renal failure on conservative and dialysis therapy *Am. J. Clin. Nutr.* 31:1615, 1978.

16. Margie, J. D., et al.: *The Mayo Clinic Renal Diet Cookbook.* New York: Goldren Press, 1974. (Available from National Kidney Foundation)

*17. Biller, D. C.: Patient's point of view: Diet in chronic renal failure. *J. Am. Diet Assoc.* 71:633, 1977.

18. Berger, M.: Dietary management of children with uremia. *J. Am. Diet. Assoc.* 70:498, 1977.

*19. Spinozzi, N. S., and Grupe, W. E.: Nutritional implications of renal disease. IV. Nutritional aspects of chronic renal insufficiency in childhood. *J. Am. Diet. Assoc.* 70:493, 1977.

20. Heuck, C. C., et al.: Serum lipids in renal insufficiency. *Am. J. Clin. Nutr.* 31:1547, 1978.

21. Abram, H. S., Moore, G. L., and Westervelt, F. B., Jr.: Suicidal behavior in chronic dialysis patients. *Am. J. Psychiatry* 127:1199, 1971.

22. Landsman, M. K.: The patient with chronic renal failure: A marginal man. *Ann Intern. Med.* 82:268, 1975.

23. Blackburn, S. L.: Dietary compliance of chronic hemodialysis patients. *J. Am. Diet. Assoc.* 70:31, 1977.

24. Perman, J. A., and Grand, R. J.: Acute and chronic hepatitis in children. *Postgrad. Med.* 63(1):191, 1978.

24a. Greenberger, N. J., et al.: The effect of vege-table and animal protein diets in chronic hepatic encephalopathy. *Am. J. Dig. Dis.* 22:845, 1977.

25. Rudman, D., et al.: Ammonia content of food. *Am. J. Clin. Nutr.* 26:487, 1973.

26. Maddrey, W., and Weber, F.: Chronic hepatic encephalopathy. *Med. Clin. North Am.* 59:937, 1975.

27. Shaw, S.: The nutritional management of liver disease. Presentation at the American Society for Parenteral and Enteral Nutrition—Third Clinical Congress, Boston, Feb. 2, 1979.

28. Fischer, J. E., et al.: Plasma amino acids in patients with hepatic encephalopathy: Effect of amino acid infusions. *Am. J. Surg.* 127:40, 1974.

29. Acosta, P. B., et al.: Methods of dietary inception in infants with PKU. *J. Am. Diet. Assoc.* 72:164, 1978.

30. Parker, C., et al.: Clinical experience in dietary management of phenylketonuria with a new phenyl-alanine-free product. *J. Pediatr.* 91:941, 1977.

*31. Wyatt, D. S.: Phenylketonuria: The problems vary during different developmental stages. *MCN* 3:296, 1978.

32. Talbott, J. H.: Treating gout: Successful methods for prevention and control. *Postgrad. Med.* 63(5):175, 1978.

* Recommended reading.

30

Alterations in blood sugar

Appropriate care and teaching of persons with altered blood sugar levels should reflect an understanding of the underlying cause and the ramifications of the particular condition involved. The term blood sugar always refers to the glucose circulating in the blood, even though small amounts of other sugars may be temporarily present.

Although several hormones may contribute to an abnormal blood sugar level, the principal problem is usually an imbalance between the supply and demand for insulin. The insulin may be *endogenous* (made within the body) or *exogenous* (administered parenterally—by injection into subcutaneous tissue or directly into a vein). Insulin deficit results in hyperglycemia (high blood sugar). Insulin excess results in hypoglycemia (low blood sugar).

Several conditions frequently associated with altered blood sugar levels are the following:
1. Diabetes mellitus: youth onset or maturity onset
2. Stress-induced hyperglycemia: severe burns, crushing injuries, major surgery, and myocardial infarction
3. Concentrated glucose infusions: total parenteral nutrition
4. Food-stimulated or reactive hypoglycemia: may occur secondary to gastrectomy, pyloroplasty, vagotomy; otherwise rare
5. Disease-related hypoglycemia: insulin-producing tumors or severe liver disease
6. Drug-related hypoglycemia: excessive dose of hypoglycemic agent (insulin or sulfonylureas) in relation to food intake or exercise; alcohol consumption without adequate food intake
7. Drug-related hyperglycemia: steroid therapy, phenytoin, thiazides

Distinguishing between normal and abnormal blood glucose levels

The laboratory values used to distinguish hyperglycemia and hypoglycemia vary depending on the choice of serum or whole blood and the particular method of determination. In general, any time a person's blood sugar concentration rises above approximately 160 mg. glucose per 100 ml. venous blood, he would be described as hyperglycemic. When the blood sugar level exceeds 160 to 180 mg. per dl., the usual renal threshold for glucose, sugar spills into the urine. This condition of sugar in the urine is called *glycosuria*. It can be readily detected by simple urine tests such as Clinitest or dipstick. A blood glucose concentration of less than about 60 mg. per dl. signals hypoglycemia. Urine tests cannot be used to identify hypoglycemia.

Blood glucose levels are most meaningful if they are related to the time and composition of the most recent meal. A "random" blood glucose determination is unrelated to food intake and provides useful information only if it falls well outside of the normal range. A normal *fasting* blood sugar (FBS), obtained after a fast of at least 8 hours, usually lies between 60 and 100 mg. glucose per 100 ml. venous blood. A very high FBS is a sign of disease and is usually accompanied by classic symptoms of diabetes mellitus.

Screening tests and sometimes glucose tolerance tests are preferable to a fasting blood sugar determination for *early* detection of abnormalities in control of blood sugar level. In a screening test the blood glucose level may be determined either 1 or 2 hours following a carbohydrate-rich meal. The meal, which should contain about 75 to 100 gm. carbohydrate, is eaten after an overnight fast. If the blood glucose level exceeds a preset level, for example 160 mg. percent 2 hours postprandial, diabetes mellitus is suspected and further testing may be done.

Tolerance for glucose is described as low, decreased, or impaired when blood glucose rises to abnormally high levels following glucose consumption. Aging is usually accompanied by a significant increase in fasting blood sugar and decrease in glucose tolerance, as described by Fagans and Freinkel.[1] Health care workers should take care not to classify an elderly client as diabetic using criteria developed for younger persons.

A new blood test, measurement of the amount of hemoglobin A_{1C} (also called glycosylated hemoglobin), indicates if the blood sugar has been abnormally high over a period of weeks to months.[2] Although not routinely used at present, it is possible that measurement of hemoglobin A_{1C} may become an effective means of evaluating ongoing control of diabetes.[3]

Hormones involved in alterations of blood sugar level

In health blood glucose levels are carefully regulated by the hormones: insulin, glucagon, and somatostatin.

INSULIN

Insulin serves as an *anabolic* hormone in addition to its roles in controlling blood sugar. Insulin exerts its many effects primarily by causing:

1. Increased glucose and amino acid uptake by the cells. By attaching to receptor sites on cell membranes, insulin apparently alters the membranes in such a way that glucose and amino acids readily enter the cell. Obesity and diabetes can both adversely affect insulin receptor sites, thus interfering with insulin activity.
2. Increased activity of cellular enzymes promoting anabolism. Without actually entering the cell itself, insulin affects specific enzymes within cells, increasing utilization of glucose for glycogenesis, lipogenesis, and glycolysis. It promotes anabolic processes of other types as well.

Some insulin must continually be present in the blood to avoid excessive catabolism of body tissue. A person who lacks insulin rapidly loses muscle tissue and fat.

GLUCAGON

Abnormal glucagon secretion may also contribute to abnormal blood sugar level. Glucagon is a hormone which increases blood sugar level. It is secreted by the alpha (α) cells of the islets of Langerhans of the pancreas. Hyperglycemia becomes more severe if insulin is lacking and excess glucagon is being secreted. Insufficient glucagon secretion prolongs hypoglycemia. Some diabetics have been found to secrete abnormally high or abnormally low amounts of glucagon in response to changes in blood sugar level.[4]

SOMATOSTATIN

Somatostatin is a newly discovered hormone produced and secreted by the D cells of the islets of Langerhans of the pancreas. Among its varied actions are *suppression* of the production of both glucagon and insulin.[5] The roles of somatostatin in normal and abnormal regulation of blood sugar levels have not yet been clearly determined.

OTHERS

Glucogenic hormones, which are released in response to stress, increase blood glucose levels. These hormones (epinephrine, glucocorticords, glucagon, and growth hormone) are sometimes called *insulin-antagonistic* hormones.

CONDITIONS ASSOCIATED WITH ALTERATIONS IN BLOOD GLUCOSE

Diabetes mellitus

Diabetes mellitus* is a group of metabolic diseases which have several commonalities and numerous differences. Elevated blood sugar level characterizes all types of untreated diabetes. All diabetics lack enough insulin for normal metabolism, but in many cases the lack is relative and may be overcome without the use of hypoglycemic agents (pharmaceutical agents which lower blood sugar levels).

For purposes of treatment it is helpful to classify diabetes mellitus according to type of onset and need for exogenous insulin.

YOUTH ONSET DIABETES MELLITUS

The most severe form of primary diabetes has a dramatic onset. Lack of ability to control and use blood sugar is often signalled by the classic signs of diabetes: extreme thirst (polydipsia), excessive hunger (polyphagia), and greatly increased urination (polyuria). An additional signal, sugar in the urine (glycosuria)

---

* The shortened but less accurate term *diabetes* will frequently be used in this chapter to refer to diabetes mellitus. Used alone, diabetes never refers to diabetes inspidus.

would be noted by the health professional. The affected individual, if untreated, loses weight, feels very ill, and soon develops a life-threatening condition called ketoacidosis. Treatment requires exogenous insulin and control of diet and exercise for the remainder of the diabetic's life.

This type of diabetes has a variety of names, including youth or growth onset diabetes,* juvenile onset diabetes, and ketosis-prone diabetes. Youth onset diabetes may first appear in older adults. About 5 percent of the diagnosed cases of diabetes are of the youth onset type.

Diabetes which is secondary to pancreatectomy has the characteristics of youth onset diabetes.

After the dramatic development of youth onset diabetes, there may be a temporary period of partial remission during which small but significant amounts of insulin are produced by the beta cells. The period of partial remission is often called the "honeymoon period"—a time which is favorable for the diabetic and his family to become acquainted with the disease and to learn how to live with it. Prompt insulin and diet treatment following diagnosis of youth onset diabetes may help preserve some B-cell activity and prolong the honeymoon period for a number of years.[6] Youth onset diabetes is described as stable when the blood sugar level is readily controlled by insulin, diet, and exercise.

A small proportion of individuals with youth onset diabetes are subject to frequent dangerously wide swings in blood glucose level for no obvious reason. These hypoglycemic and hyperglycemic episodes may seriously disrupt their lives. This unstable form of youth onset diabetes is often called *brittle* diabetes.

MATURITY ONSET DIABETES MELLITUS

A much more common form of primary diabetes mellitus—maturity onset diabetes—usually has an insidious onset. The mild symptoms associated with mild to moderate increases in blood sugar may go unnoticed for a long period of time. Diagnosis may be delayed until the person seeks medical attention for one of the complications of diabetes or for an unrelated disease or injury. Maturity onset diabetes is also called adult onset diabetes, nonketosis prone diabetes, and noninsulin dependent diabetes.

In maturity onset diabetes mellitus the ability of the pancreas to produce and secrete insulin is diminished but not absent. Insulin deficiency may be described as relative rather than absolute. A condition of insulin resistance is often present. Insulin resistance is characterized by reduced effectiveness of a given amount of insulin.

In a majority of the cases of maturity onset diabetes adequate control of blood sugar may be restored without the use of exogenous insulin or other hypoglycemic agents (drugs which lower blood sugar level) by proper

*Youth onset diabetes is the name which will be used in this book.

management of diet and exercise. This is especially true for the very large percentage of maturity onset diabetics who are above ideal body weight at the time of diagnosis. Caloric deficit facilitates control of blood sugar by several means: (1) reduction in caloric intake reduces the need for insulin, so that a balance between supply and demand is more likely; (2) reduction in caloric intake may alleviate the condition of insulin resistance so that endogenous insulin will be more effective[7]; and (3) loss of weight increases the relative amount of insulin produced in relation to body weight. Overweight individuals sometimes require exogenous insulin initially, but may lose this insulin dependence as weight is lost.

Persons with maturity onset diabetes who are at normal weight at the time of diagnosis sometimes require small doses of exogenous insulin in addition to regulation of diet and exercise. Since these people retain some activity of the B-cells of the pancreas, their blood sugar level can be stabilized fairly easily.

POINTS OF EMPHASIS
Diabetes mellitus

• *Youth onset diabetes is controlled with insulin, diet and exercise.*
• *Maturity onset diabetes has the potential of management by diet and exercise without the use of hypoglycemic agents in a majority of cases.*
• *If insulin is also required in management of maturity onset diabetes, small doses usually suffice.*

DANGERS ASSOCIATED WITH ALTERED BLOOD SUGAR LEVELS

Diabetic ketoacidosis (DKA)

Diabetic ketoacidosis is a very serious condition which is most likely to develop in individuals with youth onset diabetes. Signs and symptoms of diabetic ketoacidosis (Table 30.1) develop because of the acutely elevated blood sugar level (usually in the range of 400 to 800 mg. per dl. or more) and accumulation of acidic ketones (ketosis, accompanied by acidosis). Exogenous insulin and fluid and electrolyte replacement are essential for treatment of diabetic ketoacidosis.

A large percentage of the cases of DKA are precipitated by some type of infection. An insulin-dependent diabetic may develop mild ketoacidosis in less than a day if he misses his insulin injection(s). An occasional dietary indiscretion does not cause diabetic ketoacidosis, but continued lack of diet control increases the risk of its occurrence.

TABLE 30.1 *Signs and symptoms of diabetic ketoacidosis (DKA), hyperglycemic, hyperosmolar nonketotic coma (HHNK), and hypoglycemia*

	DKA	HHNK	HYPOGLYCEMIA
Onset	Gradual—hours or days	Gradual—hours or days	Rapid—minutes
Urine			
Output	Copious	Copious	Normal variation
Test for sugar	Strongly positive	Strongly positive	Not diagnostic
Test for ketones	Strongly positive	Negative	Not diagnostic
Appearance	Flushed		Pale, cold sweat
Respiration	May be deep and rapid (Kussmahl respiration)		Normal
GI	Nausea, vomiting		Hunger, sometimes nausea
Hydration	Dehydrated	Dehydrated	Normal
Sensorium	Drowsiness progressing to unconsciousness	Drowsiness progressing to unconsciousness	Dizziness, nervousness, staggering gait, inappropriate behavior, drowsiness progressing to unconsciousness, convulsions
Other	Fruity or actetone odor of breath		Lack of "squint reflex" (no squinting response when strong flashlight is beamed over closed eyelids of sleeping individual)

Hyperglycemic, hyperosmolar nonketotic coma (HHNK)

Hyperglycemic hyperosmolar nonketotic coma is a metabolic derangement which has a higher mortality rate (60 to 70 percent) than does diabetic ketoacidosis. Signs and symptoms of HHNK (Table 30.1) develop because of the extremely high blood sugar level (sometimes reaching 3000 mg. percent). This condition may develop in individuals with adult onset diabetes, especially if they are elderly or under stress. HHNK occasionally develops in nondiabetic individuals who are receiving total parenteral nutrition, burned individuals whose carbohydrate intake is high, and in individuals who are treated with medications which reduce glucose tolerance (e.g., certain steroids, phenytoin, thiazides, and others).

Adequate insulin dosage helps to prevent or correct this condition. Fluid replacement rather than diet gets priority when signs of impending HHNK develop. If HHNK is detected early enough, assisting a client to *greatly* increase his fluid intake may be a means of helping to correct the condition. Accurate intake and output records provide data needed for determining adequate fluid replacement.

Mild elevations of blood sugar

Effects of mild to moderate elevations of blood sugar have been and continue to be the subject of extensive research. Diabetics (both youth and adult onset) are usually susceptible to early death and to blindness primarily because of small blood vessel disease (sometimes called diabetic microangiopathy or microvascular disease). Microangiopathy may take the form of renal disease (nephropathy), damage to the nerves (neuropathy), and damage to the blood vessels of the retina of the eye (retinopathy). Evidence is accumulating that hyperglycemia contributes substantially to these and to other complications of diabetes.[9,10]

The cells which are most vulnerable to excess glucose are those into which glucose can pass freely even in the absence of insulin. Glucose can freely penetrate red blood cells, the lens of the eye, nerves, kidney cells, walls of blood vessels, and the islet cells of the pancreas.

In the past there was little evidence that control of blood sugar was really worth attempting. Hereditary influences were suspected as the cause of microvascular complications but studies are ruling them out[11] or indicating that they are not the sole cause.[12] For example, if normal kidneys are transplanted to a diabetic, the transplanted kidneys develop lesions characteristic of diabetes.[10] Now many physicians agree with the statement made by R. H. Unger and L. Orci: "Increasing evidence that hyperglycemia is a key etiologic component in the development of the microangiopathic complications of diabetes mellitus makes its improved management an urgent therapeutic goal."[13] The American Diabetes Association has accepted this position. Although precise control is impossible in diabetics, health professionals can help individuals achieve better control by improved early detection and improved education of diabetics.

Hypoglycemia

Hypoglycemia is a potentially life-threatening condition which may sometimes develop in a matter of minutes in persons receiving insulin therapy—whether they are diabetic or not. Hypoglycemia occurs when the supply of insulin (either endogenous or exogenous) is so high that practically all the glucose moves from the blood into the cells. This leaves an inadequate supply of fuel for the brain and causes the signs and symptoms of hypoglycemia listed in Table 30.1.

Severe hypoglycemia is a medical emergency. It carries the potential for causing convulsions, brain damage, and death. Hypoglycemic reactions, sometimes called insulin reactions, may be very frightening experiences. Even mild hypoglycemia can be dangerous if it causes lack of coordination and inability to think clearly sometimes, as while driving an automobile. In most cases hypoglycemia in diabetics may be quickly averted or alleviated by ingestion of rapidly absorbed carbohydrate (as in the form of fruit juice, candy, sugar, or regular carbonated beverages). Special circumstances require more intensive treatment. Fortunately hypoglycemia can generally be *prevented*.

POINTS OF EMPHASIS
*Dangers associated with altered
blood sugar levels*

• *Diabetic ketoacidosis and hyperglycemic, hyperosmotic nonketotic coma are severe but often preventable forms of hyperglycemia. They are life threatening if untreated.*

• *Mild but chronic hyperglycemia may contribute to serious forms of microvascular disease.*

• *Severe hypoglycemia, if not promptly treated, may lead to coma and death due to lack of fuel for the brain.*

CONTROLLING BLOOD SUGAR LEVEL

Relationships between feedings (enteral or parenteral), physical activity, insulin, and stress

Blood sugar concentration at any given time reflects the net balance between physical activity and insulin on one hand and feedings and stress on the other. A change in any one of these can cause the blood sugar level to change, as suggested by Fig. 30.1. Individuals who do not require exogenous insulin are not ordinarily subject to dangerous hypoglycemic reactions since they do not produce more insulin than they need.

Wide changes in blood sugar of insulin-dependent individuals can usually be avoided by making adjustments to restore balance of the opposing factors. Physical activity has an insulin-like effect in that it promotes the movement of glucose into the cell.* Thus an increase in exercise might be balanced by an increase in food intake or, if possible, a decrease in insulin dose. Too much insulin would have to be balanced by extra carbohydrate and/or a decrease in physical activity. The best adjustments to make depend on the nature of the individual's problem (maturity onset diabetes, growth onset diabetes, or stress-induced hyperglycemia).

---

* Exercise does not exert other actions of insulin and, therefore, serves only as a partial substitute for this hormone.

Controlled diabetics may suddenly become hyperglycemic in response to an increase in either psychological or physiological stress. It may be easiest to offset a temporary increase in mild *psychological* stress by an increase in exercise.

When blood sugar level is abnormally elevated, treatment may take a variety of forms, depending on the cause of the abnormality. Control of diet, reduction of stress, management of physical activity and sometimes the use of hypoglycemic agents are integral aspects of treatment.

Hypoglycemic agents

An understanding of the role of diet requires an understanding of the actions and limitations of hypoglycemic agents.

The two broad categories of hypoglycemic agents are insulin, which must be administered parenterally, and sulfonylurea compounds, which are taken orally and, therefore, are often called oral hypoglycemic agents.

INSULIN

Exogenous insulin is very similar to the insulin produced by the normally functioning human pancreas, and it has the same effects on body processes.

The types of exogenous insulin most commonly used are short-acting, such as regular insulin, and intermediate acting, such as NPH insulin. The different forms of insulin differ in rate of absorption and onset, peak, and duration of activity as shown in Figure 30.2.

Throughout the period when activity of exogenous insulin is high, it is absolutely essential to have sufficient carbohydrate in the bloodstream to avoid hypoglycemia.

Different types of insulin may be used singly or in combination. The trend is toward use of more than one injection daily since better control of blood sugar can usually be achieved by this means. If only regular insulin is used, an injection is required before each meal and possibly at night.

It is more common to give both fast acting and intermediate acting insulin. Even with this type of insulin coverage, the insulin-dependent diabetic should not expect perfect control. There is no way for the body to regulate the amount of exogenous insulin in the blood in response to changing needs.

There are numerous drawbacks to the use of exogenous insulin, including inconvenience, resistance to weight loss in obese diabetics, cost, and possible side effects such as fatty atrophy, facial edema, and peripheral edema. However, persons with youth onset diabetes must have insulin injections to maintain life.

In treatment of maturity onset diabetes it is estimated that more than 75 percent of the individuals with this disease could be controlled by management

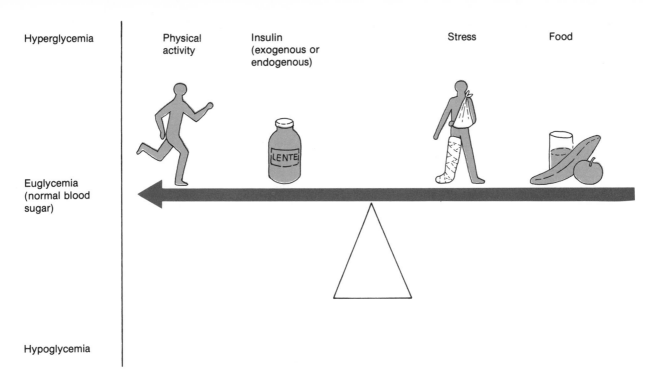

| Hyperglycemia | Physical activity | Insulin (exogenous or endogenous) | | Stress | Food |

FIGURE 30.1. Factors that must be balanced to maintain normal blood sugar level.

of three aspects of daily living—diet, exercise, and stress.[14] Management of diet, exercise, and stress is preferred since it is low in cost, generally has no serious side effects, and may offer physiological and sometimes psychological benefits. Weight loss is easier if insulin injections are not required.[15]

SULFONYLUREAS

Sulfonylurea compounds are sometimes prescribed for persons who have maturity onset diabetes mellitus. These oral hypoglycemic agents appear to help control blood sugar by stimulating the beta cells of the pancreas to produce and/or release more insulin—if these cells still retain the capacity to do so. Use of sulfonylureas is contraindicated in youth onset diabetes mellitus.

The value of oral hypoglycemic agents in the treatment of maturity onset diabetes has been seriously questioned. No well-designed prospective study has shown them to produce long term benefits.[15] A significant number of physicians have discontinued prescribing sulfonylureas, substituting intensive emphasis on weight loss (when appropriate), diet control, and, if necessary, insulin therapy.[16] Other physicians suggest that oral hypoglycemic agents may be an acceptable method of treatment in combination with diet control for carefully selected patients with maturity onset diabetes.

Oral hypoglycemic agents should never be substituted for diet control since their effectiveness depends on the capacity of the beta cells to secrete insulin. Clients look to health professionals for an explanation of why these agents are or are not used.

Sulfonylureas occasionally precipitate hypoglycemic reactions which are resistant to treatment.[17]

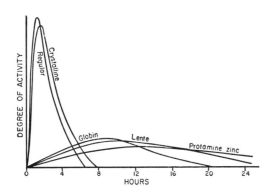

FIGURE 30.2. Time-action curves for different types of insulin. (From Guyton, A. C.: *Textbook of Medical Physiology*, ed. 5. Philadelphia: W. B. Saunders Co., 1976, with permission)

POINTS OF EMPHASIS
Use of pharmacological agents in control of diabetes mellitus

• *Whether or not pharmacological agents are used, diet control is an integral part of any plan to control diabetes mellitus.*

• *Exogenous insulin is always required for treatment of youth onset diabetes mellitus and is occasionally required for treatment of maturity onset diabetes.*

• *The value of oral hypoglycemic agents in controlling maturity onset diabetes is being questioned.*

Lack of food intake, dosage errors, or a drug which potentiates the action of the sulfonylurea may cause an imbalance between the amount of endogenous insulin produced and the amount actually needed. Chlorpropamide, the longest acting sulfonylurea, accounts for a large percentage of the cases of hypoglycemia.

Sulfonylureas are generally ineffective in controlling blood sugar level during times of increased stress.

Diet

A diabetic diet consists of every-day foods, prepared by common cooking methods, in amounts needed to attain or maintain desirable weight. Special foods are not required and may not even be desirable. Objectives for a diabetic diet differ depending on the type of diabetes involved. Table 30.2 compares the diet treatment of different types of diabetes. It should be noted that *consistency* of mealtimes, meal size, and meal composition is the key to diet modification for youth onset diabetes, whereas weight loss is the primary goal for a majority of persons with maturity onset diabetes.

Carbohydrate is an integral part of diabetic diets; therefore, diabetic diets should be viewed as *regulated* rather than restricted in carbohydrate. High carbohydrate diets may improve glucose tolerance in non-diabetics and diabetics who retain some B-cell activity as long as their total caloric intake is controlled.[18] Diabetics who use hypoglycemic agents *require* carbohydrate to avoid hypoglycemic reactions.

Both *type* and *source* of carbohydrate appear to influence postprandial blood glucose level. Glucose increases postprandial blood sugar more than does sucrose and much more than do fructose and some

TABLE 30.2 *Variations in treatment of different types of diabetes mellitus*

| | YOUTH ONSET | OBESE MATURITY ONSET | | |
| | | Insulin | | |
	Insulin dependent	dependent	Sulfonylureas	Diet and exercise only
Regularity of mealtime	*Important*			Not essential but may aid weight loss
Consistency of meal size	Client must know how to adapt for unforseen circumstances, e.g., delayed meal			Not essential but distribution of carbohydrate desirable to minimize swings in blood sugar
Consistency of meal composition				
Calorie level	Planned to achieve weight maintenance or normal growth	Reduced to result in weight loss to improve control		
Exercise	Increase carbohydrate intake prior to and during unusual exercise	Decrease insulin dose according to physician's directions prior to extra exercise if possible; otherwise increase carbohydrate intake		No diet adjustments necessary
Hypoglycemia	Client and family should recognize warning signs			Not a problem
	Carry candy Take carbohydrate each hour when driving	Weight loss often causes hypoglycemia since less insulin is needed; contact physician to have insulin dosage changed instead of continuing to increase calories to prevent hypoglycemia		
Urine testing	Usually 4 times daily		Variable	Usually once daily
Alcohol	May produce hypoglycemia			
	If allowed it should be taken with food and its exchange value should be considered in the diet	Use discouraged because of its high caloric value and its appetite stimulating effect		
			Avoid. Sulfonylureas may cause alcohol intolerance	
Stress	Likely to increase blood sugar level and insulin requirement; insulin to be taken even if food cannot be tolerated	May cause a temporary dependence on insulin for control of blood sugar		
Glucose replacements	Desirable when carbohydrate intake must be decreased			Not needed

Adapted from West, K. M.: Diet and diabetes. *Postgrad. Medicine* 60(3):210, 1976. © Copyright McGraw-Hill, Inc.

types of starch.[19,20] Starches from different foods result in different postprandial blood sugar levels.[21]

Diabetic diets are usually set up in such a way that the proportion of starch greatly exceeds the proportion of natural sugar. Refined sugar is generally excluded. Clinical evidence suggests that this division of carbohydrate favors control of blood sugar. A big advantage of starch over sugar appears to be its higher satiety value.

DIABETIC DIET ORDERS

Normally a calorie allotment is set for a diabetic diet, preferably after consultation among health team members including the client. The responsibility for this task is often the physician's but is sometimes delegated to the dietitian, nutritionist, or nurse practitioner. The caloric allowance might range from 1000 kcal. daily for an obese diabetic who is unable to increase activity to more than 3500 kcal. daily for a large adolescent male who is still growing and who participates in strenuous sports. The proportion of carbohydrate, protein, and fat is sometimes specified by the physician. However, this is often left to the dietitian/nutritionist since control of diabetes can be achieved with a wide range of intake of carbohydrate as long as calories are controlled.

"Modernized" diabetic diets specify that 50 to 60 percent of the calories come from carbohydrate, 10 to 15 percent from protein, and 30 to 35 percent from fat.[22] (This corresponds to prudent diet recommendations.) On the other hand, Joslin Clinic, a center for treatment of diabetes, feels that most diabetics achieve best control using a caloric distribution of 40 percent carbohydrate, 20 percent protein, and 40 percent fat, with a maximum of 250 gm. carbohydrate daily.[23] No matter what system is used, the long term diet is planned to allow at least the RDA for protein. The amount of insulin used, if any, is adjusted as needed.

TABLE 30.3 *Sample menus for a day for a 1650 kcal diabetic diet**

APPROXIMATE CARBOHYDRATE DISTRIBUTION	MENU PATTERN	SAMPLE MENU
2/10	*Breakfast:*	(240 cc)
	1 milk exchange	1 c skim milk
	1 fruit exchange	½ sliced banana (small)
	2 bread exchanges	¾ c wheat flakes
		1 slice toast
	2 fat exchanges	5 gm (1 tsp) margarine
		30 cc (1 oz) light cream
	free items	1 c hot free beverage
		5 gm (1 tsp) dietetic jelly, if desired
3/10	*Lunch:*	
	2 bread exchanges	2 slices rye bread
	2 lean meat exchanges	60 gm (2 oz) sliced roast turkey ⎫ turkey
	1 fat exchange	5 gm (1 tsp) mayonnaise ⎭ sandwich
	free items	lettuce
		iced tea with lemon
	1 fruit exchange	1 small orange
1/10	*Snack:*	
	1½ bread exchanges	3 graham cracker squares
	1 lean meat exchange	30 gm (2 Tbsp) peanut butter
	2 fat exchanges	
	free items	free beverage
		sour pickle, if desired
3/10	*Dinner:*	
	2 meat exchanges	60 gm (2 oz) flank steak, braised with
	2 vegetable exchanges	½ c tomato and onion
		½ c cooked greens
	2 bread exchanges	1 c cooked rice
	3 fat exchanges	1 tsp margarine
		¼ 4 inch diameter avocado sliced on
	free items	lettuce with vinegar
	1 milk exchange	240 cc (1 c) skim milk
	1 fruit exchange	1 medium peach, juice pack, drained
1/10	*Snack:*	
	1½ bread exchange	6 5.2 cm (2½ inch) square soda crackers
	1 fat exchange	with 15 gm (1 Tbsp) cream cheese

* Planned using "Exchange Lists for Meal Planning," Appendix 5I.

Insulin requirement appears to be more closely linked with caloric intake than with carbohydrate.[24] The nurse should make sure that information about the caloric level, distribution of carbohydrate, and the type and dosage of hypoglycemic agent is relayed to dietitian or nutritionist.

Some of the many ways in which diabetic diets may be ordered are indicated here:

1800 cal diab C 40% P 20% F 40%

Diet control. 1/3 1/3 1/3 with H.S. snack
(Percentage refers to percent of the calories provided by carbohydrate, protein, and fat respectively)

1800 cal   C 225 P 80 F 64

20 U Lente ⎫
10 U Regular ⎬ @ 7:30 A
8 U Lente ⎫
8 U Reg ⎬ @ 5:00 P

4/18 ±1/18 5/18 ±2/18 5/18 1/18

(The numbers following C, P, and F represent grams of carbohydrate, protein, and fat. The fractions refer to the fraction of the total carbohydrate (225 gm) which is to be provided at breakfast, midmorning, noon, midafternoon, dinner, and bedtime respectively. The ± preceeding the between meal feedings indicates that these fractions can be interchanged by the dietitian if that will help the client achieve better control.)

The dietitian translates the diet prescription into a menu pattern using an exchange system. Sometimes nurse practitioners or nurses may need to assume this responsibility, especially in nursing homes. Table 30.3 shows a sample menu pattern and examples of meals which fit the pattern. The pattern in Table 30.3 includes generous snacks in midafternoon and at bedtime because this client's insulin therapy makes him subject to hypoglycemic reactions before dinner and at night.

Several different combinations of exchanges may be used to meet a given diet prescription. This concept is illustrated in Table 30.4. This flexibilty means that the dietitian should be notified if a hospitalized client indicates that he will not find it practical or desirable to follow the same meal pattern after he goes home. In a similar vein, an ambulatory client should be referred to a nutritionist if he reports having difficulty following his diet plan at home. The diet counselor can then discuss alternatives with the client.

The checklist for meal planning in the box might be used to help make sure that the meal pattern meets the client's needs.

CHECK LIST FOR PLANNING DIABETIC DIETS

Is type and amount of carbohydrate distributed as directed (in relation to the type of hypoglycemic agent used, if any)?

Is there a source of protein and fat in each meal and snack?

Does the total number of exchanges used equal the number allowed?

Does the distribution of exchanges fit into the client's lifestyle?

Does the sample menu reflect proper use of the exchange list?

Does the sample menu provide for the client's total nutritional needs?

Does the sample menu consider the individual in relation to:
   Likes and dislikes
   Religious and ethnic background
   Condition of teeth, digestive capacity, allergy
   Cooking facilities
   Place of eating
   Amount of time client has for cooking and eating
   Amount of trouble client is willing to go to in cooking
   Season
   Cost

Does sample menu have variety of color, texture, flavor (unless client prefers otherwise)?

TABLE 30.4 *Two diet patterns meeting the same diet prescription*

1800 kcal: C 225 gm P 80 gm F 64 gm							
	C	*P*	*F*		*C*	*P*	*F*
745 ml (3 c) skim milk	36	24	—	240 ml (1 c) skim milk	12	8	—
2 vegetable	10	4	—	3 vegetable	15	6	—
3 fruit	30	—	—	5 fruit	50	—	—
10 bread	150	20	—	10 bread	150	20	—
TOTAL	226	—	—		227	—	—
5 lean meat	—	35	13	7 lean meat	—	49	18
TOTAL	—	83	—		—	83	—
10 fat	—	—	50	9 fat	—	—	45
TOTAL	—	—	63		—	—	63
For the person who wants milk with every meal and only small portions of meat				For the person who likes meat, is willing to to drink only 1 c milk, but loves vegetables and fruits			

DIABETIC DIET EXCHANGE LISTS

Use of diabetic exchange lists is meant to simplify the planning of varied diabetic diets. Foods are grouped together on the basis of their composition of carbohydrate, protein, and fat for a designated serving size. All the choices listed within an exchange group are equivalent in terms of energy nutrients and, therefore, caloric value.

Exchange systems for planning diabetic diets do not consider the fiber content of food. Recent investigations suggest that blood sugar level is apt to *decrease* if the amount of fiber in the diet is increased.[25,26] Results of these studies suggest that increased use of fiber might result in better control of diabetes. Use of high fiber rather than refined foods has been recommended for diabetics.[27] Variation in fiber intake may be responsibile for some previously unexplained fluctuations in control of blood sugar level. Thus, it might be advisable to encourage insulin dependent diabetics to be relatively consistent in use of whole grains, refined grains, and raw and cooked fruits and vegetables.

Differences among exchange lists   Although most diabetic exchange lists are similar, they have some significant differences. It is important for health care providers to become familiar with the exchange system that the client has been or is being taught. In particular, it is advisable to find the answers to the following questions:

Does one milk exchange refer to whole or to skim milk?

Is there only one group of vegetables as in "Meal Planning with Exchanges" or are there two separate groups?

Is there only one meat group or are there subdivisions according to fat content?

Are any sweets included in the exchange list?

If sweets are included, are there guidelines regarding when they may be used?

Is there more than one fruit list?

Does the list include ethnic foods preferred by the client? If not, which ones would the client like to have added?

What "free" foods and seasonings may be used in unlimited quantity, and which may be used to a limited extent?

Determining the answers to these questions in advance of working with the client should help to avoid confusion and facilitate effective diet counseling.

If a choice of exchange lists is available, the health professional will want to consider which one best meets the client's needs. The exchange system used in this chapter is "Exchange Lists for Meal Planning" (Appendix 5I). This set of exchange lists may be used for any type of diabetic.

Use of exchange lists   Reasonably accurate measurement is a key to effectiveness of the exchange system. It allows practically any unsweetened food to be worked into the diet in at least small amounts. Prunes, for example, are a source of concentrated sugar, but two medium prunes may be used since they provide 10 gm. sugar just as all fruit exchanges do. Substitution of foods between rather than within exchange groups is not recommended, especially for insulin-dependent diabetics. Even if caloric value is similar, carbohydrate content is different.

Use of the correct number of exchanges per meal, measured correctly, serves several purposes: (1) it provides the *consistency* needed by insulin-requiring diabetics in terms of total caloric intake and proportions of carbohydrate, protein, and fat; (2) it *limits caloric intake* of obese diabetics; (3) it allows choice of many normal foods, facilitating meal planning in nearly every situation; (4) it eliminates the need for clients to calculate their diets.

Usually the dietitian or nutritionist introduces the newly diagnosed diabetic to the exchange system and explains its advantages and use. The whole family is included in the "class" if possible. In some instances the nurse assumes this teaching role. Both dietitian and nurse provide these clients with opportunities for guided practice in the use of exchange lists.

The client and his family practice choosing foods for family meals from the exchange lists and specifying the amount the diabetic family member is allowed. They learn reasons for paying close attention to portion sizes. If necessary, they practice the psychomotor skills required for careful measurement or weighing. Dietitian and nurse assess the progress of the client and his family and make needed changes in the teaching plan.

Many clients want to find out how foods not included in the exchange lists, such as home-prepared casseroles, artificially sweetened homemade desserts, or frozen TV dinners, can be worked into the meal plan. Good diabetic cookbooks and references which give exchange values of commercial foods simplify the process. Some reliable references are listed at the end of Part 4. The diet counselor can guide the client in learning to use these resources effectively.

Nutritional labeling provides information which can be used by health professionals and diabetics to increase the variety of convenience foods which may be used. The process is described by the booklet "Using Nutrition Labels with Food Exchange Lists."[28] Food companies sometimes make lists available indicating the exchange value of their products.

In some circumstances, health professionals may find that the client is unwilling to learn any exchange system because he sees no pressing reason to change long established habits. Health professionals must be prepared to accomodate this point of view. If the usual diet follows a regular pattern, it may allow for satisfactory control of blood sugar with suitable adjustments of hypoglycemic agents. Compromises will also be necessary if the client cannot be motivated to lose weight and refuses to do so.

DIET ADJUSTMENTS

Consistency of mealtime, meal size, meal composition, and physical activity is not always possible for diabetics who use hypoglycemic agents, and sometimes it is not desirable. Because of this the diabetic who uses insulin or a sulfonylurea compound *must* be taught how to make appropriate diet adjustments for commonly occurring circumstances affecting blood sugar level such as delayed meals and changes in exercise. Children may benefit from guidelines for birthday parties and other special events. Diabetics of all types may want guidelines for expanding their food selection for eating away from home and drinking alcoholic beverages. All diabetics need guidelines for coping with illness. Parents may need special assistance in handling such occurrences as variations in their child's appetite and attempts by the child to use diet as a means for manipulating others. Guthrie and Guthrie present useful information regarding working with diabetic children.[29]

Adjusting for changes in food intake The diabetic who uses a hypoglycemic agent must always be prepared to deal with a delayed meal in order to avoid a serious hypoglycemic reaction. He should make sure that he always carries a supply of carbohydrate with him in anticipation of delays. Candy can be conveniently kept in pocket or purse. Crackers and peanut butter might be kept in the car in case of a mechanical breakdown or a long traffic jam. A snack might be eaten in advance of a dinner party. If for some reason the food supply is limited and the delay is long, physical exertion should be kept to a minimum.

POINTS OF EMPHASIS
Diabetic diets

• *Many variations of diabetic diets are possible; health professionals should make sure a client's diet is tailored to his particular needs.*
• *Use of an exchange system enables diabetics to eat practically any food; restricted foods are mainly those containing much refined sugar. Portion sizes, however, are carefully controlled.*
• *Diabetic exchange lists vary somewhat; those with guidelines for occasional use of sugar-rich foods may be suitable for selected clients who do not need to lose weight.*
• *Control of blood sugar level of insulin-dependent diabetics is aided by a consistent pattern of meals and physical activity and by consistent distribution and total intake of energy nutrients.*
• *Calorie restriction is more important than meal pattern or carbohydrate distribution for control of blood sugar level of obese persons with maturity onset diabetes mellitus.*

The diet counselor should advise the insulin-dependent diabetic and/or his family to be alert for signs that he needs more food because he is entering a period of rapid growth or because his prescribed diet is too low in calories for weight maintenance. If these signs develop (frequent or unexpected hypoglycemia, excessive hunger, weight loss, or growth retardation), the physician should be consulted. Consultation with the doctor is also recommended if an overweight insulin-using diabetic decides that he is ready to follow a reducing diet.

Adjusting for changes in exercise Exercise should be a regular part of the diabetic's life. When there are no contraindications, a 30-minute walk or comparable activity after each meal has been recommended as a healthful way for many diabetics to avoid high postprandial blood sugar levels.[30] If insulin-dependent individuals increase their exercise level, it will be necessary for them to ingest more carbohydrate-containing food prior to and possibly during exercise, reduce their insulin dose, or sometimes both. Injecting insulin into a nonexercised body part, such as a site on the abdomen, may reduce the likelihood of developing hypoglycemia.[31]

The general recommendation for insulin-dependent diabetics who need to maintain or gain weight is to eat at least one bread exchange and perhaps drink ½ c. whole milk or the equivalent before a fairly strenuous activity, especially if it precedes a regularly scheduled meal or occurs during a time of peak insulin activity. Extra sugar in the form of juice, fruit, sweetened beverages, or candy may need to be consumed *during* the activity to prevent hypoglycemia. During heavy exercise sugar may be needed as often as every 15 minutes. Insulin-using diabetics should always make sure that an ample supply of quick-acting carbohydrate is readily available for such occasions.

Urine or blood testing following the activity is advisable to make sure the intake of carbohydrate was not excessive. With a little practice, ongoing assessment, and the guidance of health team members, the insulin-using diabetic can determine what food intake will be best for him when he exercises at different times and in different ways. He may find that it is helpful to decrease his insulin dose in addition to increasing food intake before participating in sports, dances, or physical labor.

It is possible for diabetics to be spontaneous or inconsistent about exercising if they learn to make appropriate adjustments. They may engage in unscheduled exercise on a few moments' notice without becoming hypoglycemic if they have an adequate supply of carbohydrate available and know how to use it. One diabetic has reported about how he adjusts food intake for long distance running.[32] He has successfully completed marathons (26+ miles) in good time (some in less than 2 h. 48 min.)!

The insulin-using overweight individual with maturity onset diabetes should be guided in safe lowering of the insulin dose when exercise level is increased. Extra exercise without extra calories will greatly facilitate the weight loss which is a major goal of treatment. Of course extra carbohydrate may be *essential* to prevent a hypoglycemic reaction if the insulin dose has not been sufficiently decreased.

If an increase in energy expenditure is due to a change in occupation, as switching from being an office worker to a mail carrier, all meals and snacks will usually be made somewhat larger so that the extra fuel will be available throughout the day.

Insulin-requiring diabetics also need to be taught how to decrease caloric intake when they decrease scheduled exercise. Otherwise they will tend to become hyperglycemic and gain weight as well. It is not appropriate to adjust for decreased physical activity by keeping calories the same and increasing the insulin dosage.

POINTS OF EMPHASIS
Exercise and control of blood sugar

• *Diabetics, whether insulin dependent or not, should be encouraged to exercise daily.*

• *Insulin-dependent diabetics should be taught how to adjust diet and/or insulin as needed so that they can take advantage of opportunities to increase their level of physical activity.*

• *Overweight diabetics benefit from using exercise as part of a comprehensive weight loss program.*

Adjusting for changes in stress level   For any diabetic even mild illness or other stress has the potential for precipitating severe hyperglycemia and ketoacidosis if not managed properly. The decrease in appetite and food intake which often accompanies illness or emotional upset seldom results in hypoglycemia in those taking hypoglycemic agents because it is offset by the effect of increased stress and lack of physical activity. Many clients reason, *incorrectly*, that they should omit their insulin if they do not feel well enough to eat. The insulin-dependent client must be taught that insulin is more vital than usual when he is ill and that insulin must be used even if eating is impossible.

Sometimes the usual intake of carbohydrate, protein, and fat can be taken by substituting soft, bland foods and beverages as suggested in Table 30.5. When the usual meal plan cannot be followed because of anorexia, nausea, or vomiting, the diabetic should sip easily digested sugar-containing beverages. Apple juice, regular cola, or regular gingerale may be well tolerated. High fluid intake should be encouraged whether or not the diabetic uses insulin, especially if urine tests indicate significant glycosuria. Both insulin-dependent and non-insulin-dependent diabetics may need extra insulin when ill or under other types of stress.

EATING AWAY FROM HOME AND USING CONVENIENCE FOODS

Guidelines for eating out differ somewhat, depending on whether insulin is used or not. Guidelines for eating away from home are indicated as follows.

TABLE 30.5 *Suggestions for adapting a diabetic diet when ill*

FOODS WHICH MAY BE WELL TOLERATED WHEN APPETITE IS POOR:

Fruit exchanges: juices, fruits canned in juice or water
Bread exchanges: cooked cereal, toast, plain crackers, potatoes, rice
Meat exchanges: poached or soft cooked eggs, tender lean meat, cottage cheese
Milk exchanges: skim milk, plain yogurt
Vegetable exchanges: cooked mildly flavored vegetables
Combination: chicken noodle soup* (e.g., bread + meat) or cream soup* (e.g., bread + milk + fat + vegetable)
Follow diet plan if possible. Eat slowly; chew thoroughly.

GLUCOSE REPLACEMENTS
If you are taking insulin and are unable to eat solid food or have been vomiting, try to consume one or more of the following types of glucose replacements to "make up for" the carbohydrate missed from your usual meal. Each portion provides about 10 gm. carbohydrate.

Regular cola	100 ml (scant ½ c)
Regular gingerale	120 ml (½ c)
Regular flavored gelatin	60 ml (¼ c)
Grape juice	60 ml
Apple juice	80 ml (⅓ c)
Hard candy	10 gm.
Tea with 10 gm (2 tsp) sugar or honey	

* Exchange value varies depending on the recipe

All diabetics:
1. If you are just becoming familiar with your diet, choose restaurants serving plain foods so that you can easily order a meal which fits your menu pattern.
2. Follow your usual menu pattern as closely as possible.
3. Estimate correct portion size by eye. Set extra food aside. Request the waiter to serve salad dressing separately from the salad so that the correct amount of dressing may be used.

Insulin-dependent diabetics:
1. Be certain to eat the recommended amount of carbohydrate and total calories.
2. If no fruit is available, substitute an equivalent amount of a sugar-containing food or of bread for your fruit exchange(s). When food selection is limited, prevention of hypoglycemia must take priority over exact adherence to an exchange list.

Overweight diabetics not being treated with hypoglycemic agents:
1. Limit caloric intake as usual.
2. If skim milk and/or fresh fruit are included in your menu pattern but are unavailable, substitute another food with similar caloric value if desired, but don't feel that a substitution is essential.

When a diabetic has become familiar with exchanges, the diet counselor can provide him with guidelines for expanding his food selection.

USING SUGAR SUBSTITUTES AND DIETETIC FOODS

Because of the questions raised by the saccharin controversy, many diet counselors are discouraging recently diagnosed diabetics from beginning to incorporate this non-nutritive sweetener into their new diet. Instead diet counselors are encouraging use of fruits, as allowed by the meal pattern, to satisfy the desire for sweetness.

Many diabetics express interest in using one of the nutritive sugar substitutes such as sorbitol, xylitol, or fructose. These sweeteners do not directly cause significant elevation in blood sugar levels[18]; however, nutritive sugar substitutes should ordinarily be avoided by diabetics who are above ideal body weight because the sweeteners are high in "empty calories." Most physicians discourage use of nutritive sugar substitutes by individuals with youth onset diabetes as well but, in certain cases, limited amounts may be allowed. Corn sugar and corn syrup solids are not satisfactory sucrose substitutes for diabetics. These sugars are primarily glucose and, therefore, affect blood sugar even more than sucrose does.

Non-nutritive sweeteners have no known effect upon blood sugar level. However, if non-nutritive sweeteners are used in cooking, the caloric and exchange value of other ingredients used must not be overlooked.

It should be made clear to the client that "dietetic" food does *not* mean "diabetic" food and is not necessary for a diabetic diet. The special foods which may be most helpful to diabetics are those which are reduced in calories. If these are used it is especially important for diabetics who are taking hypoglycemic agents to find out how to exchange them correctly for "regular" foods.

DRINKING ALCOHOLIC BEVERAGES

Consumption of alcoholic beverages may pose special problems for diabetics for several reasons:

1. Alcoholic beverage consumption impedes weight loss by overweight diabetics because alcohol is high in calories and reduces control of appetite.
2. Alcohol ingestion favors development of hypoglycemia. Insulin-using diabetics may experience a hypoglycemic reaction if they consume alcoholic beverages between meals or shortly before a meal. Since erratic behavior and loss of consciousness are likely to be confused with drunkenness (especially if there is the smell of alcohol on the breath), proper treatment may be overlooked.
3. Alcohol consumption may precipitate a mild to acute toxic reaction in individuals who are taking a sulfonylurea compound. Included among the signs and symptoms are severe headaches, nausea, vomiting, tachycardia, and the appearance of drunkenness.

If diabetics wish to take an alcoholic beverage occasionally or to drink moderately, the matter should be discussed with the physician. With the doctor's approval and after the diabetes has been brought under control, the diet counselor may instruct the client in reasonably safe use of alcohol. Exchange values have been established for different types of alcoholic beverages; most alcoholic beverages are counted as fat exchanges for diabetic diets. For example, 1½ oz of 80 proof whiskey equals about 2 fat exchanges. Use of sweet wines, liqueurs, mixers, and sweet cocktails is discouraged because of high sugar content. Beer may be allowed if both its alcohol and carbohydrate content are counted.

POINTS OF EMPHASIS

Special considerations regarding foods and beverages

- *Diabetic clients can be taught to choose restaurant meals which are compatible with their diets.*
- *Food manufacturers and diet counselors can provide clients with information about the exchange value of convenience foods and mixed dishes.*
- *Fructose, sorbitol, and xylitol provide as many calories as does an equal weight of sugar, but do not significantly increase postprandial blood sugar level.*
- *Foods made with non-nutritive sweeteners may contain other high calorie ingredients; most types should not be freely used on a diabetic diet.*
- *Dietetic foods are not necessarily designed or desirable for use in diabetic diets.*
- *Suitability of light to moderate alcoholic beverage consumption depends on the client's overall condition and his drug regimen.*

APPLYING THE CLINICAL CARE PROCESS IN REGULATING DIABETES

Health professionals work with diabetic clients to develop a realistic individualized plan which, if followed, should help to minimize swings in blood glucose level. A plan may be unrealistic if it overemphasizes prevention of mild hyperglycemia. Some diabetics, especially children, experience frequent, life-disrupting episodes of hypoglycemia if they (or their parents) try to keep the blood sugar level from ever rising above normal limits. Clients who place a very high value on control of blood sugar may experience stress if their compliance fails to achieve the desired degree of control. This stress in turn makes control even more elusive.

Assisting the newly diagnosed client to learn to manage his disease on an outpatient basis has distinct advantages over requiring that he be hospitalized. Hospitalization frequently increases the level of stress, changes the pattern and decreases the level of exercise, and may cause changes in meal pattern and food intake. Since each of these affects control of diabetes, a person who is regulated in the hospital may encounter serious complications if he follows the same plan after discharge. No matter where he learns to control his diabetes, the client will benefit from skillful application of the clinical care process.

TYPES OF DATA

Determination of the desirable daily insulin dose (number of units, type(s), and time distribution) is initially a matter of trial and error. To determine dosage most efficiently and accurately, the physician must have specific information from other health team members, including the client. Pertinent types of information are listed below.[33] The time at which each event occurs must be specified.
1. Actual food intake
2. Insulin type and amount injected
3. Exercise pattern
4. Subjective sense of well-being of client
5. Objective signs of abnormal blood sugar levels including:
   a. Results of urine testing (24-hour fractional urine samples may be preferred over a record of spot tests on an outpatient basis[34])
   b. Blood sugar levels (Home monitoring of blood sugar level is reported to be associated with improved diabetic control, perhaps because it provides prompt reliable feedback to the client[35])
   c. Occurrence of diaphoresis and other visible signs
   d. Weight changes
6. Special stresses such as infection, fever, emotional upsets, or menstruation

Diaries If the client is being regulated on an outpatient basis, he may be taught to keep a diary which includes all of the above information except perhaps blood sugar level. The amount of detail and frequency of recording vary, depending on how easily the diabetes responds to treatment. Detailed records are most commonly needed when initially regulating children or when growth spurts or other circumstances complicate control of blood sugar. Any client who experiences difficulty in achieving an acceptable level of control is likely to be asked to collect data and record it in a diary.

IDENTIFYING INSULIN-INDUCED WEIGHT GAIN

The presence of a common but undesirable cycle of events may be identified using the type of data listed previously. This cycle, sometimes called the "pack-o-

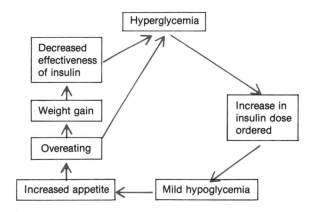

FIGURE 30.3. Series of reactions in "pack-o-derm" syndrome.

derm" syndrome,[33] may affect clients with maturity onset diabetes mellitus. The syndrome is characterized by the series of reactions shown in Figure 30.3.

If the initial cause of hyperglycemia can be ascertained (e.g., emotional upset, unscheduled eating while watching TV), health care providers may be able to make practical suggestions that will interrupt the cycle and result in better control without the use of extra insulin.

IDENTIFYING FACTORS AFFECTING COMPLIANCE

All too often the client is suspected of "cheating" on his diet when something else may be a major factor contributing to glycosuria. A review of a client's urine testing record and food diary might indicate that glycosuria correlates best with times of emotional upset. If so, the client might be encouraged to walk briskly, skip rope, ride a bicycle, scrub the floor, saw and hammer, or engage in any other vigorous activity during times of stress. Exercise serves a dual purpose in that it helps remove glucose from the blood and may help to reduce the level of stress itself. Sometimes a client needs assistance in learning how to cope with ongoing stressful situations in order to keep blood sugar level under control without excessive use of insulin.

If overeating is occurring, a behavioral approach to weight control may help overcome this problem.

The possibility exists that an insulin-dependent diabetic purposely makes himself severely hypoglycemic or hyperglycemic as a means of expressing conflicts or of escaping from unpleasant situations.[36] Adolescents sometimes equate control of their diabetes with dependence. In their struggle for independence and self-identity, adolescents may choose to eat whatever they please, change their prescribed insulin dosage, and neglect other aspects of their care. In these cases, education about diet and insulin will be of little value until the underlying conflict can be resolved or ameliorated.

POINTS OF EMPHASIS
Applying the clinical care process in regulating diabetes

• *Diaries of pertinent data (e.g., food intake, results of urine or blood testing, insulin dosage) provide the health team with information needed for optimal, realistic regulation of diabetes on an outpatient basis.*
• *Subjective data should be reviewed for signs of stress as a cause of hyperglycemia.*
• *Uncooperative behavior may be due to the client's need to assert his independence rather than because he doesn't understand his treatment program.*
• *Health professionals may need to assist clients in adjusting to their disease or in coping with other stresses to reduce inappropriate use of food or other behaviors which interfere with diabetic control.*

NUTRITIONAL CARE OF THE HOSPITALIZED DIABETIC AND OF OTHERS TREATED WITH INSULIN

Because diet plays such an integral role in the management of diabetes, health care workers must be able to assist the client in maintaining control even if the usual diet pattern is upset by hospitalization, illness, and/or injury. When making decisions about adjustments in diet, the health professional must always take hypoglycemic agents into consideration.

SUBSTITUTIONS

If a diabetic of any type is dissatisfied with a food which is served to him, it is allowable to substitute another available food if it has the same exchange value. For example, if a fresh pear (1 fruit exchange) served to the client were less ripe than he liked, he could be offered 120 ml. (½ c.) unsweetened orange juice *or* 80 ml. (⅓ c.) apple juice as a substitute.

GLUCOSE REPLACEMENTS

The health professional should be sure to facilitate ingestion of the total carbohydrate allotment if the client uses any type of hypoglycemic agent. Sometimes the client will refuse food substitutes because he feels too ill to eat. In this case, glucose replacement (a source of sugar) is offered according to the policy of the agency, if any. Commonly available glucose replacements were listed in Table 30.5.

The client is usually willing to drink a carbohy-

drate-containing beverage if small amounts are offered at frequent intervals and if the reason for the glucose replacement is understood. If the client refuses to take carbohydrate, the nursing staff must assess the client frequently for signs of hypoglycemia since onset may be sudden. Hypoglycemia itself may lead to refusal to cooperate.

Immediate action is essential if hypoglycemia develops. If the person is conscious, he is given about 10 gm. of rapidly absorbed carbohydrate immediately. Sweet juice, *regular* soft drink, or some other form of sugar should be kept at close hand in the event of such an emergency. Sugar is absorbed so quickly that it usually takes effect within 10 minutes. After the sugar is given, the client should be closely assessed to determine if additional oral carbohydrate, a glucagon injection, or intravenous glucose is needed. The physician should be notified of the hypoglycemic incident. A summary of events leading to the hypoglycemic reaction, steps taken to prevent it, and care of the client during and after the reaction should be recorded promptly in the patient's record.

Glucose replacements are *unnecessary* for diabetics controlled by diet only.

WATCHING FOR HYPOGLYCEMIC REACTIONS

Health workers should determine the times when their insulin-dependent clients are most likely to be susceptible to insulin reactions and make sure they are observed frequently during those periods. This is especially important for those clients for whom control is being established and for known brittle diabetics. Health professionals should make sure that a hospitalized client has a source of quick-acting carbohydrate, a call button within easy reach, and an understanding of how and when to use them.

Sudden reduction in stress level may unexpectedly produce severe hypoglycemia in individuals who have been requiring large doses of insulin because of the stress. Temporary discontinuation of insulin, administration of glucagon, and/or intravenous administration of a concentrated glucose solution ($D_{50}W$) may be needed to overcome hypoglycemia while the blood level of insulin remains dangerously high.

BETWEEN-MEAL FEEDINGS

Hospitalized insulin-dependent diabetics usually have at least one or two between-meal snacks included in the diet plan to prevent the development of hypoglycemia between meals and during sleep. Health professionals must make sure that these ordered nourishments are made available to the client at the specified time.

If a diabetic requests more food than has been allowed at a specified time, or requests snacks at unscheduled times, appropriate action requires additional information:

1. Is an insulin-dependent diabetic becoming hypoglycemic? If so, a carbohydrate-containing snack is essential even if unplanned.
2. If hypoglycemia is not a problem, what free foods are available which may be offered? Sugar-free beverages such as coffee or tea may be the only choices.
3. Even if hypoglycemia is not a potential problem, are there indications that the client of normal weight is experiencing hunger as a result of inadequate caloric intake? (If he has been regulated on too low a caloric intake, he may need more insulin as well as more food.)
4. If the client is obese or overweight, is he trying to comply with the caloric restriction? Will he benefit from a change in distribution of food without a change in caloric intake? Does he need extra assistance in coping with a low calorie diet? Suitable action often includes contact with other health team members to alleviate the source of the problem.

DIABETIC DIET AND DIAGNOSTIC TESTS

Hospitalized clients are often subjected to a variety of tests requiring a 12- to 14-hour fast. Such tests are usually conducted in the morning so that breakfast is the only meal missed. This poses no unusual problem for the diabetic who is controlled by diet only. However, the insulin-dependent diabetic requires special attention. Adjustments must be made to prevent hypoglycemia or hyperglycemia.

If the insulin-dependent diabetic is to be restricted the evening before the test, care must be taken to assure adequate carbohydrate intake to prevent a hypoglycemic reaction during sleep. Tests for insulin-dependent diabetics should be scheduled for early morning, if possible, in order to minimize disruption in the regular routine. The agency's guidelines should be followed regarding administration of insulin and intravenous glucose.

STUDY QUESTIONS

1. What kinds of diet adjustments for increased physical activity are recommended for an insulin-dependent diabetic? For an obese diabetic whose disease is being managed without any drugs?
2. If a normal person is under a severe stress and develops hyperglycemia, why isn't a diabetic diet prescribed?
3. An overweight diabetic claims to be taking his insulin and carefully following his diet at home. He has not lost any weight. A urine sample collected at clinic is strongly positive for glucose. What additional data should the health care worker try to obtain to find ways of helping the client achieve better control of his diabetes?
4. For a diabetic diet (any type), are foods sweetened with corn syrup solids or dextrose preferable to those sweetened with sucrose (table sugar)? Why or why not? Would fructose be more or less desirable than sucrose? Explain.
5. Discuss at least three reasons why following a diabetic diet plan may benefit a diabetic.
6. Under what circumstances might it be desirable for a diabetic to eat candy? Does this apply to all types of diabetics? Explain.
7. In what circumstances should health care workers be particularly alert for the development of HHNK? Why is this condition so dangerous?

References

1. Fajans, S. S., and Freinkel, N.: The problem of diabetes mellitus. in S. S. Fajans (ed.): *Diabetes Mellitus.* Fogarty International Center Series on Preventive Medicine, Vol. 4. Bethesda MD: National Institutes of Health, 1976. (DHEW Publ. No. (NIH) 76-584)
2. Koenig, R. J., et al.: Correlation of glucose regulation and hemoglobin A_{1c} in diabetes mellitus. *N. Engl. J. Med.* 295:417, 1976.
3. Gonen, B., et al.: Haemoglobin A_1: An indicator of the metabolic control of diabetic patients. *Lancet* 1:734, 1978.
4. Reynolds, C., et al.: Abnormalities of endogenous glucagon and insulin in unstable diabetes. *Diabetes* 20:36, 1977.
5. Taniguchi, H., et al.: Physiologic role of somatostatin. *Diabetes* 26:700, 1977.
6. Jackson, R. L., and Murthy, D. Y. N.: Importance of early insulin treatment and good regulation of children with diabetes. *Missouri Med*:173, Apr. 1974, as seen in *The Care and Teaching of the Diabetic Patient.* Boston: Education and Clinic Division of the Joslin Diabetes Foundation, Inc., March 1977.
7. Bar, R. S., and Roth, J.: Insulin receptor status in disease states of man. *Arch. Intern. Med.* 137:474, 1977.
8. Bohdan, S. T., and Jans, K.: A new diabetic with complications. *Nurs. Clin. North Am.* 12(3):393, 1977.
9. Sarji, K. E.: Vascular disease in diabetes. Pathophysiological mechanisms and therapy. *Arch. Intern. Med.* 139:225, 1979.
10. Raskin, P.: Diabetic regulation and its relationship to microangiopathy. *Metabolism* 27:235, 1978.
11. Engerman, R., Bloodworth, J. M. S., and Nelson, S.: Relationship of microvascular disease in diabetes to metabolic control. *Diabetes* 26:760, 1977.
12. Pyke, D. A.: Genetics of diabetes. *Clin. Endocrinol. Metabol.* 6(2):285, 1977.
13. Unger, R. H., and Orci, L.: Role of glucagon in diabetes. *Arch. Intern. Med.* 137:482, 1977.
14. West, K. M.: Diabetes mellitus In H. A. Schneider, C. E. Anderson, D. B. Coursin (eds.): *Nutritional Support of Medical Practice.* Hagerstown MD: Harper & Row, 1977.
15. Levine, R. and Smith, M.: Antidiabetic drugs. In W. Modell (ed.): *Drugs of Choice 1976-1977.* St. Louis: C. V. Mosby Co., 1976.
16. Davidson, J. K.: A new look at diet therapy. *Diabetes Forecast* 29(3):14, 1976.
17. Seltzer, H. S.: Drug-induced hypoglycemia: A review based on 473 cases. *Diabetes* 21:955, 1972.
18. Anderson, J. W., and Ward, K.: Long term effects of high-carbohydrate, high fiber diets on glucose and lipid metabolism. *Diabetes Care* 1:77, 1978.

*19. Brunzell, J. D.: Use of fructose, sorbitol, or xylitol as a sweetener in diabetes mellitus. *J. Am. Diet. Assoc.* 73:499, 1978.

*20. Bohannon, N. V., Karam, J. H., and Forsham, P. H.: Advantages of fructose ingestion over sucrose and glucose in humans. *Diabetes* 27(Suppl. 2):438, 1978.

21. Crapo, P. A., Reaven, G., and Olefsky, J.: Post-prandial plasma-glucose and -insulin responses to different complex carbohydrates. *Diabetes* 26:1178, 1977.

*22. West, K. M.: Diet and diabetes. *Postgrad. Med.* 60(3):209, 1976.

*23. Kaufmann, S.: Diet: Enforcing the *sine qua non.* In *Managing Diabetes Properly.* Nursing Skillbook Series. Horsham PA: Nursing 77 Books, 1977.

24. West, K. M.: Diet therapy of diabetes: An analysis of failure. *Ann. Intern. Med.* 79:425, 1973.

25. Miranda, P. M., and Horwitz, D. L.: High-fiber diets in the treatment of diabetes mellitus. *Ann. Intern. Med.* 88:482, 1978.

26. S. Anderson, J. W., and Chen, W.-S., L.: Plant fiber. Carbohydrate and lipid metabolism. *Am. J. Clin. Nutr.* 32:346, 1979.

27. Bloom, A.: Some practical aspects of the management of diabetes. *Clin. Endocrinol. Metabol.* 6(2):499, 1977.

28. Using nutrition labels with food exchange lists.

DHEW Publ. No. (FDA) 77:2072. Washington DC: U.S. Govt. Printing Office.

*29. Guthrie, D. W., and Guthrie, R. A.: *Nursing Management of Diabetes Mellitus.* St. Louis: C. V. Mosby Co., 1977.

*30. *A Guide for Professionals: The Effective Application of "Exchange Lists for Meal Planning."* American Diabetes Association, Inc. and The American Dietetic Association, 1977.

31. Koevisti, V. A., and Felig, P.: Effects of leg exercise on insulin absorption in diabetic patients. *N. Engl. J. Med.* 298:79, 1978.

32. Powers, P.: Distance for a diabetic. *Runner's World* 10, May, 1976.

*33. Myers, S. A.: Diabetes management by the patient and a nurse practitioner. *Nurs. Clin. North Am.* 12(3):415, 1977.

34. Fagan, J. E., and McArthur, R. G.: Maximizing diabetic control in children: An improved method for monitoring. *Postgrad. Med.* 63(2):58, 1978.

35. Danowski, T. S., and Sunder, J. H.: Jet injection of insulin during self-monitoring of blood glucose. *Diabetes Care* 1:27, 1978.

36. Tattersall, R.: Brittle diabetes. *Clin. Endocrinol. Metabol.* 6(2):403, 1977.

* Recommended reading.

31

Alterations in blood lipid levels

It may be that normal blood lipid levels are the exception rather than the rule in the U.S. The same holds true in many other affluent nations where usual diet is high in saturated fat and cholesterol. For example, serum lipid levels of people living in eastern Finland (the nation with the highest incidence of coronary heart disease in the world) tend to be even higher than those of Americans. Figure 31.1 contrasts typical blood cholesterol levels of Finns with those of southern Japanese (a technologically advanced population having a low fat intake and a low incidence of coronary heart disease). Typical lipid levels found in many technologically developed nations are not necessarily normal or desirable.[1] Unfortunately, optimal levels have not been determined with certainty and there is some dis-

agreement regarding when to treat elevated blood lipid levels. When treatment is indicated, however, diet modification is the principal treatment method.

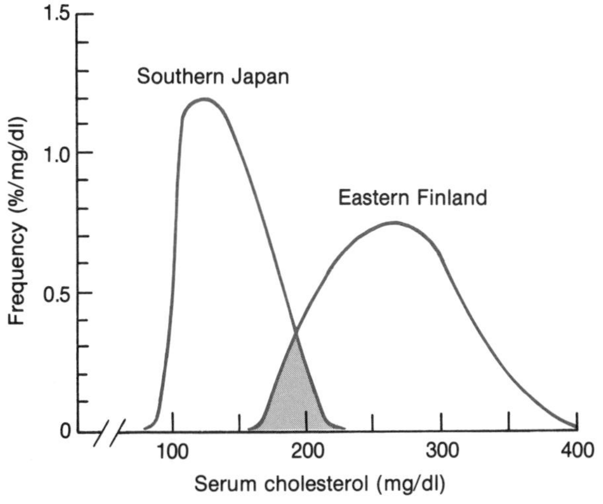

This chapter discusses common types of alterations in blood lipid levels, reasons for concern about elevated blood lipids, how dietary factors may influence lipid levels, diet modifications which have been recommended as a means of lowering blood lipid levels, and suggestions for assisting clients to follow a lipid lowering regimen.

OVERVIEW OF HYPERLIPIDEMIA AND REASONS FOR CONCERN

Hyperlipidemia is a general term referring to elevated blood lipid levels. Since altered lipid levels may arise from a number of causes, may take a variety of forms, and may be detected by several diagnostic methods, there has been a proliferation of terms referring to altered blood lipids. A few of the more common ones are defined here.

Hyperlipidemia: elevated serum levels of cholesterol and/or triglyceride

Hyperlipemic: with or causing hyperlipidemia

Hyperlipoproteinemia (HLP): elevated serum levels of lipoproteins. Since lipids travel in the blood in the form of lipoproteins, this term is more accurate than is hyperlipidemia. The abbreviation HLP is often used for simplicity

Hypercholesterolemia: elevated serum cholesterol (blood sample may be random or fasting)

Hypertriglyceridemia: elevated fasting serum triglyceride level. The fat present is primarily endogenous triglyceride (fat made in the body)

FIGURE 31.1. How nutrition influences mass hyperlipidemia and atherosclerosis. (From Blackburn, H.: How nutrition influences mass hyperlipidemia and atherosclerosis. *Geriatrics* 33:42, 1978, with permission of Raven Press, New York)

Hyperchylomicronemia: elevated fasting serum level of chylomicrons. (The fat is mainly dietary fat which hasn't been cleared from the blood)

Serum lipid levels can rise markedly without producing symptoms. Usually a hyperlipidemic individual is aware of the need for treatment of his condition only if he has his blood lipid levels checked by his physician.

Although usual forms of hyperlipidemia are symptom-free, most physicians agree that adults should have their lipid levels checked.[2-4] If lipid levels are elevated, most physicians begin corrective measures because hyperlipidemia, especially hypercholesterolemia, is linked with atherosclerosis.

Unless the dangers of elevated lipid levels and the benefits of dietary management are clearly pointed out to clients, they may be reluctant to adopt recommended changes in their eating habits. Since there is much information and misinformation about blood lipids in the general media, health professionals need to be especially well-informed on the topic in order to effectively discuss issues regarding blood lipids with clients.

Atherosclerosis and cardiovascular disease

Atherosclerosis is a disease of the intima (innermost part) of large and medium-sized arteries. It should not be confused with the more general term *arteriosclerosis*, which refers to conditions in which arteries lose their elasticity and become hardened for any one of a number of reasons. The most noticeable feature of *athero*sclerosis is the accumulation of lipids within arteries.

Atherosclerosis, like hyperlipidemia, is a common condition in adults in the U.S. and in many other affluent countries. It is believed to be a leading contributor to morbidity and mortality in technologically advanced nations. The association of atherosclerosis with coronary heart disease (CHD) is generally well recognized, but atherosclerosis may also contribute to de-

velopment of stroke (cerebral thrombosis, cerebral infarction), to aortic aneurysm (a ballooning of the wall of the aorta), or to peripheral vascular disease (impaired peripheral circulation, especially to the feet and lower legs). The only manifestations of atherosclerosis with which hyperlipidemia has been linked are CHD and peripheral vascular disease.

To understand how dietary factors may be related to the atherosclerotic process and to coronary heart disease it is necessary to be familiar with some of the features of these conditions. (Several hypotheses regarding mechanisms involved in the atherosclerotic process are reviewed by Ross.[5]) Atherosclerosis appears to begin with minor damage to the inner arterial wall (owing to any one of a variety of causes). Blood platelets, blood lipids, and other blood components may then interact with the injured vessel.

FORMS OF ATHEROSCLEROTIC DEPOSITS

At least three different forms of atherosclerotic fatty deposits have been described. Figure 31.2 illustrates some of the more serious types. One form is called a *fatty streak*. Fatty streaks consist of an accumulation of smooth muscle cells which contain and are surrounded by lipids; these streaks are not large enough to significantly decrease the diameter of arteries in which they appear. They are found in children and adolescents throughout the world. At this time, there is no evidence that they are clinically significant.

Fibrous plaque, often called plaque for short, is characteristic of advancing atherosclerosis. Plaque consists of an accumulation of smooth muscle cells in the arterial intima; in this case the cells are rather heavily laden with cholesterol and are surrounded by other lipids, collagen, elastic fibers, and other substances. Fibrous plaque protrudes into the arterial lumen, decreasing its diameter. Plaque becomes prevalent in population groups in the U.S. during the third decade of life.

Complicated lesions, as the name implies, are serious

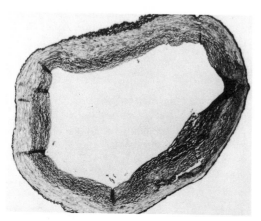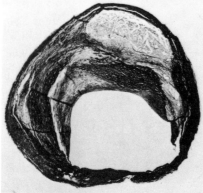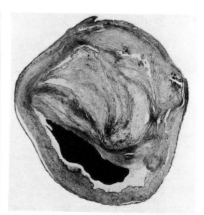

FIGURE 31.2. *Left*, Normal artery; *Middle*, Fatty Deposits in vessel wall; *Right*, Plugged artery with fatty deposits and clot. (Photo courtesy of the American Heart Association, National Center)

abnormalities; they are often associated with occlusive disease (blockage of arteries). These lesions are thought to develop when fibrous plaque is altered by hemorrhage, calcification, and arterial muscle cell necrosis (death). Complicated lesions may contribute to aortic aneurysm by weakening the arterial wall. A piece may break off from a complicated lesion, forming an embolus (mobile blood clot); the embolus may travel through blood vessels and cause thrombosis (occlusion) at a distant point. Arteries which are narrowed by raised lesions (fibrous plaque and/or complicated lesions) may become occluded more readily than would normal arteries.

The kind and degree of atherosclerotic cardiovascular disease depends on which blood vessels are obstructed and the degree of the obstruction. If an artery is partially occluded, the supply of blood may fail to meet elevated oxygen and nutrient demands of a tissue. If this occurs, the tissue is said to become *ischemic*. When coronary arteries are involved (coronary artery disease—CAD), affected persons may perceive ischemia as chest pain upon exertion, one of the classic symptoms of *angina pectoris*. If it is femoral arteries which are narrowed by fatty deposits, symptoms such as intermittent claudication (calf pain on walking) or leg ulcers might develop. In severe cases, gangrene might necessitate amputation of part or all of an extremity.

When a coronary artery is suddenly occluded, a myocardial infarction (MI) occurs. The part of the myocardium (heart muscle) ordinarily supplied by that artery suffers severe ischemia followed by cell necrosis (death of cells in the affected area). If heart damage is severe, sudden death—that is, death not preceded by any warning—may occur.

When occlusion occurs in an artery supplying the brain, the result is cerebral thrombosis (stroke).

There is strong evidence to support the suggestion that hyperlipidemia, especially hypercholesterolemia, speeds or aggravates the atherosclerotic process.[6,7] The composition of the blood (i.e., type and amount of lipids, characteristics of the platelets) and perhaps the blood pressure are believed to influence whether the process becomes pathogenic or healing occurs. Diet may influence a number of these factors. Effects of smoking are also believed to be involved in injury of the artery and/or development of plaque.

HYPERLIPIDEMIA AS ONE OF SEVERAL RISK FACTORS FOR ATHEROSCLEROSIS AND CHD

Since the principal reason for correcting hyperlipidemia is to reduce risk of cardiovascular disease, it is essential for health care workers to recognize that several factors which do not appear to influence blood lipid level may influence risk of cardiovascular disease. In fact, many individuals who have suffered an MI or sudden death have had blood lipid levels which fall within U.S. norms. When developing a plan for reducing risk of cardiovascular disease, it is desirable to consider blood lipid level along with other risk factors (Table 31.1). The greater the number of major risk factors, the more important control of hyperlipidemia becomes.

POINTS OF EMPHASIS
Hyperlipidemia and atherosclerosis

- *Arteries in a number of parts of the body are susceptible to being narrowed by plaque and complicated lesions. This process is called the atherosclerotic process.*
- *Plaque and complicated lesions contain lipid deposits as well as other substances.*
- *Narrowed arteries are more vulnerable to being occluded, as by blood clots.*
- *Hyperlipidemia is believed to contribute to the atherosclerotic process and is one of several risk factors for coronary heart disease.*
- *Blood lipid determinations are recommended as a part of routine health care, especially for adults under 55 years of age and for relatives of persons who have hyperlipidemia. Early intervention to reduce elevated lipid levels may significantly reduce risk of CHD.*

TABLE 31.1 *Classification of risk factors*

MAJOR RISK FACTORS[8]	AMENABLE TO CONTROL?	MINOR RISK FACTORS*	AMENABLE TO CONTROL?
Hypercholesterolemia	Yes	Sex (maleness)	No
Cigarette smoking	Yes	Heredity (family history of premature CHD)	No
Hypertension	Yes	Obesity	Yes
Diabetes mellitus†	Yes	Sedentary lifestyle	Yes
		Emotional stress	Usually yes
		(pattern A behavior‡)	Uncertain

* These risk factors fail to show a strong *independent* relationship to risk of CHD. However "minor" doesn't necessarily mean that these factors are unimportant. Some of them may have strong impact by influencing one or more of the major risk factors or by influencing the chance of thrombus formation. Examples: (1) Heredity factors may influence blood lipids or blood pressure, (2) attempts by individuals who have a type A personality to master uncontrollable stressful events may lead to physiological responses which increase risk of CHD, (3) obesity increases the likelihood of hypertension, hyperlipidemia, and diabetes mellitus.
    † Sometimes classed as a minor risk factor.
    ‡ Pattern A behavior is characterized by a sense of time urgency, striving hard to achieve in competitive situations, and hostility or aggression.

Risk factors do not completely account for the incidence of heart disease; therefore, other avenues are being explored. For instance, does a diet with a high P/S ratio* have a beneficial effect which is unrelated to its hypocholesterolemic (cholesterol lowering) effect? For example, changing the P/S ratio from 0.25 to 1.6 in a controlled diet fed to adult males resulted in "pronounced and significant decrease in aggregatability of blood platelets."[9] This change in platelet activity is expected to decrease the chance of thrombus formation. Further research has found that healthy people have a constant degree of platelet activation that can be significantly decreased by dietary means (i.e., increase in linoleic acid intake).[10,11]

TYPES OF BLOOD LIPID ABNORMALITIES

The forms in which lipids travel in the blood appear to have different roles in the atherosclerotic process.

Cholesterol and triglycerides are combined with protein and phospholipids to form different types of water-soluble *lipoprotein* complexes.

Five distinct types of lipoproteins have been identified: chylomicrons, very low density lipoproteins, intermediate density lipoproteins, low density lipoproteins, and high density lipoproteins. The types differ in size and in their proportions of cholesterol, triglyceride, protein, and phospholipid. They also differ in density, as their names imply. A lipoprotein profile (an analysis of how much of each type of lipoprotein is present in the blood) can be determined from density differences. The five types of lipoproteins are briefly described here.

Chylomicrons These large particles are lowest in density of all the lipoproteins because they are composed primarily of dietary fat. High fasting levels of chylomicrons are not believed to increase risk of coronary heart disease.

Very low density lipoproteins (VLDL, also called pre-beta lipoproteins) Very low density lipoproteins are triglyceride-rich particles which also contain significant amounts of cholesterol. VLDLs may be formed by either (1) partial degradation of chylomicrons or (2) hepatic synthesis from endogenous triglyceride (fat made by the liver).

A high VLDL level appears to increase risk of coronary heart disease.[12]

Intermediate density lipoproteins (IDL or lipoprotein "remnants") IDLs are formed when VLDLs undergo removal of part of the triglyceride and other compo-

nents. These remnant lipoproteins then give rise to low density lipoproteins. There is little information regarding risk associated with elevated IDL's.[13]

Low density lipoproteins (LDL, also called beta-lipoproteins) Low density lipoproteins are cholesterol-rich particles which are formed from IDL. A majority of the cholesterol present in serum is typically contained in low density lipoproteins. An elevated LDL level (which could also be called hypercholesterolemia) is believed to accelerate the atherosclerotic process and to increase risk of coronary heart disease. Evidence suggests that the degree of atherosclerosis is proportional to the degree of hypercholesterolemia.[1]

High density lipoproteins (HDL, also called alpha-lipoproteins) These are small protein-rich and phospholipid-rich particles which also contain cholesterol. HDLs appear to have several functions in *retarding* the atherosclerotic process. For example, HDL may serve to remove early cholesterol deposits and to transport cholesterol back to the liver for processing.

To date, HDL cholesterol level is claimed to be the strongest predictor of risk of CHD, at least in affluent nations.[14] (In diabetics, however, low density lipoproteins appear to be better correlated with risk of CHD than are high density lipoproteins.[15]) The amount of cholesterol in high density lipoproteins (HDL cholesterol) is inversely correlated with risk of CHD. That is, the higher the level of HDL cholesterol, the *lower* the risk of CHD.

Serum lipid levels are subject to fluctuation; therefore, if hyperlipidemia is found it is generally recommended that three determinations of serum lipid levels be made at 2-week intervals to establish a baseline level. Occasionally a lipoprotein profile is a useful supplementary diagnostic tool.

Fredrickson at NIH[16] has classified blood lipid abnormalities into five major categories of hyperlipoproteinemia (HLP), as shown in Table 31.2. A *modified diet is the mainstay of treatment of any type of HLP.*[16] It is important for health professionals to recognize that HLP classifications are somewhat arbitrary and that errors in interpretation of test results are possible.

Evaluation of the client's compliance with and response to treatment is essential to a satisfactory plan of nutritional care. Within 6 weeks following initiation of treatment, a 15 percent or greater reduction in

---

TABLE 31.2 *Categories of hyperlipoproteinemia*

C high; TG normal	Type IIa
C high; TG 150–400	Type IIb, III, or IV
C high; TG 400–1000	Type III, IV, or V
C high; TG >1000	Type I or V
C normal; TG high	Type IV (I or V)

Source: *The Dietary Management of Hyperlipoproteinemia.* DHEW, NIH, National Heart and Lung Institute. Bethesda MD: DHEW Publ. No. (NIH) 76-110, 1976, p. ix.

---

* The amount of polyunsaturated fat divided by the amount of saturated fat in the diet.

TABLE 31.3 *Summary of diets for treatment of hyperlipoproteinemia*

	TYPE I	TYPE IIa	TYPE IIb & TYPE III	TYPE IV	TYPE V
DIET PRE-SCRIPTION	Low fat 25–35 gm	Low cholesterol polyunsaturated fat increased	Low cholesterol Approximately: 20% cal pro 40% cal fat 40% cal CHO	Controlled CHO Approximately 45% of calories Moderately restricted cholesterol	Restricted fat 30% of calories Controlled CHO 50% of calories Moderately restricted cholesterol
CALORIES	Not restricted	Not restricted	Achieve and maintain "ideal" weight, i.e., reduction diet if necessary	Achieve and maintain "ideal" weight, i.e., reduction diet if necessary	Achieve and maintain "ideal" weight, i.e., reduction diet if necessary
PROTEIN	Total protein intake is not limited	Total protein intake is not limited	High protein	Not limited other than control of patient's weight	High protein
FAT	Restricted to 25–35 gm Kind of fat not important	Saturated fat intake limited Polyunsaturated fat intake increased	Controlled to 40% calories (polyunsaturated fats recommended in preference to saturated fats)	Not limited other than control of patient's weight (polyunsaturated fats recommended in preference to saturated fats)	Restricted to 30% of calories (polyunsaturated fats recommended in preference to saturated fats)
CHOLESTEROL	Not restricted	As low as possible; the only source of cholesterol is the meat in the diet	Less than 300 mg —the only source of cholesterol is the meat in the diet	Moderately restricted to 300–500 mg	Moderately restricted to 300–500 mg
CARBO-HYDRATE	Not limited	Not limited	Controlled—concentrated sweets are restricted	Controlled—concentrated sweets are restricted	Controlled—concentrated sweets are restricted
ALCOHOL	Not recommended	May be used with discretion	Limited to 2 servings (substituted for carbohydrate)	Limited to 2 servings (substituted for carbohydrate)	Not recommended

Source: *The Dietary Management of Hyperlipoproteinemia.* DHEW, NIH, National Heart and Lung Institute. Bethesda MD: DHEW Publ. No. (NIH) 76-110, 1976.

serum lipids indicates that the diet treatment is effective.[16]

Only two types of hyperlipoproteinemia are common, namely type II (subtypes IIa and IIb) and type IV. In most cases it is sufficient for health care workers to know that an elevated cholesterol level usually signals type II HLP and that an elevated triglyceride level usually signals type IV HLP. Type II HLP appears to carry considerable risk of coronary heart disease. Type IV HLP may also carry a risk of CHD.

Distinct diet plans have been developed for treating the different types of HLP. They are available to qualified health professionals through the National Institutes of Health and are summarized in Table 31.3. Diet plans for HLP IIa and IV are discussed later in the chapter.

Causes of hyperlipidemia

There are numerous causes for development of hyperlipidemia. *Environmental factors* (e.g., high fat diet with a low P/S ratio, excessive alcohol intake, sedentary lifestyle) are believed to contribute substantially to the high incidence of hyperlipidemia in affluent countries.

Certain *genetic defects* lead to familial hyperlipidemia. The principal means of distinguishing familial from environmental forms of hyperlipidemia is examining other family members. If a person is diagnosed to have hyperlipidemia, his relatives should have their blood lipid levels monitored so that abnormalities can be detected and treated early.

Hyperlipidemia can be *secondary to disease* conditions which affect lipid metabolism, such as diabetes mellitus, nephrosis, obstructive liver disease, and hypothroidism. If a person has a disease affecting lipid metabolism, treatment of the disease often brings lipid levels under control. Hyperlipidemia may also be secondary to certain types of drugs, such as oral contraceptive agents.[17] Discontinuation of the drug may promptly result in lowering of serum lipid levels.

Degrees of hyperlipidemia

It is useful for health professionals to be able to distinguish between different degrees and types of hyperlipidemia. They should recognize that there are no cutoff points for blood lipid levels at which risk disappears or suddenly becomes worse.

HYPERCHOLESTEROLEMIA

Grundy[7] classifies hypercholesterolemia into three separate groups.

Mild hypercholesterolemia (plasma cholesterol of 225 to 275 mg%) This range of cholesterol is very common for Americans. Diet treatment, usually by moderate fat modified diet recommendations, has excellent potential for bringing serum cholesterol down to a more desirable level (see Appendix 5K).

Moderate hypercholesterolemia (plasma cholesterol of 275 to 350 mg%) Within this cholesterol range risk of CHD may be two to several times higher than it would be if cholesterol level were below 200 mg%. Treatment may involve close adherence to a fat modified diet. In some cases drug therapy (usually cholestyramine or colestipol) may be combined with diet modification in an attempt to bring cholesterol closer to the desired level.

Severe hypercholesterolemia (levels above 350 mg%) When hypercholesterolemia is severe, genetic factors usually play a major role. *Familial hypercholesterolemia* (type IIa HLP) is a very serious condition which is sometimes resistant to treatment. Cholesterol levels have been found to average 750 mg% in untreated children believed to be homozygous for the defective gene.[13] Treatment involves long term diet modification and drug therapy and remains somewhat investigational.

HYPERTRIGLYCERIDEMIA

The upper limit of normal for serum triglyceride is usually considered to be 150 mg% in this country. Levels can rise many times this value, occasionally reaching 1000 to 2000 mg%. At this extreme, symptoms may develop (e.g., marked intolerance to dietary fat, eruptive xanthamatosis, enlarged liver and spleen,

neuromuscular problems, and perhaps even pancreatitis). Diet treatment may be very effective in managing hypertriglyceridemia.

Value of treatment of hyperlipidemia

The value of treating unsymptomatic hyperlipidemia in older adults, especially those over 55 or 60 years of age, is quite uncertain. If atherosclerosis is well developed in a senior citizen, correction of hyperlipidemia might make little difference to his health. Health professionals should weigh disadvantages against possible advantages when considering placing an elderly person on a fat and cholesterol controlled diet. Some elderly individuals would find the diet so unpalatable or so unlike their customary intake that they might greatly reduce their food intake rather than make suitable substitutions. For example, many elderly individuals use eggs as their principal source of protein because eggs are so easy to prepare and chew. It might sometimes be advisable to encourage this practice in order to help prevent malnutrition.

The value of treating hyperlipidemia is probably much greater for younger adults. There are reports that early atherosclerosis may regress in femoral arteries in humans if serum cholesterol and triglyceride levels are lowered.[18,19]

Reduced coagulability of the blood is another poten-

POINTS OF EMPHASIS
Diet, blood lipids, and cardiovascular disease

• *There are a number of types of blood lipid abnormalities.*

• *Some types of blood lipid abnormalities appear to predispose an individual to atherosclerosis, coronary heart disease, and other forms of cardiovascular disease. Some uncommon blood lipid abnormalities lead to severe noncardiovascular illness if untreated.*

• *Blood lipid abnormalities may be caused by environmental factors, genetic defects, and/or disease conditions.*

• *Diet is the primary means of correcting blood lipid abnormalities unless they are secondary to disease conditions.*

• *Effectiveness of diet treatment varies considerably. In some cases drugs are used in conjunction with diet to help control blood lipid levels.*

• *It is not known how much protection is afforded by lowering high blood lipid levels. Treatment is believed to be most beneficial if initiated in young people and continued throughout life. Benefits of reducing serum lipid levels have been questioned for persons over about 55 years of age.*

tial benefit of a diet with a high P/S ratio. For reasons such as these, old and young alike may wish to try to follow a fat modified diet.

If health professionals expect to have clients follow through with measures to reduce serum lipid levels, they must be able to provide clients with some motivation for doing so. Clients need to believe in effectiveness of treatment. Treatment can almost always cause significant lowering of blood lipid levels. There is no reason to believe that elevated lipid levels are benign and there is much reason to believe that they are harmful. Freedom from heart disease cannot be promised, but health professionals have a responsibility to make a strong case for taking action to reduce risk, especially in the younger age groups.

DIETARY EFFECTS ON BLOOD LIPID LEVELS

Numerous dietary factors may influence blood lipid levels. These include the amount and type of dietary fat, P/S ratio, dietary cholesterol, amount and type of dietary fiber, source of dietary protein, alcohol, and perhaps sugar and less well-studied non-nutritive components of food. When combined in the diet, some components of food may interact to produce a greater lipid lowering effect than would be anticipated on the basis of their known independent effects.

Weight reduction if overweight or obese   Weight reduction is a major goal for overly-fat individuals with hyperlipidemia. It may be achieved through caloric restriction and/or increase in physical activity (with the physician's approval). According to Heyden,[20] weight loss appears to have no predictable effect on serum cholesterol; however, caloric deficit and loss of excess weight usually result in rapid fall of serum triglyceride level.[21]

Since weight loss may also significantly reduce an elevated blood pressure and help in management of maturity onset diabetes mellitus, the combined effects of weight loss may greatly reduce risk of coronary heart disease.

Altering the type and amount of dietary fat   It has been well established that blood cholesterol level tends to fall when the proportion of polyunsaturated fat in the diet is increased and the proportion of saturated fat is decreased. The effect of saturated fat in raising serum cholesterol level is about two times greater than the cholesterol-lowering effect of polyunsaturated fat, as illustrated in Figure 31.3.[6]

Dietary cholesterol intake   There are conflicting reports about how dietary cholesterol influences blood cholesterol levels. In a number of controlled studies participants have been fed carefully formulated diets which varied primarily in cholesterol content; their serum cholesterol levels increased or decreased in relation to the amount of dietary cholesterol ingested.[6,22] Decreasing daily cholesterol intake from about 700 mg. to 100 mg. is expected to produce about a 30 mg% drop in serum cholesterol.[11] In contrast, studies which have involved changing cholesterol intake of persons who were selecting their own diets at home have failed

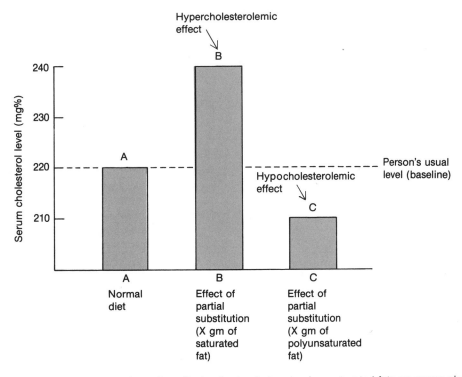

FIGURE 31.3. Opposing effects of saturated and polyunsaturated fats on serum cholesterol levels.

to show that cholesterol intake significantly influences blood cholesterol levels.[23-25]

Not all individuals who consume a diet high in saturated fat and cholesterol have high serum cholesterol levels. Different people may absorb and metabolize cholesterol differently. However, serum cholesterol level appears to be highly correlated with cholesterol intake when the diet is *very low* in cholesterol.[26]

Carbohydrate intake Since circulating triglycerides can be made from dietary sources of carbohydrate, controlling carbohydrate intake may help to correct some forms of hypertriglyceridemia. However, serum triglyceride level can usually be controlled if the diet (1) does not contain excess calories and (2) had a moderate to fairly high content of complex carbohydrate (with very little added sugar). Many individuals can achieve an acceptable triglyceride level with this pattern even if 50 percent or more of the calories are provided by carbohydrate.

Alcohol Alcohol ingestion changes liver metabolism in such a way that production of very low density lipoproteins is usually increased. This is most often seen in persons who already have hypertriglyceridemia. In these individuals even moderate consumption of alcohol readily increases serum triglyceride.[27] Restricting or eliminating alcohol causes a dramatic lowering of serum triglyceride in some hyperlipemic individuals.

Although moderate alcohol intake (5 to 6 oz. of alcohol per week) has been correlated with increase in HDL cholesterol and decreased risk of CHD,[28] Castelli recommends a cautious approach to basing advice on these findings. Known adverse physiological effects of alcohol should be considered.

Other factors Certain types of food, protein, and fiber have been reported to affect blood lipid levels. Legumes have been found to lower serum cholesterol levels even when included in a diet high in saturated fat.[29] This effect might be related to effects of indigestible residue (fiber and carbohydrate) from the beans and/or to the protein they contain.

Substitution of soybean-textured protein (meat analogs) for animal products has been suggested for lowering serum cholesterol level in individuals with HLP II.[30] Studies with healthy young women also report a lowering of serum cholesterol level when soy protein is used in place of animal protein.[31]

Effects of fiber on serum cholesterol are still under investigation. Generally, bran has not been found to have a hypocholesterolemic effect whereas pectin (a component of raw apples, oranges, and some other fruits and vegetables) may significantly reduce serum cholesterol level.[32]

When a single food is found to affect blood lipid levels, it is important to note under what circumstances this is so. For example, yogurt and even milk have been reported to have hypocholesterolemic effects when consumed in large quantity.[33] Results of other studies, however, suggest that this effect is not significant when smaller amounts of whole milk are consumed.

In folklore onion and garlic have been described as having the ability to retard the development of atherosclerosis (and a number of other ills). Brief reports[34,35] suggest that these vegetables may decrease serum triglyceride levels and increase fibrinolytic activity of blood if consumed in high amounts (e.g., 5 gm. crushed garlic daily). There are no contraindications to such a practice as long as it doesn't interfere with adherence to other aspects of a nutritional plan of care.

Vegetarian diets have many features which have been identified as having antilipemic effects. Many types of vegetarian diets are low in cholesterol, have a high P/S ratio, provide less than 30 to 35 percent of calories as fat, include considerable fiber of a variety of types, include legumes and/or soy protein, and seldom provide excess calories. It is not surprising, therefore, that vegetarians tend to have lower serum lipid levels than do nonvegetarians.[36,37] Below the age of 65, *male* vegetarian Seventh-Day Adventists (SDAs) have lower incidence of fatal coronary heart disease than do nonvegetarian SDAs.[38] As a result of his findings, Sanders has suggested that a vegan type of diet may be desirable for treatment of certain kinds of hyperlipidemia.[36]

Trans-fatty acids Hydrogenation (hardening) of vegetable oils is a common practice in food processing. Hydrogenation changes part (about 5 to 45 percent) of the polyunsaturated fatty acids into monounsaturated trans-fatty acids.[39] Trans-fatty acids are not naturally present in foods. Some work suggests that trans-fatty acids may contribute to development of atherosclerosis.[40] The issue is far from resolved.

Meal size and frequency of eating Large fatty meals can result in a temporary marked increase in nonfasting triglyceride level. If the fat in the meal is mainly saturated, the blood may coagulate more readily.[41] Moderation in meal size is recommended.

POINTS OF EMPHASIS
Dietary effects on blood lipid levels

• *Weight reduction is a major means of decreasing serum triglyceride level.*

• *Changing diet by increasing the P/S ratio (usually to the range of 1.0 to 2.0) and limiting total fat intake to less than 35 percent of calories is a practical means of lowering serum cholesterol level.*

• *Restricting dietary intake of cholesterol to less than 300 mg. daily may help correct hypercholesterolemia.*

• *Restriction of alcohol intake may help lower serum triglyceride levels.*

• *A vegan diet or generous use of legumes, certain other unrefined plant foods, and meat analogs have a hypocholesterolemic effect.*

ASSISTING CLIENTS TO CONTROL HYPERLIPIDEMIA

Clients who are strongly urged to modify their diets in an attempt to correct hyperlipidemia are likely to need considerable assistance in altering their behavior to achieve that goal. Before trying to provide this assistance, the health professional needs to try to identify how the diet modifications may affect a client emotionally and she also needs to be aware of other restrictions imposed on the client, such as calorie restriction, sodium restriction, and abstinence from cigarettes.

Health team members, including the client, decide together when the time is right for taking action to correct hyperlipidemia. Care is taken to avoid asking so much from the client that he resorts to cancelling appointments and avoiding contact with health care providers.

Diet treatment does require a change in food selection that may be objectionable to many people, especially when first tried; however, diet treatment is preferable to exclusive use of drug treatment.

Diet instruction should include information on menu planning, shopping, food preparation, and eating away from home. Ideally the whole family will support the client and simplify food preparation by following most of the diet recommendations. For example they might follow a prudent diet.

Meal planning

Fat and cholesterol modified meals can be tasty, varied, and nutritious. Competent health care providers try to present the features of the diet in a positive light. They may, for example, draw the client's attention to "allowed foods" on the diet plan. Nevertheless, many clients first look at the list of foods to be avoided and become understandably dismayed by finding that it includes some of their favorite foods. A health professional can foster a more positive attitude by helping the client identify acceptable substitutes for favorite foods. (Attractive pictures often help.) Some suggestions for substitutions are given in Table 31.4.

Fat modified diets are usually set up so that the client can exchange one source of saturated fat for another only within the meat group. The help of a dietitian or nutritionist should be sought if a client wants to find out if and how an unusual substitution might be made.

TABLE 31.4 *Some suggested substitutions for well-liked foods that are to be omitted from a low cholesterol fat modified diet*

MENU ITEMS OF CONCERN	POSSIBLE SUBSTITUTIONS (Client's diet form is used to double check on allowed foods and ingredients)
Traditional Sunday breakfast: bacon and eggs	1 egg (if allowed) with imitation bacon bits,* french toast made with part of egg allotment for the week or with egg white; pancakes made from "scratch" using allowed ingredients; omelet made with egg substitute and flavored with herbs or preserves
Daily breakfast or coffee break: donuts, danish pastry	English muffins with allowed margarine, jam or jelly; raisin toast with allowed margarine; homemade muffins,† biscuits,† or coffee cake†
Brown bag lunch: cold cut or cheese sandwich	A variety of allowed sandwiches: thinly sliced chicken, turkey, or lean roast beef; tuna salad*; egg salad made from egg substitute or allowed egg; home-prepared meatloaf,† peanut butter (with many possible "extras,") spreads made from seasoned cooked legumes or tofu. (Those who try these spreads often discover that they are surprisingly tasty)
Dinner: meat and potatoes with gravy	Fat-free gravy
hot dogs	Lean ham*
casseroles made with cheese	Casseroles made with cottage cheese or with special "filled" cheeses* (skim milk cheese with added corn oil made to resemble a cheese food such as Velveeta). A bit of romano or parmesan cheese, if allowed, adds a lot of cheese flavor with little saturated fat
Commercially fried foods	Home fried foods† (Limit the number of foods prepared in this way to avoid excessive fat intake)
Creamed dishes	Sauce† made with skim milk and polyunsaturated margarine
Ice cream	Sherbet, fruit ice
Cake, cookies, pie	Angel food cake, home-prepared baked goods† (limit servings of desserts to promote weight control and to avoid crowding out more valuable sources of nutrients)
Potato and corn chips	Pretzels,† corn popped in polyunsaturated oil, plain crackers with peanut butter
Sour cream	Yogurt made from skim milk
Whipped cream	Whipped instant nonfat dry milk or evaporated skimmed milk

* Very high in sodium, probably not appropriate for hypertensive clients.
† Made following special recipe which uses only allowed ingredients.

Some of the details of type IIa and type IV HLP diets follow. These two diets (or minor variations of them) are commonly prescribed.

DIET FOR TYPE IIa HLP—LOW CHOLESTEROL (<200 MG), MODIFIED FAT (INCREASED POLYUNSATURATED FAT) DIET

The type IIa HLP diet is a fairly strict version of a low cholesterol, modified fat diet. A P/S ratio of about 2 is recommended. Cholesterol intake is kept below about 200 mg. daily. With the exceptions noted here, foods allowed are those allowed in the diet in Appendix 5K.
1. No egg yolks or whole eggs are allowed, even in cooking, because of their cholesterol content.
2. Servings of lean red meat (beef, pork, ham, lamb) are limited to three 85 gm. (3 oz.) cooked weight servings per *week.* Up to 225 gm. (9 oz.) cooked weight of fish, poultry (skinless), shellfish (except shrimp) and veal are allowed daily.
3. To keep the P/S ratio favorable, 5 gm. (1 tsp.) of polyunsaturated fat is to be consumed for each 30 gm. of meat, fish, or poultry. If more red meat is desired, (1) limit all meat to 255 gm. (9 oz.) cooked weight daily and consume 10 gm. (2 tsp.) of polyunsaturated fat for each 30 gm. of meat.
4. The only butterfat allowed is from creamed cottage cheese. If creamed cottage cheese is used, it should be substituted for meat (60 ml. or ¼ c. cottage cheese = 30 gm. meat).
5. Margarine used should have the highest P/S ratio available (usually soft safflower or sunflower oil type).
6. Safflower, sunflower, and corn oil are the only recommended vegetable oils.

DIET FOR TYPE IV HLP (CONTROLLED CARBOHYDRATE, MODIFIED FAT, MODERATELY RESTRICTED CHOLESTEROL DIET)

A type IV HLP diet is very similar to a diabetic diet plan for a person with maturity onset diabetes mellitus. A low calorie diet is likely to be emphasized for both. "Exchange List for Meal Planning" (Appendix 5I) is suitable to use for this type of diet, using the items in **bold type.** For example, the lean meat exchange group would be the principal meat exchange group used. The type IV HLP diet developed by the National Institutes of Health allows some additional substitutions, which are listed in Appendix 5J.

A modified fat diet is usually more enjoyable if many foods are prepared at home from basic ingredients. This allows the family to enjoy certain sauces and fried foods, homemade muffins and other quick breads, and many desserts (if excess calorie intake is not a problem). A reliable fat-controlled cookbook such as the *American Heart Association Cookbook*[42] can help the cook learn to prepare well-liked foods that are

acceptable for the diet. Even some French chefs are admitting that food doesn't have to be rich in cream, butter, and eggs in order to be tasty.[43]

A client may not recognize that many recipes in fat-controlled cookbooks and leaflets are high in calories and/or sodium. If there is a need to reduce weight or to reduce sodium intake, clients should be referred to a diet counselor to learn how to determine which recipes should be bypassed and which recipes can be altered to make them lower in calories or sodium.

Shopping for foods for a fat-controlled diet

With all of the publicity regarding the desirability of controlling intake of fat and cholesterol, a wide variety of "low cholesterol" products has been promoted. The family member who purchases food needs to know how to find out if specific "low cholesterol" products are acceptable for the prescribed diet. Label reading can be an invaluable part of this process if the item is not specifically mentioned on the diet form.

Statements made in advertisements or on labels can be confusing. Here are ways to interpret a few common statements or phrases:
1. "Low in cholesterol." If the product is a *plain* food obtained from a plant (e.g., cereal, nuts, fruits, vegetables), any brand is essentially free of cholesterol even if that fact is not stated on the label. Clients should remember that saturated fat content is probably more important than cholesterol content. Some low cholesterol products such as hard margarine and hydrogenated shortening are high in saturated fat and should be avoided even though they are free of cholesterol.
2. "Margarine made from 100% corn oil." If the first ingredient in the margarine is *partially hydrogenated* corn oil, the P/S ratio of the product should be checked. If no information is given regarding the number of grams of polyunsaturated and saturated fat, the P/S ratio is probably lower than desirable. If, on the other hand, the label states that the product contains 5 gm. (or more) of polyunsaturated and 2 gm. of saturated fat, it has a favorable P/S ratio for most fat modified diets.
3. "Contains no animal fat" or "Made of pure vegetable oils (or fats)." This offers no advantage if the product is made with coconut oil, palm oil, or with partially hydrogenated vegetable oil. None of these oils is polyunsaturated even though they are of vegetable origin.
4. "Nondairy product." Many people erroneously believe that nondairy creamers, whipped toppings, and imitation cheeses are fine for fat modified diets. Most of these products substitute coconut oil (a highly saturated fat) for butterfat. The listing of ingredients should be checked. A few nondairy creamers containing primarily polyunsaturated fat are available; these indicate their P/S ratios on the label.

It also may be helpful to ask some of the following questions before purchasing a product:

Is the sodium content excessive? The sodium content of many specially prepared "low cholesterol" products is much higher than desirable for clients who are trying to control hypertension as well as hyperlipidemia. This is especially true of most meat analogs (such as imitation bacon, ham, sausage) and of low cholesterol filled cheeses (skim milk cheese with added vegetable oil).

Has processing seriously affected the nutritive value of the product? Many "low cholesterol" foods are engineered foods containing few micronutrients other than those added in processing. Imitation cheeses and other nondairy products and meat analogs are in this category.

Does the product have advantages which make it worth the extra money it costs? For example, many people like the increase in variety and convenience which egg substitutes make possible. Margarine with a high P/S ratio usually costs considerably more than do more saturated forms of margarine, but adequate control of hyperlipidemia is usually not achieved with the less expensive spreads. The quality of some low cholesterol products is decidedly inferior even though the price might be high. Health professionals should make sure that the client understands that no fabricated low cholesterol food is essential to the success of a fat-controlled diet.

Eating out

When eating out, a person may be able to comply with a fat modified diet by choosing plain, low fat foods. The client's diet form is used for checking if a specific food is allowed.

The degree to which a person should adhere to his diet at an infrequent party or other special event is a matter which should be discussed with the health professional. Consideration should be given to the seriousness of the condition, its responsiveness to diet treatment, and the effect of occasional "splurging" on overall adherence to the diet and other aspects of treatment. The Inter-Society Commission for Heart Disease Resources states "It is the reduction in average fat intake over a period of time that matters. Exceptions can be made for special occasions."[44]

COORDINATING NUTRITIONAL CARE WITH OTHER ASPECTS OF TREATMENT

PHYSICAL ACTIVITY

When working with a client to develop a plan of nutritional care, health professionals should recognize possible beneficial effects of physical activity on blood lipid levels and cardiovascular fitness, and they should consult with the physician regarding safe exercise levels. Ideally a progressive aerobic exercise program will be planned. Such a program may result in measurable decrease in total serum cholesterol level, but the effect is usually small. In contrast, physical activity comparable to brisk walking on a treadmill for 30 minutes per day or a regular jogging program may result in marked decrease in serum triglyceride level.[45] Increased physical activity may also be beneficial by increasing the blood level of HDL cholesterol.

Appendix 4F gives an indication of how different forms of exercise contribute to physical fitness and caloric expenditure. It can be useful to point out to clients that increased activity allows them to consume somewhat more food without gaining weight.

DRUG TREATMENT

In this age of reliance on drugs as a means of curing disease, it is appropriate to emphasize that drug treatment is not generally considered to be an acceptable *substitute* for diet treatment of hyperlipidemia. Rather, the use of drugs may be needed in *addition* to dietary modifications. The value of drugs in preventing or retarding developing of cardiovascular disease is still under investigation.

Use of antilipemic agents has a number of potential disadvantages which vary with the drug being used. Possible nutrition-related problems are summarized in Table 31.5. These may gain significance because the drugs are used daily for long periods of time (years).

TABLE 31.5 *Potential nutrition-related problems associated with anti-lipemic agents*

DRUG	POTENTIAL NUTRITION-RELATED EFFECTS
Cholestyramine (Cuemid, Questran)—a resin	Nausea, vomiting, occasionally steatorrhea
	Constipation a common complaint
	As a resin it binds bile salts, intrinsic factor, some minerals
	May seriously interfere with absorption of calcium and of vitamins A, D, K, B_{12}, and folate
Aluminum nicotinate, a relative of the vitamin niacin	May decrease glucose tolerance; may lead to severe GI upset
	Prolonged treatment may lead to liver disease
Clofibrate (Atromid-S)	May cause numerous GI symptoms including stomatitis, gastritis, abdominal distress, loose stools, and flatulence. (Incidence of symptoms in patients in a 6-yr trial in Scotland was insignificant when compared with incidence in patients receiving placebo.[46])
	May impair taste perception
	Decreases absorption of a number of nutrients, but the significance of this is undetermined

Antilipemic drugs are costly and may be unpleasant to take. For example, the usual dose of cholestyramine for an adult is a hefty 16 to 20 gm. per day; most clients find it quite unpalatable and are bothered by the constipation it commonly causes. Competent health professionals anticipate these problems and make suggestions to prevent or alleviate them (e.g., mixing the drug with applesauce or other suitable foods, increasing fiber content of the diet).

ASSISTING HOSPITALIZED CLIENTS ON FAT AND CHOLESTEROL MODIFIED DIETS

People who are being treated for hyperlipidemia generally want or are advised to continue following their modified diet if they are hospitalized for an illness, injury, or surgical procedure. Sometimes the fat modified diet order is overlooked since other matters may have higher priority. Sometimes the slipup will be noticed by an alert health care provider who overhears the client commenting on the lack of acceptable menu choices or expressing confusion about why "forbidden" foods are included on his menu or tray. Some clients assume that the diet order is correct just because they are under a good doctor's care in the hospital. On the other hand, a client who has been on a more moderate fat and cholesterol controlled diet than is routinely used in the health agency may become upset if his request for an egg is consistently ignored. Competent health team members take action to provide continuity of care and make appropriate explanations to the client.

STUDY QUESTIONS

1. What benefit(s) should a young adult with hypercholesterolemia expect if he complies with his fat-controlled diet?
2. Is avoiding all high cholesterol foods the best way to lower blood cholesterol level? Explain.
3. List several changes in a diet which help to increase the P/S ratio of the diet.
4. Describe a restaurant meal which would be a good choice for a person who has HLP IV, and explain why you named those foods. What changes would be desirable for a person with HLP II?
5. Several brands of cookies are labeled "made with 100% vegetable oil." Are they good choices for a person who is following a moderate fat- and cholesterol-controlled diet? Explain.
6. Under what circumstances is compliance with a fat- and cholesterol-controlled diet most apt to be ineffective in correcting hyperlipidemia?

References

1. Kannel, W. B.: The role of cholesterol in coronary atherogenesis. *Med. Clin. North Am.* 58(2):363, 1974.
2. Diet and coronary heart disease. Food and Nutrition Board, NAS, NRC and Council on Foods and Nutrition, A.M.A. *Nutr Rev.* 30:223, 1972.
3. Norum, K. R.: Some present concepts concerning diet and prevention of coronary heart disease. *Nutr. Metabol.* 22:1, 1978.
*4. Diet and coronary heart disease. Nutrition Committee of the Steering Committee for Medical and Community Program of the American Heart Assoc. Dallas: American Heart Assoc., 1978.
5. Ross, R., and Glomset, J. A.: The pathogenesis of atherosclerosis. *N. Engl. J. Med.* 295:369, 1976.
*6. Blackburn, H.: Coronary risk factors. How to evaluate and manage them. *Eur. J. Cardiol.* 2/3:249, 1975.
*7. Grundy, S. M.: Treatment of hypercholesterolemia. *Am. J. Clin. Nutr.* 30:985, 1977.
*8. Fact sheet: Diabetes and cardiovascular disease. DHEW, NIH, National Heart, Lung and Blood Institute Public Inquiries and reports Branch, OPEC. DHEW Publ. No. (NIH) 77-1212. Washington DC: U.S. Govt. Printing Office.
9. Hornstra, G., et al.: Influence of dietary fat on platelet function in men. *Lancet* 1:1155, 1973.
10. O'Brien, J. R., et al.: Effect of a diet of polyunsaturated fats on some platelet function tests. *Lancet* 2:995, 1976.
11. *Dietary Fats and Oils in Human Nutrition. Report of an Expert Consultation.* FAO Food and Nutrition Paper 3. Rome: Food and Agricultural Organization of the United Nations, 1977.
12. Heyden, S.: Risk factors of ischemic heart disease. As seen in *Dietary Goals for the United States—Supplemental Views.* Senate Select Committee on Nutrition and Human Health. Washington DC: Superintendent of Documents, 1977. p. 327.
13. Khachadurian, A. K.: Hyperlipoproteinemia. *Diet. Currents* 4(4):19, 1977.
14. Castelli, W. P., et al.: HDL cholesterol and other lipids in coronary heart disease. *Circulation* 55:767, 1977.
15. Reckless, J. P. D., et al.: High-density and low-density lipoproteins and prevalence of vascular disease in diabetes mellitus. *Br. Med. J.* 1:883, 1978.
16. *The Dietary Management of Hyperlipoproteinemia.* DHEW, NIH, National Heart and Lung Institute. Bethesda MD: DHEW Publ. No. (NIH) 76-110, 1976.
17. Wallace, R. B., et al.: Altered plasma-lipids associated with oral contraceptive or oestrogen consumption. *Lancet* 2:11, 1977.
*18. Gotto, A. M.: Is atherosclerosis reversible? *J. Am. Diet. Assoc.* 74:551, 1979.
19. Blankenhorn, D. H., et al.: The rate of atherosclerosis change during treatment of hyperlipoproteinemia. *Circulation* 57:355, 1978.
20. Heyden, S.: The workingman's diet. II. Effect of weight reduction in obese patients with hypertension, hyperuricemia and hyperlipidemia. *Nutr. Metabol.* 22(3):141, 1978.
21. Kudchodkar, B. J., et al.: Effects of acute caloric restriction on cholesterol metabolism in man. *Am. J. Clin. Nutr.* 30:1135, 1977.
22. Anderson, J. T., Grande, F., and Keys, A.: Independence of the effects of cholesterol and degree of saturation of the fat in the diet on serum cholesterol in man. *Am. J. Clin. Nutr.* 29:1184, 1976.
23. Porter, M. W., et al.: Effect of dietary egg on serum cholesterol and triglyceride of human males. *Am. J. Clin. Nutr.* 30:490, 1977.
*24. Flynn, M. S., Nolph, G. B., and Flynn, T. C.: Effect of dietary egg on human serum cholesterol and triglycerides. *Am. J. Clin. Nutr.* 32:1051, 1979.
25. Slater, G., et al.: Plasma cholesterol and triglycerides in men with added eggs in the diet. *Nutr. Reports Int.* 14:249, 1976.

26. Connor, W. E., et al.: The plasma lipids, lipoproteins, and diet of the Tarahumara Indians of Mexico. *Am. J. Clin. Nutr.* 31:1131, 1978.

27. Nestel, P. J., Simons, L. A., and Homma, Y.: Effects of ethanol on bile acid and cholesterol metabolism. *Am. J. Clin. Nutr.* 29:1007, 1976.

28. Castelli, W. P., et al.: Alcohol and blood lipids: The Cooperative Lipoprotein Phenotyping Study. *Lancet* 2:153, 1977.

*29. Hellendoorn, E. W.: Beneficial physiologic action of beans. *J. Am. Diet. Assoc.* 69:248, 1976.

30. Sitori, C. R., et al.: Soybean protein diet in the treatment of type-II hyperlipoproteinemia. *Lancet* 1:275, 1977.

31. Carroll, K. K., et al.: Hypocholesterolemic effects of substituting soybean protein for animal protein in the diet of healthy young women. *Am. J. Clin. Nutr.* 31:1312, 1978.

32. Anderson, J. W., and Chen, W.-J. L.: Plant fiber, carbohydrate and lipid metabolism. *Am. J. Clin. Nutr.* 32:346, 1979.

33. Hepner, G., et al.: Hypocholesterolemic effect of yogurt and milk. *Am. J. Clin. Nutr.* 32:19, 1979.

34. Jain, R. C.: Effect of garlic on serum lipids, coagulability and fibrinolytic activity. *Am. J. Clin. Nutr.* 30:1381, 1977.

35. Sainani, G. S., Desai, D. B., and More, K. N.: Onion, garlic, and atherosclerosis. *Lancet* 2:575, 1976.

36. Sanders, T. A. B., Ellis, F. R., and Dickerson, J. W. T.: Studies of vegans: the fatty acid composition of plasma choline, phosphoglycerides, erythrocytes, adipose tissue, and breast milk, and some indicators of susceptibility to ischemic heart disease in vegans and omnivore controls. *Am. J. Clin. Nutr.* 31:805, 1978.

37. Simons, L. A., et al.: The influence of a wide range of absorbed cholesterol on plasma cholesterol levels in man. *Am. J. Clin. Nutr.* 31:1334, 1978.

38. Phillips, R. L., et al.: Coronary heart disease among Seventh-Day Adventists with differing dietary habits: a preliminary report. *Am. J. Clin. Nutr.* 31:S191, 1978.

39. Nazir, D. J., Moorecroft, B. J., and Mishkel, M. A.: Fatty acid composition of margarines. *Am. J. Clin. Nutr.* 29:331, 1976.

40. Kummerow, F. A.: Symposium: Nutritional perspectives and atherosclerosis. Lipids in atherosclerosis. *J. Food Sci.* 40:12, 1975.

41. O'Brien, J. R., Etherington, M. D., Jamieson, S.: Acute platelet changes after large meals of saturated and unsaturated fats. *Lancet* 1:878, 1976.

42. *The American Heart Association Cookbook.* New York: David McKay Co., 1975.

43. Guerard, M.: *Michel Guerard's Cuisine Minceur.* (Chamberlain, N., and Brennan, F., trs.). New York: William Morrow and Company, 1976.

44. Report of Inter-Society Commission for Heart Disease Resources: Primary prevention of the atherosclerotic diseases. New York: Intersociety Commission for Heart Disease Resources, 1972.

45. Gyntelberg, F., et al.: Plasma trigylceride lowering by exercise despite increased food intake in patients with type IV hyperlipoproteinemia. *Am. J. Clin. Nutr.* 30:716, 1977.

46. Ischaemic heart disease: A secondary prevention trial using clofibrate. Report by a research committee of the Scottish Society of Physicians. *Br. Med. J.* 4:775, 1971.

* Recommended reading.

32

Alterations in ingestion

NUTRITIONAL SUPPORT AND CONDITIONS CALLING FOR ITS USE

Clients who *will* not, *can*not, or *may* not take adequate nourishment by the usual means need individualized nutritional support. Nutritional support entails use of one or more alternate methods or approaches to feeding. These include selected modifications in consistency and flavor of foods, use of special formulas or other nutritive supplements, tube feedings, feedings via peripheral vein, and feedings via a central vein. Behavior modification techniques, psychiatric counseling, and/or use of drugs are sometimes essential components of effective nutritional support.

Nutritional support promotes the client's health and sense of well-being and often saves him money by shortening his hospital stay. It can provide a septic patient with increased ability to fight his infection, help prevent development of decubitus ulcers, and promote wound healing. Nutritional support can help prevent muscle wasting and can actually restore lean body mass even if an individual is unable to eat for a period of several weeks or longer. Sometimes measures such as surgical intervention, chemotherapy, or radiation therapy are both feasible and therapeutic only if a client receives intensive nutritional support. Because of the positive impact of nutritional support on effectiveness of therapeutic measures, nutritional support may be called "adjunctive therapy."

Ideally, nutritional support is initiated at the first indication of a serious problem with ingestion, *before* nutritional status has deteriorated. This approach provides maximum benefit to the client from the standpoint of his health and well-being and from a financial point of view. Nutritional *rehabilitation* re-

quires time and, in the interim, the client remains at increased risk of developing complications.

Ambulatory clients can carry out most types of nutritional support for themselves following appropriate teaching. However, clients who require nutritional support are often debilitated, acutely ill, or psychologically disturbed and, therefore, depend on health team members for adequate nourishment.

Nutritional support is apt to entail actually delivering or assisting with the delivery of nutrients *into* the intestinal tract or the bloodstream. Providing adequate nutritional support is a responsibility taken seriously by knowledgeable health professionals. The care they provide greatly influences morbidity and mortality of their clients.

Early detection of nutrition-related problems is facilitated by familiarity with conditions which commonly interfere with adequate ingestion of nutrients. Following is one classification of general types of conditions health professional might consider when planning for nutritional care. The groupings are arbitrary and may overlap.

1. The client avoids feeding himself adequately. He is often unwilling to eat enough to maintain satisfactory nutritional status even if he knows it is important to his health. Conditions which contribute to this problem include impaired sense of taste or smell, anorexia associated with disease, pain accompanying ingestion of food, psychological and psychiatric problems, and the attitude that foods should be selected according to their taste rather than according to their nutritive value.

2. The client cannot feed himself adequately. Conditions preventing adequate self-feeding include coma, debilitating conditions, senile dementia, severe neurological disorders, severe mental retardation, and paralysis.

3. The client requires special types of feedings because of altered structure and/or function of his gastrointestinal tract or because nutritional demands are greater than can be met by customary feedings. Among conditions included in this category are obstructions of the alimentary canal, inflammatory bowel disease, intestinal fistulas, resections of the small bowel, and severe hypermetabolic conditions such as sepsis, extensive burns, or crushing injuries. Some clients in this category *are not allowed* to eat because it is necessary for them to rest the gastrointestinal tract.

4. The client has any combination of the above conditions. For example, a client with cancer may be anorexic and have nutritional needs which cannot be met by ordinary feeding methods.

THE CLIENT WHO WILL NOT EAT

Anorexia

Anorexia or aversion to food is apt to be one of the first symptoms of illness or other stress. Prolonged anorexia, in the absence of adequate nutritional support, leads to life-threatening protein-energy malnutrition. When dealing with clients who will not eat, professionals assess whether refusal is primarily for physiological or psychological reasons. No medication has been found which is generally useful for stimulating the appetite.

Alteration in taste and smell perception The disease condition which is most notorious for its adverse effects on taste perception is cancer. Specific means of treating cancer such as chemotherapy with 5-fluorouracil, radiation of the head and neck, and surgical interventions in the head and neck region can seriously compound problems of taste perception. Taste abnormalities appear to be most marked in persons with extensive disease, such as metastatic cancer.[1] Persons with cancer may experience decreased ability to taste salt, sugar, and/or acid. Perception of bitterness is sometimes increased, sometimes decreased. A profound aversion to certain types of food, especially meat and poultry, has been reported by many individuals who have cancer. They may describe meat as tasting "rotten." Just the smell of the food may cause nausea. Sense of smell may also be adversely affected by cancer.[2]

Gradual loss of the senses of taste and smell accompanies aging; this may impair appetite of the elderly. Alterations in taste and smell perception are commonly exhibited in a number of diseases, including colds, liver disease, Bell's palsy, chronic rhinitis, olfactory and glossopharyngeal nerve paralysis, or basal skull fracture. An easily treatable condition—zinc deficiency—causes impaired sense of taste. Many medications adversely affect taste perception and may contribute to anorexia.

Persons whose food intake has fallen below acceptable levels because their sense of taste and/or smell is altered benefit from individualized attention. One or a combination of the following suggestions may be helpful in combatting the anorexia associated with altered sense of taste or smell:

1. Provide a wide selection of foods.
2. Encourage the client to intensify the flavor of his food if not contraindicated. Use of extra salt, extra sugar, and/or lemon or other tart flavorings may be helpful. Cured meats such as ham or cold cuts may be enjoyed more than other types of meat. Depending on the nature of the problem, use of herbs and spices may make the food taste either better or worse. It is helpful for the client to keep a record of his responses when he experiments with particular seasonings.
3. Suggest that the client try meat, fish, poultry, and eggs in cold rather than hot forms. Meat sandwiches, tuna or chicken salad, and deviled eggs may be acceptable in taste.
4. Encourage use of dairy products, legumes without meat flavoring, and nuts when there is an aversion to meat. Combine acceptable high protein foods with other flavorful well-liked foods (fresh fruit with cottage cheese, celery stuffed with peanut butter or cheese spread, ground nuts in bread products) to improve their taste appeal.
5. Take advantage of times of the day when sense of taste is least impaired.

Early satiety A poorly understood finding in cancer and some other disease conditions is the ease with which a person becomes uncomfortably full even if he was quite hungry at the start of the meal. When this occurs the person severely limits his food intake. Small meals and frequent snacking may help to maintain adequate intake, but more intensive nutritional support is often required.

PAIN, DISCOMFORT, OR FEAR ASSOCIATED WITH ORAL FEEDING

Some clients are willing to take an adequate diet by mouth if steps can be taken to reduce the pain or discomfort they experience during eating. Pain is apt to be associated with inflammatory conditions, ulceration, or structural defects in the mouth, throat, or esophagus. If any of these conditions is present, it may be useful for the client to avoid acidic, salty, spicy, dry, and very hot foods. Very cold foods either may irritate or may help to numb the painful area. Very moist foods, those with a smooth consistency, and those without the irritants mentioned previously are apt to be tolerated well. Most clients prefer a combination of pureed and liquid foods rather than a full liquid diet.

If pain medication has been ordered for a client, oral intake may be promoted by administering the drug at a suitable interval prior to the meal. In some cases, application of a local anesthetic such as viscous xylocaine or Tylenol elixir to the affected area of the oral cavity or pharynx prior to the meal may decrease pain and increase oral food intake. Measures to stimulate flow of saliva may also serve to prevent unnecessary pain or discomfort.

Frequent, thorough mouth care helps maintain the integrity of the oral tissues, partly because it helps stimulate salivation. Thorough mouth care helps prevent complications such as parotitis (inflammation of the parotid glands) by helping to maintain the normal function of the salivary glands. If mouth care is carried out before, after, and between meals, its beneficial effects may result in more adequate food intake since eating will be more pleasurable. Maurer presents an excellent description of means of promoting optimal oral health in clients with oral problems.[3]

If radiation treatments of the head and neck region damage the salivary glands so that saliva cannot be produced, a saliva substitute (artificial saliva) can be used whenever the mouth feels dry. The client can keep a plastic squeeze bottle with him for use throughout the day. Artificial saliva is helpful in relieving soft tissue discomfort and in reducing the incidence of dental caries. (Rampant caries are very common and serious following radiation of the head and neck.) The mineral content of artificial saliva resembles that of natural saliva and has been found to help maintain normal remineralization of the teeth.[4]

Whether or not artificial saliva is used, a person whose mouth is dry usually enjoys normal food served with extra liquids, sauces, and fats to aid chewing and swallowing.

Tooth extraction and periodontal surgery are common reasons for temporary interference with oral intake. The client should be encouraged to resume a normal diet as soon as possible, even if he seems reluctant to do so. Oral tissues need to be used to maintain optimal health.

Dysphagia (swallowing problems) People tend to voluntarily decrease food intake when it is difficult for them to swallow. They avoid pain or discomfort in preference to nourishing themselves adequately. Dysphagia may be caused by inflammation, as in pharyngitis, by an obstruction in the oral cavity or esophagus, by head and neck surgery, or by lack of normal control of voluntary or involuntary muscles. Swallowing is impaired by achalasia, a condition which involves decreased motility of the lower two thirds of the esophagus. Radiation treatment of the head and neck or mediastinal area is likely to cause local inflammation, edema, and, therefore, partial obstruction of the pharynx or esophagus.

The site and cause of a swallowing problem influence recommended feeding methods and the possibility of rehabilitation. Different approaches are used depending on whether the problem is in the oral, pharyngeal, or esophageal phase of swallowing. When partial obstruction or achalasia is the problem, a change to a full liquid or a pureed food plus liquid diet may temporarily make adequate food intake possible; however, supplemental feeding by a different route is often indicated.

Sometimes adults need to relearn to swallow. This is likely to be the case if surgical resection is responsible for major anatomical changes, such as removal of much of the tongue or of the larynx, or if neurological disorders impair swallowing. In some health agencies a "deglutition therapist" is a member of the health team. This health professional is a speech pathologist who has had training in teaching swallowing skills. With the assistance of a deglutition therapist a client who has undergone a supraglottic laryngectomy may be able to learn to take food safely by mouth rather than remain dependent on tube feeding. Many clients can relearn to swallow starting with textured foods that slip down easily. Custard, plain gelatin, and pureed fruit, for example, have less tendency to spill into the laryngeal inlet than do thin liquids.[5] Hot and cold foods provide more stimulation than do tepid foods, but hot foods especially may need to be avoided if inflammation is part of the problem. Deglutition therapist, dietitian, and nurse work cooperatively so that food of the proper consistency and temperature is available and so that the client can practice skills during the therapist's absence. Strategies for assisting a person to regain control of the mouth and to relearn how to swallow are presented by Gaffney and Campbell and by Dobie.[6,7]

CONDITIONED AVERSION TO FOOD

If a person repeatedly experiences pain, choking, or other disturbing symptoms as a result of eating, he is likely to develop a *conditioned aversion* to food. He learns to shun food even if his stomach and brain signal to him that he is very hungry. A conditioned aversion to a specific food may develop if an unpleasant experience, such as certain types of chemotherapy, follows the ingestion of that food.[8] A conditioned aversion often persists long after the underlying problem has been corrected. The person will not eat even though there is no physiological problem. Behavior modification therapy may provide such a person with the support he needs to gradually resume normal eating habits.

PSYCHOLOGICAL PROBLEMS OR DISTURBED PATTERNS OF FAMILY INTERACTION

Anorexia nervosa A person who has had anorexia nervosa for an extended period of time appears emaciated. It is a serious illness characterized by severe disruption in eating behavior but not by loss of appetite. Self-inflicted starvation appears to be used as a means to establish a sense of identity and control. It is a life-threatening psychiatric illness found principally among adolescent females and less frequently among prepubescent males. Generally a problem with family dynamics contributes to the development of this condition. Anorexia nervosa is difficult to treat successfully, particularly if diagnosis is delayed, and can result in tragic death from starvation.

A person with anorexia nervosa *will not* eat adequate amounts of foods. Occasionally the person may go on eating binges, followed by excessive use of cathartics, self-induced vomiting, or enemas. Vital aspects of treatment include "(1) resolution of underlying psychological problems, (2) correction of disturbed patterns of family interaction, and (3) restitution of normal nutrition."[9,10] A vicious cycle complicates treatment: very poor nutritional status interferes with the effectiveness of psychotherapeutic work and psychological problems interfere with improvement in nutritional status. Nutritional rehabilitation in the hospital, sometimes including intensive nutrition support, may be necessary.

All team members should be unusually well-informed of the methods of treatment being used for a client with anorexia nervosa so that care provided will be consistent. All team members need to know, for example, how to interact with the client at mealtime. Are they to apply specific behavior modification techniques, set limits, remind the client that tube feeding will be employed if weight is not maintained, or use other strategies? Consistency in care reduces the chance that the person with anorexia nervosa can successfully manipulate those providing care. Sometimes when more than one physician is involved, the health team may need to insist on agreement among the doctors regarding desirable forms of interaction with the client and the specific way in which nutritional support is to be provided.

Persons with anorexia nervosa may take ingenious steps to make it appear that food intake is satisfactory. They might secretly water plants with their beverages or give food to others. Sometimes they actually consume the food and then surreptitiously (secretly) cause themselves to vomit. Parenteral or tube feeding may be difficult because of lack of cooperation. Devious means may be used to increase apparent body weight.[10]

It is desirable to prevent anorexia nervosa from progressing to this difficult stage. Health professionals who have contact with families may be able to identify the problem in its early stages and refer families for treatment. Significant warning signs in a young person include[11] (1) excessive preoccupation with weight loss, (2) extraordinary attempts on the part of the youth to comply with unrealistic parental demands for "perfection," (3) a tendency to become isolated from peers and friends in conjunction with weight loss, and (4) *excessive* involvement in solitary physical activity such as jogging, calisthenics, or skipping rope.

Improved nutrition is not a cure for anorexia norvosa. Adequate psychiatric care by health professionals and/or a health agency with expertise in treating anorexia nervosa is essential.

Other psychological disorders A number of psychiatric problems can seriously interfere with food intake. Persons may refuse to eat anything because they fear that food is poisoned or is harmful to them in some other way. Depression is a well-known cause for failure to eat. Individuals in a catatonic state refrain from eating just as they do not participate in other activities of daily living. Satisfactory nourishment of individuals in such extreme states requires definitive intervention such as tube feeding. This "violation" of the disturbed person's body can, in turn, result in his becoming more disturbed, especially if health professionals are too rushed to be supportive. Fortunately, these extreme psychiatric conditions are less common than they used to be. Use of psychotropic drugs allows most individuals with psychiatric problems to function fairly normally, especially if they have an effective support system. However, aberrant eating behavior may be quite apparent at mealtime, sometimes arousing the concern of the health professional. Safety is a major concern if a client swallows without chewing or if he is liable to aspirate as a result of hysteria. Those working with clients with psychiatric problems are encouraged to refer to references listed at the end of Part 4 for principles and practical suggestions.

Unfortunately, the same drugs which promote more normal behavior in persons with psychiatric problems may have adverse pharmacological effects upon ingestion and nutrient use in the body as indicated in Table 32.1. Since these medications are usually used for prolonged periods of time, their effects upon ingestion and nutritional status should be assessed periodically.

Failure to thrive Failure to thrive is a general term used to describe a child whose weight and/or height is below the third percentile of standard growth charts. In some cases there is an obvious physical reason for the child's growth failure; however it ap-

TABLE 32.1 *Effects of some psychotropic drugs on the GI system, food intake*

TYPE OF DRUG	EFFECTS
Antidepressants	Anorexia, nausea, vomiting, dysgeusia, epigastric distress are symptoms associated with several types
Monoamine oxidase inhibitors (MAOI)	Require: abstinence from many types of aged cheese (e.g., cheddar, Gruyere, Stilton, Emmanthaler, and Brie), pickled herring, and chianti wine.[12] Ingestion of these foods by a person taking a MAOI may precipitate a severe headache and a hypertensive crisis that could lead to death
Lithium	Dysgeusia (unpleasant, persistent metallic taste), anorexia, nausea, diarrhea (also affects fluid and electrolyte balance)

pears that environmental deprivation may be the most common cause.[13] The child's apparent malnutrition, growth failure, and delayed development may be a result of parental neglect. The neglect might take the form of failing to provide the child with enough food, or it might involve failing to provide pleasurable physical contact, failing to respond to the child's needs, and failing to communicate with the child in other ways. Because of its association with neglect, the term "failure to thrive" should be used judiciously. Similar symptoms may occur as a result of certain disease conditions (e.g., serious congenital heart defects) in children who receive plenty of attention and love.

When growth failure and malnutrition are present, an attempt should be made to obtain a detailed psychosocial history from the parents. Health care workers who closely observe and document the way a child with failure to thrive interacts with his parents and other persons may help identify or clarify the nature of the problem. If upon being hospitalized a child eats well and starts to gain weight within 10 to 14 days, it is likely that the problem is psychosocial in origin.

If failure to thrive is due to parental neglect, parents may be given specific guidance and support in practicing successful "parenting."

POINTS OF EMPHASIS
Assisting clients who will not eat

• *If physical problems make eating unpleasant for a client and result in unwillingness to eat, health team members should work cooperatively to develop strategies for making the client more comfortable during eating and/or for relearning eating skills which have been lost or impaired.*

• *Clients need support and encouragement if they have little appetite or they experience discomfort upon taking food by mouth.*

• *If psychosocial problems lead to unwillingness to eat, the plan of care should be very clearly delineated and should be implemented consistently by all health team members.*

• *Careful documentation of the client's responses to care (positive or negative, psychological and physical) can play a key role in guiding effective treatment.*

THE CLIENT WHO CANNOT EAT NORMALLY

Many different conditions may make it impossible for a person to ingest food independently. If a person is in a coma, acutely ill, or in some other crisis situation,

having health professionals assume full responsibility for feeding is indicated. However, it may be possible for persons with chronic conditions to learn to feed themselves and, thus, gain a sense of independence, self-confidence, and self-worth. Often the health professional must determine which approach will be most beneficial for the client. The approach is subject to modification as the client's condition changes.

ADULTS WITH FEEDING DISABILITIES

Adults who have a feeding disability because of recent blindness, injury or loss of hands or arms, crippling conditions such as rheumatoid arthritis, or partial paralysis can often be assisted in regaining ability to feed themselves.. Many self-help devices can be purchased or improvised. Sometimes a simple step such as preventing the dish from slipping and having a vertical edge to push the food against may greatly simplify self-feeding.

Adults who are suddenly faced with a loss of independence have many psychological adjustments to make. They may feel frustrated, embarrassed, isolated, deprived, socially unacceptable, or too proud to ask for assistance. Health care workers provide an invaluable service by reassuring these persons of their worth, accepting them as they are, and by providing encouragement and appropriate guidance or other support when a seemingly simple task turns out to be surprisingly difficult.

Ideally, an occupational therapist or physical therapist who is trained and experienced in dealing with feeding disabilities assesses a disabled client's needs. Then, together with the client and other health team members, the therapist develops a feeding care plan including realistic short and long term goals.

If initial consultation with the therapist must be delayed, the health professional caring for a person with a feeding disability can plan and implement adequate care. In lieu of special equipment the nurse or dietitian might improvise by bending a spoon, securing foam around the outside of a glass, fashioning a long straw out of suitable tubing, or changing the height of the table. References listed at the end of Part 4 include information about self-help devices and guidelines for helping with self-feeding. No matter what the feeding disability, the health professional tries to create an environment in which the client can retain a sense of self-esteem.

CLEFT LIP AND CLEFT PALATE

Cleft lip and cleft palate are congenital anomalies which have marked effects on an infant's ability to eat. Cleft palate, an opening in the roof of the mouth, is the more serious condition because it makes normal sucking impossible. If not surgically corrected, the cleft will also interfere with normal growth of the jaw, facial form and appearance, speech, hearing, and chewing. Surgical rehabilitation often requires a series of operations over a period of years. In the meantime parents need guidance to deal with the day-to-day aspects of care of their child.

Since normal sucking is impossible, it has been thought that infants with cleft palate cannot be breast fed. Most mothers who have tried have been unsuccessful; however, a mother of twins, one of whom had cleft palate, has reported on how she successfully nursed both babies.[14] If a mother wishes the baby to have the benefits of breast milk and is unable to nurse successfully, she can use a breast pump and then feed the milk from a bottle. Feeding must be a slow process. The time required for a bottle feeding is usually 30 minutes to an hour, but 1½ hours is not unusual.[15]

During a feeding, milk may spill out of the infant's nose. Feeding the infant in an upright position and directing the flow of milk to the back or side of the mouth, away from the cleft, helps minimize choking. If choking occurs, feeding is temporarily stopped until the infant's airway is cleared and he has regained his composure. Special feeders such as a Beniflex cleft palate nurser or bulb syringe with rubber tubing may make the feeding process simpler and more enjoyable for both infant and mother. An ordinary nursing bottle with a nipple with an enlarged cross-cut opening may also be used. Early introduction to the use of a cup may be desirable. (The 2 to 3 oz. size of paper cup seems to work well.) Use of a bottle is contraindicated for a while after surgery since it may disrupt the suture line. Some doctors recommend use of a Brecht feeder for a specified time following surgery. (This is an ascepto syringe with a catheter tip.)

An infant or toddler with a cleft palate can be introduced to solid foods at the usual stages of development, but a few foods may need to be avoided if they tend to get caught in the cleft. These include peelings on fruits; leafy vegetables (especially if raw); nuts; and sticky foods such as peanut butter, cooked cheese dishes, and foods in a heavy cream sauce. Thickened food, such as fruit thickened with precooked baby cereal, is less apt to run out of the nose than are the unthickened strained fruits and vegetables.

Since successful feeding usually requires small bites and slow eating, adequate intake is promoted by more frequent feeding than is common for young children. It may be helpful to avoid acidic, spicy, and salty foods, because food may come in contact with the sensitive tissues of the nose because of the cleft. If citrus fruits are avoided, better tolerated sources of vitamin C should be included in the diet. Fortunately, surgical repair eventually eliminates the need for restrictions and special care.

Parents appreciate detailed information about care and treatment of cleft lip and palate. A number of states have parents' groups (e.g., Prescription Parents, Inc.) which offer supportive services and resource materials to health professionals and to parents of children with this condition. A few helpful publications are listed at the end of Part 4.

DEVELOPMENTALLY DELAYED CHILDREN

Conditions associated with delayed development of children commonly result in feeding problems. Among the problems which may be encountered are difficulty in sucking, biting, chewing, swallowing, holding up the head, and using the hand and arm for self-feeding. Developmentally delayed children may chronically exhibit inappropriate mealtime behavior such as tantrums, throwing food, regurgitation, food refusal and cramming food into the mouth. Many times the problems can be overcome by an effective training program for both parents and children.

Special attention should be directed toward the caloric requirements of developmentally delayed children. For example, the continual movement which is characteristic of the athetoid type of cerebral palsy increases the child's caloric requirement. Since feeding may be quite difficult, tube feeding is sometimes necessary, at least temporarily, to assure adequate intake. When food is given by mouth, concentrated sources of nutrients are encouraged so that nutritional requirements can be met by normal feeding methods. Adequate provision of fluid is emphasized as well.

Some severely mentally retarded children move very little, especially if their condition is accompanied by a degree of paralysis. Because of their limited activity they may easily gain excess weight. Parents must be cautioned against feeding practices which lead to obesity since excess fat further impedes the child's movement and development. Health professionals can provide anticipatory guidance and discuss with the parents ways of rewarding their children and providing pleasure which do not involve food.

Feeding a child who is developmentally delayed provides nourishment and may, at the same time, provide valuable opportunities for the child to learn to use muscles of the mouth, tongue, throat, arms, and hands. Finger foods may be helpful for developmentally delayed children long after most children have learned to skillfully manage eating utensils.

POINTS OF EMPHASIS
Assisting clients with feeding disabilities

• *Work cooperatively with health team members to devise a plan of care based on assessment of the client's nutritional needs, customary food intake, feeding skills, mealtime behavior, support system, and potential for learning self-feeding skills.*

• *Gear assistance toward helping the client achieve his potential, taking care not to set overly optimistic goals.*

• *Provide genuine encouragement and praise for any behaviors which will help the client along the path toward a desired end result.*

Foods which stick to a spoon without being too stiff to swallow easily may promote success in self-feeding. Some developmentally delayed children are very intelligent and thrive on feeding experiences which help them learn about their environment. Table 32.2 offers suggestions for assisting handicapped children in developing self-feeding skills.

An occupational or physical therapist assists parents in planning activities to improve the child's coordination, choosing eating equipment, adjusting the chair used during meals, and instituting other measures which foster the child's independence and self-reliance.

Serious behavior problems exhibited by behaviorally delayed children may be exceedingly distressing to the family and very difficult to overcome. Thompson and Palmer describe a behavioral approach which they have found to be successful.[16]

Children who are mentally retarded may pose special problems. Limited ability to learn in combination with physical disability accentuates feeding problems and may be a source of frustration to parents. The child's potential for learning self-feeding skills should be assessed by experts and thoroughly discussed with parents to aid them in establishing realistic expectations and providing suitable care.

FEEDING METHODS USED IN NUTRITIONAL SUPPORT

Feeding methods used for nutritional support include special feedings by mouth, tube feedings, nutrient solutions via peripheral veins, and nutrient solutions via a catheter inserted into a central vein (total parenteral nutrition). Micronutrients can of course also be provided by injection. These feeding methods may be used singly or in combination, depending on the client's condition and individual nutrient requirements.

Enteral feeding

Inability to ingest or tolerate conventional foods is not a sufficient reason to abandon the enteral route. Enteral feeding is preferred unless there are serious contraindications.

ADVANTAGES

Enteral feeding has many advantages, some of which are described here.
1. The presence of nutrients within the intestinal tract

TABLE 32.2 *Suggested strategies for developing feeding skills*

AREAS OF CONCERN		SUGGESTED STRATEGIES
Inability to suck, chew, and swallow	Suck:	Use cold substances around lips to stimulate sucking
		Use a cloth soaked with water for the child to suck
		Try different types of nipples
		As child begins to improve in ability, change to nipple with smaller hole
	Chew:	Place a small amount of food between back teeth and move jaw up and down. A mirror may help demonstrate and point out various body parts
		Wash with tongue—place foods such as peanut butter on lips, to allow tongue to be used. Gradual transition from pureed foods to solid foods (sprinkle crackers in soup, etc)
	Swallow:	Swallowing easiest when mouth closed
		Close jaw and lips of child together
		Stroke throat upward under chin
		Offer next bite of food only after child swallows
		Demonstrate—let child feel *you* swallow
Inability to grasp: hand-mouth coordination		To assist grasping coordination:
		Allow child to finger food
		Guide child in exploring mouth
		Cut food into small pieces
		Place your hand over child's hand and help him or her grasp spoon
		Use adaptive equipment (plastic spoon, etc)
		Make sure bowl is stabilized (suction, tape)
		Use plates with high straight sides, or build higher edge using aluminum foil
		Develop activities which will help child with coordination:
		Pour sand, etc
		Play with ball
		Push-pull objects
		Study body parts with child
		Visually impaired:
		Place meats and vegetables consistently in same areas of plate so child can find

From Calvert, S., and Davis, F.: Nutrition of children with handicapping conditions. *Public Health Currents* 18:6, 1978. First part of table, used with permission of Ross Laboratories, Columbus OH.

has an "intraluminal effect" which helps maintain the integrity of the gut mucosa.[17] This means that food has a beneficial effect on the mucosa even before it is absorbed.

2. It is much *safer* to feed enterally than by total parenteral nutrition. Risk of infection and of fluid and electrolyte imbalance is less if the gastrointestinal tract can be used. Sepsis is a possible complication of feeding via a central vein. Catheter-related complications are obviously avoided by enteral feeding.

3. It may be much more pleasant for the client to provide for adequate intake by the enteral route, especially if some conventional foods can be tolerated.

4. It is much *less costly* to feed enterally from the standpoint of the feeding itself, the equipment required, and the amount of staff time required. This holds true even when specially prepared formulas are fed.

Many ingestion problems can be circumvented by changing the method of delivering food to the gastrointestinal tract and/or by changing the composition of the formula. Use of a straw often allows food to be taken by mouth even if there is ulceration within the oral cavity or serious obstruction such as wiring of a fractured jaw.

TUBE FEEDING

If inability to swallow, severe debilitation, or an obstruction or a lesion in the upper part of the alimentary canal interferes with food intake, one of several methods of gavage or tube feeding is likely to be an acceptable way to nourish the client. Figure 32.1 shows different routes by which tube feedings may be administered. The nasogastric (NG) route (intragastric route) is most commonly utilized for short term feeding since no incision is required. It carries risks for comatose patients in that it increases the possibility of regurgitation and aspiration. (The presence of a tube interferes with the functioning of the lower esophageal sphincter.) For long term use, the nasogastric route is *least* apt to be acceptable. A gastrostomy is a common alternative. Keeping a nasogastric tube in place for a prolonged period may cause irritation of the mucous membranes of the nose and throat or more serious

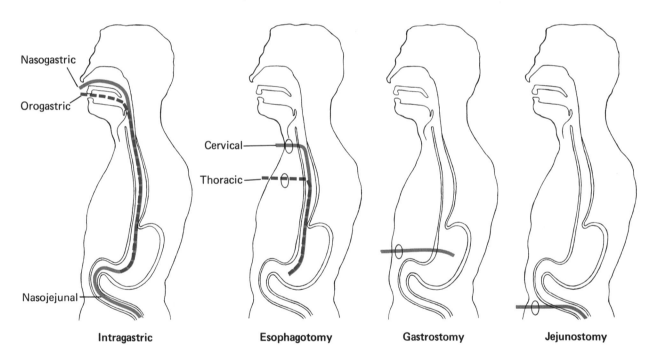

FIGURE 32.1. Types and sites of gastric feeding.
Intragastric (nasogastric, NG): A tube is passed through the nose or mouth into the stomach and secured in place. (A tube passed through the mouth is more correctly called an orogastric tube. An orogastric tube is ordinarily inserted at mealtime and removed following the meal.) Intragastric tube preferred for short term gavage feeding; easily inserted by physician or trained nurse, remains in place between feedings. (Some clients are taught to insert their own tube; they may remove the tube between meals.) Variations include nasopharyngeal and nasojejunal feeding tubes.
Esophagotomy: A temporary or permanent opening (stoma) is constructed at one of several sites to allow a tube to be introduced through the skin into the esophagus. Feeding tube is usually removed between meals. Advantages: dependable for long term feeding, allows concealment of apparatus, easy to handle.
Gastrostomy: A temporary or permanent stoma is constructed allowing food to be introduced through the skin directly into the stomach. Preferred for long term gavage feeding of children and for long term feeding of adults when use of esophagus is contraindicated. Disadvantages: partial undressing necessary at mealtime; skin care may pose problems.
Jejunostomy: A stoma is constructed which gives direct access to the jejunum. This method of feeding may be used when the stomach must be bypassed. Disadvantages: high incidence of dumping syndrome and diarrhea; adequate nutrient intake difficult to maintain.

problems. Use of flexible tubes of small diameter helps to prevent or delay the onset of these complications. Tubes of larger diameter can be used for orogastric feeding. For clients with impaired swallowing ability, swallowing an orogastric tube several times a day may hasten return of ability to swallow food.[17]

Depending on the circumstances, the tube feeding formula may be fed intermittently as meals (sometimes called bolus feeding) or it may be fed continuously at a very slow rate, sometimes around the clock. Usually, force of gravity is used to get the formula into the body, but sometimes a pump is needed to assure a satisfactory rate of flow. Excessive force should be avoided when giving a tube feeding since it may result in damage to the gastrointestinal tract.

SPECIAL PRODUCTS FOR ENTERAL FEEDING

The physician, often in consultation with the dietitian, bases her choice of formula on the client's medical diagnosis, the reason for giving nutritional support, the composition of available products, the agency's or client's capacity to prepare noncommercial formulas, and cost. The dietitian and nurse collect data regarding the client's responses to the formula. When indicated they may make recommendations for changes in type or amount of feeding.

Feeding formulas, either commercial or prepared "from scratch," are sometimes made from conventional foods blended together to a suitable consistency. Blenderized conventional foods simulate a normal, well-balanced diet. Outpatients sometimes prefer to prepare their own blenderized formulas to reduce cost and, if taken by mouth, to increase variety and palatability. Unfortunately, blenderized foods may pose problems in certain situations. If particle size is not sufficiently small, they may clog feeding tubes or necessitate tedious prolonged cleaning of a mouth wired to treat a fractured jaw.[18] For this reason strained baby foods are sometimes used for preparing liquid formulas at home. This does, however, add considerably to the cost and some people find the odor less appetizing than that of freshly cooked food. If certain ingredients are mixed, such as acidic foods plus milk, the mixture may curdle and be unsuitable for use. Blenderized conventional foods may tend to separate. If this happens during a tube feeding, the rate of flow may be affected. Frequent agitation of the container during the feeding may be necessary to prevent separation.

COMMERCIAL PRODUCTS FOR ENTERAL NUTRITIONAL SUPPORT

Commercial formulas are widely used by health agencies for tube feeding and special oral feeding. They come as ready-to-use liquids, dry mixes, or liquid concentrates. Advantages of commercial products in general include consistent nutrient content for any given brand, sterility before the containers are opened, ease of preparation, and low risk of mixing error. The fact that commercial formulas can be altered only by *adding* ingredients limits their flexibility. For some hospitalized clients specially designed formulas may be preferable to standard commercial formulas for optimal nutritional support.[19]

Because of the wide range of commercial enteral nutritional products available, it is helpful to categorize them into three groups: incomplete supplements, balanced "complete"* formulas containing intact protein, and balanced "complete"* formulas containing hydrolyzed (predigested) protein or chemically pure amino acids.

Incomplete supplements Types of incomplete supplements are the following: *protein supplements:* hydrolyzed protein (e.g., EMF, Promix, Liquid Predigested Protein; *vitamin and mineral supplements; essential fatty acid source:* fat emulsions (e.g., Lipomul, Microlipid); and *calorie supplements:* carbohydrate such as glucose (e.g., HyCal) or glucose polymers (dextrins) (e.g., Polycose, Sumacal), medium chain triglycerides, and mixtures of the above (e.g., Controlyte). These supplements may be used in combination with a diet of normal foods or in conjunction with formula feeding.

Balanced "complete" formulas containing intact protein* These formulas are used for clients who are able to digest and absorb nutrients reasonably well. They may be used as the only source of nourishment or they may be fed between meals to increase the client's intake of calories and all nutrients. Examples include Meritene, Nutri-1000, Sustagen, Isocal, Osmolite, Compleat B, Formula 2, Ensure, Precision, and Meatbase Formula 142.

Balanced "complete" formulas containing hydrolyzed (predigested) protein or chemically pure amino acids These formulas are commonly called defined formula diets,[20] chemically defined diets, or elemental diets. These "predigested" formulas allow adequate nourishment of many clients who have limited ability to chemically digest foods or to absorb nutrients. Chemically defined diets differ from other liquid formulas in the following ways:
1. They contain a balanced mixture of amino acids or short chain peptides rather than intact protein.
2. They require little digestion (in fact some ingredients require no digestion).
3. They allow rapid absorption of nutrients in the proximal small intestine.

---

* Formulas are complete in that they contain all nutrients for which USRDA's have been established plus certain other micronutrients know to be required. To date, chromium content has not been declared on these products. Adequacy of a formula depends on the client's nutritional needs (requirements have not been well-defined for diseases states) and on the amount of formula consumed and retained by the client.

4. They may allow adequate nutrient absorption even if bowel length is significantly shortened by surgical resection.
5. If properly administered they leave little or no unabsorbed residue in the colon.
6. They are hypoallergenic.

For these reasons, defined formula diets have been useful in the treatment of short bowel syndrome and chronic pancreatic insufficiency, in management of gastrointestinal fistulas, in preoperative feeding to minimize residue without compromising nutrition, and in postoperative feeding following surgery on the colon or rectum. Examples of defined formulas include Flexical, Vipep, Vital, and Vivonex.

Clients who require nutritional support may have their special nutritional requirements met by combining incomplete supplements with a basic balanced formula. Innumerable combinations are possible. In this way, for example, a concentrated formula could be prepared to provide needed nutrients in a small volume feeding. Concentrated formulas may be particularly beneficial for clients who must be fluid restricted and for those who are anorexic and limit their intake to a very low volume of food. "Modular feeding" is the term used to describe this individualized approach to formula feeding.[21]

CHARACTERISTICS OF FORMULAS INFLUENCING THEIR USE

The following are important variables to note when comparing nutritionally complete products.

Concentration   Standard concentration is 1 kcal. per ml. More concentrated formulas allow unusually high caloric demands to be met without the need for an excessively high volume of formula. However, when concentrated formulas are used, extra care must be taken to make sure that fluid requirements are met.

Taste   Formulas come in a limited choice of flavors. Exclusive use of one or two flavors by the oral route can lead to "flavor fatigue" and reduced formula consumption. Objectionable taste is also likely to interfere with optimal formula intake by mouth. Even tube-fed clients may request a change in flavor.

Lactose content   Formulas containing significant amounts of lactose are not recommended for individuals who are suspected of being lactose intolerant. Some formulas contain lactose in such a low concentration that symptoms of lactose intolerance are unlikely.

Osmolarity   Physiologic osmolarity is about 280 mOs per L. The osmolarity of many commercial formulas is much higher. The higher the osmolarity the greater the chance that the formula will be poorly tolerated unless the client is gradually adapted to it. Formula with high osmolarity is apt to cause the dumping syndrome and diarrhea. The dumping syndrome is characterized by a feeling of distention, weakness, nausea, tachycardia (rapid heartbeat), dizziness, and a cold sweat.

Protein (N), sodium, and fat content   Formulas high in protein (more than 16 percent protein) have the potential of causing the client to become dehydrated, especially if he is not sufficiently alert to request additional fluid. On the other hand, some formulas are too low in nitrogen to permit accelerated anabolism. A formula selected for a client with congestive heart failure or some other form of fluid retention should be suitably low in sodium. High fat content may pose a problem if a client has impaired gastrointestinal function, unless much of the fat is in the form of medium chain triglycerides. If tolerated, fat may be useful since it may increase the palatability of formulas taken orally.

Amount of digestion required (presence of intact protein vs. predigested (hydrolyzed) protein or synthetic amino acids)   The formulas requiring least digestion (defined formula diets) have several disadvantages which make their use inadvisable when other formulas can be well tolerated and utilized. For instance, (1) the distinctive "chemical" taste is objectionable to many people; (2) the cost is high compared to that of formulas containing intact protein; and (3) usually the osmolarity is high compared to that of other formulas. Some chemically defined diets contain dipeptides and tripeptides rather than amino acids. Dipeptides and tripeptides can be absorbed without further digestion, sometimes more readily than are free amino acids.

Amount of residue (material left following digestion)   Low residue formulas are beneficial in a few circumstances, but increased residue may be desirable to promote normal bowel function.

NUTRITIONAL CARE OF CLIENTS RECEIVING SPECIAL ENTERAL FEEDINGS

This section gives guidelines for promoting optimal intake of defined diets by mouth and of any type of formula by tube.

Guidelines for giving defined formula diets by mouth follow:
1. Assist client in working out a plan to enable him to ingest the prescribed amount of formula each day. The plan should allow for a period of adaptation to the high osmolarity of the formula.
   a. Inform client of the maximum rate at which the formula should be consumed and why. A glass of chemically defined formula should be sipped slowly over a period of an hour to prevent gastric retention, the dumping syndrome, and diarrhea. Taking extra fluid along with the formula helps avoid these symptoms.

b. If appropriate, inform client of the total amount to be consumed in a day.

c. Jointly develop a realistic feeding pattern allowing for rest periods, scheduled treatments, and other essential aspects of care. If additional fluids are allowed, such as coffee or tea, find out how the client wants them incorporated into the plan. Some clients benefit from recording the fact that they have finished a feeding.

d. If possible encourage use of socialization periods (with visitors or other patients) as a favorable time for eating.

2. If the client objects to the taste, minimize taste perception by serving formulas at a *very cold* temperature (except beef flavor) and/or having the client sip the formula with a bent straw placed well at the back of the tongue. (If there are contraindications to feeding very cold liquids to the client, tube feeding may be necessary.)

3. Adapt the client to the formula by initially serving it diluted (¼ to ½ normal strength)

4. Monitor intake and response to feeding. Gradually increase volume of formula served to equal the volume prescribed. Then gradually increase concentration of the formula to achieve the prescribed concentration.

5. Take corrective action if intake remains inadequate. This may mean conferring with other health team members to decide if an alternate method of feeding, such as continuous intragastric feeding, would be more appropriate. The question is not just whether the client is getting the special feeding, but whether he is consuming *enough* and tolerating it well.

Achieving prescribed intake may be impractical because the client is too ill to be fully cooperative or because he finds the formula exceedingly objectionable in taste. Few clients who feel quite ill or who are seriously debilitated will be able to consume adequate amounts by mouth. Since these clients are at serious nutritional risk, prompt corrective action may be life saving.

The following are general guidelines for tube feedings:

1. Check the diet and fluid order:
   a. Note the type and amount of formula and the rate at which it is to be administered.
   b. If increases in the amount and concentration of the formula are not specified by the physician, follow guidelines for adaptation such as those given on pages 370 and 371.

2. Check and prepare the formula:
   a. Date: Usually an expiration date and time is marked on the container. If opened can or other nonsterile container has been refrigerated more than 24 hours, it should be discarded. (Opened formula which has been left at room temperature for several hours should also be discarded.)
   b. Consistency: smooth, lump free, uniform. If necessary to mix, follow directions exactly.
   c. Temperature: warm the required amount of formula to room temperature right before use by setting in warm water bath. Do not heat on the stove since this may cause destruction of vitamins and formation of curds or clumps.
   d. Store unused formula in covered container in refrigerator, labeled with date and time it was opened.

3. Check equipment for cleanliness. Obtain new equipment and request a tubing change if indicated.*

4. Determine the position of the tube and amount of gastric residua.*

5. Check the patency of tubing.*

6. Try to appear unhurried, provide for a pleasant environment, and adjust client's position if necessary.*

7. Administer feeding at appropriate rate.

8. Properly clean and store equipment after use.*

If use of the oral route is not contraindicated, a client who is tube fed may derive considerable pleasure from a cup of an allowed hot beverage or a favorite food. The presence of a nasogastric tube does not, in itself, preclude oral intake. If the tube is small in diameter and flexible (such as a #8 French silastic tube), there is little interference with swallowing and little likelihood of aspiration.

Sometimes tube feeding is used to supplement oral feeding. The combination is planned to provide total nutritional needs. If this is the case, maximum appetite for oral feeding is promoted by having oral intake precede a meal to be fed by tube. If tube feeding is by continuous drip, timing of oral intake is less important.

If a client is being fed by continuous drip, keeping blocks under the head of the bed to achieve a 30 degree angle helps to minimize danger of aspiration. In addition, the physician may choose to pass the tube into the duodenum to reduce the risk of gastroesophageal reflux and aspiration.[22]

ADAPTATION OF CLIENT TO TUBE FEEDING

Successful adaptation of a client to tube feeding is apt to be a challenge if the client has previously been fed nothing by mouth, has been on standard clear liquids, and/or if the osmolarity of the tube feeding formula is high. The following principles should be observed when adapting a client to the feeding:

1. Initially administer small, dilute feedings. If formulas with high osmolarity are being introduced, a concentration of ⅓ kcal. per cc. may be recommended. Quarter strength is preferable for individuals known or suspected of being osmotically sensitive and for initiating jejunal feeding. When the formula used has a more nearly physio-

---

* Guidelines for these exceedingly important measures can be found in nursing fundamentals textbooks and in hospital procedure manuals.

logic osmolarity, half strength formula may be sufficiently dilute.

2. If possible use continuous drip for chemically defined (elemental) diets rather than feeding the formula intermittently as a meal.
3. Observe the client for signs of intolerance such as gastric retention, diarrhea, glycosuria.
4. If the formula is tolerated, gradually increase the size of the feeding (rate of delivery for continuous drip) to approach the prescribed rate and volume. This facilitates meeting fluid requirements.

5. If the increased volume is tolerated, increase the concentration, usually in one or two steps. *Never increase the volume (rate) and concentration at the same time!*

Adaptation may require three to five days. Rushing this adjustment period in an attempt to more completely meet nutritive needs is likely to have the opposite effect. Lack of adaptation is accompanied by diarrhea and increased nutrient losses. If diarrhea develops because of inadequate adaptation, treatment requires starting the adaptive process over again.

TABLE 32.3 *Some problems which may be encountered in tube-fed clients and examples of corrective measures*

FACTORS TO ASSESS TO DETERMINE HOW INDIVIDUAL IS TOLERATING THE FEEDING	POSSIBLE CAUSES OF PROBLEMS	CORRECTIVE MEASURES
1. Gastrointestinal function		
a. Vomiting	Feeding too soon after intubation	Allow patient time to relax and rest after tube is inserted
	Improper location of tip of feeding tube	Repositioning of tube by qualified health professional
	Rapid rate of infusion	Administer slowly
	Excessive volume	Be sure tube feeding container does not run dry before feeding is completed
	1) Air	
	2) Formula	Check with doctor regarding number and size of feedings
	Position of patient	Position on right side for ½ hr following feeding—reverse Trendelenberg or semi-Fowlers
Applies to both vomiting and diarrhea {	Food infection or poisoning	Check sanitation of formula and equipment
	Anxiety	Explain procedures. Provide reassurance and other needed types of support. Provide privacy.
b. Diarrhea	Rapid rate of infusion	Administer slowly—very slowly if formula is cold
	High osmolarity of formula or high concentration of formula	Adapt patient to formula gradually
	Lactose intolerance	Contact physician regarding change of formula
c. Constipation	High content of milk in formula	Contact physician regarding:
	Lack of fiber	1) change in formula
	Inadequate fluid intake	2) laxatives
		3) increasing fluid
2. Fluid and electrolyte balance		
a. Dehydration	Rapid infusion of carbohydrate → hyperglycemia → osmotic diuresis → dehydration	Administer slowly. Exogeneous insulin sometimes needed
	Excess protein and electrolytes in formula	Change formula and/or increase fluid according to physician's orders
	Inadequate fluid intake	
b. Edema	Excessive sodium in formula	Check with physician about change in formula
3. Nutritional adequacy		
a. Undernutrition (gradual weight loss)	Inadequate number of calories to meet energy requirements	Check to see if patient is receiving prescribed amount of formula. Estimate client's caloric intake
		Check with physician regarding increasing the volume, concentration or number of feedings given
b. Overnutrition (gradual gain of undesirable weight)	Excessive caloric intake	Check with physician regarding decreasing the volume, concentration, or number of feedings given
c. Undernutrition (inadequate intake of protein and/or micronutrients leading to biochemical or clinical signs of deficiency)	Amount of standard formula needed to maintain weight is too low to meet requirements for essential nutrients	Check with physician regarding providing appropriate nutrient supplements

Gradual adaptation also helps prevent development of glycosuria. If glycosuria develops despite proper adaptation, the formula need not be discontinued. Instead the client is given insulin coverage and enough extra fluid to prevent dehydration and hyperglycemic hyperosmolar nonketotic coma (HHNK), a life-threatening condition characterized by polyuria, increased thirst, and impairment of consciousness.[23]

NUTRITION-RELATED PROBLEMS ASSOCIATED WITH TUBE FEEDINGS

It is not unusual for clients who are being tube fed to develop problems despite suitable adaptation. Table 32.3 lists potential problems and suggests possible causes and corrective measures.

Parenteral feeding

There are numerous occasions when it is desirable for hospitalized clients to be given nutrients parenterally. This section gives special attention to the provision of energy nutrients by peripheral or central vein.

PERIPHERAL VEIN

Uses and limitations   When enteral feeding is contraindicated, supplying nutrients via peripheral veins rather than by a central vein is preferred from the standpoint of safety. Unfortunately, there are limitations on the quantity of nutrients which can be infused via peripheral vein.

Most solutions which are high in calories are hyperosmotic and, therefore, tend to rapidly cause phlebitis and sclerosis of the vein into which they are infused. Isotonic solutions are less likely to disrupt the integrity of the veins, but they are so dilute that danger of fluid overload severely restricts input of energy. For example, it would require almost 9 L. of isotonic (5%) glucose solution to provide about 1500 kcal.!

Sometimes use of peripheral infusions can adequately augment oral or tube feedings so that the *combination* provides recommended intake.

A limited variety of nutrient solutions is used for feeding by peripheral vein. They are listed in Table 32.4. Each of them, given alone, is *unbalanced* nutritionally. Each has advantages and disadvantages, also listed in the table.

Estimating adequacy of parenteral feeding by peripheral vein   It is possible to estimate the amount of calories provided by nutrient solutions. The procedures for the calculations are given here.

Glucose or Amino Acid Solutions:

$$\begin{array}{ccc} \text{ml of solution} & \text{concentration of} & \text{no. of gm} \\ \text{infused} & \times \text{ nutrient in} = & \text{of glucose or} \\ & \text{solution} & \text{amino acid} \\ & & \text{infused} \end{array}$$

TABLE 32.4 *Nutrient solutions for use via peripheral vein*

NUTRIENT SOLUTION	ADVANTAGES	DISADVANTAGES
D₅W (5% dextrose in water)	Partially spares protein Nearly isotonic Inexpensive	Negative nitrogen balance Permits extensive loss of lean body mass Caloric deficit
D₁₀W (10% dextrose in water)	Provides more calories than D₅W Inexpensive	Hyperosmolar Other disadvantages the same as for D₅W
Amino acid solution (crystalline amino acids) 3.5%	Nearly isotonic	Expensive

	Provides source of N to help
	    achieve nitrogen balance
	Few adverse physiological
	    effects
		Since the solution fails to provide adequate
		    calories, it is particularly unsuitable as the
		    exclusive nutrient solution for individuals with
		    limited fat stores

Higher concentrations	Provide more N	Hyperosmolar

Protein hydrolystates	Lower in cost than are
	    synthetic amino acids
		Some nitrogen is in the form of dipeptides and
		    tripeptides which may be less efficiently used
		    than are amino acids
		May precipitate an allergic reaction
		Same limitations as crystalline amino acids

10% Fat emulsion (Intralipid)	Isotonic
	Concentrated source of kcal
	    (1.1 kcal/cc)
	A source of linoleic acid
		Ability to promote nitrogen balance, especially in
		    stressed clients, is unclear
		Contains no nitrogen. Cannot be mixed with
		    amino acids
		Expensive. Elevates serum cholesterol level[24]
		Contraindicated in marked liver disease and in
		    marked hyperlipidemia. Clients with preexisting
		    pulmonary or vascular disease may be at high
		    risk[25]

$$\begin{array}{l}\text{no. of gm} \\ \text{of nutrient} \\ \text{infused}\end{array} \times \begin{array}{l}\text{physiological} \\ \text{fuel factor}\end{array} = \begin{array}{l}\text{no. of kcal} \\ \text{delivered to} \\ \text{client}\end{array}$$

Physiological fuel factor for dextrose in water = 3.4 kcal/gm

Physiological fuel factor for amino acids in water = 4.0 kcal/gm

sample calculations

A. 2500 cc of D_5W were given in 24 hr. How many kcal were provided?

$$2500 \text{ cc} \times \frac{5 \text{ gm glucose}}{100 \text{ cc}} = 125 \text{ gm glucose} \times \frac{3.4 \text{ kcal}}{\text{gm}}$$
$$= 425 \text{ kcal}$$

B. 2000 cc of 3.5% amino acid solution were given in 24 hr. How many gm of amino acid were given? How many kcal were provided?

$$2000 \text{ cc} \times \frac{3.5 \text{ gm aa}}{100 \text{ cc}} = 70 \text{ gm amino acid (equivalent to 70 gm protein in nutritive value)}$$

$$70 \text{ gm aa} \times \frac{4 \text{ kcal}}{\text{gm}} = 280 \text{ kcal}$$

10% Fat Emulsion (Intralipid):

1 ml of 10% fat emulsion provides 1.1 kcal

\# ml × 1.1 = no. of kcal provided.

(When a rough estimate will suffice, the number of ml. [cc.] given to patient approximately equals the number of kcal. provided.)

Various combinations of peripheral amino acids with glucose and/or fat emulsion may be used to more nearly meet nutritional requirements by peripheral vein. There is lack of agreement as to the most effective combinations for particular conditions. In particular there is disagreement as to whether or not glucose should be given with amino acids if caloric needs cannot be met.[26-28]

Because of its high caloric density, fat emulsion increases the chance that caloric requirements can be met by peripheral feeding. Total parenteral feeding (IV feedings of amino acids, glucose, fat emulsion, electrolytes, and other micronutrients) may be achieved peripherally in carefully selected clients who can tolerate a relatively high fluid volume.

When clients are nutritionally depleted or have greatly increased nutritional needs because of hypermetabolic states, parenteral feeding via peripheral vein ordinarily should not be expected to maintain, much less improve, their status. If the gastrointestinal tract cannot be used, total parenteral nutrition is a means of providing normal or unusually high amounts of nutrients.

TOTAL PARENTERAL NUTRITION (TPN)

Description and uses The most sophisticated and dramatic method of nutritional support is total parenteral nutrition (TPN). It involves the feeding of a sterile solution of glucose, crystalline amino acids (or hydrolyzed protein), and micronutrients, usually via an indwelling catheter inserted into a large central vein (i.e., the superior vena cava). A central vein must be used to allow rapid dilution of exceedingly hyperosmotic solutions. Because the solution is hyperosmotic, this method of feeding is also called intravenous hyperalimentation, IVH, or simply hyperalimentation. Occasionally the term hyperalimentation is mistakenly taken to mean that a client is receiving an excessive number of calories. As TPN is increasingly used as a preventive therapeutic measure, it is more apt to provide only the amount of calories needed for tissue maintenance (usually in the range of 1800 to 3000 kcal. daily). For unusual circumstances involving severe stress, TPN has the potential for providing up to 7000 kcal. per day.[29] Table 32.5 lists some of the conditions for which TPN may be indicated.

TPN can be used to maintain a person's weight, to achieve normal growth or catch up growth in children, and to restore lean body mass and adipose tissue in

TABLE 32.5 *Conditions for which parenteral nutrition via central vein may be indicated*

TOTAL FEEDING	SUPPLEMENTAL FEEDING*
Gastrointestinal fistulas	Burns, crushing injuries, sepsis, and other highly catabolic conditions
Crohn's disease (inflammatory bowel disease)—allows the bowel to rest	Limited gastrointestinal function (as when resection of part of the small intestines prevents adequate nutrient absorption)
Congenital anomalies of the gastrointestinal tract	
Acute renal failure†	
Hepatic failure†	
Any condition in which the gastrointestinal tract is not functioning and is not expected to promptly regain function	
Cancer—if client may benefit from further treatment (e.g., surgery, chemotherapy, radiation treatments). When treatment is possible, any disadvantage of increasing supply of nutrients to the tumor is believed to be outweighed by beneficial effects of adequate nourishment of person with cancer[30]	

* Used in conjunction with enteral feeding to allow total nutrient requirements to be met.
† Under investigation using special amino acid solutions.

wasted individuals. With modifications, it can be used for infants, even premature ones.

TPN entails either a continuous infusion of the same nutrient solution around the clock or a *cyclic* pattern of infusion in which there is a set period of time when no glucose is infused. In cyclic TPN, the glucose infusion is started and discontinued gradually to avoid dangerous changes in blood sugar level.

Cyclic TPN has definite physiological advantages.[31] By allowing a period during which blood sugar level falls, insulin level also falls. This promotes mobilization of glycogen and fat which were stored during the glucose infusion, preventing excessive buildup. Cyclic TPN helps avoid development of a fatty liver, a possible side effect of continuous glucose infusion. Cyclic TPN also retards development of essential fatty acid deficiency by allowing mobilization of stored linoleic acid.

Many clients are surprised to learn that this unusual feeding method can be used to meet their nutritional needs for a prolonged period of time (years if necessary). Carefully selected individuals who are permanently without small bowel function (short bowel syndrome) have learned how to feed themselves parenterally at home and have thus been able to resume their former roles in the community.[17,32,33] However, cost and inconvenience are major drawbacks of home hyperalimentation.

Inadequacies of TPN formulas   TPN solutions are not truly "total." Health professionals should be aware of inadequacies of TPN formulas, measures used to prevent development of deficiency states, and signs and symptoms of deficiencies.

Essential Fatty Acids (EFA). Since TPN formulas are fat free, the development of essential fatty acid deficiency in persons of any age is likely unless preventive measures are instituted. Linoleic acid deficiency has been reported in infants maintained on TPN for as little as one week. Adults are affected with EFA deficiency even if they have large stores of this nutrient in their adipose tissue. The continual infusion of glucose keeps circulating insulin at such a high level that mobilization of fat stores (and hence of linoleic acid) is inhibited.

Administration of IV fat emulsion (Intralipid) via a peripheral vein or enteral feeding of a source of polyunsaturated oil (if tolerated) are the most reliable means of preventing essential fatty acid deficiency.[17]

Trace Minerals. Total parenteral nutrition has precipitated trace mineral deficiencies which were previously rare or unknown in this country. In particular, severe deficiencies of zinc, copper, and chromium have been reported.[34] Signs of these deficiencies are listed in Appendix 4G.

Standard TPN solutions vary widely in their concentrations of trace minerals. Variation appears both from brand to brand and among samples of any one brand. Trace metal solution or plasma must be given to prevent trace metal deficiency. Monitoring of serum levels of these trace metals followed by needed supple-

mentation is urged if TPN continues for a prolonged period.[35] Routine supplementation with trace minerals is practiced in some health agencies.

Vitamins. Multivitamin preparations may be added to TPN solutions. Vitamins B_{12}, K, and folic acid are usually administered separately, about once weekly. A careful check should be made to ascertain that all vitamins have been appropriately ordered. Recently a question has been raised about the need for unusually high amounts of vitamins B_6 and E and for supplemental biotin.[33]

Nutritional care of clients receiving total parenteral nutrition   The success of TPN depends on meticulous attention to detail. Because of this a special nutritional support or hyperalimentation team is often responsible for technical aspects of care including determination of the contents of the nutrient solution, insertion of the catheter, and dressing changes. Nonetheless, staff nurses actively participate in the nutritional care of clients receiving TPN.[36-38] Staff nurses are responsible for safely delivering nutrient solution and supplemental nutrients, monitoring the client's responses, and initiating corrective action when indicated. Prompt identification and reporting of problems associated with this feeding method may be lifesaving. The nursing staff and dietitians assist clients in adjusting to this unique feeding method—explaining, allaying fears, and providing suitable forms of stimulation of the oral cavity when oral intake is completely contraindicated. In cooperation with physical therapists they encourage and facilitate the client's participation in an exercise program designed to promote maintenance and/or rebuilding of muscle tissue. Nurses and dietitians provide invaluable assistance to clients during the gradual transition (weaning) from TPN back to enteral feeding. Guidelines for each of these areas of intervention, along with brief descriptions of the rationale for action, are given in Table 32.6.

Nutrition-related concerns of clients receiving TPN   Clients express many concerns when introduced to this drastically different method of meeting their nutritional needs. They are likely to need a great deal of emotional support. Health professionals who anticipate that the client will have concerns can provide an environment in which the client feels free to ask questions and express feelings. Family members will be better able to cope with the situation themselves and to support the client if they also are given explanations regarding this feeding method. Table 32.7 gives some frequently expressed concerns and measures which may assist clients in dealing with them.

Weaning from TPN to enteral feeding   Plans for the weaning process must consider the amount and type of enteral intake during TPN and medical-surgical influences on gastrointestinal function. To prevent setbacks in use of the enteral route and in total nutrient intake, weaning must be a gradual process, a tapering off. Close contact between nursing and dietary per-

TABLE 32.6 *Guidelines for safe delivery of nutrients*

INTERVENTION	RATIONALE
Check composition of the TPN solution against orders before administering it	TPN solutions vary in composition of energy nutrients and of micronutrients such as potassium
Check orders for micronutrients to make sure they are complete	If vitamin B_{12}, vitamin K, and folic acid are not included in the TPN solution, IM injections will be required periodically to meet the client's needs for these nutrients. If trace minerals are not administered, carefully assess for signs of deficiency
If ordered, administer fat emulsion via peripheral vein following established procedure. Monitor the client's condition closely	Side effects including allergic reactions may occur[39]
Check date and time of expiration of solution and policy of agency. Refrigerated solutions are generally kept no more than 24 hr. Unrefrigerated solutions (those hanging) are usually considered safe for no more than 12 hr.	TPN solutions support rapid growth of fungi and certain bacteria
Maintain the prescribed rate of flow of nutrient solution. If intake falls behind, *do not try to catch up.* The rate should not be increased more than 10% above the prescribed rate.[38,40] Take special care during cyclic TPN to change the rate as ordered at the beginning and end of the cycle	Too slow a rate deprives the client of needed nutrients and may precipitate hypoglycemia. Too fast a rate may precipitate hyperglycemia. Too rapid an increase or decrease in rate may precipitate hyperglycemia or hypoglycemia, respectively
Monitor urine sugar	Early detection of hyperglycemia signals the need for interventions to prevent osmotic diuresis and HHNK
Promptly report any sign of infection	Infection is the most frequent serious complication of TPN
If food is allowed by mouth, determine restrictions (if any), and whether intake is to be encouraged, as desired by the client, or small designated amounts to fill specific functions	Goals of p.o. feeding vary with the client's condition. Some physicians specify small (100 cc q 8°) feedings of elemental diet when possible to reduce incidence of problems associated with refeeding.[17] Specified fat-containing mixtures may be ordered to be given p.o. to supply linoleic acid.
If, by accident, no more TPN solution is immediately available and a new bottle needs to be hung, temporarily substitute $D_{10}W$ (10% dextrose in water) and obtain TPN solution as soon as possible	A supply of glucose should be maintained to minimize danger of hypoglycemia

sonnel permits development of a comprehensive plan of nutritional care which facilitates the weaning process.

Guidelines for weaning from TPN include the following:

1. Encourage the client to take small (or increased) amounts of easily digested liquids *even though he is not apt to be hungry.* Among those generally well tolerated are clear liquids (including defined formula diets) and complete formulas with low lactose content and low osmolarity. Products containing milk may precipitate problems since temporary lactase deficiency may be present following TPN. Some clients object to liquid feedings and do well when weaned directly to solid foods such as toast and jelly. Young infants who have been maintained on TPN for a period of time may need to learn or relearn how to suck and swallow from breast or bottle. A medicine dropper or rubber-tipped syringe may be used during the transition

TABLE 32.7 *Nutrition-related concerns of clients receiving TPN*

CONCERN	POSSIBLE MEANS OF ASSISTING THE CLIENT
Fear that he cannot be adequately nourished in this manner	Explanation of what the TPN solution is and what it can do
Fear of being unable to eat again or of a permanent loss of appetite	Reassurance; explanations
Dreaming about, hallucinating about, and/or craving for certain foods	Reassurance that this is a normal reaction. Provide the food p.o. if allowed. Provide oral stimulation
Sense of deprivation owing to lack of oral stimulation (e.g., taste, texture, chewing, salivation)	Frequent mouth care. (Encourage the client to participate.) Use of a variety of flavors of lip balm, mouthwash, toothpaste. Sugarless chewing gum if allowed. Intake by mouth as allowed. Diversional activities at mealtime. Change in client's location at mealtime if indicated and possible
Concern about changes in bowel pattern	Reassurance that small, infrequent stools are normal; explain why
Fear that physical activity will cause injury (due to the catheter)	Explanation regarding placement of catheter and what keeps it in place

period. Care must be taken to avoid the possibility of the infant's aspirating milk.

2. Recognize that the client may be *afraid* to resume normal intake since he may associate eating with pain.

3. If indicated, maintain desirable intake by using supplemental intragastric feedings.

4. *Document all enteral intake.* As enteral intake increases, the physician orders a decrease in the infusion rate. If intake is not documented, continuing high intravenous intake is apt to seriously impair appetite and may even contribute to development of nausea and vomiting, thus interfering with further increases in enteral intake.

5. Gradually progress the client as tolerated to the type of diet prescribed by the physician.

ONGOING NUTRITIONAL ASSESSMENT OF A CLIENT RECEIVING SPECIAL FEEDINGS

The goals of special feeding for a given client guide the ongoing assessment of the client's response to treatment. The plan of care should clearly state whether the nutritional support is meant to maintain a client's satisfactory nutritional status, to nutritionally rehabilitate the client to a specified extent, or to keep deterioration in nutritional status above a preset level. The health professional should realize that, since a client's nutritional requirements are not definitely known, there is a chance that the special feeding will not meet all of his needs. Therefore, ongoing assessment is of great importance.

If nutritional rehabilitation is a goal, the client is likely to be the first person to perceive beneficial effects. He may report that he has a greatly improved sense of well-being days before there are any overt signs of change. Weight increases represent gain of both muscle and of fat. Weight gain should be gradual; the usual goal is 120 to 240 gm. (4 to 8 oz.) per day. A sharp increase represents fluid retention and warns of danger of fluid overload.

Electrolyte levels should receive close attention. Levels of three of the electrolytes—potassium, magnesium, and phosphate—may fall rapidly and, therefore, should be monitored frequently. If they are provided in insufficient quantity, anabolism will be impaired and the imbalances may interfere with other cellular functions as well.

Indicators of lean body mass other than weight change slowly. Restoration of immunocompetence, as measured by delayed sensitivity reactions to skin testing, usually requires 2 to 3 weeks. Significant increases in serum transferrin levels or total iron-binding capacity generally appear at about the same time, if not sooner. Albumin responds more slowly than does transferrin. If salt-poor albumin has been admin-

istered as a plasma expander, this will interfere with interpretation of serum albumin levels.

Lack of improvement; signs of deterioration of the skin, mucous membranes, or nails; and abnormal wound healing should be brought to the physician's attention. Deficiencies of various single nutrients, particularly those not included in Recommended Dietary Allowances, may occur as a result of the combination of increased nutritional demands and an "artificial" diet.

STUDY QUESTIONS

1. Mr. A. is currently in satisfactory nutritional status, but he is about to begin radiation therapy of the head and neck region. What kinds of measures would:
   a) help Mr. A maintain oral intake?
   b) prevent unnecessary deterioration of teeth and oral tissues?

2. If TPN solution runs out and no replacement is immediately available, would a 3.5 percent amino acid solution be the best substitute? Explain?

3. Mr. B. is to be maintained on a defined formula diet by mouth, but his intake has fallen far short of the goal. He is alert and oriented. What could you do to try to help him voluntarily increase his intake?

4. Ms. P. has received 1400 cc. of half strength commercial formula (Ensure) for the past week. There is no record of vomiting, diarrhea, or other signs of intolerance. This amount is the last order written in the doctor's order book. What change in nutritional status do you anticipate? What action should you take?

5. Mr. N. is a 20-year old receiving the following solutions by vein daily: 500 cc. Intralipid, 1000 cc. 3.5% amino acid solution and 1000 cc. $D_{10}W$. What is his daily intake of amino acids? Of calories? Compare these amounts to his estimated need for protein and energy.

6. Arthritis prevents Ms. C. from lifting a glass to her mouth and from firmly gripping cutlery/eating utensils. What approach would you use in assisting her? Explain your rationale.

References

1. DeWys, W. D.: Changes in taste sensation and feeding behavior in cancer patients: A review. *J. Human Nutr.* 32:447, 1978.
2. Shils, M. E.: Nutritional problems in cancer patients. *Nutrition in Disease.* Columbus OH: Ross Laboratories, August 1976.
*3. Maurer, J.: Providing optimal oral health. *Nurs. Clin. North Am.* 12(4):671, 1977.
4. Shannon, I. L., Trodahl, J. D., and Slarcke, E. N.: Remineralization of enamel by a saliva substitute designed for use by irradiated patients. *Cancer* 41:1746, 1978.
5. Fleming, S. M., Weaver, A. W., and Brown, J. M.: The patient with cancer affecting the head and neck: Problems in nutrition. *J. Am. Diet. Assoc.* 70:391, 1977.
6. Gaffney, T. W., and Campbell, R. P.: Feeding

techniques for dysphagic patients. *Am. J. Nurs.* 74:2194, 1974.

7. Dobie, R. A.: Rehabilitation of swallowing disorders. *Am. Fam. Physician* 17(5):84, 1978.

8. Bernstein, I. L.: Learned taste aversions in children receiving chemotherapy. *Science* 200:1302, 1978.

9. Bruch, H.: Anorexia nervosa: A review. *Diet. Currents* 4(2):10, 1977.

10. Schmidt, M. P., and Duncan, B.A.B.: Modifying eating behavior in anorexia nervosa. *Am. J. Nurs.* 74:1646, 1974.

11. Bruch, op. cit., p. 8.

*12. Visconti, J. A. (ed.): Drug-food interaction. *Nutrition in Disease.* Columbus OH: Ross Laboratories, May 1977.

*13. Sills, R. H.: Failure to thrive: The role of clinical and laboratory evaluation. *Am. J. Dis. Child.* 132:967, 1978.

14. Grady, E.: Breast feeding the baby with a cleft of the soft palate. *Clin. Pediatr.* 16:978, 1977.

15. MacDonald, S. K. (ed.): *Caring for Your Newborn with Cleft Lip and/or Cleft Palate.* Quincy MA: Prescription Parents, Inc., 1977.

16. Thompson, R. J., and Palmer, S.: Treatment of feeding problems—A behavioral approach. *J. Nutr. Educ.* 6:63, 1974.

17. Driscoll, R. H., and Rosenberg, I. H.: Total parenteral nutrition in inflammatory bowel disease. *Med. Clin. North Amer.* 62(1):185, 1978.

18. Boucher, M.: Broken jaw guide and cookbook. *Am. J. Nurs.* 77:831, 1977.

19. Chernoff, R., and Bloch, A. S.: Liquid feedings. Considerations and alternatives. *J. Am. Diet. Assoc.* 70:389, 1977.

20. Shils, M. E., Bloch, A. S., and Chernoff, R.: Liquid formulas for oral and tube feeding. *Clinical Bulletin* 6(4), 1976. New York: Memorial Sloane-Kettering Cancer Center.

21. Blackburn, G. L., and Bistrian, B. R.: Curative nutrition: Protein-calorie management. In H. A. Schneider, C. E. Anderson, and D. B. Coursin (eds.): *Nutritional Support of Medical Practice.* Hagerstown MD: Harper & Row, 1977, p. 88.

22. Dobbie, R. P., and Hoffmeister, J. A.: Continuous pump-tube enteric hyperalimentation. *Surg. Gynecol. Obstet.* 143:273, 1976.

23. Witt, K.: HHNK. *Nursing '76.* 6:66, 1976.

24. Broviac, J. W., Riella, M. C., and Scribner, B. H.: The role of Intralipid in prolonged parenteral nutrition. I. As a caloric substitute for glucose. *Am. J. Clin. Nutr.* 29:255, 1976.

25. Greene, H. L., Hazlett, D., and Demaree, R.: Relationship between Intralipid-induced hyperlipemia and pulmonary function. *Am. J. Clin. Nutr.* 29:127, 1976.

26. Blackburn, G. L., et al.: Peripheral intravenous feedings with isotonic amino acid solutions. *Am. J. Surg.* 125:447, 1973.

27. Howard, L., et al.: A comparison of administering protein alone and protein plus glucose on nitrogen balance. *Am. J. Clin. Nutr.* 31:226, 1978.

28. Greenberg, G. R., et al.: Protein-sparing therapy in post-operative patients. *New Engl. J. Med.* 294:1411, 1976.

29. Dudrick, S. J.: Total intravenous feeding: When nutrition seems impossible. *Drug Therapy.* 1(2):11, 1976.

30. Deitel, M., Vasic, V., and Alexander, M. A.: Specialized nutritional support in the cancer patient: Is it worthwhile? *Cancer* 41:2359, 1978.

31. Maini, B., et al.: Cyclic hyperalimentation: An optimal technique for preservation of visceral protein. *J. Surg. Res.* 20:515, 1976.

32. Shils, M. E.: A program for total parenteral nutrition at home. *Am. J. Clin. Nutr.* 28:1429, 1975.

33. Jeejeebhoy, K. N., Longer, B., Tsalles, G.: Total parenteral nutrition at home: Studies in patients surviving 4 months to 5 years. *Gastroenterology* 71:943, 1976.

34. Jeejeebhoy, K. N., et al.: Chromium deficiency, glucose intolerance, and neuropathy reversed by chromium supplementation, in a patient receiving long-term total parenteral nutrition. *Am. J. Clin. Nutr.* 30:531, 1977.

35. Hauer, E. C., and Kaminski, M. V.: Trace metal profile of parenteral nutrition solutions. *Am. J. Clin. Nutr.* 31:264, 1978.

*36. Colley, R., and Wilson, J.: Meeting patients' nutritional needs with hyperalimentation. *Nursing '79.* 9:76, 1979.

*37. Rapp, M. A. et al.: Hyperalimentation: Special nutrition therapy for the cancer patient. *RN.* 39:55, 1976.

*38. Borgen, L.: Total parenteral nutrition in adults. *Am. J. Nurs.* 78:224, 1978.

39. Organ, C. H., and Finn, M. P.: The importance of nutritional support for the geriatric surgical patient. *Geriatrics* 35(5):77, 1977.

40. MacFayden, B. V., and Dudrick, S. J.: Total parenteral nutrition of the critically ill patient. *Diet. Currents* 5(1):1, 1978.

* Recommended reading.

33

Alterations in digestion and/or absorption

Inadequate digestion and malabsorption are two separate entities, both of which may lead to inadequate absorption of nutrients and to serious nutritional problems. *Maldigestion* usually refers to any condition which interferes with the chemical (hydrolytic) breakdown of energy nutrients to a form which can be absorbed by the gut. In a broader sense it refers to conditions in which there is disturbed passage of nutrients along the alimentary canal or in which gastrointestinal (GI) pain or other unpleasant GI symptoms are present. *Malabsorption*, in the strict sense, refers to any condition in which the actual absorption of any nutrient is impaired; however, the term malabsorption often refers to maldigestion as well, since energy nutrients are not absorbed unless they are adequately digested.

A number of conditions may be responsible for abnormal digestion and/or absorption. Inflammation is a common example. If the mucosa is inflamed, it becomes edematous (swollen with fluid) and sensitive to irritation; it functions less efficiently. Other conditions which may lead to maldigestion or malabsorption include ulceration, impaired secretion of digestive substances, trauma, ischemia, cancer, neurogenic disorders, and obstruction. Obstruction may be either partial or complete.

Maldigestion usually leads to malabsorption of one or more types of energy nutrients since nutrients can be absorbed only if broken down to relatively small molecules. Physical and physiological changes caused by the abnormal presence of undigested food in the GI tract may lead to impaired absorption of certain micronutrients as well.

Primary types of malabsorption (malabsorption resulting from a disorder of the small intestines rather than from maldigestion) may be general or specific.

That is, the intestines may poorly absorb most nutrients or they may fail to absorb just a few nutrients.

Health professionals should take care to determine just what types of nutritional problems are likely to develop in a client with a particular type of GI disorder. Anticipating possible problems or detecting them early may improve nutritional care.

Some problems are common to many types of GI disorders. These are presented first in this chapter because the information influences care of clients with many types of digestive disease. Causes and treatment of maldigestion and malabsorption of fat are discussed next. A description of how specific disease conditions influence client care follows. This organization should help health care workers focus on dealing with individual client's nutritional problems.

FACTORS WHICH MAY AGGRAVATE NUTRITIONAL PROBLEMS IN CLIENTS WITH GI DISORDERS

In many GI disorders, one or more of the following conditions may be present. Each may have strong impact on the kind of nutritional care most suited to the client.

Reduced food intake

Persons with GI disorders commonly avoid discomfort by eating very selectively or by eating little or nothing. A reduction in food intake or ongoing omission of valu-

378

able nutrient sources, especially in combination with malabsorption, may quickly lead to nutrient deficiencies. In turn, nutrient deficiencies may further impair absorption. In some cases, such as complete intestinal obstruction, a person may not be able to tolerate any food in his GI tract and may require intensive nutritional support to maintain satisfactory nutritional status until the underlying problem can be corrected. In many other cases diet modifications which eliminate or reduce symptoms associated with eating may promote adequate intake.

Persistent vomiting and/or diarrhea

Persistent vomiting for any reason requires that nutritional care first be directed toward achieving and maintaining fluid, electrolyte, and hydrogen ion balance. If oral fluids can be tolerated, broth may be a good choice because of the electrolytes it contains. Other clear liquids may also be given. However, if losses are acute, intravenous fluid and electrolyte replacement is often required.

Diarrhea can be of a variety of types. *Acute* diarrhea owing to a mild infection or ingestion of a food toxin is usually self-limited; attention is directed toward the client's comfort and to maintenance of fluid, electrolyte, and hydrogen ion balance. *Intractable* diarrhea (diarrhea which is persistent and/or is severe) may be broken down into various categories (Table 33.1) and may result in serious nutritional disturbances in addition to fluid, electrolyte, and hydrogen ion imbalances.

Health care workers provide information useful to diagnosis and treatment by documenting volume, nature, and frequency of stools; time of bowel movements in relation to food or fluid consumption; presence or absence of cramping or other types of pain; and the relationship of ingestion of specific foodstuffs to symptoms.

When a client has persistent vomiting and/or diarrhea, careful ongoing assessment of his response to treatment is necessary. As soon as fluid and electrolyte balance has stabilized, more attention can be directed toward meeting the client's other nutrient needs.

Bleeding

Bleeding is a chronic, unnoticed complication in many disorders of the GI tract. Chronic loss of small amounts of blood (occult blood loss) anywhere along the alimentary canal significantly increases the need for iron and for other nutrients involved in blood formation. One of the dangers of occult (insidious) blood loss is that a person may become severely anemic and weakened before recognizing that medical attention should be sought.

Severe hemorrhage develops in a substantial number of cases of GI disease or injury. Severe hemorrhage at any point along the gut is a medical emergency; care is initially directed toward stopping the bleeding. Later, when the client's condition has stabilized, more attention is directed toward his overall nutritional status.

When a client is convalescing from a GI disorder that involved chronic or acute blood loss, nutritional care includes an attempt to rebuild body stores of iron and of other nutrients which were lost. Supplemental iron (usually ferrous sulfate) is often viewed as the most practical way of repleting iron stores; a well-balanced diet should be encouraged also. Health professionals who recognize that iron supplements may lead to GI side effects can recommend measures to minimize symptoms and promote the client's cooperation. For example, advising the client to take iron supplements *with* rather than between meals may reduce the chance of GI upsets. To promote iron absorption at mealtime, the health care worker can recommend that any of the following be included with the meal[1]:

At least 75 mg. vitamin C (e.g., 180 cc. (¾ c.) orange juice, or a supplement)
or
At least 90 gm. (3 oz.) meat, fish or poultry
or
At least 25 mg. vitamin C *and* at least 30 gm. meat, fish, or poultry

It is advisable for the health care worker and client to jointly develop a plan for including one of these "enhancers" of iron absorption at each meal.

TABLE 33.1 *Categories and subgroupings of intractable diarrhea*

TYPE	DESCRIPTION	EXAMPLES OF DISEASE WITH WHICH IT MAY BE ASSOCIATED
Watery	Large volume liquid stools	
Secretory	Increased secretion of water and electrolytes from the mucosa into the lumen of the intestines; persists during fasting	Inflammatory bowel disease; cholera
Osmotic	Movement of water into the intestines in response to an increased solute load within the lumen of the intestines; not present if a person is fasting	Dumping syndrome following gastric resection; some malabsorption syndromes
Fatty (steatorrhea)	Foul smelling, greasy, large volume floating stools	
	Secondary to maldigestion	Cystic fibrosis
	Secondary to malabsorption	Gluten-induced enteropathy
Small volume	Frequent passage of small volume stools	Carcinoma of the colon

Some clients refuse to take iron supplements because unabsorbed iron colors the stool black. This may worry them if previous GI bleeding had a similar effect on the appearance of the stool. When this is the case, motivating a client to increase his intake of iron rich foods and absorption enhancers may be a particularly valuable aspect of his care.

Nutritional anemia

The term nutritional anemia is used for those types of anemia which are caused by a nutrient deficiency or which may be gradually corrected by administration of a particular nutrient. Nutritional anemias may develop under many circumstances (e.g., pregnancy, poor eating habits) but are considered here since many types are commonly associated with GI disturbances. The principal types of nutritional anemia include iron deficiency anemia and megaloblastic anemias caused by deficiency of folic acid and/or vitamin B_{12}. Lack of certain other trace minerals may also lead to anemia.

IRON DEFICIENCY ANEMIA

Iron deficiency anemia is by far the most common form of nutritional anemia. It is characterized by small (microcytic) pale (hypochromic) erythrocytes. Severe cases are more apt to be due to blood loss than to poor diet; however, many GI disorders lead to impaired absorption of iron. Since iron is absorbed best from an acid medium, iron absorption may be seriously decreased by treatments which decrease gastric acidity (e.g., use of antacid therapy) or by surgical procedures which remove or denervate parietal cells (acid secreting cells in the stomach). Absorption of iron may also be impaired by rapid movement of intestinal contents (chronic diarrhea) and by resection of part of the proximal small intestine (a common practice in gastric surgery). Avoidance of food sources of vitamin C is a common finding in GI diseases; this may further limit absorption of ingested iron.

When iron absorption is impaired, increasing oral intake by use of supplements plus absorption "enhancers" usually allows absorption of enough iron to meet normal needs.

MACROCYTIC MEGALOBLASTIC ANEMIA

Changes in the blood which are characteristic of macrocytic megaloblastic anemia resulting from folic acid deficiency are indistinguishable from those caused by vitamin B_{12} deficiency. In both types the red blood cell count is relatively lower than the hematocrit. Macrocytic red blood cells may be detected in blood, and megaloblastic changes in bone marrow can be identified. Data about customary food intake, data about the client's physical condition, and results of tests of vitamin B_{12} absorption (Schilling test) are used to distinguish between the two types of anemia. Treatment with folic acid may correct either type of anemia at least temporarily, but it is not a satisfactory substitute if vitamin B_{12} deficiency is present. By masking or correcting anemia caused by vitamin B_{12} deficiency, folic acid supplements might delay accurate diagnosis. Such a delay could lead to serious irreversible neurological complications (another symptom of vitamin B_{12} deficiency).

In GI diseases, folic acid deficiency may be due to abnormally low intake, especially if accompanied by lack of vitamin C. (Vitamin C helps convert folic acid to its active form.) However, in many instances, malabsorption of folic acid is believed to be responsible for deficiency. Some drugs used for GI disorders may also lead to folic acid deficiency. Oral folic acid supplements are usually well tolerated and can make up for decreased percent absorption.

Inadequate intake of vitamin B_{12} is unlikely except for vegans or individuals with food habits which include few animal products. Deficiency may be due to lack of intrinsic factor (the substance produced by the stomach which is needed for absorption of vitamin B_{12}). Individuals with *pernicious anemia* have an abnormality in the gastric mucosa which prevents them from producing intrinsic factor. Persons whose stomachs have been resected are likewise unable to produce intrinsic factor and, therefore, cannot absorb vitamin B_{12}. Other reasons for reduced absorption of vitamin B_{12} include ileal disease or resection (the ileum is the site of absorption of this vitamin) and bacterial destruction of vitamin B_{12} (e.g., in conditions of bacterial overgrowth of the small bowel).

If vitamin B_{12} absorption is impaired, the vitamin is usually given intramuscularly at regular intervals (e.g., once monthly).

Gastrointestinal-cutaneous fistulas

Occasionally GI disorders are complicated by fistula formation. A gastrointestinal-cutaneous fistula is a narrow inflammatory tract which connects a part of the alimentary canal with an opening on the skin. Drainage of stomach or intestinal contents can lead to serious fluid, electrolyte, and hydrogen ion disturbances, protein loss, and other nutritional problems. If good nutritional status can be achieved when a person has a fistula, spontaneous healing of the fistula may occur. Surgical correction of a fistula, if necessary, may be successful only if satisfactory nutritional status has been maintained.

Since oral intake usually increases drainage from a gastrointestinal fistula, adequate nourishment poses a challenge. Defined formula diet can sometimes be used successfully in treatment of a fistula,[2] but total parenteral nutriton may be preferred. Either feeding method may be life saving.

MALDIGESTION AND MALABSORPTION OF FAT

Many GI disturbances and a number of surgical procedures used to correct such disturbances are associated with maldigestion and/or malabsorption of fat (Table 33.2). The term malabsorption is generally used to include either type of problem. It is important for health professionals to be knowledgeable about effects of fat malabsorption and of ways to achieve adequate nutrient intake despite fat malabsorption.

Identifying fat malabsorption and its effects

A 100 gm. fat diet (or some other amount of fat) might be ordered as a part of a diagnostic test to estimate a client's ability to absorb fat. It is not necessary for the client to consume all of the fat which is served, but it is essential for health care workers to accurately record the type and amount of food which is eaten. If vomiting occurs, this should be brought to the dietitian's attention.

The presence of an abnormally high amount of unabsorbed fat in the intestinal tract may cause one or more of the following problems:
1. Steatorrhea (fatty diarrhea). Steatorrhea may be accompanied by cramps and other unpleasant symptoms. One possible reason for the cramps and diarrhea is the effect which bacteria may have on unabsorbed fatty acids. Bacteria can change fatty acids into compounds similar to castor oil.[3]
2. Loss of an important source of calories and essential fatty acid.
3. Loss of weight and wasting of muscle tissue owing to caloric deficit. Cessation of growth in children.
4. Impaired absorption of calcium and magnesium, which may form insoluble "soaps" with unabsorbed fatty acids.
5. Impaired absorption of fat soluble vitamins, which may remain dissolved in the unabsorbed fat.
6. Increased absorption of oxalate, a non-nutritive component of a number of foods, which may lead to formation of oxalate stones in the kidneys.

Diet modifications useful in treatment of fat malabsorption

When maldigestion and malabsorption of fat are problems, diet modifications are indicated. The diet modifications are geared toward (1) avoiding unpleasant symptoms, (2) helping correct the source of the problem, if possible, and (3) meeting the person's nutritional needs.

AMOUNT OF FAT

Reducing dietary intake of fat generally helps avoid symptoms; therefore, diets reduced in fat content are often ordered or recommended for individuals with any of the conditions listed in Table 33.2.

Diet manuals usually provide guidelines for diets containing a specified amount of fat, such as 50 gm. or

TABLE 33.2 *Examples of conditions interfering with the digestion and/or absorption of fat*

PROBLEM	CAUSE OF PROBLEM
Incomplete digestion	
Lack of bile	Obstruction of common bile duct due to gallstones
	Excessive loss of bile due to disease or resection of the ileum
	Bile bound by a drug, such as cholestyramine
	Inadequate synthesis of bile due to severe liver disease
Deconjugation of bile salts (Chemical change of bile salts to a form which has reduced ability to emulsify fats)	Bacterial action in the small intestine due to bacterial overgrowth (blind loop syndrome)
Lack of pancreatic lipase	Cystic fibrosis
	Chronic pancreatitis
	Severe protein-energy malnutrition
	Carcinoma of the pancreas
Incomplete mixing	Stasis, hypomotility (scleroderma); subtotal gastrectomy
Impaired absorption	(All conditions listed above since undigested fat cannot be absorbed)
Loss of integrity of intestinal mucosa	Gluten-induced sensitive enteropathy (celiac disease)
	Drug induced (e.g., by colchicine or by antineoplastic agents which decrease cell renewal)
	Tropical sprue
	Protein-energy malnutrition
	Radiation enteritis
	Ileitus (Crohn's disease, regional enteritis)

80 gm. fat. An example is found in Appendix 5L. It should be noted that a small amount of visible fat can be included in a 50 gm. fat diet. Such a diet is often prescribed for a person being medically managed for disorders of the biliary tract, such as cholelithiasis (gallstones). Boosting protein and calorie intake while keeping fat intake low is likely to be desirable for treatment of a person who has malabsorption but is seldom necessary for a client with gallstones (many clients with gallstones are overweight). Appendix 5L gives guidelines for increasing intake of protein and calories without significantly increasing fat intake.

DISTRIBUTION AND TYPE OF FAT

Usually when a gastrointestinal problem is the reason for a fat-restricted diet, more attention should be given to the distribution and type of fat than to the exact amount of fat allowed daily. The most desirable distribution of fat depends on the origin of the problem. Fairly even distribution of fat between three meals is usually recommended in management of disease of the gallbladder or pancreas. This pattern may reduce the chance of overstimulation of these organs and, therefore, may decrease the chance that the client will experience intense pain after eating. Omitting fat from breakfast and lunch in order to have a big dinner would defeat the purpose of a low fat diet.

In contrast, if a client's problem involves a decreased supply of bile salts in the bile salt pool (common following ileal resection), more fat may be tolerated at breakfast than at any other meal. Practically all available bile (both reabsorbed and newly synthesized) is stored in the gallbladder overnight. This may be sufficient to promote normal fat absorption during breakfast.[3] At other meals the supply of bile is much lower (owing to loss of bile in the feces) and, consequently, fat is less well tolerated and absorbed.

Advantages and disadvantages of medium chain triglycerides Type of fat makes a difference in how well the fat is tolerated because chemical composition affects the ease with which fat is hydrolyzed and absorbed. Long chain triglycerides, the most common type of dietary fat, require an ample supply of lipase and bile for their digestion and absorption.

If extra calories are needed, medium chain triglycerides (MCT) may be a satisfactory supplement to incorporate into the diet. They offer the advantage of providing about 9 kcal. per gm. in a form which may be well tolerated by persons who cannot efficiently digest or absorb ordinary fat. Medium chain triglycerides are very readily hydrolyzed by both gastric and pancreatic lipase. MCT can also be rapidly absorbed into the musoca without first being hydrolyzed, even if little or no bile is available to emulsify it. Hydrolysis may then occur within the mucosa. Medium chain fatty acids travel via the portal vein to the liver where they are readily metabolized—an advantage in certain disease conditions. There is no fat or oil available in super-markets which is high in medium chain triglycerides. They must be obtained from a pharmacy.

MCT looks similar to vegetable oil. Its taste is sometimes described as "fishy" but this can be disguised. Medium chain triglycerides can be successfully used in preparing baked goods, salad dressings, puddings, and sautéd foods. References about cooking with MCT are found at the end of Part Four.

Primarily because of its very high cost, MCT is not appropriate for use by members of the family who do not have a problem of fat digestion and absorption. This means that some foods would need to be specially prepared for the affected family member.

If MCT is to be used, care must be taken to distribute the recommended amount fairly evenly throughout the day, using it in meals and snacks because it may cause osmotic diarrhea if given in large amounts.

Medium chain triglycerides contain only saturated fatty acids. Thus MCT cannot help to meet the need for linoleic acid. Neither does it improve absorption of fat-soluble vitamins or of ordinary fat.

USEFUL NUTRIENT SUPPLEMENTS

When fat malabsorption is a problem, use of vitamin supplements is generally recommended, with special consideration given to the fat-soluble vitamins. Even if fat absorption is only mildly impaired, severe malabsorption of fat-soluble vitamins (A, D, E, and K) may develop. Deficiency of vitamin K is apt to appear first, since stores of this vitamin are limited. To facilitate an adequate supply of fat-soluble vitamins they may be given in a water-soluble form or, if necessary, by injection.

Since fat malabsorption increases the need for calcium and magnesium, an oral calcium supplement and perhaps a parenteral magnesium supplement may be needed. (Oral magnesium supplements may cause diarrhea.) When fat malabsorption is a chronic condition, as would be the case following ileal resection or jejunoileal bypass surgery, twice yearly monitoring of serum calcium, phosphorus, and alkaline phosphatase is recommended. If these values cannot be maintained within reasonably normal limits, the person is likely to develop osteomalacia.[4] Supplemental vitamin D helps prevent this problem.

MODIFICATIONS TO REDUCE INCIDENCE OF OXALATE KIDNEY STONE FORMATION

Another common complication of fat malabsorption is the formation of oxalate renal stones. Oxalate is a nonnutritive component of many common foods. Spinach, chard, rhubarb, and tea are notable sources. Others are listed in Appendix 5F. Oxalate normally forms an insoluble salt with calcium ions in the intestinal tract. This prevents absorption of most dietary oxalate. However, when extra fatty acids are present in the gut because of fat malabsorption, calcium ions tend to bind to the fatty acids rather than to oxalate. When calcium is tied up in this way, oxalate is readily absorbed. The kidneys remove oxalate from the blood, increasing the concentration of oxalate in the urine. This predisposes an individual to oxalate stone formation.

Certain dietary measures reduce oxalate absorption. Limiting fat intake is more useful than reducing intake of foods high in oxalates. Greatly *increasing oral calcium intake* (i.e., taking large doses of calcium supplement) helps tie up oxalate in the gut, reducing the amount of oxalate that can be absorbed.

POINTS OF EMPHASIS
Fat malabsorption

• *Fat malabsorption may have far-reaching adverse effects on absorption of micronutrients and other food components.*

• *Reducing fat intake and distributing fat appropriately (according to the disease state) provides symptomatic relief of fat malabsorption.*

• *Medium chain triglycerides may be used to boost caloric intake of persons who do not tolerate other types of fat.*

• *Nutrient supplements such as fat-soluble vitamins, calcium, and magnesium are often advisable.*

NUTRITIONAL CARE ASSOCIATED WITH DISTURBANCES IN SPECIFIC PARTS OF THE ALIMENTARY CANAL AND ACCESSORY ORGANS

Various parts of the GI tract are discussed separately in this section to show how malfunctioning of a specific part of the digestive tract may influence nutritional care of clients. Health care workers should note that malfunctioning of even one small part of the alimentary canal can have far-reaching effects on ingestion, digestion, absorption, elimination, and on other body systems.

Esophagus

The esophagus serves mainly as a passageway; it is not truly involved in active digestion of food. However, under certain circumstances, the esophagus itself is subjected to digestive activity. Although the esophagus normally withstands the insults of such items as peppery foods, alcohol, and poorly chewed crackers, it is susceptible to damage from gastric juice.

GASTROESOPHAGEAL REFLUX

The esophagus is exposed to gastric juice if a person experiences gastroesophageal reflux, a backflow of gastric contents into the esophagus. Reflux is most apt to occur if there is decreased tone of the lower esophageal sphincter (LES). Regurgitation and heartburn are symptoms of reflux. The mucous lining of the esophagus provides only limited protection against digestion by gastric juice; therefore, frequent episodes of reflux may lead to inflammation of the distal end of the esophagus. When irritating foods or gastric contents come in contact with the inflamed area, a person experiences pain. If contact of gastric juice with the esophagus is frequent and prolonged, serious ulceration and even perforation of the esophagus may develop.

The likelihood of reflux may be increased if a person has a hiatal hernia. Hiatal hernia involves an anatomical abnormality in which part of the stomach protrudes (herniates) through the diaphragm, sometimes forming a pouch next to the esophagus. Fortunately, although it is estimated that about half of the American population has at least a minor form of hiatal hernia, only a small percentage of people are symptomatic with reflux.[5]

Nutritional care of clients with gastroesophageal reflux
Several aspects of nutritional care may help prevent or alleviate symptoms of reflux and help to reduce the chance of developing complications[5]:
1. Decrease pressure within the stomach:
   a. Reduce weight if overweight or obese.
   b. Eat enough fiber to avoid constipation. (Straining during defecation increases intraabdominal pressure.)
   c. Keep meal size small. Take most liquids between rather than with meals.
   d. Avoid strenuous exercise after eating.
   e. Avoid lying flat for about 2 hr. after eating.
2. Decrease the acidity of gastric contents. (Use of prescribed antacids is the principal means of achieving this goal.)
   a. Omit coffee (regular or decaffeinated,[6] strong tea, and alcoholic beverages, all of which are potent *secretagogues* (stimulators of gastric acid secretion).
   b. Omit spicy foods and carbonated beverages if they cause distress. (Many persons find that it also helps to avoid rich pastries and frosted cakes.[7])
3. Avoid foods/ingredients which *decrease* lower esophageal sphincter pressure.
   a. Avoid chocolate[8] and alcohol.[9]
   b. Limit fat intake.[5]
4. Consume a well-balanced diet using a variety of foods. Skim milk may be helpful since it *increases* LES pressure.[8]

These measures promote comfort and help avoid more serious problems.

Stomach and duodenum

NUTRITIONAL PROBLEMS ASSOCIATED WITH GASTRITIS AND PEPTIC ULCERS

Chronic inflammation of the stomach (gastritis) and ulceration of the stomach or duodenum (peptic ulcers) are fairly common problems in America, and they can have detrimental effects upon food intake and digestive processes. Gastritis may be an acute condition precipitated by an infection but, more often, it is associated with alcohol abuse. A peptic ulcer can become a very serious condition if untreated since it actually involves digestion of a part of the wall of the stomach or duodenum. Abnormally low resistance of the mucosa to attack by acid and/or abnormally high acid production may be responsible for development of peptic ulcers. (The disease process differs somewhat for gastric and duodenal ulcers.) If not treated, an ulcer can lead to life-threatening complications, such as massive hemorrhage or perforation and peritonitis. Many of the surgical means of treating peptic ulcers result in malabsorption of fat and some micronutrients.

In both gastritis and peptic ulcer, self-treatment by exclusion of many types of food is common and may lead to nutrient deficits. For example, a milk-based diet is a common home remedy; this diet may result in inadequate iron intake. Abuse of aspirin accompanies some cases of ulcers; this may lead to occult blood loss and, thus, may increase the chance of anemia. Narayanan[10] reports that some elderly individuals with "chronic stomach upset" have treated themselves with magnesium-aluminum hydroxide compounds and have developed phosphate depletion syndrome (anorexia, weakness, bone pain) as a result.

NUTRITIONAL CARE OF CLIENTS WITH GASTRITIS OR PEPTIC ULCER

Traditionally a person with an ulcer or gastritis has been prohibited from eating many types of foods. Emphasizing restrictions increases the chance that a diet will be nutritionally inadequate. This emphasis appears to be unjustified since there is no concrete evidence that special "ulcer diets" (also called bland diets) promote healing of an ulcer.[11,12] In fact, there is no scientific basis for most of the restrictions traditionally imposed by bland diets for the treatment of duodenal ulcer.[13]

Nevertheless, an extreme version of a bland diet (a Stage 1 Bland Diet or "milk routine") is still sometimes prescribed.[12] The patient on a milk routine is given 60 to 120 ml. of milk every hour during the day and perhaps every 2 hours during the night. Sometimes milk is given every other hour alternating with an antacid. The continuing prescription of this type of diet may help perpetuate the lay person's erroneous belief that milk "coats the stomach" and is protective or soothing when, actually, milk forms curds upon contact with gastric acid.

There appears to be justification, however, for restricting the following items on a bland diet:

1. Alcohol. Alcohol can be a direct irritant to the gastric mucosa, especially if present in high concentration (as when alcoholic beverages are taken on an empty stomach). A combination of alcohol and aspirin is particularly damaging to the mucosa. Alcohol also stimulates increased secretion of gastric juice.

2. Caffeine and related compounds (theobromine, theophylline). These stimulants increase secretion of acidic gastric juice. Beverages containing these compounds are listed in Table 24.1, p. 266.

3. Coffee (including decaffeinated). Coffee of any type contains one or more unidentified substances which stimulate secretion of gastric juice.[14] The effect is large in comparison to that of caffeine. Therefore, decaffeinated coffee offers little advantage when gastric secretion needs to be controlled. Coffee is most likely to cause excessive acid secretion if taken between meals.

4. Specific spices. Pepper and chili, as in chili powder and chili peppers, may be chemically irritating to the gastrointestinal mucosa. It is not clear how much effect these seasonings have if small amounts are used, especially if their concentration is decreased by incorporating them into a meal.

Eating any kind of food stimulates acid production, as does the sight or smell of appetizing food. Consequently some physicians question the advisability of small frequent feedings as opposed to three normal meals daily.[11,12] Choice of meal pattern is best made on an individual basis. Frequent feedings of protein-containing foods are often suggested as beneficial in the treatment of peptic ulcers and gastritis because of protein's ability to neutralize acid. This advantage is offset, however, by protein's ability to stimulate gastric acid secretion. Recommended protein intake should be based primarily on protein requirements and individual food preferences.

Nutritional care should emphasize assisting the client to meet nutrient needs using foods which he tolerates well. Nutrient needs are apt to be increased because of the demand imposed by wound healing and possibly by previous nutritional depletion. If certain foods caused the client distress or discomfort prior to his illness, they are likely to continue to do so. If the client feels uneasy about resuming his usual diet, a soft or bland diet may provide a psychological advantage during his recovery.

Foods allowed on a bland diet (Appendix 5C) are likely to be well tolerated by most people (with the notable exception of milk products in lactose intolerant individuals). The list of allowed foods may include one or more foods which the client claims to tolerate poorly. Orange and tomato juice are good examples. Clients often describe these juices as "acidy." They may be tolerated better if diluted with water and taken at the end of the meal. Health professionals should recognize that individual tolerance to different foods can vary widely.

Some clients may be upset by being asked to follow some type of bland diet or by being asked to abstain from coffee and alcoholic beverages. Since stress may stimulate excessive gastric secretion, those providing care might initiate action on behalf of an upset client to liberalize his diet. Sometimes the physician will agree to allow an *occasional* cup of coffee or glass of wine *with meals*. A conference with the physician and perhaps with other health team members will often result in liberalization of the diet order.

The use of antacids or Cimetidine is a major aspect of treatment of peptic ulcers. These drugs may have significant effects on nutritional status, as described in Table 33.3.

SURGERY INVOLVING THE STOMACH/DUODENUM

Surgical procedures may be used in the treatment of carcinoma of the stomach or peptic ulcer. Stomach cancer usually requires excision of part or all of the stomach, whereas a vagotomy (severing of the vagus nerve) and/or gastric resection may be used in the treatment of severe peptic ulcers.

Vagotomies with and without drainage procedures Vagotomy eliminates vagal stimulation of both hydrochloric acid and pepsin. Since some types of vagotomies may seriously impair gastrointestinal motility, a surgical procedure to promote drainage may be used in conjunction with it. Drainage procedures involve surgical enlargement of the pylorus (pyloroplasty) or the surgical formation of a second opening between the stomach and a part of the small intestines.

A selective vagotomy or a truncal vagotomy is sometimes followed by fatty diarrhea, bilious vomiting, and other undesirable consequences which influence nutritional care.[16] Small, frequent, low fat meals may promote the client's comfort and nutritional status.

Gastroduodenal resection Following gastroduodenal resection, such as Bilroth I and II and gastrectomy, eating a moderate amount of food may cause considerable discomfort because of the small size of the stomach. In perhaps 10 percent of those who undergo gastric resection, food may be rapidly "dumped" from the stomach into the intestines. If food with high osmolarity is dumped into the jejunum, the dumping syndrome may develop shortly after eating. This syndrome is characterized by shocklike symptoms (associated with vasodilation of peripheral blood vessels) and marked abdominal distention (owing to a rapid shift of water from the blood to the intestinal lumen). Cramps and watery diarrhea may follow. Although the symptoms are self-limited (they usually fade within 30 minutes to an hour), they may be frightening and lead to food aversions.

TABLE 33.3 *Nutritional effects of selected drugs used to decrease gastric acidity*

TYPE OF DRUG	EXAMPLES OF NUTRITION-RELATED EFFECTS
Histamine H$_2$-receptor antagonist (Cimetidine)	May decrease absorption of vitamin B$_{12}$[15]
Antacids Nonabsorbable* Aluminum hydroxide	Chronic use may lead to phosphate depletion. Commonly causes constipation
Magnesium carbonate or trisilicate	Commonly causes diarrhea. Some is absorbed; therefore it may lead to elevated blood magnesium level and toxic effects in persons with impaired renal function
Absorbable Sodium bicarbonate	Incompatible with a sodium restricted diet Metabolic alkalosis is possible with prolonged high intake
Calcium containing antacids	May cause constipation. Prolonged use may lead to hypercalcemia and hypercalcinuria. Decreases absorption of iron

* Combinations of nonabsorbable antacids are marketed; these may help avoid undesirable changes in bowel patterns.

Nutritional care of a client after gastric surgery A plan of care for a client who has undergone gastric surgery should detail how and when appropriate small, frequent feedings are to be provided so he can ingest enough food to maintain his weight. During the adaptation period following gastric surgery, the client needs to be observed closely for symptoms of the dumping syndrome, especially 5 to 30 minutes following meals. When observation of the client is not possible, the client should be instructed to signal immediately if symptoms develop following ingestion of food. Shortly after oral intake is resumed, clients may appreciate having a list of recommended foods and of foods which should be used cautiously, if at all (Table 33.4).

Clients who have undergone gastric resection should receive ongoing medical attention to prevent and correct potentially serious nutritional problems such as weight loss, steatorrhea, and nutrient deficiencies.

Pancreas

Since the pancreas is the accessory organ of the GI tract which is the major producer of digestive enzymes and of bicarbonate rich secretions, disorders of the pancreas can markedly impair chemical digestion of food.

Production of pancreatic enzymes may be reduced by cystic fibrosis, prolonged chronic pancreatitis,

TABLE 33.4 *Diet guidelines following gastric surgery*[17]

FOODS USUALLY WELL TOLERATED
Meat, fish, poultry, eggs, cheese, refined breads and cereals (unsweetened)
Unsweetened canned fruits and juices
Cooked mild vegetables, including potatoes
Fats and oils

FOODS TO ADD AS TOLERANCE IMPROVES
Sweetened canned fruits*
Whole grains

*FOODS FREQUENTLY POORLY TOLERATED**
Sugar, candy, syrup, sweetened desserts (cake, cookies, pie, pudding, ice cream)

FOODS AND BEVERAGES TO AVOID
Cold high carbohydrate items such as milkshakes, slush, fruit ice
Coffee and tea (unless allowed by physician)

SPECIAL CONSIDERATIONS
Begin with *very* small portions; eat 5 to 6 times daily
Take most liquids between rather than with meals
Milk: include in early stages unless poorly tolerated
Fresh fruits and vegetables: gradually include after 2 to 3 wk; chew thoroughly

---

* Add *gradually* to diet if desired unless bothered by symptoms of dumping.

protein-energy malnutrition,[18] or carcinoma of the pancreas. Pancreatectomy not only eliminates pancreatic enzymes entirely but also removes the body's source of insulin and glucagon, thus complicating nutritional care. If the pancreas is inflamed or obstructed (as due to chronic alcohol abuse), hormonal stimulation of pancreatic secretion may be a source of excruciating pain. In this case a client views pain avoidance as a major goal of treatment. In contrast, normal growth and maintenance of body tissue might be central concerns of a person with cystic fibrosis. It is important for health care workers to consider the type of pancreatic problem when planning nutritional care.

NUTRITIONAL CARE WHEN PANCREATIC ENZYME PRODUCTION IS INADEQUATE

When production of pancreatic enzymes is abnormally low, fat digestion is likely to be impaired more than is digestion of protein and starch. Thus, when there is a deficiency of pancreatic enzymes, the proportion of calories coming from ordinary dietary fat is usually decreased, and the proportion of calories from carbohydrate and protein is increased. If enzyme production is low because of protein-energy malnutrition, nutritional repletion usually improves exocrine pancreatic function.[18]

Ingestion of pancreatic extracts *at mealtime* and snack time is a major means of improving digestion when there is deficiency of endogenous pancreatic en-

zymes, as in cystic fibrosis* and, sometimes, in chronic pancreatitis. Unfortunately these enzyme extracts are much less effective than are normal pancreatic secretions, leaving digestion somewhat impaired. Mild malabsorption usually persists and worsens if fat intake is high. A smaller dose of extract is needed if MCT replaces part of the fat.[19]

Elliott and coworkers[20] have observed that deficiency of linoleic acid may either contribute to the development of cystic fibrosis or aggravate symptoms. Because of impaired fat digestion in cystic fibrosis, deficiency of linoleic acid is not readily corrected by oral means. Therefore, Elliott administered fat emulsion parenterally to children with cystic fibrosis and found that it had beneficial effects on their health. This work suggests that it might be advisable for health professionals to carefully assess clients with any type of chronic fat malabsorption for deficiency of essential fatty acid.

NUTRITIONAL CARE TO MINIMIZE STIMULATION OF PANCREATIC SECRETION

In order to avoid pain associated with acute pancreatitis, an attempt is made to minimize pancreatic secretions. Although elemental diets are sometimes given, the surest way to rest the pancreas is to keep a person from taking any food by the enteral route.[21]

Since nutrient needs are usually great in a person with pancreatitis, TPN may be needed to maintain or improve nutritional status. Using only dextrose in water plus electrolytes for an extended period may place the client at great nutritional risk. His nutritional status is likely to be poor, especially if he has been abusing alcohol.

PROBLEMS WITH THE BILIARY SYSTEM

A common but potentially serious abnormality of the biliary system is cholelithiasis (gallstones in the gall bladder). In cholelithiasis, the supply of bile may be normal, but its entry into the duodenum may be prevented (temporarily or permanently) because of one or more obstructing gallstones. Sometimes cholecystitis (inflammation of the gallbladder) is associated with gallstones even if they are not obstructive. Contraction of an inflamed gallbladder may result in mild to acute pain.

Abnormal loss of bile salts from the body is one condition which makes bile more lithogenic (likely to form stones). Thus gallbladder disease may gradually develop secondary to ileal disease or resection, both of which interfere with normal reabsorption of bile salts.

---

* Individuals with cystic fibrosis have an increased salt requirement which becomes very high in hot weather. This is due to increased loss of salt in sweat and is unrelated to lack of pancreatic enzymes.

Heredity appears to have a major influence on development of gallstones, but diet may influence the lithogenicity of bile to some extent. In particular, incidence of gallstones may *increase* if the total amount of polyunsaturated fat in the diet is greatly increased.[22] Populations with low intake of fat may be less vulnerable to cholesterol gallstone formation.

Medical management of gallbladder disease may be used at least temporarily. An attempt may be made to dissolve gallstones using the drug chenodeoxycholic acid (a bile salt). Management may be directed toward making the client a better surgical risk—losing fat if obese or building up lean body mass and stores of micronutrients if nutritionally depleted. A low fat diet (Appendix 5L) is an integral part of medical management.

Cholecystectomy (removal of the gallbladder) has less effect on ongoing nutritional care than many people suspect. The surgical procedure allows bile to enter the small intestine, essentially on a continuous basis. Initially, clients may be most comfortable if they limit their intake of fat and distribute it between small meals but, with time, adaptation occurs so that some bile may be temporarily stored between meals in an enlarged portion of the duct. Because of this adaptation, many clients can gradually resume a normal diet (within a month or two) following a cholecystectomy.

Small intestine

DAMAGE TO OR LOSS OF INTESTINAL MUCOSA

Loss of integrity of the small intestine or literal loss of functioning intestine as a result of surgical resection or bypass may seriously interfere with normal absorptive processes. The types of problems which develop depend on the part of the intestine involved, since the duodenum, jejunum, and ileum are somewhat specialized in function.

Acute gastroenteritis owing to microorganisms or toxins is usually self-limited. The resulting watery (secretory) diarrhea helps to rid the body of offending substances. Accompanying temporary malabsorption is of little consequence in previously well-nourished individuals if fluid and electrolyte balance can be maintained. However, gastroenteritis may be life threatening to a child with protein-energy malnutrition. Severe protein-energy malnutrition itself results in loss of mucosal integrity and malabsorption; the problem may be intensified when an inflammatory condition is superimposed. The need for nutritional support during acute gastroenteritis depends upon the circumstances.

Loss of integrity of the intestinal mucosa may result in a decrease in production of disaccharidases. Production of lactase in particular may sharply decrease, resulting in an acquired but usually temporary form of lactose intolerance. If drinking milk precipitates cramps and diarrhea during convalescence from gastrointestinal disorders, reduction or sometimes complete elimination of lactose from the diet may be necessary. The lactose content of milk can be appreciably reduced by mixing milk with a commercially available form of active lactase and allowing the mixture to stand for a specified period of time.[23] The resulting partially digested milk tastes slightly sweeter than usual. Lactase-treated milk is less expensive and lower in lactose content than is commercial yogurt.

GLUTEN-INDUCED ENTEROPATHY (CELIAC DISEASE, CELIAC SPRUE)

Celiac disease is characterized by a flattening of the intestinal mucosa (shortening of villi). The decreased absorptive area results in generalized malabsorption. A modified diet is used to correct the underlying problem and improve absorption. If deficiencies of vitamin B_6 and of trace metals such as zinc and copper are present, they should be corrected to enhance the effectiveness of diet modification.

A food protein called *gliadin* causes the mucosal damage in sensitive individuals[24] but the culprit is usually called gluten. Gliadin is a part of wheat protein (gluten) and is also found in rye, oats, and barley. If *all* gluten (gliadin) is removed from the diet of a person who has celiac disease, the mucosa gradually regains normal structure and function. Children with celiac disease may respond positively to removal of gluten within a few days, but improvement usually takes longer. Lack of improvement may be due to the presence of an unsuspected source of gluten in the diet. Restricting fat intake for the first month or two following diagnosis may hasten improvement.[25] Adults with gluten-induced enteropathy (sometimes called celiac sprue or just sprue in adults) may respond to treatment more slowly.

A person with celiac disease does not outgrow his sensitivity to gluten; the prohibition against this food component should be permanent. Reintroduction of even small amounts of gluten causes histological damage to the mucosa. This may result in unsymptomatic malabsorption and development of serious nutritional deficiencies.[26]

A gluten-free diet is expensive and can be difficult to plan and follow. Foods containing even small amounts of wheat, rye, oats, or barley are eliminated. Since these grains are used in the preparation of many staples and convenience foods, careful label reading becomes essential. Some of the less obvious sources of gluten are (1) hot dogs and bologna if made with added cereal, (2) soups containing barley, noodles, or flour (for thickening), (3) malted milk (contains barley), (4) meatloaf, (5) salad dressing, (6) ice cream, (7) gravy, sauces, and puddings if thickened with wheat flour, (8) foods containing hydrolyzed vegetable or plant protein. Because wheat starch and products made with wheat starch are not strictly gluten free, their use is not endorsed by the American Celiac Society.[27] In some situations, as when eating out, certain foods should be avoided because they *might* contain gluten.

The family needs detailed guidelines regarding foods which are allowed and foods which must be *eliminated* from the diet. Appendix 5M provides such a listing. There are no "grey areas" of foods which are allowed in limited amounts. Recipes for suitable bread products may be especially helpful additions to the diet plan since gluten-free baked goods are not generally available. Cornmeal or rice flour are used for making baked goods. Special gluten-free "sandwich loaf" and other baked products can be purchased by mail order or can sometimes be obtained from health food stores, but they are costly. The American Celiac Society is a good resource for persons needing help in dealing with celiac disease.

Unfortunately, the mucosal damage characteristic of untreated celiac disease often leads to development of lactase deficiency and lactose malabsorption. Lactose intolerance may persist throughout the early stages of treatment. If lactase deficiency is secondary to the disease rather than acquired, lactase activity should gradually return. In the meantime, limitations on milk intake and substitution of low lactose dairy products may be helpful.

Defined formula diet is lactose free; it may be useful during celiac crisis, that is, in an early stage of treatment or during a flare-up of the disease. If solid foods are tolerated, a meal and snack such as the ones shown in Table 33.5 might be acceptable during celiac crisis.

Diet can be liberalized somewhat with regard to fat content, lactose, and other sugars after the mucosa regains its normal structure. When the disease is under control it is said to be in remission, but it is never cured. Possible diet changes during remission are also shown in Table 33.5. If the disease becomes apparent toward the end of the first year of life rather than at a later age, initial adaptation of diet is simpler. A formula such as Probana might be given as the basis of the diet, with gluten-free solid foods added as appropriate for the stage of development. Baby food companies are glad to send individuals lists of their gluten-free products.

ILEITIS (CROHN'S DISEASE, REGIONAL ENTERITIS)

Ileitis, an inflammatory bowel disease, is a very serious chronic condition, most commonly seen in children and young adults. Abdominal pain, watery (secretory) diarrhea, weight loss, and fever are usual symptoms. Obstruction, ulceration, abscesses, fistulas and bacterial overgrowth may complicate the disease. An affected person is likely to eat much less than a healthy person of similar size and activity; malabsorption may develop rapidly because of high metabolic needs, general malabsorption, and leakage of serum protein from the mucosa into the intestinal lumen (exudative enteropathy).

A low or minimum residue diet of conventional foods (Appendix 5C) may be recommended for times when symptoms are relatively mild. One purpose of a residue restricted diet is to reduce fecal output. Thus, foods used are low in indigestible fiber. For example, refined rather than whole grain cereals are recommended. The diet also restricts other substances with low digestibility (e.g., lactose if lactase deficiency is suspected). Use of nonfibrous food ingredients which stimulate increased peristalsis (e.g., coffee, prune juice) and irritating seasonings such as pepper may be discouraged.

Guidelines for use of fruits and vegetables (cooked, strained, juice, or none) should depend on the client's response to these different food forms. Individual food intolerances are common. Care should be taken to assure adequate intake of folic acid[28]; supplements may be required, especially if few vegetables and fruits are consumed. The most satisfactory meal pattern (small frequent feedings versus three larger meals daily) cannot be determined without data about the client's response to different feeding strategies. Unfortunately, for persons with Crohn's disease a low residue diet seldom allows satisfactory food intake and relief from symptoms.

Intensive nutritional support is frequently indicated in severe cases, perhaps in conjunction with anti-inflammatory drugs (corticosteroids) and immuno-suppressive drugs.

Total parenteral nutrition (TPN) is the type of nutritional support which has most consistently given good results in severe attacks of Crohn's disease. TPN may be called a "definitive treatment" because in many cases it has allowed self-healing of fistulas, clearing of obstructions, and return to a relatively normal state of health.[29] Treatment with TPN often eliminates or postpones indefinitely the need for surgery[30]—a very big advantage since recurrence of the disease following surgery occurs about 50 percent of the time.[31] Use of defined formula diet for long term nutritional support in Crohn's disease has also been reported to improve the condition of many clients.[32]

Because of the chronic and disabling nature of Crohn's disease, those affected may need much psychological support. If oral feedings of any type are prescribed, it may be particularly helpful to promote a relaxed environment and to encourage the person to eat slowly.

Radiation enteritis (inflammation of the bowel following radiation therapy) can be just as serious as Crohn's disease and can involve a large portion of the intestinal tract. Like Crohn's disease, radiation enteritis may result in extensive loss of serum protein through the damaged intestinal wall. Obstruction is a common complication. Dietary treatment parallels that of Crohn's disease.

RESECTION OF THE SMALL INTESTINE

The most common surgical procedure involving resection of a part of the small intestine is appendectomy (removal of the appendix). Since appendicitis is usually a short term acute condition, it is seldom

TABLE 33.5 *Sample meal and snack for a child with celiac disease (gluten-induced enteropathy)*

MENU* DURING CELIAC CRISIS	POSSIBLE CHANGES DURING REMISSION
LUNCH OR DINNER	
Sliced roast turkey or chicken (no skin)	More frequent use of meats which are higher in fat (e.g., beef, lamb, and pork) if desired
Mashed potato with added MCT†	With butter or margarine
Cooked vegetable salad with MCT† salad dressing	Raw vegetable salad if desired, with any salad dressing that is free of added flour
Low lactose skim or low fat milk	Low fat or whole milk
SNACK	
Homemade 100% corn muffin (made with MCT)†	Corn muffin may be made with vegetable oil and eaten with butter or margarine
Low lactose skim or low fat milk	Low fat or whole milk
	(Larger meals and smaller snacks may now be better tolerated)

* Portion sizes vary with nutritional needs and appetite of the child.
† Gradual adaptation to MCT is recommended.

accompanied by malnutrition. Recovery of normal gastrointestinal function is expected to proceed rapidly following an appendectomy. Nutritional care is usually straightforward; it involves gradual progression of the client from a clear liquid to a normal diet.

Resection or bypass of a larger part of the intestinal tract for any reason causes reduced absorption of the nutrients normally absorbed in the particular area involved. Fortunately, if resection is not too extensive (40 percent or less of the total length) adaptive processes may gradually restore normal absorption. The functioning gut which remains gradually hypertrophies, increasing the absorptive surface.[33] If the resection or bypass is very extensive, absorption gradually improves but may never allow for meeting nutrient needs completely by the enteral route.

Following extensive intestinal resection, clear liquids are the first nourishment offered by mouth; progression to a normal diet is likely to be a slow process. Use of TPN and/or chemically defined diets may be necessary to permit maintenance of satisfactory nutritional status. Once normal food can be tolerated in small amounts, it can be offered while intensive nutritional support measures are still being used. If the gut is very short, some type of nutritional support measure might need to be continued indefinitely on an outpatient basis. Following jejunoileal bypass operations an attempt is made to achieve a balance so that weight will be lost without precipitating serious malnutrition. However, serious nutritional problems such as osteomalacia[4,34] and oxalate kidney stones occur with disturbing frequency.[35]

Large intestine

Although the colon is not involved in digestion and is usually considered to have a minor absorptive function, its condition can strongly influence food intake and fluid and electrolyte balance. Problems in the colon usually have a major impact on nutritional status. Partial or complete obstruction of the bowel (e.g., by a tumor) call for major change in diet, such as defined formula diet or total parenteral nutrition.

Even constipation may interfere with nutritional status if it leads to loss of appetite, use of mineral oil at mealtime, or abuse of laxatives.

IRRITABLE BOWEL

Irritable bowel, a condition characterized by recurrent attacks of abdominal pain and diarrhea (sometimes alternating with constipation), is one of the more common disorders of the colon. Irritable bowel is called a "functional disease;" this means that damage or disease of the colon is not believed to be the source of the problem. Many physicians believe that emotional stress is a major precipitating factor for irritable bowel syndrome.

If constipation is a frequent symptom of irritable bowel, an increased intake of fiber may be helpful. However, controlled studies indicate that use of supplemental fiber does not bring significant improvement.[36,37] Those who are troubled by diarrhea may benefit from avoiding cold liquids, carbonated beverages, and coffee.[37,38] Health professionals should respect individual food intolerances but, if the number is so large as to interfere with nutritional adequacy, it may be advisable to test for intolerance during a period of remission (adding only one test food at a time).

Assisting a person who has irritable bowel to improve his ability to cope constructively with stress may be more beneficial than directing excessive attention to diet.

DIVERTICULOSIS AND DIVERTICULITIS

If conditions are right, tiny pockets of the membrane lining the colon can be pushed out through weak spots in the muscular wall to form small sacs or diverticula. The resulting condition is called diverticulosis. Fortunately most people who have diverticulosis have only mild symptoms or no symptoms at all. Abdominal cramps, flatus, and diarrhea alternating with constipation are the most common complaints. In perhaps 15 percent of the persons, diverticulosis progresses to the inflammatory condition called diverticulitis.

Dietary treatment of persons with diverticulosis and diverticulitis is very different. The diet which is most apt to be prescribed for diverticulosis is a high fiber diet, often with supplemental bran (seeds are avoided since it is thought that they might lodge in a diverticulum and become a site for infection.) A low residue diet (Appendix 5C) is indicated during an attack of diverticulitis. Health professionals should make sure that clients with diverticulosis understand that a high fiber diet is to be used only when there are no acute abdominal symptoms and when body temperature is normal. If a client should develop severe abdominal pain and fever, he should discontinue use of high fiber foods and contact his doctor promptly.

There is considerable disagreement about the effectiveness of a high fiber diet in the treatment of diverticulosis. Connell suggests that there is little good evidence that high fiber intake helps persons with diverticular disease.[39] The American Digestive Disease Society, on the other hand, takes a strong stand recommending high fiber intake, especially bran, as an effective treatment. Broadrib reports that several months are required for a high fiber diet to produce a maximal therapeutic response.[40] If intake of bran is recommended, unpleasant symptoms can be minimized by taking small amounts at first and gradually increasing intake up to the specified "dose."

DISEASES OF THE COLON

Colitis is a serious form of inflammatory bowel disease which, like Crohn's disease, is most commonly seen in young people. Signs and symptoms of severe cases include grossly bloody diarrhea, fever, and a low serum albumin (≤3.0 gm. per 100 ml.); nutrition-related problems are common. Treatment with a low residue diet and with drugs is usually attempted, but this often fails to prevent malnutrition. Even if diet is closely followed, diarrhea and weakness may seriously interfere with participation in activities of daily living. In severe cases, TPN may be needed to restore satisfactory nutritional status. Defined formula diet is sometimes a suitable alternative. Colitis differs from Crohn's disease in that nutritional rehabilitation almost never induces remission. Surgery is often required in serious cases; it almost invariably cures the disease.

Surgical treatment and nutritional care Ileostomies. It is difficult for most people to agree to surgical treatment of colitis since surgery may involve removal of the entire colon and rectum and creation of a permanent ileostomy. An ileostomy is an opening formed by cutting across the ileum and bringing the proximal cut end to the skin through an opening (stoma) in the abdominal wall. Waste material from an ileostomy is in a liquid state. Drainage into an attached pouch is continual. Diet cannot alter this situation.

When oral feedings can be resumed following surgery, a person who has had an ileostomy is placed on a progressive diet (starting with clear liquids) and gradually is encouraged to take a normal mixed diet. The person should be reminded to drink plenty of fluid —at least 2 L. (2 qt.) daily. It may help to motivate the client to take extra water if it is explained that fluid needs are increased because of reduced ability to absorb water. The client may need reassurance that the extra fluid will not make care of his ostomy more difficult.

Since many clients who were ill enough to require an ileostomy are nutritionally depleted, they should be encouraged to select a variety of nourishing foods. If a client is concerned that a food might bother him, he might want to try just a small amount to see how well he tolerates it. If it causes a problem shortly after surgery, it won't necessarily always do so and can be tried again at a later date. Since many persons who have undergone an ileostomy had to restrict their diet during their illness, they may be delighted to be able to eat foods that had previously been a source of distress.

Anticipatory guidance can help assure adequate intake and prevent unnecessary worry or problems. Some foods have a tendency to block the stoma. The most common offenders are dried fruit, corn, popcorn, mushrooms, coconut, and the membranes of citrus fruit.[41] The chance of blockage is greatly reduced if food is thoroughly chewed. If there are no contraindications because of other illnesses, usually all foods are allowed. The client can determine for himself if he wishes to avoid a food because it causes him discomfort, diarrhea, excessive flatus, or other problems.

Lack of a sphincter may make flatus a major concern for the client with an ostomy. The only diet-related remedies which can be suggested are the usual measures for reducing gaseousness—avoiding excessive swallowing of air and limiting intake of foods which the individual has found cause excessive flatus or a particularly offensive odor. Unfortunately, no foolproof treatment is available.

Permanent and temporary colostomies. Treatment of serious diseases of the large bowel or rectum (e.g., cancer and diverticulitis) often requires surgical removal of the affected area (most commonly the sigmoid colon). Depending on the disease condition, either a permanent or temporary colostomy is constructed.

Colostomies differ from ileostomies in the larger size of the stoma and in the nature of the fecal output. The more distal the point in the colon where the resection is made, the more solid the fecal output.

A person who has a colostomy can usually progress rapidly to a completely normal diet—hopefully one which will make up for deficits associated with his illness and surgery. Intake of 1½ to 2 L. of fluid (6 to 8 c.) is recommended. The stoma is large enough that blockage by undigested food is not a common problem. Foods which might cause GI problems are those (if any) which caused problems prior to the illness requiring the ostomy. If the client would like to eat foods which formerly caused problems, he might want to try them cautiously, one at a time, to see if they can be tolerated satisfactorily.

STUDY QUESTIONS

1. Why is avoidance of chocolate sometimes helpful in treatment of esophageal reflux?
2. Mr. P. is being discharged from a health care agency following treatment for a bleeding duodenal ulcer. His physician has ordered discharge diet instruction for a bland diet. Mr. P. has complained about the tasteless hospital food, has lost weight during his hospitalization, and seems upset that he won't be able to eat many of his favorite Italian foods. What action would be appropriate for the nurse to take? Why?
3. Following a selective vagotomy and pyloroplasty, Ms. T. is troubled by gastric retention and diarrhea. What diet modifications might help alleviate these symptoms?
4. If a person is on a 50 gm. fat diet because of cholelithiasis, what foods would be good choices when eating in a restaurant?
5. Jane has been diagnosed to have celiac disease. What kinds of snacks would be suitable for her to have in nursery school? What could her parents do so that Jane would not feel too different from the other nursery school children?

References

1. Mertz, W.: Provisional recommendations and calculations of available iron. Presentation at the 61st Annual Meeting of The American Dietetic Association, New Orleans. Sept. 26, 1978.
2. Rocchio, M. A., et al.: Use of chemically defined diets in the management of patients with high output gastrointestinal cutaneous fistulas. *Am. J. Surg.* 127: 148, 1974.
*3. Holt, P. R.: Malabsorption. *Nutrition in Disease* Columbus OH: Ross Laboratories, Aug. 1977.
4. Short bowels. *Brit. Med. J.* 1:737, 1978.
5. Fisher, R. S., and Cohen, S.: Gastroesophageal reflux. *Med. Clin. North Am.* 62(1):3, 1978.
6. Cohen, S., and Booth, G. H.: Gastric acid secretion and lower esophageal sphincter pressure in response to coffee and caffeine. *N. Engl. J. Med.* 293:897, 1975.
7. About hiatal hernia. *Person to Person.* New York: American Digestive Disease Society.
8. Babka, J. C., and Castell, D. O.: On the genesis of heartburn: the effects of specific foods on the lower esophageal sphincter. *Digest. Dis.* 18:391, 1973.
9. Kaufman, S. E., and Kaye, M. D.: Induction of gastroesophageal reflux by alcohol. *Gut* 19:336, 1978.
10. Narayanan, M., and Steinheber, F. U.: The changing face of peptic ulcer in the elderly. *Med. Clin. North Am.* 60(6):1159, 1976.
11. Chapman, M. L.: Peptic ulcer: A medical perspective. *Med. Clin. North Am.* 62(1):39, 1978.
12. Walsh, J. D.: Diet therapy of peptic ulcer disease. *Gastroenterology* 72:740, 1977.
13. Position paper on bland diet in the treatment of chronic duodenal ulcer disease. *J. Am. Diet. Assoc.* 59:244, 1971.
14. Review. Coffee drinking and peptic ulcer disease. *Nutr. Rev.* 34:167, 1976.
15. Barbezat, G. O., and Bank, S.: Effect of prolonged Cimetidine therapy on gastric acid secretion in man. *Gut* 19:151, 1978.
16. Rudick, J.: Peptic ulcer: Surgical alternatives. *Med. Clin. North Am.* 62(1):53, 1978.
17. Behm, V., Murchie, G., and King, D. R.: Nutritional care of the patient following gastric surgery. *Diet. Currents* 1:1, Mar./Apr. 1974.
18. Viteri, F. E., and Schneider, R. E.: Gastrointestinal alterations in protein-calorie malnutrition. *Med. Clin. North Am.* 58(6):1487, 1974.
19. Smalley, C. A., et al.: Reduction of bile acid loss in cystic fibrosis by dietary means. *Arch. Dis. Child.* 53:477, 1978.
20. Elliott, R. B.: A therapeutic trial of fatty acid supplementation in cystic fibrosis. *Pediatrics* 57:474, 1976.
21. Soergel, K. H.: Medical treatment of acute pancreatitis: What is the evidence? *Gastroenterology* 74:620, 1978.
22. Sturdevant, R. A. L., Pearce, M. L., and Dayton S.: Increased prevalence of cholelithiasis in men ingesting a serum cholesterol lowering diet. *N. Engl. J. Med.* 288:24, 1973.
23. Turner, S. J., et al.: Utilization of a low-lactose milk. *Am. J. Clin. Nutr.* 29:739, 1976.
24. Evans, D. J., and Patey, A. L.: Chemistry of wheat proteins and the nature of damaging substances. *Clin. Gastroenterol.* 3(1):199, 1974.
25. Stewart, J. S.: Clinical and morphologic response to gluten withdrawal. *Clin. Gastroenterol.* 3(1):109, 1974.
26. McNeish, A. S., and Anderson, C. M.: The disorder in childhood. *Clin. Gastroenterol.* 3(1):127, 1974.
27. Wilson, E.: Guide for the celiac. Jersey City NJ: American Celiac Society, 1975.
28. Gerson, C. D., and Cohen, N.: Folic acid absorption in regional enteritis. *Am. J. Clin. Nutr.* 29:182, 1976.
29. Abbott, W. W.: Indications for parenteral nutrition. In J. E. Fischer (ed.): *Total Parenteral Nutrition.* Boston: Little, Brown & Co., 1976.
30. Rault, R. M. J., and Scribner, B. J.: Treatment of Crohn's disease with home parenteral nutrition. *Gastroenterology* 72:1249, 1977.
31. About inflammatory bowel disease. *Person to Person.* New York: American Digestive Disease Society.
32. Nelson, L. M., et al.: Use of an elemental diet (Vivonex) in the management of bile acid-induced diarrhoea. *Gut* 18:792, 1977.
33. Sherman, C. D., Faloon, W. W., and Flood, M. S.: Revision operations after small bowel bypass. *Am. J. Clin. Nutr.* 30:98, 1977.
34. Compston, J. E., et al.: Osteomalacia after small bowel resection. *Lancet* 1:9, 1978.
35. Stauffer, J. Q.: Hyperoxaluria and calcium oxalate nephrolithiasis after jejunoileal bypass. *Am. J. Clin. Nutr.* 30:64, 1977.
36. Søltoft, S., et al.: A double-blind trial of the effect of wheat bran on symptoms of the irritable bowel syndrome. *Lancet* 1:270, 1976.
*37. Almy, T. P.; Wrestling with the irritable colon. *Med. Clin. North Am.* 62(1):203, 1978.
38. Wald, A., Back, C., and Bayless, T. M.: Effect of caffeine on the human small intestine. *Gastroenterology* 71:738, 1976.
39. Connell, A. M.: Wheat bran as an etiologic factor in certain diseases: Some second thoughts. *J. Am. Diet. Assoc.* 71:235, 1977.
40. Brodribb, A. J. M.: Treatment of symptomatic diverticular disease with a high-fibre diet. *Lancet* 1:664, 1977.
*41. Watson, P. G., et al.: Comprehensive care of the ileostomy patient. *Nurs. Clin. North Am.* 11(3):427, 1976.

* Recommended reading

34

Care of clients with other special nutritional needs Part 1

Some individuals are at increased risk of developing nutrition-related problems at particular stages of life. Others are at great nutritional risk because of disease or trauma or because of certain types of long term drug therapy. This chapter and the following discuss examples of special nutritional problems. Topics, though not necessarily related, have been selected to illustrate how various components of nutritional care can be effectively integrated to promote optimal nutrition and health of clients. This chapter focuses on special needs of mothers and children.

DURING PREGNANCY

Early nutritional assessment of pregnant women is recommended to identify those needing *special* nutritional care. The sooner appropriate nutritional care is begun, the higher its potential may be for promoting optimal health and well being of both mother and infant. However, prenatal nutritional care can be of great benefit whenever it is initiated. Nutritional risk during pregnancy is related to age, socioeconomic status, and a history of medical and obstetrical problems.

Age Adolescent girls belong to one of the most poorly nourished groups in the U.S. Since wide variation exists in any group, some teens enter pregnancy in superb nutritional status; however, there appears to be a sizable number of teens who enter pregnancy in a state of poor nutrition. Women over 30 to 35 years of age who are beginning to experience effects of the aging process are also at increased risk.

Socioeconomic factors Income, occupation, and education are some of the interwoven variables often adversely affecting a woman's nutritional status dur-

ing pregnancy. When low socioeconomic status is coupled with another factor such as young age, the chance of a nutritional problem increases. Maternal Infant Care (MIC) clinics have been established in some low income areas to provide comprehensive perinatal and infant care, including emphasis on sound nutrition.

Obstetrical history High parity (a high number of live or stillborn infants delivered by a woman), frequent pregnancy, and multiple births deplete a mother's nutritional stores. Complications of pregnancy such as toxemia, miscarriage, and premature labor are sometimes associated with a mother's nutritional status.

Medical problems Diabetes mellitus and cardiovascular and pulmonary disease are among the medical problems for which a mother requires close attention during pregnancy. Sound nutritional care to meet special needs posed by these and other conditions may help to improve the chance of a favorable course and outcome of pregnancy.

Among the potentially serious conditions which sometimes develop during pregnancy are anemia, toxemia, undesirable pattern of weight gain, and pica.

Most anemias in pregnancy are nutritional in nature. Iron deficiency anemia is most common; megaloblastic anemia associated with folic acid deficiency is seen to a lesser extent. An adequate diet and supplements of iron and/or folic acid are important to prevent and correct nutritional anemia.

Toxemia is a term used to describe hypertensive states of pregnancy including preeclampsia (hypertension with edema and/or proteinuria) and eclampsia (convulsions in a woman with preeclampsia). Pathophysiological changes which occur in toxemia are complex; some of them may be related to nutritional factors. Low protein intake, for example, may contribute to the development of toxemia.[1] Data from one study indicated that a sizable number of women with preeclampsia had hypoglycemia; the hypoglycemia was directly related to perinatal infant death.[2] Emphasis on sound eating habits throughout pregnancy may help prevent the occurrence of complications such as toxemia.

The incidence of low birth weight babies is higher in women who have a low prepregnant weight and women who gain less than 5 kg. (11 lb.) during pregnancy.[3] Thus, pregnant women should be counseled to strive for a desirable pattern of prenatal weight gain regardless of their prepregnancy weight.

Pregnant women who gain weight rapidly as a result of fluid retention sometimes greatly decrease their caloric intake because they think the gain is due to overeating. Health care providers should take steps to prevent this practice since adequate intake of calories and nutrients remains important to the health of both mother and fetus.

Pica, ingestion of nonfood items, is a practice admitted to by some teens and women.[4,5] Excessive pica may result in decreased intake of essential nutrients. A small study conducted by Snow and Johnson identified that a few women were likely to follow cultural food practices such as pica even when the women knew the practice was in direct conflict with a health professional's view of good nutrition.[6] For this reason, it is important that health care workers attempt to identify the cultural basis of food behaviors in order to discuss them with clients in a constructive manner.

The special needs of the pregnant adolescent and of the pregnant diabetic are discussed in the following section. Many of the principles of care discussed in relation to the adolescent might be applied in caring for pregnant women of any age.

Pregnancy during adolescence

Pregnancy during adolescence is an increasingly common event. In 1974 nearly one million teenagers became pregnant. Of the 608,000 teens who gave birth, 12,529 were under 15 years of age.[7]

Nutrition may be overlooked among the many other pressing concerns of pregnant teens. Many teens are only just developing skills to cope with sociologic, emotional, and physical stresses. Emotional and/or economic deprivation more commonly affect teenage mothers than women who are older when they first become pregnant. Some adolescents attempt to hide the fact that they are pregnant; consequently, prenatal care is not obtained until late. If they do not want a baby, a few mothers may not make an effort to maintain health and nutritional status during pregnancy.

A pregnant adolescent's nutritional needs depend on her own stage of growth and development, her current nutrient stores, and on fetal demands (based on the trimester of pregnancy). Total recommended intake can be roughly estimated by using values from the Table of Recommended Dietary Allowances (see inside back cover). This table specifies amounts to be added to cover the needs of pregnancy. These amounts are added to the RDAs for an adolescent. Estimates should be adjusted to fit the individual girl's needs. For example, some girls who continue to be fairly active throughout their pregnancy have high energy needs; however, if a girl becomes less active, her energy needs may be similar to those of a nonpregnant adolescent.

A few studies indicate that a considerable number of pregnant adolescents are at nutritional risk because of inadequate intakes of iron, calcium, vitamin A, and energy.[4,8] Since most studies of nutritional status of adolescents have assessed adequacy of intake of a limited number of nutrients, many adolescents might also be at increased risk with regard to other nutrients as well.

NUTRITIONAL CARE OF THE PREGNANT ADOLESCENT

Personalized nutritional care and counseling is recommended as a way of improving the nutritional status of pregnant adolescents.[9] Careful assessment of a pregnant teen's home situation is essential to develop effective means of providing nutritional care. Health professionals must take care not to make assumptions since the possibilities for living and eating arrangements are very numerous. It may be necessary to take steps to resolve conflicts among family members as a means of promoting improved food intake of a pregnant teen.

Concerned health professionals provide concrete information about what consitutes a nutritionally sound diet while allowing the teen freedom to make informed decisions for herself and her baby. Clear explanations of why and how to change may increase the teen's willingness to try to cooperate with recommended nutritional care measures. This should be considered when recommending specific nutritional supplements to augment a pregnant teen's food intake. Supplements are beneficial only if taken and studies have found that many adolescent girls do not like to take pills.[8,10] A pregnant girl needs to appreciate the importance of taking nutritional supplements and at the same time understand that supplements do not lessen the value of a well-balanced diet. After explaining the importance of supplements and food for both mother and growing fetus, the health professional might work with the client to develop a reminder system to increase the girl's compliance.

Some teenagers' erratic food habits might contribute to an undesirable pattern of weight gain. One study identified that some pregnant teens continued to eat as they did before they were pregnant.[8] This often means skipping meals and eating snack foods, many of which are high in calories and low in nutrients. Depending on what she learns during assessment, the nutrition counselor might suggest nutritious snack foods which could be kept on hand, appropriate selections of fast foods, or quick yet adequate low cost breakfasts. She would encourage the teen to identify practical ways of improving her own diet.

Some adolescents find it difficult to follow diet guidelines. In this case a gradual approach may be essential to maintain the client's cooperation and to keep her from avoiding prenatal care appointments. A team approach in which all health professionals stress the value of sound nutrition and acknowledge the client's progress may motivate the teen to make further improvements in her diet.

A pregnant adolescent may appreciate receiving written material such as the government publication "Food for Teens during Pregnancy."[11] Audiovisual materials can be a particularly effective means of stimulating an adolescent's interest in nutrition. For example, the slide tape presentation "Inside My Mom" which uses a cartoon character to discuss the importance of maternal nutrition to the developing fetus might be appropriate for use with some expectant mothers.[12] Teaching aids used should be carefully screened to be sure they do not instill a feeling of guilt or hopelessness if a person's food intake has previously been low in nutritive value.

Pregnancy complicated by diabetes

Appropriate health care of a pregnant woman who has diabetes mellitus greatly increases the chances of immediate survival of the mother and decreases morbidity and mortality in the newborn to about 2 percent.[13] Dietary management is essential to promote and maintain adequate nutritional status and to control blood glucose levels throughout pregnancy. Control of diabetes during pregnancy is so important that it is advisable to refer a woman whose pregnancy is complicated by diabetes to health professionals who are especially competent in this field of care.[13] There are two forms of diabetes which could complicate pregnancy: *pregestational* diabetes, that is diabetes mellitus which is present before pregnancy occurs, and *gestational* diabetes, that is disease which develops during and is limited to pregnancy. Pregestational diabetes is usually of the youth onset type.

Women who develop diabetes in the childbearing years (or before) should be carefully counseled regarding the risks of their disease during pregnancy and the increased importance of careful control if they should become pregnant. Health care workers encourage diabetic women to plan pregnancies only when their diabetes is well controlled; this increases the chance of effective control during pregnancy.

An important goal of care is to keep blood sugar levels within the normal ranges for the particular stage of pregnancy. This is even more important to the health of the developing fetus than it is to the mother. An understanding of the changes in glucose utilization during pregnancy serves as a basis for adapting care for a pregnant woman who has diabetes.

Changes in glucose metabolism and utilization help assure that the growing fetus has enough glucose, his primary fuel source. Consequently during the first half of pregnancy, diabetic and nondiabetic women may develop hypoglycemia, especially during periods of fasting. Maternal blood glucose level is lowered since glucose moves rapidly across the placental membrane by diffusion and active transport. (Insulin is not required for movement of glucose across the placental membrane.) Nausea and hyperemesis (excessive vomiting) decrease food intake and aggravate hypoglycemia.

Lowered maternal blood glucose level is accompanied by an elevation in plasma free-fatty acids and ketone bodies and by a decrease in plasma amino acids.[14] If hypoglycemia occurs, ketosis may develop as fat is used for fuel. Ketonuria (presence of ketones in the urine) in diabetic mothers has been associated with fetal brain damage.[15]

In managing ketosis, it is important to differentiate between starvation ketosis and ketosis resulting from inadequate levels of insulin. Both types may be harmful to the fetus, but they are managed in different ways. During starvation ketosis, the blood glucose level is low. This can be corrected by oral intake of a rapidly absorbed carbohydrate such as fruit juice or candy or by intravenous administration of dextrose and water. In diabetic ketoacidosis (ketosis caused by lack of insulin), the blood sugar level remains high. Insulin is needed so that the body can utilize the glucose already present. It has been suggested that diabetic ketoacidosis is the single most significant cause of intrapartal fetal death.[16] Ketoacidosis affects the fetus most severely during the second trimester of pregnancy.

During the second half of pregnancy the placenta secretes increasing amounts of several hormones, some (e.g., placental lactogen) act antagonistically toward insulin.[14] The antagonistic effects of placental hormones markedly increase the mother's need for insulin around the 20th to 28th week of pregnancy. At this time all mothers, whether diabetic or not, need more insulin; the need may be as much as two to three times greater than normal.[16] Although gestational diabetes may develop any time during pregnancy, it is most likely to develop about or after the 28th week because this is when the pancreatic reserve may be exceeded.

When maternal diabetes is not well controlled and the mother becomes hyperglycemic, the fetus is exposed to either continuous or meal-related hyperglycemia. The fetal pancreas, in response to hyperglycemia, steps up its production of insulin. (Maternal insulin does not cross the placental membrane.) Fetal hyperglycemia and hyperinsulinemia develop. The elevated insulin level in the fetus does not necessarily keep his blood sugar level within normal limits. High blood sugar and high insulin level probably account for many fetal complications.[16] Excessive insulin in the fetus acts as a fetal growth factor producing a characteristically large infant. Excessive growth, viceromegaly (excessive enlargement of visceral organs), and obesity may all occur in infants of diabetic mothers.

After the infant is born, flow of maternal glucose across the placenta ceases; however, the baby's pancreas does not immediately slow down insulin production. Thus, infants of diabetic mothers are at great risk of developing severe hypoglycemia shortly after delivery. This can be minimized by giving these infants intravenous glucose.

After delivery of the infant and placenta, the mother's level of placental hormones gradually drops. Correspondingly her need for insulin decreases to a prepregnancy or even lower level by the fourth to sixth postpartum week. The woman who developed gestational diabetes can usually expect blood sugar levels to normalize by the sixth postpartal week.

Felig and Tyson suggest that diabetic mothers should be encouraged to breast feed their infants. Preliminary studies indicate the breast feeding has a positive effect on the mother's utilization of glucose. This may be because glucose is used in the production of milk and because of endocrine changes which accompany lactation.[16]

CARE OF PREGNANT DIABETICS

Blood sugar levels of women with gestational diabetes can often be controlled by diet without insulin therapy since these women continue to secrete some insulin. Women with *gestational* diabetes may need more diet counseling than women who have pregestational diabetes since they are not likely to be familiar with the components of a diabetic diet.

When insulin is needed, the type, amount, and frequency of administration is planned in conjunction with the mother's meal and activity pattern. Since most women tend to be hypoglycemic during the first half of pregnancy, insulin doses are usually lowered to about two thirds of the prepregnancy amount.[16] During the second half of pregnancy the amount of insulin administered is increased considerably to control hyperglycemia which would otherwise develop. Close daily monitoring of blood sugar levels (as by a daily Dextrostix) is recommended for women who require insulin therapy during pregnancy.

DIETARY MANAGEMENT

Nutrient needs of pregnant diabetics are similar to those of nondiabetic pregnant women. However, since careful control of blood glucose levels is desirable, particular attention needs to be paid to several aspects of dietary management.

Diabetics are urged to gain weight according to the pattern and amount specified for pregnant women by the Committee on Maternal Nutrition—about 1 kg. (2 to 3 lb.) during the first trimester and 350 to 400 gm.

(0.8 lb.) per week during the second and third trimesters. Close adherence to these guidelines is stressed more strongly than it is for nondiabetic women.

Emphasis must be placed on a fairly even distribution of caloric intake throughout the day. A mother who skips breakfast is placing herself and her fetus in jeopardy since starvation hypoglycemia and ketosis may develop quickly.

Food intake may be distributed among three daily meals and two snacks. Some women also need a midmorning snack. This is especially likely to be the case if regular and intermediate acting insulin are mixed in the morning insulin dose. A food exchange list such as "Exchange Lists for Meal Planning" (Appendix 5I) may be used by the pregnant diabetic to plan varied meals.

Written instructions relating to nutritional care of diabetes might include specific information regarding the following points:

1. The diet plan, including reminders to follow the plan closely and to avoid skipping meals or leaving foods out of one meal and adding them to the next
2. Guidelines for what to do if daily blood tests reveal hypo- or hyperglycemia or daily urine tests reveal ketonuria
3. Special guidelines for dealing with morning sickness, especially if the woman is taking insulin
4. Guidelines for what to do if activities of daily living (especially activity level) change significantly

POINTS OF EMPHASIS
Management of pregnancy complicated by diabetes

• *Close cooperation among the client and other health team members contributes to a successful outcome of pregnancy.*
• *Important goals of care are to keep blood sugar levels within a normal range for the stage of pregnancy and to prevent ketosis.*
• *As a result of changes in glucose metabolism during the first half of pregnancy, hypoglycemia may develop; during the second half, hyperglycemia is more likely.*
• *Close monitoring of blood glucose and urinary ketones and an even distribution of food intake throughout the day are essential components of care.*

THE HIGH RISK INFANT

Nutritional care is essential to help control many of the problems confronting high risk infants and to supply adequate energy and nutrients for their growth. In order to plan appropriate nutritional care it is necessary to have an understanding of the nutrition-related problems these infants face.

Classification of high risk infants

Infants are described as term, preterm, or post-term. Preterm infants are infants who are younger than 38 weeks gestation at birth. Newborns are also classified by their weight in relation to fetal age; they may be large for gestational age (LGA), appropriate for gestational age (AGA), or small for gestational age (SGA). Infants classified for gestational age may be term, preterm, or post-term infants. Preterm and SGA infants are also described as low birth weight (LBW) (those weighing 2500 gm. or less) and very low birth weight (VLBW) (those weighing 1500 gm. or less). *Stressed* newborn is a term used to describe an infant who is ill or who faces stress of any type which he cannot easily handle unaided.

Preterm infants face predictable neonatal problems which influence their nutritional needs. These problems include (1) immaturity of all body systems (notably respiratory, cardiovascular, and gastrointestinal), (2) difficulty regulating body temperature, (3) various metabolic problems (e.g., hypoglycemia), (4) alterations in fluid and electrolyte balance, (5) hyperbilirubinemia (jaundice), and (6) congenital anomalies.

The infant who is small for gestational age faces some problems which are similar to those faced by the preterm infant. However, a SGA infant may be developmentally more mature than a pre-term of the same weight. Because of developmental superiority the SGA infant may tolerate certain stresses better than does the preterm infant. The majority of SGA infants are undernourished. (This may be due to a placental abnormality rather than to the mother's prenatal diet.) They are likely to develop hypoglycemia after birth owing to lack of glycogen stores.

Despite their large size, LGA infants are subject to problems which may confront LBW infants; actually some LGA infants are preterm. The best known condition leading to infants who are large for gestational age is the infant of a diabetic mother.

Nutrition-related problems

Some of the nutrition-related problems high risk infants face are briefly discussed here.

CARDIOVASCULAR AND RESPIRATORY PROBLEMS

Cardiovascular and respiratory problems make it difficult for high risk infants to ingest adequate amounts of food. These infants tire readily. Rapid breathing interferes with sucking and swallowing. Respiratory distress such as seen in hyaline membrane disease predisposes an infant to acidosis. Close attention to maintain acid-base balance and fluid and electrolyte balance may be life saving.

GASTROINTESTINAL IMMATURITY

Immaturity of the gastrointestinal tract limits ingestion, digestion, and absorption of nutrients. Sucking and swallowing reflexes and peristaltic movement are not fully coordinated in preterm infants. Initially the total volume of each feeding must be small because of small stomach capacity. Delayed stomach emptying limits the frequency of feedings for these infants. Preterm infants lose some ingested nutrients as a result of their immature digestive and absorptive systems. Fat absorption may be poor; transitory lactose intolerance may be present. A further complicating problem is an apparent delay in healing of the gastrointestinal tract following trauma to it.[17]

ALTERED METABOLISM

Basal metabolic needs are greater in preterm and SGA infants than in normal newborns. SGA infants also usually show an increase in overall metabolic rate postnatally. The response is similar to that seen in starved infants.[18] Preterm and SGA infants do not have adequate adipose tissue to insulate their bodies from heat loss. Normally deposition of adipose tissue increases after the 34th week of gestation. Thus the younger a preterm infant is, the less likely he is to have adequate fat stores.

Preterm and SGA infants often have very limited glycogen and fat stores to draw on for energy metabolism. After birth energy stores are rapidly expended to maintain body functions. Output of glucose from the neonate's liver depends on adequate glycogen stores and effective activity of enzymes and hormones. Inadequate stores pose a serious threat to the newborn. Hypoglycemia has been linked with damage to the central nervous system. SGA infants also have a relatively increased demand for glucose as a fuel. This is because the brain (which has an absolute requirement for glucose) is more likely to be near normal weight than are other tissues.[19] Utilization of glucose is increased by the neonate's response to cold, stress, acidosis, and hypoxia (inadequate supply of oxygen to body tissues).

Management of hypoglycemia All infants should be closely observed for hypoglycemia. When hypoglycemia is suspected the infant's blood glucose level should be monitored closely since symptoms of hypoglycemia in a neonate are similar to symptoms of many other conditions which may affect these infants. Normal blood glucose levels for term infants are 30 to 125 mg. per 100 ml.; for pre-term infants they are 20 to 100 mg. per 100 ml. If an infant is hypoglycemic, treatment should be initiated promptly. Intravenous administration of glucose is recommended for some infants (such as those of diabetic women). It is important to avoid too fast an infusion rate since it may stimulate increased insulin production which could aggravate the problem. It is helpful to start oral feedings as soon as a hypoglycemic infant can tolerate them. Blood glucose level is very frequently monitored to evaluate the infant's response and to adjust treatment.

FLUID AND ELECTROLYTE BALANCE

The state of fluid and electrolyte balance in high risk infants depends on the maturity of renal function and other regulatory mechanisms. The glomerular filtration rate is lower in pre-term than in term infants. Immature kidneys also have a relatively limited ability to concentrate urine. Thus, excessive amounts of fluid may be lost if the pre-term infant's kidneys are presented with a high renal solute load (an excessive amount of electrolytes and urea which must be excreted). However, LBW infants who are *growing* may tolerate higher protein and electrolyte intake than term infants since some of the "potential" load from intake is diverted into new tissue growth.[20]

Hypocalcemia Hypocalcemia may develop in stressed pre-term infants and in infants of diabetic mothers. It is thought that lowered calcium levels are due to depressed function of the parathyroid gland. After about the fifth to tenth day, neonatal tetany (hypocalcemia) may occur because of the calcium-phosphorous balance in some infant formulas. Low magnesium level frequently accompanies hypocalcemia. Therefore, magnesium level should also be closely monitored.

If required, intravenous calcium should be administered very slowly to prevent bradycardia (slowed heart beat). When oral feedings are possible calcium chloride or calcium lactate may be added to feedings.[19]

Hyperbilirubinemia Hyperbilirubinemia frequently occurs in preterm infants and in infants with hemolytic diseases such as ABO or Rh incompatibility. Level of serum bilirubin may remain elevated longer in preterm than in term infants. Kernicterus (irreversible brain damage) results when bilirubin level remains elevated (16 mg. per 100 ml. or more for preterm infants). Early and adequate gastric feeding is helpful to decrease bilirubin levels. Feeding increases gastrointestinal motility and promotes excretion of bilirubin (a bile pigment) via feces.[21]

Studies such as one conducted by Fisher and co-workers indicate some breast fed infants have higher bilirubin concentrations than bottle fed infants.[22] This is thought to be due to a substance in breast milk which interferes with enzyme activity needed to change (conjugate) bilirubin to an excretable form. Most babies can continue to breast feed. If bilirubin level rises too high, breast feeding may be withheld for a brief period until the bilirubin level drops. The mother who has maintained her supply of breast milk by use of a breast pump or manual expression should have little difficulty resuming breast feeding.

Feeding the high risk infant

Specific techniques of feeding preterm and SGA infants are controversial; data for relative success of various methods is limited. Early and adequate provision of calories and water is an important aspect of therapy for preterm, SGA, and stressed newborns. These infants must be promptly adapted to an adequate supply of nutrients in some form. Their nutrient reserves are often so low that they tolerate even short periods of deprivation poorly.

Many pre-term and SGA infants tolerate oral feedings. Smaller preterms and SGAs or infants who are stressed may need to be fed by tube or parenterally. In some instances, combining various feeding methods is beneficial. Principles for providing nutritional support to the adult apply to the high risk infant; however, details of feeding differ considerably. Each infant should be individually assessed to determine which feeding method is most appropriate for him. Indications that a LBW infant can tolerate gastric feedings include[23] (1) regular, adequate respirations and absence of respiratory distress; (2) adequate bowel sounds and absence of abdominal distention; and (3) acceptance of feedings by the infant with a minimal residual volume on pre-feeding aspiration.

Bottle feeding Infants must have an adequate sucking and swallowing reflex to tolerate bottle feedings. An infant who sucks on a gavage feeding tube may be indicating his readiness to try oral feedings. For the first oral feeding infants are usually given sterile water to minimize problems in case aspiration occurs. After that formula concentration and volume are selected and gradually advanced on an individual basis. Close observation of the infant's toleration of feeding is essential. Use of a soft "preemie" nipple decreases the infant's energy expenditure when sucking. A change in feeding behavior should be reported since it is often an early indication of illness.

If a formula is used for feeding a high risk infant it should be carefully customized to fit the infant's nutritional needs. Commercially prepared formulas are satisfactory for some infants; other infants need specially prepared formulas. Careful attention must be given to the type and distribution of protein, carbohydrates, and fat. In addition, vitamin and mineral supplementation may be critical.

Breast feeding The use of human milk for feeding high risk infants has both advantages and disadvantages. The advantages[24] are (1) protection against infection and necrotizing enterocolitis; (2) low potential renal solute load; (3) high digestibility of fat; and (4) specific composition of proteins and other nitrogenous compounds. Disadvantages[23] are that the protein and mineral content of breast milk may be inadequate to meet the nutritional needs of VLBW infants.

Human milk might be supplemented to provide adequate amounts of nutrients. A recent study suggests that the nitrogen concentration in milk from mothers of preterm infants is higher than that from mothers of term infants. The higher nitrogen intake may be of advantage to a rapidly growing preterm infant.[25] This area needs further investigation.

Another advantage of using breast milk is that it gives the mother an opportunity to participate in her infant's care. Participation in the infant's care may increase a mother's sense of self-worth and her feelings of attachment to the infant.[26]

If an LBW infant is not able to suck and swallow, a mother can express milk from her breast. It is preferable to refrigerate freshly expressed milk and use it within 24 hours. When this is not possible, milk may be frozen. However, both freezing and pasteurization destroy many of the protective components of human milk.[3]

Gastric feeding via gavage   When an infant is unable to suck and swallow, formula or expressed breast milk may be introduced directly into the stomach via gavage. Ziemer and Carrol outline an acceptable method for feeding an infant by gavage.[27] Indwelling nasogastric catheters are not recommended since they are a foreign material and their constant presence stimulates mucus production. Excessive mucus can block the neonate's small airway.

Nasojejunal feeding   Very weak or sick infants who do not tolerate gavage feedings may benefit from naso-jejunal (transpyloric) feedings. A feeding tube is passed through the pylorus into the jejunum and a constant infusion pump is used to provide a small steady supply of formula.[28]

Parenteral feeding   Parenteral feedings are indicated for infants with severe medical and/or surgical problems (e.g., severe respiratory distress, complicated surgical procedures) and for infants who do not tolerate gastric feedings. Peripheral alimentation is safer than total parenteral nutrition but is limited in terms of meeting the infant's nutrient needs. Peripheral intravenous therapy is difficult to initiate and maintain in small babies; an intravenous site may not last much longer than 24 hours. Total parenteral nutrition is still considered investigational when used with VLBW infants. Babson and coworkers recommend that neonates who require extended parenteral alimentation be cared for in regional neonatal centers.[23]

Planning to meet needs   Planning to meet the long term needs of the high risk infant should begin at the time of birth. Encouraging parents to visit their infant and participate in his care promotes parent attachment to the infant. As the infant grows parents can participate in care activities such as feeding. If parents have an opportunity to feed and care for their infant while he is hospitalized, the transition home may be easier.

FOOD ALLERGY AND FOOD SENSITIVITY

Food allergy and food sensitivity are common chronic problems of children, but they can occur at any age. Food allergy may place a child at nutritional risk for several reasons. The allergic reaction imposes a stress on the body. Food intake may be decreased because of avoidance of certain foods or because of malabsorption which sometimes develops secondary to food allergy. Early identification and avoidance of offending foods is an important component of management.

Allergy has an immunological basis. If eating a food causes an allergic reaction, something in the food triggers increased production of antibody (especially immunoglobulin E) in the gut and/or bloodstream. Ordinarily antibodies are viewed as protective but, when allergy is involved, the antigen-antibody combination results in an inappropriate inflammatory response.

The most common signs and symptoms of food allergy include urticaria (skin rash); eczema; rhinitis (runny nose); severe swelling of face, mouth, and throat; and asthma. A life-threatening condition called anaphylactic shock is the most serious type of allergic reaction, but anaphylaxis is rarely associated with food allergy. There may be many nonspecific signs and symptoms of food allergy, including gastro-intestinal problems, headache, and irritability. The vagueness of these symptoms sometimes makes it difficult to determine if they are really caused by an allergy.

If a food causes a person to experience adverse reactions but no immunological disturbance is involved, the term "food intolerance" (e.g., lactose intolerance) or food sensitivity is more appropriate.[29]

There are several distinctive features of allergy and allergic reaction which influence diagnosis and treatment:

1. Allergic reactions may appear at different rates.

POINTS OF EMPHASIS
Nutritional care of high risk infants

• *Many body systems of the pre-term are immature and limit normal intake and utilization of food.*

• *High risk infants often have inadequate energy stores and high metabolic demands.*

• *Body surface area and immaturity of the kidneys place some neonates at risk of becoming dehydrated.*

• *Early and adequate provision of nutrients, energy, and water is an important aspect of nutritional care for the high risk infant.*

• *High risk infants may be fed orally, by gavage, nasojejunally, or parenterally.*

• *Feeding options for the high risk infant include customized formula and human milk.*

Sometimes the effect of an antigen is immediate (immediate hypersensitivity) and sometimes it is delayed for hours or even several days (delayed hypersensitivity). The frequency and severity of allergic manifestations may be influenced by physical and emotional stress.

2. The amount of antigen required to stimulate an observable adverse reaction varies. In some people allergy becomes apparent only if a larger-than-normal serving of the food or ingredient is eaten.

3. Foods which belong to the same botanical group may contain the same or similar antigens; therefore, related foods may trigger the same allergic response in the same person. For example, onions, garlic, leeks, and asparagus are among members of the lily family. If a child is allergic to one, he may be allergic to all. When this is true, eating two related foods together might cause an allergic reaction, whereas eating a small serving of either food alone might not.

4. The same food may cause different signs and symptoms in different allergic individuals.

5. Since immune responses are genetically controlled, allergy tends to run in families.

6. The amount and combining power of antibodies which are formed by exposure to antigens may change over time. Thus, it is possible for a child to lose his allergy to a food as he grows older.

If food allergy is suspected, the recommended diagnostic procedure includes food history, elimination of suspected foods, and challenge with suspected foods.

FOOD HISTORY

A careful, detailed food history often provides strong clues regarding foods or ingredients which are responsible for allergic reactions. The client or parents are asked to keep a diet diary during a period of normal food intake. This diet diary includes a listing of every food eaten, the amount consumed, and the time it was eaten. Clients should record brand names and they should be prepared to provide the health professional with recipes which were used. The client also keeps a chart of adverse reactions, specifying date, time of onset, intensity, and duration of symptoms. When instructing a client or his family about keeping these records, it is essential for the health care worker to emphasize the importance of including every detail and to teach individuals to record the information in an understandable manner. Guided practice in using the forms is sometimes desirable. Children who have independent access to food need to be involved in the data collection process.

A health professional experienced in allergy reviews the records and determines what type of elimination diet will be most appropriate for the client. If the records are strongly suggestive that one or two foods or ingredients are involved they may be the only foods eliminated from the diet.

ELIMINATION OF SUSPECTED FOODS

If no foods can be singled out as probable allergens despite the history, a more restricted elimination diet such as one of Rowe's elimination diets[30] might be used. Some elimination diets are nutritionally incomplete because of the large number of foods which are eliminated. Health professionals may need to recommend appropriate nutritional supplements to assure adequate intake; it may take quite a while before the client can advance to a more normal varied diet.

An allergic person has to follow an elimination diet very carefully if it is to be of any value. Health professionals may need to spell out what definitely can be eaten. They should also teach about label reading to make sure that the client does not inadvertently eat an ingredient which is supposed to be eliminated. Use of fresh foods simplifies food selection. Parents appreciate assistance in planning nutritionally adequate, satisfying meals, particularly if the food to be avoided is commonly found in many prepared foods. Written instructions about foods which can be eaten and foods to avoid are helpful. A diet counselor can provide recipes for items which will allow increased variety, for example egg-free or milk-free baked goods. She may also identify brands or types of foods which are safe.

Ideally, if the client follows the elimination diet, there will be relief from symptoms within a week or two. If relief is not prompt, doesn't last, or is questionable for other reasons, a search for another cause usually is in order.[31]

CHALLENGE WITH SUSPECTED FOODS

If an elimination diet has brought relief to the client, the client is systematically challenged by adding foods which are suspect. The client remains on the elimination diet and one food is added at a time, initially in small amounts but working up to a normal portion if no signs or symptoms develop. The period of observation when a new food is added ranges from 4 days to 1 week. If signs and symptoms develop, the challenging food is no longer eaten. If the food was to blame, the symptoms should subside once more. Before this food is definitely identified as an allergen, it should be given two more times in a similar manner, with intervals between each challenge period. (Caution is necessary if the reaction is severe.)

TREATMENT

After an allergy-causing food or ingredient has been identified, treatment involves eliminating that substance from the diet. The family may need more assistance with planning a varied, well-balanced diet and with dealing with food-related behavior problems. Health professionals can develop teaching tools and techniques to aid children in learning to identify and

TABLE 34.1 *Types of food and food ingredients most commonly associated with allergic reactions and examples of hidden sources of these foods*[31-35]

FOOD TYPE	POSSIBLE HIDDEN SOURCES
Milk in any form	Bread, pudding, cream soups, most bakery products, sherbet, some gravies, many mixes, butter, margarine, some hot dogs and bologna
Eggs, especially egg white	Mayonnaise, breaded foods, cakes, cookies, custard, some ice cream, noodles, noodle soup, meatloaf, spun soybean protein used in meat analogs, candies, meringue
Wheat, sometimes other small grains	Bakery products, breaded foods, pasta, many soups, some puddings and gravies, mixes, stuffing, some hot dogs and bologna, some textured vegetable protein
Citrus fruit, especially oranges	Some fruit desserts, some types of punch
Kola nut family	Chocolate, cocoa, cola beverages
Corn	Corn cereals including hominy and grits, Cracker Jacks, corn chips and other corn snack foods, tortillas, and certain other Mexican foods. Foods containing refined corn products such as corn syrup, corn starch, corn flour, corn oil may cause problems in persons allergic to corn
Legumes	Peanut butter; foods containing soy protein, soy flour or perhaps soybean oil; assorted soups; licorice
Tomato	Meatloaf, stews, and other prepared dishes
Spices, especially cinnamon	Catsup, baked goods, candy, chewing gum, various prepared dishes
Food colors, especially tartrazine (FD & C Yellow No. 5)	Soft drinks, candy, pudding, frosting, colored breakfast cereals, and other artificially colored foods; many medications
Nuts	Candy, bakery products, granola
Fish, meat, bananas	Identity is usually apparent

gracefully refuse foods which might harm them.[32] In some cases, all traces of the allergen must be avoided if the client is to remain symptom-free, but this is not always necessary. For example, a child may need to avoid eating a whole egg but not a bakery product made with egg. Some people who develop relatively mild allergic reactions to a well-liked food choose to eat the food occasionally and suffer the consequences.

There is general agreement that milk (excluding human milk) is the leading cause of food allergy.

POINTS OF EMPHASIS
Dietary management of food allergy and sensitivity

- *Allergy is the result of an inappropriate antibody-antigen reaction.*
- *Parents and/or clients can keep an accurate diet history to aid in diagnosis.*
- *If the diet history indicates particular foods appear to be allergenic, these foods are eliminated from the diet for a week or more.*
- *If on three occasions reintroduction of the food produces allergic manifestations, diagnosis is confirmed.*
- *Once allergy-causing foods are identified, treatment requires avoidance of the food.*
- *Clients and family often need detailed instructions to plan nutritious meals while avoiding offending foods.*

There is little sound evidence upon which to rank other causes of food allergy. Table 34.1 lists foods which one or more allergists have reported to be common food allergens and identifies possible hidden sources of these ingredients.

Hyperactivity

Hyperactive or hyperkinetic children are described as restless, emotionally labile, and having a short attention span. Parents of hyperactive children are eager to find a cure because the children pose serious management problems and may be slow learners in school. Health professionals should realize that accurate diagnosis of hyperactivity is difficult and that some people confuse the normal activity of healthy children (especially of boys) with hyperactivity.

In 1973, Feingold[36] proposed a method of treating hyperactive children by dietary means. He claimed that about 40 percent of hyperactive children would improve if they followed his diet recommendations. In brief, the Feingold diet eliminates artificial color, artificial flavor, the food additives BHA and BHT, and a number of foods (such as orange juice, apples, and tomatoes) which are reported to contain natural salicylates. As long as the Feingold diet is carefully planned to contain adequate amounts of vitamin C and folic acid, food restrictions should not interfere with meeting nutrient requirements.

The Feingold diet has been the subject of considerable controversy, especially since the original claims were not supported by conclusive evidence of its effectiveness. Many parents who use the diet for a hyperactive child strongly feel that the diet works. The suggestion has been made that the placebo effect is at work when parents place a hyperactive child on the diet.[37,38]

Results of double-blind crossover tests indicate that the diet may benefit a small proportion of hyperactive children, especially preschoolers, but there is no known way to predict which children will benefit.[39,40] Even though there is no convincing evidence of the Feingold diet's widespread effectiveness, there seems to be no pressing reason to advise families to discontinue the diet if they think it is helpful.[37]

Some hyperactive children are treated with stimulant drugs such as dextroamphetamine and methylphenidate. Special attention to nutrition may be beneficial. Stimulant drugs may interfere with normal growth in children,[41] probably because of decreased caloric intake.[42] Serving small frequent meals and offering breakfast in the morning before medication may improve food intake.

STUDY QUESTIONS

1. Nancy J., a 16-year old, just delivered an infant in a health care facility. This is her first contact with health care workers. List several ways of establishing a positive relationship with Nancy. Identify several topics for nutritional counseling which might be of benefit to Nancy and her infant. Why would it be desirable to assess Nancy's nutrition-related needs before providing diet counseling?

2. Why is early and close nutritional care an essential component of health care for a pregnant woman who has diabetes mellitus?

3. Ms. J., the mother of a preterm infant, states she wishes she could breast feed her infant. The physician states her infant could be fed breast milk by gavage now, and later (when the infant is bigger and stronger) he could breast feed. Outline a plan to help Ms. J. successfully provide breast milk for her infant now and breast feed her infant when he is larger.

4. John, who is allergic to strawberries, asks why he can eat some foods which contain strawberry flavoring. What would you tell him?

5. List guidelines you would give to a school-aged child and his parents who are being asked to keep a food diary to help determine whether or not the child has any food allergies.

References

*1. Worthington, B., Vermeersch, J., and Williams, S.: *Nutrition in Pregnancy.* St. Louis: C. V. Mosby Co., 1977.

2. Long, P. A.: Importance of abnormal glucose tolerance (hypoglycaemia and hyperglycaemia) in etiology of preeclampsia. *Lancet* 1:923, 1977.

*3. Moore, M. L.: *Realities in Childbearing.* St. Louis: C. V. Mosby Co., 1978.

4. Snowman, M.: Nutrition component in a comprehensive child development program, Part II. Nutrient intakes of low-income, pregnant women and the outcome of pregnancy. *J. Am. Diet Assoc.* 74:124, 1979.

5. Chachere, N.: The diet of pregnant teenagers. *J. Home Econ.* 68:43, 1976.

6. Snow, L. F., and Johnson, S. M.: Folklore, food and female reproductive cycle. *Ecol. Food Nutrition* 7:41, 1978.

7. Teenage Pregnancy Everybody's Problem. DHEW Public Health Service, Health Services Administration DHEW Pub. No. (HSA) 77-5619. Washington DC: U.S. Govt. Printing Office, 1977.

8. King, J., et al.: Assessment of nutritional status of teenage pregnant girls. 1. Nutrition intake and pregnancy. *Am. J. Clin. Nutr.* 25:916, 1972.

9. Huyck, N.: Nutrition Services for pregnant teenagers. *J. Am. Diet Assoc.* 69:60, 1976.

10. Seiler, J. A., and Fox, H. M.: Adolescent pregnancy: Association of dietary and obstetric factors. *Home Econ. Res. J.* 1:188, 1973.

*11. Phillips, M.: Food for the teenager during pregnancy. DHEW Public Health Service Administration, Bureau of Community Health Services, Office of Maternal and Child Health. DHEW Pub. No. (HSA) 77-5106, Rockville MD 1977.

*12. Rees, J.: *Inside My Mom.* Audiovisual with teaching manual, White Plains NY: National Foundation March of Dimes, 1975.

13. Felig, P., and Tyson, J.: Diabetes in pregnancy—Discovering gestational diabetes. *Patient Care* 9(15): 26, 1975.

14. Mintz, D., Skyler, J., and Chez, R.: Diabetes mellitus and pregnancy. *Diabetes Care* 1:49, 1978.

15. Churchill, J. A., Berendes, H. W., and Nemrore, J.: Neurophysiological deficits in children of diabetic mothers. *Am. J. Obstet. Gynecol.* 105:257, 1969.

*16. Felig, P., and Tyson, J.: Managing diabetes and pregnancy together, *Patient Care* 9(15):36, 1975.

*17. Richard, K., and Gresham, E.: Nutritional considerations for the newborn requiring intensive care. *J. Am. Diet Assoc.* 66:592, 1975.

*18. Sinclair, J. C., et al.: Supportive management of the sick neonate. *Pediatr. Clin. North Am.* 17(1):863, 1970.

*19. Korones, S.: *High Risk Newborn Infants,* ed. 2. St. Louis: C. V. Mosby Co., 1976.

20. Ziegler, E. E., and Ryw, J. E.: Renal solute and diet in growing premature infants. *J. Pediatr.* 89:609, 1976.

*21. Neonatal jaundice. *Pediat. Nurs. Currents* 23(2): 1, 1976.

22. Fisher, A., et al.: Jaundice and breast feeding among Alaskan Eskimo newborns. *Am. J. Dis. Child* 132:859, 1978.

*23. Babson, S. G., et al.: *Management of High-Risk Pregnancy and Intensive Care of the Neonate.* St. Louis: C. V. Mosby Co., 1975.

24. Fomon, S. J., Ziegler, E. E., Vasquez, H. D.: Human milk and the small premature infant. *Am. J. Dis. Child.* 131:463, 1977.

25. Atkinson, S. A., Bryan, M. H., and Anderson, G. H.: Human milk: Difference in nitrogen concentration in milk from mothers of term and premature infants. *J. Pediatr.* 93:67, 1978.

26. Choi, M.: Breast milk for infants who can't breast feed. *Am. J. Nurs.* 78:852, 1978.

*27. Ziemer, M., and Carroll, J.: Infant gavage reconsidered. *Am. J. Nurs.* 78:1543, 1978.

*28. Price, E., and Gyotoker, S.: Using the nasojejunal feeding technique in a neonatal intensive care unit. *MCN* 3:361, 1978.

* Recommended reading

29. May, C. D.: Food allergy: A commentary. *Pediatr. Clin. North Am.* 22(1):217, 1975.

30. Rowe, A. H.: *Food Allergy. Its Manifestations and Control and the Elimination Diets. A Compendium.* Springfield IL: Charles C Thomas Co., 1972.

31. May, C. D.: Food allergy. In S. Foman (ed.): *Infant Nutrition.* Philadelphia: W. B. Saunders Co., 1974.

32. Bergner, M., and Hutelmyer, C.: Teaching kids how to live with their allergies. *Nursing '76* 6(8):11, 1976.

33. Speer, F.: Food allergy: The 10 common offenders. *Am. Fam. Phys.* 13:106, 1976.

34. Eade, O. E., and Wright, R.: Dietary hypersensitivity: the gastroenterologist's view. *J. Human Nutr.* 30:157, 1976.

35. Zlollow, M. J., and Settipane, G. A.: Allergic potential of food additives: A report of a case of tartrazine sensitivity without aspirin intolerance. *Am. J. Clin. Nutr.* 30:1023, 1977.

36. Feingold, B. F.: *Why Your Child is Hyperactive.* New York: Random House, 1975.

*37. Wender, E. H.: Food additives and hyperkinesis. *Am. J. Dis. Child.* 131:1204, 1977.

38. Larkin, T.: Food additives and hyperactive children. *FDA Consumer* 11(2):19, 1977.

39. Harley, J. P., et al.: Hyperkinesis and food additives: Testing the Feingold hypothesis. *Pediatrics* 61:818, 1978.

40. Bierman, C. W., and Furukawa, C. T.: Food additive and hyperkinesis: Are there nuts among the berries? *Pediatrics* 61:932, 1978.

41. Safer, D. J., and Allen, R. P.: "Factors influencing the suppressant effects of two stimulant drugs on the growth of hyperactive children. *Pediatrics* 51:660, 1973.

42. Lucus, B., and Sells, C. J.: Nutrient intake and stimulant drugs in children. *J. Am. Diet. Assoc.* 70:373, 1977.

* Recommended reading.

35

Care of clients with other special nutritional needs Part 2

The topics discussed in this chapter—nutritional care of clients with burns, cardiac disorders, neurological disturbances, and mental disturbances—have no strong connecting links. Each of the conditions affects many Americans; each condition benefits from different kinds of nutritional care measures. The topics covered serve to illustrate various ways the nutritional care process can be applied to meet the sometimes complex needs of clients in different settings. It is important for health professionals to note that, in several of the examples, special attention to nutrition is desirable even though there may be no need for a modified diet. By being alert for conditions which alter nutritional needs and by dealing with them knowledgeably, health professionals can improve the quality of health care.

THERMALLY INJURED PERSONS

Effects of burns on nutritional status

Of all the stresses that humans may experience, *extensive* thermal injury has the most dramatic and sustained impact on nutritional status. Other forms of severe trauma (e.g., crushing injuries or major surgical procedures if they are followed by sepsis) may have similar effects on nutritional status. Therefore, many nutritional care measures which are recommended for burned clients are appropriate for clients experiencing other forms of trauma.

Burns produce a hypermetabolic state characterized by (1) increased heat production and elevated body temperature, (2) increased energy (calorie) expendi-

ture, (3) heightened protein catabolism with negative nitrogen balance and rapid loss of lean body mass, and (4) an above-normal rate of anabolism (once the healing process begins). Without good nutritional care, even a previously well-nourished person with extensive burns may quickly develop severe protein-energy malnutrition.

The degree to which metabolic rate increases is proportional to the total body surface (TBS).[1] The deeper the burn the greater the increase in metabolic rate and the longer a hypermetabolic state is sustained. The metabolic rate reaches its peak 6 to 10 days postburn and remains high for several weeks or longer. Coverage of burned surface by grafting and healing results in gradual return to normal metabolic rate.

The amount of calories required by a thermally injured person can be estimated using any one of several formulas. (Most health agencies have approved the use of a specific one.) A suggested formula for estimating calorie requirements is shown below.[2]

$$\text{Total energy requirement} = (25 \times \text{ideal body weight}) + (40 \times \% \text{ TBS burned})$$

The hypermetabolic state is not the only cause for nutritional concerns in thermally injured persons. Losses and shifts of fluid and electrolytes demand immediate attention to prevent life-threatening hypovolemia. Exudates from open wounds result in loss of protein, fluid, and electrolytes from the body.

Estimation of protein requirement of thermally injured persons is based on usual protein requirements with an adjustment made for the extent of injury, the amount of exudation, and (if indicated) the need to correct preexisting malnutrition. Usually the recommended protein intake falls within the range of two to four times the individual's RDA for protein.[2] It is important for health care providers to remember that the protein supplied is of limited value unless caloric needs are also met.

Adequate intake of protein and calories is essential for reasons unique to thermal injury. In particular, it favors formation of healthy granulation tissue (of third degree burns), normal epithelialization of second degree burns, "taking" of grafts, and healing of donor sites.[2] Protein is also necessary to maintain body defenses against infection, a serious and frequent complication of burn wounds. If infection develops, the nutritional stress experienced by the burned person is magnified and intensive nutritional support becomes even more essential to the client's survival. Since recovery is slow (requiring many weeks) under the best of conditions, every effort should be made to provide enough protein and fuel to promote the healing process.

The health team should also give attention to the burned client's need for micronutrients. An elevated metabolic rate increases requirements for many of the B complex vitamins. These vitamins are needed to act as coenzymes to promote optimal use of protein and fuel. Thermal injury appears to increase excretion of some micronutrients (e.g., zinc).[3] Anabolic processes, including wound healing, increase the need for vitamin C and for a wide variety of other vitamins and of mineral cofactors. It is customary to give supplements of vitamins (including perhaps 1 to 2 gm. of vitamin C daily[4]), iron, and perhaps zinc. Calcium and phosphate supplements are seldom needed unless the person receives all nourishment parenterally.

Just when the body is faced with extraordinary nutrient requirements, gastrointestinal function is initially impaired by the extreme stress posed by thermal injury. Narcotics and sedatives may contribute to impaired appetite and depressed intestinal function.

In time, appetite and food tolerance usually improve, but spontaneous food intake is not likely to exceed the client's usual intake during health; this is generally insufficient to maintain satisfactory nutritional status unless the burn is quite small. Supplemental oral or tube feedings are usually needed to prevent excessive weight loss. Intravenous feeding may be required as well. If 40 percent or more of TBS is burned, intensive nutritional support including parenteral feedings is almost always desirable.[7]

Planning and monitoring nutritional care of burned persons

Nutritional care of a thermally injured person must be carefully planned and monitored and not left to chance. A team approach is essential. All team members should be aware of how their own responsibilities fit into the total scheme of nutritional care and of how the client is responding to different care measures.

A realistic weight goal should be set for the client. Although weight maintenance would seem to be desirable, in most cases it is impossible to achieve. Usually the aim is to prevent the client from losing more than 10 percent of his body weight.[5] If more weight is lost, the chance of complications accelerates. If the client was malnourished at the time of injury, it may be advisable to go to greater effort to limit weight loss.

Routine weighing of the client under *uniform* conditions is of utmost importance in making sure that the amount of nourishment provided is adequate to prevent the client's weight from falling below his weight limit. However, weighing a burned person may give deceptive results, especially in the early postburn period, because fluid retention often masks loss of lean body mass. Thus other means of nutritional assessment are also employed.

Careful recording of all food intake is of value for at least two reasons. (1) The dietitian uses food intake records to calculate actual caloric intake (calorie count) and compares this value to weight status and to recommended calorie intake. If the client is losing weight despite consuming the recommended amount, increased food or some other form of nutritional support is required. If food intake is well below recommended intake, improved nutritional care measures need to be instituted. (2) The dietitian uses food intake records to calculate the client's nitrogen intake. By comparing actual nitrogen intake with 24-hour urine urea nitrogen output for the same period of time, the state of nitrogen balance can be roughly estimated.

Standard measures for detecting the development of protein-energy malnutrition may be inappropriate for ongoing assessment of the nutritional status of thermally injured persons. Serum albumin level is likely to be a poor indicator of the adequacy of nutrient intake because blood transfusions are commonly given and because fluid balance often shifts when a person is burned. Anthropometric measures other than height/weight may be impossible to obtain or they may be highly inaccurate. Thus, weight and food intake records are of great importance.

ACHIEVING ADEQUATE NUTRIENT INTAKE BY MOUTH

When the oral route can be used, competent health professionals make every effort to assist burned persons to meet their increased nutritional needs in a comfortable and enjoyable manner. The health team tries to obtain a complete list of the client's food preferences and to record observations of the client's response to different foods. Adjustments in menu are made when indicated. If possible, health care workers enlist the aid of the burned person's family and friends when his intake of hospital food is low but his gastrointestinal function is relatively normal. A favorite homemade casserole or a big cheeseburger from a fast food chain may help to spark his appetite. The health team plans to make well-liked food available any time the burned person might be able to eat it. Commercial supplements may be useful for providing lots of calories and protein in a small volume, but some clients eat better if offered nutrient-rich, high calorie foods to which they are accustomed. (A burned person should be warned to drink rich beverages slowly, since digestion may be subnormal.)

If eating is painful because of burns of the face, adjustment of consistency of foods may be helpful. If a thermally injured person cannot use his hands or arms, it is especially important for health care workers to make pleasant, unhurried arrangements for feeding him. Health professionals may need to encourage the client to use his arms, hands, and facial muscles during mealtime even though the movement is painful. Movement is an important means of maintaining joint function. A firm but understanding approach is helpful.

Adults and children may have much trouble coping with painful or otherwise stressful treatment measures such as debridement (removal of necrotic tissue from the wound), dressing changes, physical therapy to prevent contractures, and immobilization of a body part to restrict motion after grafting. These necessary procedures may lead to manipulative behavior. For example, adults and children alike may refuse to eat unless they "get their way." Clients may be less likely to manipulate through food if they are allowed control over other aspects of their care. They might be allowed to set the time when the dressing change is to be done. If a client tries to be manipulative about food anyway, health team members all try to handle the problem with consistent firmness.

The stress associated with a distorted body image may result in severe depression and may further interfere with appetite. Because nurses are in close, frequent contact with a burned client, they are in a good position to communicate with the client in ways which contribute to a sense of self-esteem and of being accepted by others. Nurses and other health team members may help family and friends deal with their discomfort in looking at the burned person. Team conferences may be a good means of developing improved strategies of nutritional care.

Burned children may not feel hungry or may not begin to follow a relatively normal eating pattern for a considerable period of time. They are likely to regress behaviorally (act much younger than their age) shortly after being burned. This regressive behavior may persist for weeks—until skin coverage is nearly complete.[6]

Because so many features of thermal injury and its treatment interfere with adequate food intake, nurses contribute to the client's nutritional support by organizing care to minimize these problems. They arrange schedules so that meals will not be missed and so that the most painful periods do not coincide with mealtime. They take steps to be sure that the prescribed exercise program is followed, not only to prevent contractures but also to promote positive nitrogen balance. This is especially important if an air fluidized bed or water bed is being used. By reducing weight bearing, use of these beds may hasten loss of lean body mass unless exercise is used to compensate.[1]

When thermally injured persons are given high calorie liquid supplements, tube feedings, or parenteral nutrient solutions they may be quite vulnerable to problems such as dumping syndrome, osmotic diarrhea, and glucose intolerance, especially when special feedings are first introduced. Often it takes about ten days to safely work up to adequate nutrient intake. Stress-induced hyperglycemia is frequently seen in thermally injured persons; it usually requires treatment with insulin. Burned persons should be very carefully monitored to guard against development of serious fluid and electrolyte imbalances and hyperglycemic hyperosmotic nonketotic coma (HHNK).

POINTS OF EMPHASIS
Nutritional care of persons with thermal injury

- *Extensive burns greatly increase requirements for calories and protein. Failure to meet these needs rapidly results in serious complications.*
- *Increased requirements for micronutrients are met by food and by selected supplements.*
- *Lack of appetite and/or impaired gastrointestinal function often seriously limits food intake of burned clients.*
- *Routine weighing and recording of food intake are essential for determining the need to adjust nutritional care. Intensive nutritional support should be used to prevent weight loss from exceeding 10 percent of ideal or preburn weight.*

CLIENTS WITH CARDIAC DISORDERS

When any condition seriously impairs the heart's ability to function, diet modifications are an important part of overall client care. This section of the chapter identifies diet modifications which may be useful in treating persons with cardiac conditions. More importantly, it highlights reasons *why* specific modifications are used and ways in which care might be adapted to meet the unique psychological needs of clients with cardiac disorders.

Priority goals of treatment of a person with an acute heart condition include reducing the workload of the heart, improving cardiac output, restoring or maintaining a balance of electrolytes which favors coordinated heart muscle activity, and promoting the client's comfort and relieving his anxiety. During the subacute and rehabilitative phases, additional goals also become important. These include maintenance of adequate nutrient intake and perhaps dietary control of hypertension and hyperlipidemia. Measures used to achieve goals of treatment vary according to the client's immediate clinical condition, any accompany-

TABLE 35.1 *Possible diet progression for a 40-year-old male of desirable body weight who has had a myocardial infarction*

ACUTE PHASE
First day of oral feedings
  Clear liquids and skim milk
  No caffeine*
  Limit fluids to 1200 ml
  Avoid extremes of temperature
  Sodium restriction if needed

SUBACUTE PHASE
Beginning the second day of feedings, if arrhythmias are not a problem
  1000 to 1200 kcal, fat and cholesterol controlled, 5 small meals, soft (caffeine restricted, sodium restriction if needed)
Gradual increase in intake

REHABILITATION PHASE
Diet order for discharge instruction
  Moderate fat and cholesterol controlled diet (pending blood lipid determinations)—3–4 gm sodium
  Caffeine restricted

*Decaffeinated coffee may be allowed.

ing disease conditions, the type and extent of damage to the heart, and the type of drug therapy used. Guidelines for nutritional care postmyocardial infarction and in severe congestive heart failure are illustrated in Tables 35.1 and 35.2.

Specific details of nutritional care are presented in the following section. Some nutritional care measures have been arbitrarily placed under a particular goal of care; health care workers should realize that many measures serve more than one purpose.

REDUCING THE WORKLOAD OF THE HEART

Although absolute rest for the heart is impossible, several nutritional care measures may substantially reduce the workload of the heart. The three most effective ways are to keep the size of meals small, to reduce

TABLE 35.2 *Example of progression of diet for an obese person in severe congestive heart failure (CHF) (Drugs include Digoxin and Lasix)*

Initial diet order:
  500 mg Na, 1000 cc fluid restriction
  ±4 gm K,* small feedings, soft (as tolerated)
Diet order following diuresis and stabilization of condition:
  1000 mg Na, ±4 gm K,* soft, caloric intake to achieve weight loss of 0.5 kg (1#) per week
Diet order for discharge instruction:
  2 gm Na, high potassium
  Referral to clinic for behavior modification program for weight reduction

*This notation is used to signify increased potassium intake. Exact amount is not rigidly controlled.

to ideal body weight (if necessary), and to eliminate excess body fluid. Small meals also minimize the chance of abdominal distention. Increased pressure on the heart (which might result from stomach or intestinal distention) could perhaps interfere with cardiac activity and output.

In order to avoid distention, cardiac clients are usually advised to avoid high fiber foods. It is also advisable for a person with a heart condition to avoid constipation and straining at stool. Frequent use of cooked fruits and vegetables may be a satisfactory compromise.

Loss of excess body weight gradually reduces cardiac workload by (1) decreasing the amount of tissue that must be supplied with blood and by (2) decreasing the amount of work required to move the body. Any sound low calorie diet which is used to accomplish weight loss also has an immediate beneficial effect because it reduces the need for extra cardiac output to cover the processes of digestion and absorption.

Loss of excess body fluid reduces the workload on the heart by reducing the amount of fluid which must be pumped and by decreasing body weight.

IMPROVING (OR AVOIDING INTERFERENCE WITH) CARDIAC OUTPUT

One aspect of diet that may interfere with normal cardiac output is the consumption of caffeine-containing beverages. The type of stimulation provided by caffeine and related compounds might contribute to spontaneous ventricular fibrillation in a damaged heart, especially early in the convalescent period following a myocardial infarction.[7] Decaffeinated coffee, cereal-based hot beverages, or herb tea can be substituted for coffee if desired. Gingerale, other noncola carbonated beverages, or fruit juices could be substituted for cola. The extent of the caffeine restriction should be specified by the physician.

Temporarily limiting the diet to fluids may help clients who have had a myocardial infarction, especially if they are subject to arrhythmias. There is less chance of choking on liquids. Choking may reflexively stimulate the vagus, triggering arrhythmias.[8]

A controversial aspect of care involves the temperature at which foods and beverages are served to persons who have had a myocardial infarction. It has been common practice when caring for patients post-MI to avoid offering foods or fluids which are very cold or very hot. By avoiding extremes of temperature it is hoped that risk of developing arrhythmias is lessened. However, a controlled study by Houser[9] indicates that ice water can be safely given on the third and fourth days post-MI. Similarly, Cohen and associates[10] report that hot decaffeinated coffee (70° C.) and cold water (7° C.) appear to cause no physiological problems in the first 36 hours following admission for an acute MI. Nevertheless, health care workers should check the agency's policy regarding extremes of temperature.

RESTORING AND MAINTAINING ELECTROLYTE BALANCE

Care directed toward restoring and maintaining electrolyte balance should be highly individualized. Many people automatically associate sodium restriction with heart disease, but heart disease is not always accompanied by edema or hypertension. In fact, persons who have experienced a myocardial infarction sometimes lose excessive amounts of sodium and may be vulnerable to hypovolemic shock if sodium intake is restricted. Thus, competent health professionals accurately collect and record data needed to determine the appropriate level of sodium intake. Correction of hyponatremia in persons with congestive heart failure usually requires fluid restriction rather than an increase in sodium intake.

When there is a problem with cardiac function, health professionals must remain on the alert for signs of potassium imbalance. Too high or too low a level of serum potassium may seriously impair the activity of the heart, especially if the client is being treated with digitalis.

PROMOTING COMFORT AND RELIEVING ANXIETY

If a person's heart is not pumping normally, he is likely to experience many distressing and frightening symptoms. Dyspnea (shortness of breath) is one of the more common problems experienced by clients with cardiac disorders. Eating and/or abdominal distention worsen dyspnea. Eating itself is a chore if a person is very short of breath (e.g., a result of pulmonary edema). Nutritional care is adjusted as necessary to allow breathing to remain as normal as possible. This usually involves serving small, easy-to-eat meals. Ideally, care is planned so that energy is conserved for self-feeding and so that a rest period can follow the meal.

Although self-feeding expends energy, clients are usually allowed to feed themselves, even during the first meals after a myocardial infarction. Most clients prefer to feed themselves, and evidence suggests that this activity has no ill effects.[11] It is less anxiety-provoking for most clients to be allowed some control over their body activities than being made completely dependent on others. If a client's activity must be quite restricted, health care workers can simplify self-feeding by opening cartons and cutting meat. A person with congestive heart failure may be encouraged to perform simple tasks such as self-feeding as a means of promoting venous return to the heart.

People who have a cardiac problem are likely to become very worried if they experience pain in the epigastric region. It can be difficult (and dangerous) to try to distinguish indigestion from chest pain that is related to heart disease. For this reason persons who have had a myocardial infarction or have severe angina are usually encouraged to temporarily avoid foods which have caused them digestive problems.[12] This is a highly individual matter; it is inappropriate to use one list of food restrictions for all clients.

A fat controlled diet may help to relieve anxiety of some clients who have cardiac disorders associated with coronary artery disease. Following such a diet might help them feel that they are taking a positive step to slow the atherosclerotic process and to reduce the coagulability of their blood. A limited study is suggestive that a vegan diet may help reduce symptoms of angina.[13] Actual benefits of either a fat controlled or vegan diet for clients with coronary heart disease are uncertain. If prescribed, care should be taken that the diet itself does not result in a high anxiety level.

The anxiety which is commonly felt by persons who have a cardiac condition needs to be considered when providing them with food and when counseling them about recommended dietary adjustments. If the meal pattern is unusual (e.g., five very small meals daily) or a restriction is new to a client (e.g., sodium restriction), it helps to let the client know ahead of time and to give both a simple verbal and written explanation. Psychological reactions to a severe cardiac disorder influence how and when teaching is instituted. Even if the affected person appears to be calm and states that he is feeling fine, he may be experiencing physiological changes associated with the stress response. Teaching often needs to be delayed until the client is receptive.

POINTS OF EMPHASIS
Nutritional care of persons with cardiac disorders

• *Keeping meal size small and losing excess weight and fluid help to ease the workload of the heart.*

• *Avoiding caffeine may help to prevent undesirable stimulation of the heart following a myocardial infarction.*

• *Avoiding extremes of temperature and taking liquids rather than solid foods may help avoid arrhythmias in the acute phase following a myocardial infarction.*

• *Restoring and maintaining electrolyte balance promotes optimal cardiac function. Safe use of digitalis preparations requires careful regulation of serum potassium level.*

• *Avoiding indigestion, distention, and constipation helps relieve possible sources of anxiety and may help keep cardiac function stable.*

• *Nutritional care should include measures to provide cardiac clients with extra reassurance and emotional support.*

• *Diet instruction should include recommendations for adjustments needed because of drug therapy.*

TABLE 35.3 *Relationships of nutrition with drugs commonly used for treating cardiac patients*

TYPE OF DRUG	EXAMPLES OF RELATIONSHIPS TO NUTRITION AND NUTRITIONAL STATUS	RECOMMENDED NUTRITIONAL CARE MEASURES
Cardiac drugs		
Digitalis and its glycosides (Digoxin, Digitoxin)	May promote diuresis. May increase urinary excretion of magnesium.	Promote adequate intake of potassium and magnesium.
	May become toxic if serum potassium level is abnormally high or low.	Monitor serum potassium and magnesium levels.
	Produces gastrointestinal symptoms when potentially toxic levels accumulate in serum	Promptly report gastrointestinal symptoms
Propranolol (Inderal)	May cause nausea, vomiting, mild diarrhea, or constipation	Report symptoms
Anticoagulants		
Heparin	Long term therapy may lead to osteoporosis.	Special attention appears to be generally unnecessary. Occasionally special mouth care and soft diet needed
	Mucous membranes lining GI tract may bleed easily	
Coumarins such as warfarin (Coumadin)	Competes with vitamin K.	Avoid large servings of vitamin K rich foods such as dark-green leafy vegetables, cauliflower. Avoid high fat intake and excessive alcohol consumption[14]
	May occasionally result in nausea, vomiting, diarrhea, ulcers of the mouth	
Aspirin	Frequently causes gastrointestinal irritation, occult blood loss	Take with meals. Avoid taking aspirin with alcohol or with megadoses of vitamin C[15]
Hypotensives (antihypertensives)		
Clonidine	Dry mouth, constipation, fluid retention	Increase bulk as needed. Limit sodium intake according to physician's advice.
Methyldopa (Aldomet)	Dry mouth, fluid retention	Limit sodium intake according to physician's advice
Guanethidine (Ismelin)	May result in diarrhea	Reduce intake of high residue foods, if necessary. Report serious symptoms
Prazosin (Minipress)	Nausea is common. Occasionally leads to vomiting, diarrhea, constipation, abdominal discomfort	Take usual measures for alleviating nausea. Report serious symptoms

There is a wide array of medications which may be used for persons with cardiac problems. Table 35.3 includes a partial listing and some of their nutrition-related effects. Certain combinations of drugs may increase the need for attention to adequate nutrient intake. For example, Digitoxin used in combination with a diuretic such as Diuril is dangerous if potassium intake is low. Coumadin may lead to hemorrhage if a person eats very little food and, consequently, ingests and absorbs little vitamin K. Health care workers need to be sure to advise clients about how to achieve desirable intake of critical nutrients.

PERSONS WITH NEUROLOGICAL DISTURBANCES

PARKINSONISM

Parkinsonism is a progressive neuromuscular disorder associated with a *low* concentration of the neurotransmitter dopamine in the basal ganglia of the brain. Drugs are used to treat the condition. The level of dopamine in the basal ganglia can be increased by giving the drug levodopa, an immediate precursor of dopamine. Levodopa may be given alone or in combination with α-methyldopa hydrazine (Carbidopa).

Several drug-nutrient interactions should be considered for clients receiving either levodopa or the levodopa-carbidopa combination. A high protein diet *reduces* the effectiveness of levodopa. Persons who are on levodopa therapy can be controlled more easily and with a lower dose of levodopa if they limit their dietary intake of protein and if they avoid taking the drug with meals. A detailed protein restricted diet plan is not necessary, but distributing protein into four small meals and decreasing consumption of high protein foods is recommended.[16] A variable intake of protein is objectionable since high intake may result in loss of control of symptoms and low intake may result in an increase in involuntary movements (choreiform dyskinesia). Overweight individuals often have difficulty regulating the dose of levodopa; therefore, moderation (or restriction) of caloric intake complements the decreased protein intake. Use of alcoholic beverages may be discouraged since alcohol can antagonize the action of levodopa.

When levodopa is given alone some of it is transformed to dopamine before it reaches the brain. Vitamin B_6 increases this extracerebral transformation. It is, therefore, suggested that clients avoid dietary *supplements* of vitamin B_6. (If multivitamins are needed, a pyridoxine-free form may be used.) Foods which are naturally good sources of vitamin B_6 may be used, but vitamin B_6 fortified foods (e.g., fortified cereals) are usually avoided.[17]

CHRONIC SEIZURE DISORDERS

The symptoms of a seizure disorder are sufficiently disruptive that the affected person and his family are usually very eager to control the condition. Medication (anticonvulsant therapy) is the major means of controlling seizures. Since medication is used regularly for an indefinitely long period of time, the possible nutritional effects listed in Table 35.4 may become serious. Risk of calcium imbalance (perhaps followed by rickets in children or osteomalacia in adults) may increase with increases in drug dosage and with duration of drug usage.[20] This risk is associated with each of the drugs named in Table 35.4. Folic acid deficiency may develop early in some types of anticonvulsant therapy. Children may be especially vulnerable to nutritional problems associated with anticonvulsant therapy because of nutritional demands related to growth. Careful monitoring of nutritional status should be included in routine care of clients being treated with anticonvulsants.

Guidance in selection of a well-balanced diet may also be advisable to help assure adequate intake of all nutrients. If vitamin supplements (especially vitamin D, folic acid, and perhaps riboflavin) are prescribed, health professionals should guide clients in using them safely and consistently. Guidelines for use of alcoholic beverages by adults with seizure disorders should be individualized according to the person's response to alcohol consumption. Alcohol tends to reduce the effectiveness of anticonvulsants. Drinking to excess is strongly discouraged.[21]

MENTALLY DISTURBED CLIENTS IN THE COMMUNITY

Mentally disturbed individuals living in the community may be in great need of nutritional services. Some clients have been abandoned by their families and must fend for themselves for the first time. Many are poor. Frequently these clients have little experience or skill in buying and preparing food, especially at low cost and with limited equipment.[22] Eating out is seldom a realistic alternative because of its expense. Some formerly hospitalized mental patients live in privately owned boarding homes where the food served is monotonous and low in nutritive value and fiber. They may not even be allowed to heat water for tea or instant soup.[23]

Day treatment centers have the potential for helping mentally disturbed individuals gain practical skills which will benefit them nutritionally. At the same

---

POINTS OF EMPHASIS
Nutritional care of persons with neurological disturbances

• Treatment of parkinsonism with levodopa therapy may be more effective if high intake of dietary protein and vitamin B$_6$ supplements are avoided.

• Anticonvulsant therapy may have serious nutritional effects including calcium imbalance and folic acid deficiency. Ongoing nutritional care measures are needed to prevent or correct drug-induced nutrient deficiencies.

TABLE 35.4 *Nutritional effects of drugs used in anticonvulsant therapy*

TYPE OF DRUG	POSSIBLE NUTRITIONAL EFFECTS	SUGGESTED NUTRITIONAL CARE MEASURES
All types listed below	May interfere with metabolism of vitamin D and lead to calcium imbalance, bone demineralization, possibly rickets or osteomalacia, with long term use (lack of serious effects has been noted in one study[18]	Vitamin D supplement recommended as a preventive measure; the active form (25-hydroxy vitamin D) may be needed for satisfactory results[19]
Succinimides, e.g., ethosuximide (Zarontin) Trimethadione Primidone Phenobarbitol Phenytoin (Dilantin)	May cause distressing gastrointestinal symptoms and weight loss	Routinely assess weight, growth of children, and adequacy of food intake Urge clients to report recurring gastrointestinal symptoms
	Decreases serum levels of several B vitamins (e.g. folic acid, B$_{12}$, B$_6$) May result in megaloblastic anemia May result in gastrointestinal symptoms and in gingival hyperplasia of the gums May result in carbohydrate intolerance and (rarely) HHNK	Guide clients in use of folic acid supplements, if indicated Dosage must be regulated since folic acid may antagonize action of phenytoin, primidone Warn against self-treatment with unprescribed vitamin supplements to avoid toxicity or antagonism (Vitamin B$_{12}$, for example, may antagonize phenobarbitol[19]) Give with meals to reduce gastrointestinal symptoms Practice thorough mouth care Monitor serum glucose levels

time, the learning experiences may help clients develop social skills and an improved sense of self-esteem and self-confidence. Food can be a good topic to include in therapeutic activities since most people are interested in it and feel comfortable talking about it, working with it, and eating it.

Health care workers need to be able to build and maintain a sense of trust and rapport with mentally disturbed clients if they hope to be able to promote learning. Progress is usually slow; pushing clients to meet objectives may result in withdrawal, resentment, or other negative responses.[23]

It is desirable for health team members to jointly plan the kinds of learning experiences which will be best suited to a particular group of mentally disturbed clients. Formal classes are avoided since attention span is usually short. Activities are planned so that clients do not have to be attentive to the leader for more than a few minutes. Health professionals try to create a relaxed atmosphere which provides opportunities for social interaction.

Structured, active experiences which incorporate basic learning principles may facilitate the client's learning and performance.[22] For example, participants might learn to prepare a simple but tasty food with basic equipment and then share the experience of eating their creations in pleasant surroundings. Group leaders might give priority to encouraging cleanliness, safety, and appropriate social interaction. Another practical activity might be a trip to the supermarket to learn how to select fresh produce that can be eaten raw and to learn how much it is safe to buy if the food has to be stored at room temperature.

Some clients may try to use a new skill at home and be eager to tell the group about the complements received from family or significant others. Time needs to be available for this as well as for more structured learning.

In some situations health professionals need to take action on the client's behalf, as by showing a boarding house owner how he could easily serve more satisfactory meals at no extra cost or by helping the client to find more satisfactory living arrangements.

If a client has family or friends who are concerned about him, they may raise questions about whether the client would benefit from the therapeutic use of nutrients. For example, they may wonder if he should avoid carbohydrates (especially any food containing natural or added sugar) or they may inquire about the use of megavitamin (orthomolecular) therapy. Unless the client is diagnosed to have reactive hypoglycemia (a rare condition), a varied diet based on the Basic Four food groups is most appropriate for mentally disturbed persons. Affirming the family's belief that it is desirable to limit intake of added sugar may help them to accept advice about a balanced diet. Megavitamin therapy (that is, pharmacological use of certain vitamins) may pose hazards; it should only be used under the guidance of a qualified psychiatrist. Some psychiatrists prescribe megavitamin therapy for schizophrenics.[24] Others state that there is no good evidence

of its effectiveness except in rare cases of vitamin dependency involving genetic defects.[25] If megavitamin therapy is used, the client should be regularly monitored for signs of vitamin toxicity.

ALCOHOLICS

There is a large population of Americans who abuse alcohol, and the number has increased sharply since 1945.[26] Accurate estimates of the incidence of alcoholism are impossible because of the frequency with which this illness is hidden or overlooked, but the rate may be more than 4200 per 100,000 American adults.[26] Studies suggest that an increasing number of youth are at risk of becoming alcoholics and that a significant number of teens (5 to 23 percent) are already problem drinkers.[27]

There is very great concern about pregnant women who are alcoholics. A large body of evidence indicates that maternal alcoholism can lead to the fetal alcohol syndrome. Babies who are born live to alcoholic mothers may have serious birth defects because of the effects of alcohol on the developing fetus.[28]

Persons who abuse alcohol are subject to nutritional problems, no matter whether they are young or old, rich or poor. There are numerous reasons why this is so. Alcohol is a source of "empty" calories and tends to crowd nutritious foods out of the diet when used to excess. A person who drinks about 500 ml. (1 pt.) of whiskey daily (a common amount for some alcoholics) obtains about 900 kcal. daily just from the alcoholic beverage. Drinking a sweet wine often results in a much higher caloric intake.

High alcohol consumption tends to curb the appetite and interferes with normal functioning of the gastrointestinal tract. Vomiting and diarrhea often prevent utilization of some of the consumed food. Alcohol may directly irritate the intestinal tract, causing inflammation of the stomach and/or small intestines and impaired absorption of thiamine, folic acid, vitamin B_{12}, fat soluble vitamins, fat, and some minerals. In time, alcohol may directly damage the liver and pancreas. Alcoholic hepatitis (inflamed liver), cirrhosis of the liver, and pancreatitis are serious complications which may result from prolonged abuse of alcohol.

Alcohol abuse has additional effects on the body which contribute to malnutrition. Alcohol alters the metabolism of certain nutrients. For example it retards gluconeogenesis (formation of glucose from protein), affects the metabolism of fat in the liver, and appears to interfere with the utilization of some of the B complex vitamins. By damaging tissues, alcohol increases the need for synthesis of DNA and RNA, increasing the requirement for folic acid, vitamin B_{12}, and other nutrients. Changes in the liver limit that organ's ability to store nutrients.[29] Alcohol also increases the urinary excretion of some water soluble nutrients, especially magnesium, potassium, and zinc. Thus, alcohol abuse can readily lead to deficiency of a wide variety of nutrients.

It can be difficult to predict what type of nutritional deficiencies may be present in an alcoholic client since patterns of eating are quite variable and many alcoholics are poor historians. Deficiencies of zinc, magnesium, B complex vitamins, vitamin C, electrolytes, and protein are not uncommon.[29,30] Nutritional deficiencies are unusually serious when combined with the toxic effects of alcohol.

When working with alcoholics who are unwilling to quit drinking, health professionals should be careful to avoid practices which place false emphasis on nutrition.[31] If the client improves his diet and takes a vitamin supplement but does not stop drinking, damage to the body is likely to continue. If a pregnant woman eats well but continues to drink, her baby remains in danger. These things should be made clear to clients. Nevertheless, the client must understand the necessity of eating well in order to avoid such serious consequences as Wernicke's syndrome (a serious, progressive mental disease which is due to deficiency of thiamine). Consultation with other health team members may be helpful in arriving at the best approach to use with a particular client.

Once an alcoholic agrees to treatment, he is apt to be an inpatient in an alcohol rehabilitation center for a period of time. It is desirable to begin nutritional rehabilitation and teaching while the client is in this therapeutic environment. Nutritional care should include strategies to help the client develop an increased sense of responsibility for his own actions. The client should be educated away from looking for an easy way out, such as use of vitamin supplements as a substitute for developing sensible food behaviors.

Restoration of good nutritional status cannot prevent a return to alcoholism, but it may help reestablish a sense of well being which, in turn, may have a positive impact. If abuse of alcohol has already led to serious health problems such as liver disease, a former alcoholic will probably need to follow a modified diet to help restore and/or maintain a satisfactory state of health.

Ideally, a rehabilitated alcoholic returns to his family and begins to take meals with them on a regular basis. This may help to meet the client's psychosocial needs. If this option is not open to a client, health professionals should help him make practical arrangements for regular meals. This may be particularly important for indigent persons.

FORMER DRUG ADDICTS

Once a person has made a decision to try to "kick the habit," nutritional care can play a significant role in his rehabilitation. Some form of malnutrition is a common finding in drug abusers. Abuse of amphetamines, for example, may seriously interfere with appetite and increase energy expenditure, resulting in marked weight loss. Heroin users are noted for having a poor appetite but a moderate to intense craving for sweets.[32] Sweet desserts (e.g., prepackaged cakes and cookies)

and sweetened beverages may make up a large share of their diets. (This practice may persist during methadone maintenance.) The heroin addict may fail to be concerned about food; rather, getting money for the next "fix" demands his attention. Abuse of other drugs may have more subtle effects on eating habits and nutritional status.

Health care professionals who work with former addicts need to be aware of the high incidence of hepatitis among this group. By increasing nutritional requirements and dulling appetite, hepatitis makes these clients even more vulnerable to malnutrition. Careful assessment is advised before malnutrition is ruled out.

A major goal of overall treatment of former addicts is psychosocial growth of the client. Nutritional care can contribute to this growth very early in treatment. Rapport established between the client and the health care worker is important to the growth process. If a client can be encouraged to become interested in nutrition, he may become more interested in his own well being. Nutrition counseling provides the addict with a concrete, nonthreatening method to do something constructive for himself. Frankle suggests that the exaddict may respond positively to the idea of "getting high" by living in harmony with the body.[33]

A diet history interview can be an experience which helps the client to view himself in a more positive manner and to feel comfortable giving important details about his situation. Some drug rehabilitation clinics use special diet history forms which include pattern of eating before, during, and after the addiction; patterns of drug use; employment history; and legal history.

Halfway houses and other residences have been established to help former addicts become well-functioning members of the community. These community resources are sometimes in need of guidance with regard to food service. The provision of safe, well-balanced meals can be a real challenge when facilities and funds are limited.[34] Ideally, a dietitian or nutritionist will be available to serve as a consultant. If not, other health professionals such as nurses can provide concrete suggestions regarding hygiene, safe food storage, and balanced meals. They can also provide some reliable resource materials.

STUDY QUESTIONS

1. Suggest several ways in which health care workers might encourage a burned child to substantially increase oral food intake.
2. Why might a badly burned person develop cramps and diarrhea after rapidly drinking a large milkshake?
3. Discuss three reasons why thermal injury greatly increases nutritional requirements.
4. Discuss several reasons why keeping meal size small may benefit persons who are recovering from a myocardial infarction.

5. Why is it advisable for a person who is taking levodopa to avoid skipping meals?

6. Health professionals should look for what potential nutritional problems when assessing clients who are taking Dilantin?

7. Discuss several reasons why abuse of alcohol or other drugs may lead to malnutrition.

8. What is a potential problem associated with strongly emphasizing the importance of an adequate diet for alcoholics who continue drinking?

References

1. Witmore, D. W., and Pruitt, B. A.: Parenteral nutrition in burn patients. In J. Fischer (ed.): *Total Parenteral Nutrition*. Boston: Little, Brown & Co., 1976.

2. Curreri, P. W., et al.: Dietary requirements of patients with major burns. *J. Am. Diet. Assoc.* 65:415. 1974.

3. Cohen, I. K., Schecter, P. J., and Henkin, R. I.: Hypogeusia, anorexia and altered zinc metabolism following thermal burn. *JAMA* 223:914, 1973.

4. Pearson, E., and Soroff, H. S.: Burns. In H. A. Schneider, C. E. Anderson, and D. B. Coursin (eds.): *Nutritional Support of Medical Practice*. Hagerstown MD.: Harper & Row, 1977.

*5. Pennisi, V. M.: Monitoring the nutritional care of burned patients. *J. Am. Diet. Assoc.* 69:531, 1976.

6. Herrin, J.: Care of the critically ill child: Major burns. *Pediatrics* 45:449, 1970.

*7. Hemzacek, K. I.: Dietary protocol for the patient who has suffered a myocardial infarction. *J. Am. Diet. Assoc.* 72:182, 1978.

8. Christakis, G., and Winston, M.: Nutritional therapy in acute myocardial infarction. *J. Am. Diet. Assoc.* 63:233, 1973.

9. Houser, D.: Ice water for MI patients? Why not? *Am. J. Nurs.* 76:432, 1976.

10. Cohen, I. M., et al.: Safety of hot and cold liquids in patients with myocardial infarction. *Chest* 71:450, 1977.

11. Merkel, R., and Brown, C. M.: Evaluating feeding activities in a cardiac care unit. *Am. J. Nurs.* 70:2348, 1970.

12. Haldeman, J., and Olson, P. T.: Classes for coronary care patients. *J. Am. Diet. Assoc.* 63:648, 1973.

13. Ellis, F. R., and Sanders, T. A. B.: Angina and vegan diet. *Am. Heart J.* 93:803, 1977.

14. Moore, K., and Maschak, B. J.: How patient education can reduce the risks of anticoagulant therapy. *Nursing 77.* 7(9):24, 1977.

15. Lo, G. Y., and Konishi, F.: Synergistic effect of vitamin C and aspirin on gastric lesions in the rat. *Am. J. Clin. Nutr.* 31:1397, 1978.

16. Langan, R. J., and Cotzias, G. C.: Do's and don'ts for the patient on levodopa therapy. *Am. J. Nurs.* 76: 917, 1976.

*17. Visconti, J. A.: Drug-food interaction. *Nutrition in Disease.* Columbus OH: Ross Laboratories, May 1977.

18. Winnacker, J. L., et al.: Rickets in children receiving anticonvulsant drugs. *Am. J. Dis. Child.* 131: 286, 1977.

*19. March, D. C.: *Handbook: Interactions of Selected Drugs with Nutritional Status in Man,* ed. 2. Chicago: The American Dietetic Association, 1978.

20. Roe, D.: *Drug-Induced Nutritional Deficiencies.* Westport CT: Avi Publishing Co., 1976.

21. Conway, B. L.: *Carini and Owens' Neurological and Neurosurgical Nursing,* ed. 7. St. Louis: C. V. Mosby Co., 1978.

22. Johnson, C. A., et al.: Dietitians help mental patients "make it on the outside." *J. Am. Diet. Assoc.* 70: 513, 1977.

23. Schneggenburger, C., and Nolan, B. S.: Diet teaching at Dustin House. *J. Psychiatr. Nurs.* 15:18, 1977.

24. Hoffer, A.: Orthomolecular treatment of schizophrenia. *Can. J. Psychiatr. Nurs.* 14:11, 1973.

25. Kity, S. S.: Nutrition and psychiatric illness. In G. Serban (ed.): *Nutrition and Mental Functions.* New York: Plenum Press, 1975.

26. Haglund, R. M. J., and Schucket, M. A.: The epidemiology of alcoholism. In N. J. Estes and M. E. Heinemann (eds.): *Alcoholism: Development, Consequences and Interventions.* St. Louis: C. V. Mosby, 1977.

27. Globetti, G.: Teenage drinking. In N. J. Estes and M. E. Heinemann (eds.): *Alcoholism: Development, Consequences and Interventions.* St. Louis: C. V. Mosby Co., 1977.

28. Erb, L.: The fetal alcohol syndrome (FAS). *Clin. Pediatr.* 17:644, 1978.

*29. Thomson, A. D.: Alcohol and nutrition. *Clin. Endocrin. Metab.* 7(2):405, 1978.

30. Shaw, S., and Lieber, C. S.: Nutrition and alcoholic liver disease. *Nutrition in Disease.* Columbus OH: Ross Laboratories, March 1978.

31. Leevy, C. M., Tamburro, C., and Smith, F.: Alcoholism, drug addiction and nutrition. *Med. Clin. North Am.* 54(6):1567, 1970.

32. Gambera, S. E., and Clarke, J. A. K.: Comments on dietary intake of drug-dependent persons. *J. Am. Diet. Assoc.* 68:155, 1976.

33. Frankle, R. T., et al.: The Door, a center of alternatives. The nutritionist in a free clinic for adolescents. *J. Am. Diet. Assoc.* 63:269, 1976.

34. Washburn, A. B.: Nutrition counseling for drug addicts in rehabilitation. *J. Nutr. Ed.* 6:13, 1974.

* Recommended reading.

Part 4

Bibliography and additional recommended readings

Acosta, P. B., and Elsas, L. J.: *Dietary Management of Inherited Metabolic Disease: Phenylketonuria, Galactosemia, Tyrosinemia, Homocystinuria, Maple Syrup Urine Disease.* Atlanta: ACELMU Publishers, 1976.

Aponte, H., and Hoffman, L.: The open door: A structural approach to a family with an anorectic child. *Family Process* 12(1):1, 1973.

Barnard, M., and Wolff, L.: Psychosocial failure to thrive: Nursing assessment and intervention. *Nurs. Clin. North Am.* 8(3):557, 1973.

Brown, Z.: Diabetes in pregnancy. *Family Community Health* 1(3):43, 1978.

Bruch, H.: *The Golden Cage: The Enigma of Anorexia Nervosa.* Cambridge MA: Harvard University Press, 1978.

Bush, J.: Cervical esophagostomy to provide nutrition. *Am. J. Nurs.* 79:107, 1979.

Cosper, B.: Physiological colostomy. *Am. J. Nurs.* 75:2014, 1975.

(Diabetes) *Nurs. Clin. North Am.* 12(3), 1977.

Feldtman, R. W., and Andrassy, R. J.: Meeting exceptional nutritional needs. 2. Elemental enteral alimentation. *Postgrad. Med.* 64(3):65, 1978.

Harris, C.: Helping the breast-feeding mother whose baby refuses to suckle. *Nursing '79* 9(5):96, 1979.

Hathcock, J. N., and Coon, J.: *Nutrition and Drug Interrelations.* New York: Academic Press, 1978.

Jones, A. M.: Overcoming the feeding problems of the mentally and physically handicapped. *J. Human Nutr.* 32:359, 1978.

Luke, B.: Guide to better evaluation of antepartal nutrition. *JOGN Nurs.* 5(4):37, 1978.

McConnell, E.: 10 problems with nasogastric tubes . . . and how to solve them. *Nursing 79.* 9(4):78, 1979.

McElroy, D. B.: Nursing care of patients with viral hepatitis. *Nurs. Clin. North Am.* 12(2):305, 1977.

Mikkelsen, C., Waechter, E., and Crittenden, M.: Cystic fibrosis: A family challenge. *Children Today* 7(4):22, 1978.

Roe, D.: *Alcohol and the Diet.* Westport CT: Avi Publishing Co., 1979.

Schreier, A. McB., and Lavenia, J.: The nurse's role in nutritional management of radiotherapy patients. *Nurs. Clin. North Am.* 12(1):173, 1977.

Shakert, J.: Nutrition and cancer. In P. Burkhalter and D. Donley (eds.): *Dynamics of Oncology Nursing.* New York: McGraw-Hill Book Co., 1978.

Smelo, L. S.: The recognition and care of hypoglycemic reactions. *ADA Forecast* 26(1):1, 1973.

Smith, M. A. H. (ed.): *Feeding the Handicapped Child.* Memphis: Child Development Center, Dept. of Nutrition, 1971.

Tzagournis, M.: Triglycerides in clinical medicine. A review. *Am. J. Clin. Nutr.* 31:1439, 1978.

Watt, R. C.: Ostomies: Why, how and where. *Nurs. Clin. North Am.* 11(3):393, 1976.

Wilson, H. S., and Kneisl, C. R.: *Psychiatric Nursing.* Menlo Park CA: Addison-Wesley, 1979.

HELPFUL RESOURCES FOR CLIENTS WITH HEALTH PROBLEMS*

Allergy

Baking for People with Food Allergies. by L. H. Fulton and C. A. Davis. Consumer and Food Economics Institute, ARS, USDA, 1975.

Coping with Food Allergy. by C. A. Frazier. New York: Quadrangle/The New York Times Book Co., 1974. (General information, detail regarding labeling information and dietary modifications, many recipes)

Creative Cooking Without Wheat, Milk and Eggs. by R. R. Shattuck. Cranbury NJ: A. S. Barnes and Co., 1974. (Valuable because of its recipes and cooking tips)

Diabetes mellitus

Controlling Diabetes with Diet. by A. Gormican. Springfield IL: Charles C Thomas Co., 1971.

Diabetes Guidebook. by J. K. Davidson and M. P.

---

* For other sources of information, see Appendix i.

Goldsmith. Atlanta: Emory University School of Medicine, 1972. (Geared to be used by professionals and their clients; includes visual aids for persons with limited reading ability; features some Southern ethnic foods)

Exchanges for Special Occasions. by M. Fruin, M. Hargrave, and M. Lavelle. Diabetes Education Center, 4959 Excelsior Blvd., Minneapolis 55416. (Other titles are available from this source)

Guide to Self-Care in Diabetes. by G. Stamm. American Diabetes Association, Nebraska Affiliate, 921 Dorcas St., Room 915, Omaha 68108. 1974. (Good teaching tool regarding all aspects of diabetic care)

The Art of Cooking for the Diabetic. by K. Middleton and M. A. Hess. Chicago: Contemporary Books, 1978. (Includes expanded exchange lists, recipes, practical ideas)

The Diabetic Diet in Spanish. California Dietetic Assoc., 1609 Westwood Blvd., Suite 101, Los Angeles, 90024. 1975.

The Diabetic Gourmet. by A. Bowen. New York: Harper & Row, 1970.

The Peripatetic Diabetic. by M. Bennett. New York: Hawthorne Books, 1969. (Practical suggestions regarding management of diabetes, written in a very readable style)

Gastrointestinal diseases and malabsorption

Cooking for Your Celiac Child—Dietary Management in Malabsorption Disorders. New York: Dial Press, 1969.

Low Gluten Diet with Tested Recipes. by M. Hjortland and A. B. French. Ann Arbor MI: Clinical Research Unit, University Hospital.

Using MCT Oil and Portagen. Evansville IN: Mead Johnson & Co., 1974.

Handicapping conditions

A Guide for Feeding Children with Cerebral Palsy. Bureau of Public Health Nutrition, California State Dept. of Public Heaht, rev. 1966.

Gallender, D.: *Eating Handicaps: Illustrated Tech-* *niques for Feeding Disorders.* Springfield IL: Charles C Thomas, 1979.

Mealtime Manual for People with Disabilities and the Aging. by J. L. Klinger. (Available from Campbell Soup Co., Box (MM) 56, Camden NJ 08101)

Self-Help Manual for Arthritis Patients. by J. L. Klinger. New York: The Arthritis Foundation, 1974.

Modified fat, low cholesterol, and sodium restricted diets

A Change for Heart: Your Family and the Food You Eat. by J. M. Ferguson, C. B. Taylor, and P. Ullman. Palo Alto CA: Bull Publishing Co., 1978. (Incorporates a behavioral approach; self-instructional)

Fat-Controlled and Sodium-Restricted Cooking. Toronto: Doubleday Canada Ltd., 1971.

Living with High Blood Pressure: The Hypertension Diet Cookbook. by J. D. Margie and J. D. Hunt. Bloomfield NJ: HLS Press, 1978. (Includes practical suggestions in addition to explanations, menus and recipes)

The American Heart Association Cookbook. by R. Eshleman and M. Winston. New York: M. David McKay Co., 1975. (Includes tips for menu planning, shopping, cooking fat controlled meals)

The Fat and Sodium Controlled Cookbook, ed. 4. Boston: Little, Brown & Co., 1975. (Also includes information about control of carbohydrate intake)

Phenylketonuria

Low Protein Cookery for Phenylketonuria. by V. E. Shuett. Madison: The University of Wisconsin Press, 1977. (Comprehensive)

Renal disease

Dietary Management of Renal Disease. by J. S. Cost. Thorofare NJ: Charles B. Slack, 1975. (Includes recipes)

Fun Food Recipes for Renal Diets. Illinois Council on Renal Nutrition, Kidney Foundation of Illinois, Inc., 127 N. Dearborn St., Chicago 60602. 1977. (Includes helpful hints about the diet)

Appendices

Appendix 1

Sources of nutrition information and federal consumer services

Government sources of nutrition related materials

CONSUMER INFORMATION CATALOG

Free catalog. Lists publications which have been particularly popular; more than 150 of those listed are free.

Write to Consumer Information Center
Pueblo, CO 81009

SELECTED UNITED STATES GOVERNMENT PUBLICATIONS

Free. Each issue lists 150 to 200 popular sale publications (10 issues per year)

Write to Superintendent of Documents
Washington, DC 20402

DHEW PUBLICATIONS

Relating to health and disease, some are geared toward health professionals, others toward consumers.

NIH Office of Information, OD
Rm. 2310, Bldg. 31
9000 Rockville Pike,
Bethesda, MD 20014

FDA PUBLICATIONS

Relating to food labeling, additives, safety, nutrition.

FDA
5600 Fishers Lane
Rockville, MD 20852

STATUTORY DISTRIBUTION

Some publications are available free of charge from one's Congressperson.

Information can be obtained about some of the publications available by writing to one of the following addresses:

USDA
Office of Governmental and Public Affairs
Washington, DC 20250

DHEW
Office of Child Development
Box 1182
Washington, DC 20013

STATE AGRICULTURAL EXTENSION PUBLICATIONS

Lists of state publications are available free of charge.

Write or call your Cooperative Extension Service (listed in the white pages of the telephone directory).

Additional sources of nutrition education materials*

ORGANIZATIONS

Allergy Information Association, 3 Powburn Pl., Weston, Ontario, M9R2C5 Canada

American Academy of Pediatrics, Box P, P.O. Box 1034, Evanston, IL 60204

American Cancer Society (contact your local cancer association)

American Celiac Society, Inc., 45 Gifford Ave., Jersey City, NJ 07304

American Dental Association (Bureau of Dental Health Education), 211 E. Chicago Ave., Chicago, IL 60611

The American Dietetic Association, 430 N. Michigan Ave., Chicago, IL 60611

American Digestive Disease Society, Inc., 420 Lexington Ave., New York, NY 10017

*For a more complete listing, see *Index of Nutrition Education Materials* (rev. ed.). Washington DC: The Nutrition Foundation, Inc., 1977.

American Health Foundation, 1370 Avenue of the Americas, New York, NY 10019 (materials relating to diet in prevention of cardiovascular disease, many geared toward teens)

American Heart Association (contact your local heart association)

American Medical Assoc., Order Dept., 535 N. Dearborn St., Chicago, IL 60610

Cornell University, Division of Nutritional Sciences, Media Services B-10, Martha van Rensselaer Hall, Ithaca, NY 14853

La Leche League International, Inc., 9616 Minneapolis Ave., Franklin Park, IL 60131

National Dairy Council, 6300 N. River Rd., Rosemont IL 60018

National Foundation-March of Dimes, Box 2000, White Plains, NY 10602

National Kidney Foundation, 2 Park Ave., New York, NY 10016 (or contact your local kidney foundation)

National Library of Medicine, Literature Search Program Reference Section, 8600 Rockville Pike, Bethesda, MD 20014

The Nutrition Foundation, Inc., Office of Education and Public Affairs, 888 17th St., N.W., Suite 300, Washington, DC 20006

Prescription Parents, Inc., P.O. Box 855, Quincy, MA 02169 (regarding cleft lip and cleft palate)

Society for Nutrition Education, 2140 Shattuck Ave., Suite 1110, Berkeley, CA 94704

United Fresh Fruit and Vegetable Association, 1019 19th St. N.W., Washington, DC 20036

United Ostomy Association, Inc. 1111 Wilshire Blvd, Los Angeles, CA 90017 (contact your local ostomy association)

JOURNALS

Journal of The American Dietetic Association (includes monthly reviews, mainly of printed nutrition education materals)

Journal of Nutrition Education (includes quarterly reviews of print and audiovisual nutrition education materials)

FOOD COMPANIES

Write to address given on food labels for specific nutritional information about their products and for nutrition education materials. (Specify audience)

Federal consumer services

CHILDREN AND YOUTH

Special Assistance for Consumer Affairs
Office of Human Development Services
DHEW
Washington, DC 20201

CONSUMER AFFAIRS/COMPLAINTS

Director
Office of Consumer Affairs
DHEW
621 Reporters Building
Washington, DC 20201

CONSUMER EDUCATION AND PROTECTION, COOPERATIVES

U.S. Community Services Administration
Room 318-B
1200 19th St., N.W.
Washington, DC 20506

ELDERLY

Information on Social Security, SSI, Food Stamps, Medicaid and Medicare, jobs, housing, homemakers, and home health aides.
Administration on Aging
Washington, DC 20201

ENERGY

Department of Energy
Washington, DC 20461

ENVIRONMENT

Information on environmental contaminants of food and water.
Office of Public Affairs
EPA
Washington, DC 20460

FISH AND WILDLIFE

Information on safety of specific types of fish and wildlife.
Fish and Wildlife Service
Office of Public Information
Washington, DC 20240

FOOD

Assistant Secretary for Food and Consumer Service
USDA
Washington, DC 20250

FOOD LABELING, ADDITIVES, SAFETY, NUTRITION

Consumer Inquiry Section
FDA
5600 Fishers Lane
Rockville, MD 20852

Appendix 2

Federal programs to prevent and relieve hunger

Appendix 2A
FOOD STAMPS (FOOD STAMP ACT OF 1977)

PURPOSE: "... to promote the general welfare and to safeguard the health and well being of the Nation's population by raising the level of nutrition among low income households." §271.1 Food Stamp Act of 1977 *Fed. Reg.* 43(85):18905 May 2, 1978.

ELIGIBILITY:

• Monthly net income of household* after allowed deductions must be less than monthly income eligibility standards.
• Resources (money in savings accounts, recreational property, certain licensed vehicles, etc.) must not exceed a pre-set amount.
• Household members are required to register to work unless:
    –under 18 years
    –over 65 years
    –incapacitated
    –caring for children or incapacitated adults
    –attending school
    –working full time
• U.S. citizen or eligible alien.
• Permanent residence is *not* required, e.g., migrant workers can make arrangements for receipt of food stamps to be uninterrupted in spite of moves.
• Recipients of Supplemental Security Income (SSI) in "cash-out" states (California and Massachusetts) are ineligible. (Value of SSI in cash-out states is reported to include the value of food stamps.)

* A household can be one person or a group of persons, not necessarily related, who meet(s) specified requirements.

• Recertification is required at intervals.
• Processing of applications requires 30 days, with benefits retroactive to date of application. *Expedited* (1 to 2 days) service is available for destitute households (those without any income).

FEATURES:

• As of 1979 Food Stamps are issued free each month to certified households. (Previously they had to be purchased for less than their retail value.)
• Stamps are used like money for buying:
    –Food—any type *except pet food*
    –Beverages—any *except alcoholic*
    –Seeds/plants for growing *food.*
    –Specific types of hunting & fishing equipment in Alaska
• Value of stamps issued depends on:
    –size of household (maximum coupon allotment increases with each additional household member)
    –resources of household
• *Maximum* allotment is equivalent to current value of U.S.D.A.'s Thrifty Food Plan, adjusted for family size.†
• Applicants or recipients who suspect an error has been made (e.g., if the household has been determined ineligible) may request a *fair hearing* to air their complaint and seek corrective action.

† Determined by a prescribed procedure.

POTENTIAL AND ACTUAL PROBLEMS:

• Freedom of choice may result in use of food coupons for foods low in nutritive value. The program does not assure that households will be better fed.

• Maximum effectiveness of program requires an accompanying nutrition education program, but this is generally very limited except in areas served by the Expanded Food and Nutrition Education Program (EFNEP).

• There is potential for fraud (e.g., selling stamps to uncertified individuals at a profit), but this has been reduced by the Food Stamp Act of 1977.

• Despite improvements in the new Act, some administrative details remain confusing to recipients. This may prevent some households from participating or receiving all the benefits to which they are entitled.

• Funding is a continuing problem. The program cost more than $5.5 *billion* in FY 1977.[1]

FOR FURTHER INFORMATION:

Food and Nutrition Service
U.S.D.A.
Washington, DC 20250

USDA Food and Nutrition Service Regional Office (Call Federal Information Service under U.S. Government in the white pages of the telephone directory for the nearest address.)

Local: State or city welfare office
Advocacy groups: See pages 282 and 423

Appendix 2B
SPECIAL SUPPLEMENTARY FOOD PROGRAM FOR WOMEN, INFANTS AND CHILDREN (WIC)

PURPOSE: To improve nutrient intake of women prenatally and postnatally, lactating mothers, infants, and young children who are at high nutritional risk.

FEDERAL AGENCY RESPONSIBLE:

Food and Nutrition Service, USDA

ELIGIBILITY REQUIREMENTS:

• Developmental Stage
Pregnant
Less than 6 months postpartum *or*
Up to 1 year lactating
Children under 5 years
• "At nutritional risk"—examples:
Poor dietary habits
Previous history of miscarriage or preterm birth
Nutritional anemia
Abnormal growth pattern (e.g., stunting, underweight, obesity)
• Eligible for low cost medical care
• Residence in neighborhood served by the local program

FEATURES OF PROGRAM:

• Participants receive "WIC Food Packages" (specific supplemental foods)
–directly from clinic *OR*
–via vouchers which can be used like money in a grocery store to purchase the designated foods
• Contents of WIC Food Package for women:
Milk and/or cheese
Eggs
Vitamin C-rich fruit or vegetable juice
Iron fortified cereal

• Contents of WIC Food Packages for infants and children: Foods similar to above in appropriate forms, e.g., iron-fortified infant formula

• Brands of some types of foods (e.g., infant formula) may be specified to guarantee meeting preset nutritional requirements.

• Simple monitoring of health status and nutrition education are mandatory components of program.

• WIC must be affiliated with an established health clinic.

• Participation in WIC does not reduce benefits from Food Stamp Program.

POTENTIAL AND EXISTING PROBLEMS:

• Sharing of food package with other family members may minimize benefits to participants.

• Participant may not know how to make effective use of the food package.

• Program is unavailable to many individuals who meet certification requirements.

• Lack of funds and administrative problems hamper many programs.

• Legislation does not specifically allocate funds for nutrition education.

FOR FURTHER INFORMATION:

(Your State) Department of Health
State Capital, Your State

Supplemental Food Programs
Food and Nutrition Service
USDA
Washington, DC 20250

Appendix 2C
NUTRITION PROGRAM FOR THE ELDERLY

(Formerly Title VII of the Older American's Act, now merged with Title III)
PURPOSE: To improve the nutrition of citizens sixty years of age and older.

FEDERAL AGENCY RESPONSIBLE:

Administration on Aging (AoA), DHEW.

ELIGIBILITY REQUIREMENTS:

• Sixty years of age or older, or spouse of someone who is
• No consideration of financial or health status.
(A contribution toward the cost of the meal is encouraged but *not* required.)

FEATURES OF PROGRAM:

• Lunches served at least five days per week in congregate meal site (often a church, school, or other community building)
• Lunches should provide at least one third of the RDAs for elderly individuals. (Some have been found to provide about one half of the RDA for some nutrients[2])
• A fixed percentage of the meals can be home delivered to individuals who are truly homebound.
• Programs must provide services to increase socialization and improve self-reliance of senior citizens:
　　–Transportation and escort services to and from the meal site
　　–Nutrition education
　　–Information and referral services
　　–Shopping assistance
　　–Recreational activities
• A Project Council influences operation of each local program:
　　–More than one half of members of council must be participants in the program
　　–Council influences menus, fee guidelines, days and hours of operation of meal site, environment of meal site
• Participation in the program does not reduce food stamp allotment.

POTENTIAL AND EXISTING PROBLEMS:

• Many programs have long waiting lists since expansion is limited by lack of funds.
• Required services may be of a token nature owing to lack of funds.

FOR FURTHER INFORMATION:

Nutrition Program for the Elderly
(State) Department on Aging
　or Bureau
　or Commission
State Capital, Your State

Administration on Aging
330 C. Street, S.W.
DHEW
Washington, DC 20201

Area Agency on Aging (names and locations available from the state agency)

Advocacy groups: see page 423

Appendix 2D
CHILD NUTRITION PROGRAMS (All programs under USDA)

National School Lunch and Breakfast Programs

PURPOSE:

• School Lunch, as stated in the National School Lunch Act:
"as a measure of national security to safeguard the health and well-being of the nation's children, and to encourage domestic consumption of nutritious agricultural commodities and other foods." (42 U.S.C. § 1751) Passage June 4, 1946.
• School Breakfast
"As a national nutrition and health policy, it is the purpose and intent of the Congress that the school breakfast program be made available in all schools where it is needed to provide adequate nutrition for children in attendance." Section 4(g) of the Child Nutrition Act as amended by Public Law 94-105 (as quoted in *Guide to American Food Programs*, p. 40[3])

ELIGIBILITY REQUIREMENTS:

• Attendance at a participating school and payment of price set by the school.
• Children from families whose income is less than 195 percent of poverty level are eligible for reduced price meals.
• Children from families whose income is less than 125 percent of poverty level are eligible for *free meals*.

FEATURES OF SCHOOL LUNCH AND
BREAKFAST PROGRAMS:

- "Type A" school lunch is supposed to provide one-third of RDA for nutrients.
  - For children 10- to 12-years old it includes:
    - 2 oz. meat or equivalent
    - ¾ c. (combined) vegetables and/or fruits (minimum of two)
    - 1 serving whole or enriched grain product
    - ½ pt. (245 ml.) fortified fluid milk (flavored milk is approved federally, but not by all states)
    - 1 tsp. butter or fortified margarine in some states (not a federal requirement)
  - High school students may choose to take only three of these five components if they wish.
  - Serving sizes may be decreased for younger children, increased for older youth, in relation to nutritive needs.
- School breakfast includes:
  - ½ pt. fortified fluid milk
  - ½ c. fruit or juice
  - 1 serving whole or enriched grain product
  - Protein-rich food as often as possible
- Substitutions may be made for verified medical reasons (e.g., allergy to wheat).
- USDA has approved some variations which meet specified nutrient standards.
- Nutrition education is to be included in the program.

Special Milk Program

ELIGIBILITY:

Same as for school lunch

FEATURES OF PROGRAM:

½ pt. fluid milk is offered at lunch and/or snack time

Child Care Food Program

ELIGIBILITY:

Children (≤ 18-years old) attending an organized child care program

- Free and reduced cost meals available as in National School Lunch Program

FEATURES OF PROGRAM:

Nutritious breakfasts, lunches, suppers and snacks. Meals and snacks must meet USDA guidelines.

Summer and Holiday Food Program

PURPOSE: Similar to school lunch and breakfast programs.

ELIGIBILITY:

Free for all children (≤ 18 years old) attending regardless of income

Available only for low income communities or for programs serving a high percentage (33⅓ or more) of children eligible for free or reduced cost meals (see National School Lunch Program)

FEATURES:

- Camps may serve three meals daily plus a snack
- Other programs may serve up to two meals and a snack
- Meals and snacks must meet USDA guidelines

Potential and actual problems of child nutrition programs

- Lack of availability of the programs, especially the newer child feeding programs such as School Breakfast, Summer and Holiday Food Program (due primarily to lack of local initiative or administrative problems rather than lack of federal funds)
- Poor operation of some existing programs:
  - Excessive plate waste owing to poor menu planning, low quality ingredients, substandard food preparation, and/or too short a time period for eating
  - Menus which set a poor example for development of good eating habits (e.g., (1) Use of fortified high sugar foods such as "astro-cakes," "super-donuts," and presweetened cereals (advantages versus disadvantages of these foods is a controversial subject) and (2) food selection very high in fat content such as 50 percent or more of the calories from fat[4])
  - School lunches which are low in several nutrients when compared to the goal of one third the RDA (a wide variation is found among schools)[4-6]
  - The School Lunch Program has occasionally been criticized for failing to use nutritional risk as an independent criterion for eligibility for free school lunches. It has been estimated that there are many middle and upper income children at nutritional risk who would benefit from participation in the lunch program but who do not participate because their parents do not give them money to cover the cost.[7]

FOR FURTHER INFORMATION:

Child Nutrition Programs
Food and Nutrition Service USDA
Washington, DC 20250

or

Regional Office (of above)
Call Federal Information Service for address

Food and Nutrition Service
(Your State) Dept. of Education
State Capital, Your State

Advocacy groups: See page 423

Appendix 2E
FOOD DISTRIBUTION PROGRAM (COMMODITY ASSISTANCE)

ELIGIBILITY:

Primarily for food programs, e.g., school lunch and breakfast, Title III, charitable institutions, disaster relief agencies, and needy family programs on some American-Indian reservations.

FEATURES:

• Commodities are *donated* foods, usually acquired under price support and surplus removal legislation.
• Examples of donated foods: frozen chicken, turkey, and ground beef and pork; canned applesauce, green beans, and tomato paste; peanut butter; raisins; flour; dried beans.
• Commodities which have been processed under government contract may be available, e.g., turkey rolls, pizza shells.

• By law some federal feeding programs must receive a minimum annual level of commodity food assistance.
• In some cases federal feeding programs are entitled to receive cash in lieu of commodities.

POTENTIAL AND ACTUAL DRAWBACKS:

• Local programs may find it difficult to make effective use of available commodities.
• Types and amounts of commodities fluctuate.

FOR FURTHER INFORMATION:

FNS
USDA
Washington, DC 20250

or
Regional office of FNS

Appendix 2F
ADVOCACY GROUPS WHICH CAN GIVE ASSISTANCE WITH QUESTIONS OR PROBLEMS RELATING TO FEDERAL FOOD PROGRAMS

Food Research and Action Center (FRAC)
2011 Eye Street, N.W., Suite 700
Washington, DC 20006

Community Nutrition Institute
1910 "K" Street, N.W.
Washington, DC 20006

The Food Law Center
1029 Connecticut Avenue, N.W.
Washington, DC 20036

} All federal food programs and the Food Stamp Program

The Children's Foundation
1420 New York Ave., N.W.
Suite 800
Washington, DC 20005

WIC and all child nutrition programs

National Senior Citizens Law Center
1709 West Eighth Street
Los Angeles, CA 90017

Nutrition Program for the Elderly under Title III of the Older American's Act

References

1. Barclay, R. W.: Legislative highlights. *J. Am. Diet. Assoc.* 71:653, 1977.

2. Greger, J. L., and Sciscoe, B. S.: Zinc nutriture of elderly participants in an urban feeding program. *J. Am. Diet. Assoc.* 70:37, 1977.

3. Fulmer, S., Gill, M., and Teets, R. M., Jr.; *Guide to American Food Programs.* San Francisco: Food Law Center, 1977.

4. Head, M. K., Weeks, R. J., and Gibbs, E.: Major nutrients in the Type A lunch. 1. Analyzed and calculated values of meals served. *J. Am. Diet. Assoc.* 63:620, 1973.

5. Voichick, J.: School lunch in Chicago. *J. Nutr. Ed.* 9:102, 1977.

6. Jansen, G. R., et al.: Comparison of Type A and nutrient standard menus for school lunch. III. Nutritive content of menus and acceptability. *J. Am. Diet. Assoc.* 66:254, 1975.

7. Emmons, L., Hayes, M., and Call, D. L.: A study of school feeding programs. I. Economic eligibility and nutritional need. *J. Am. Diet. Assoc.* 61:262, 1972.

Appendix 3

Tables of food composition

Key and explanatory notes for Appendices 3A, B, and C

* Weight and measure includes uneaten parts (e.g., peel, seeds).

† Data unavailable for item as described, but nutrient is probably present in measurable amount.

‡ Nutrient content depends on amounts of nutrients added, as by enrichment or fortification. Check nutritional labeling of the product in question.

§ Values given by Perloff and Butrum are used if possible.

Numbers represent averages. Water and energy nutrient content are rounded off to the nearest whole number, except for amounts of protein less than 5 gm which are indicated to the nearest 0.1 gm. A zero (0) does not necessarily mean that the food is completely free of the nutrient, but the amount present is probably too small to be significant for the serving size indicated. Other tables of food composition should be used if greater accuracy is required.

Sources of data

DAIRY PRODUCTS AND EGGS

Composition of Foods. Dairy and Egg Products. Consumer and Food Economics Institute, Agricultural Research Service, USDA. Agriculture Handbook No. 8-1. Washington DC: Superintendent of Documents, 1976.

ALL OTHER FOODS IN TABLES

Adams, C. F.: *Nutritive Value of American Foods.* Agriculture Handbook No. 456. Washington DC: Superintendent of Documents, 1975.
Nutritive Value of Foods. Home and Garden Bull. No. 72. USDA. Washington DC. 1970.
Young, E. A., Brennan, E. H., and Irving, G. L.: Perspectives on fast foods. *Diet. Currents* 5(5):24, 1978.

MAGNESIUM, FOLACIN, AND PANTOTHENIC ACID

Pennington, J. A.: *Dietary Nutrient Guide.* Westport CT: Avi Publishing Co., 1976.
Perloff, B. P., and Butrum, R. R.: Folacin in selected foods. *J. Am. Diet. Assoc.* 70:161, 1977.
Robinson, C., and Lawler, M. R.: Mineral and vitamin content of foods, Table A-2. *Normal and Therapeutic Nutrition,* ed. 15. New York: Macmillan Publishing Co., 1977.

Appendix 3A
FOOD COMPOSITION OF A SELECTION OF FOODS FROM THE BASIC FOUR FOOD GROUPS

	Household measure	Weight gm	Water %	Food energy kcal	Protein gm	Fat gm	Carbo-hydrate gm	Calcium mg	Iron mg	Magne-sium mg	Vita-min A value IU	Thiamine mg	Ribo-flavin mg	Niacin mg	Folacin§ µg	Panto-thenic acid mg	Ascorbic acid mg
Apple, raw, unpared	1 med 2¾" diam	150*	84	80	0.3	0	20	10	0.4	8	120	0.04	0.03	0.1	13	0.15	6
Apple juice, canned or bottled	½ c	124	88	59	0.1	0	15	8	0.7	5	†	0.01	0.03	0.1	0	0.12	1
Applesauce, canned, sweetened	½ c	128	78	116	0.3	0	30	5	0.7	5	50	0.02	0.01	0	2	0.13	2
Apricots, raw	3 (12 per lb)	114*	85	55	1.1	0	14	18	0.5	12	2890	0.03	0.04	0.6	3	0.24	11
Apricots, canned, heavy syrup	3 halves; 1¾ Tbsp liq	85	77	73	0.5	0	19	9	0.3	†	1480	0.02	0.02	0.3	†	†	3
Apricots, dried, sulfured, uncooked	10 med halves	35	25	91	1.8	0	23	23	1.9	22	3820	0	0.06	1.2	5	†	4
Asparagus, cooked green spears	4 med	60	94	12	1.3	0	2	13	0.4	12	540	0.10	0.11	0.8	7	†	16
Avocado, raw	⅛ med	25*	74	42	0.5	4	2	3	0.1	9	72	0.03	0.05	0.4	15	0.28	4
Banana, raw	1 sm (7¾")	140*	76	81	1.0	0	21	8	0.7	30	180	0.05	0.06	0.7	22	0.30	10
Beans, green snap, cooked	½ c	65	92	16	1.0	0	3	32	0.4	14	351	0.05	0.06	0.3	25	0.13	8
Beans, lima (Fordhook), froz cooked	½ c	85	74	84	5	0	16	17	1.5	†	195	0.06	0.05	0.9	25	0.20	15
Beans, red kidney, cooked	1 c	185	69	218	14	1	40	70	4.4	†	10	0.20	0.11	1.3	68	†	0
Bean sprouts, mung, raw	½ c	53	89	19	2.0	0	4	10	0.7	†	10	0.07	0.07	0.4	†	†	10
Beef chuck, cooked, trimmed choice	3 oz	85	57	212	25	12	0	11	3.1	20	20	0.05	0.19	3.8	3	0.34	0
Beef, corned canned	3 oz	85	59	245	29	14	0	22	2.3	23	†	0.02	0.27	3.9	3	0.51	0
Beef, round steak, cooked, trimmed	3 oz	85	61	161	27	5	0	11	3.1	24	10	0.07	0.20	5.1	3	0.43	0
Beets, red, canned drained	½ c	80	89	32	0.8	0	8	15	0.6	12	16	0.01	0.02	0.1	16	0.08	2
Beet greens, cooked	½ c	73	93	13	1.3	0	2	72	1.4	†	3700	0.05	0.11	0.2	†	†	11
Biscuits, baking powder, made from mix	1 med 2¼" diam	35	29	114	2.5	3	18	24	0.8	8	0	0.09	0.09	0.7	3	0.14	0
Blueberries, fresh cultivated	½ c	73	83	45	0.5	0	11	10	0.8	†	75	0.02	0.05	0.4	5	†	10
Bologna	1 slice (1 oz)	28	56	86	3.4	8	0	2	0.5	†	†	0.05	0.06	0.7	1	†	0
Bran cereal	½ c	30	4	72	3.8	1	22	25	‡	50	‡	‡	‡	‡	‡	†	‡
Bread, French enriched	1 slice 1" thick	35	31	102	3.2	1	19	15	0.8	7	0	0.10	0.08	0.9	3	0.14	0

Food	Measure																
Bread, rye (American)	1 slice	25	36	61	2.3	0	13	19	0.4	10	0	0.05	0.02	0.4	6	0.12	0
Bread, white enriched	1 slice	25	36	68	2.2	1	13	21	0.6	6	0	0.06	0.05	0.6	10	0.10	0
Bread, whole wheat	1 slice	25	36	61	2.6	1	12	25	0.8	10	0	0.06	0.03	0.7	16	0.18	0
Broccoli, raw	1 sm stalk	114	89	38	4.1	0	7	117	1.3	+	2835	0.10	0.23	0.9	78	+	102
Broccoli, cooked drained	1 sm stalk	140	91	36	4.3	0	6	123	1.1	27	3500	0.13	0.28	1.1	96	0.69	126
Brussels sprouts, froz cooked drained	½ c	78	89	26	2.5	0	5	17	0.6	+	440	0.06	0.08	0.5	+	+	63
Buttermilk, cultured	1 c	245	90	99	8	2	12	285	0.1	27	81	0.08	0.38	0.1	+	0.67	2
Cabbage, raw, chopped	½ c	45	92	11	0.6	0	3	22	0.2	6	60	0.03	0.03	0.2	30	0.06	21
Cabbage, boiled, drained wedge	½ c	85	94	16	0.9	0	3	36	0.3	10	100	0.02	0.02	0.1	15	0.17	21
Cantaloupe	¼ melon 5" diam	239*	91	41	1.0	0	10	38	0.6	14	4620	0.06	0.04	0.8	41	0.15	45
Carrots, raw	1 carrot 7½" long	81	88	30	0.8	0	7	27	0.5	13	7930	0.04	0.04	0.4	26	0.23	6
Carrots, cooked, drained	½ c	73	91	23	0.7	0	5	24	0.5	5	7615	0.04	0.04	0.4	19	0.23	5
Cauliflower, cooked, drained	½ c	63	93	14	1.5	0	3	13	0.5	+	40	0.06	0.05	0.4	21	+	35
Celery, green, raw	1 outer stalk 8" long	40	94	7	0.4	0	2	16	0.1	+	110	0.01	0.01	0.1	5	+	4
Cheese, American	1 oz slice	28	39	106	6	9	0	174	0.1	6	343	0.01	0.10	0	2	0.08	0
Cheese, blue	1 oz	28	42	100	6	8	1	150	0.1	7	204	0.01	0.11	0.3	10	0.49	0
Cheese, cheddar	1 oz	28	37	114	7	9	0	204	0.2	8	300	0.01	0.11	0	5	0.10	0
Cheese, cottage, creamed	4 oz	113	79	117	14	5	3	68	0.2	6	184	0.02	0.18	0.1	14	0.08	0
Cheese, cream	1 oz	28	54	99	2	10	1	23	0.3	2	405	0.01	0.06	0	4	0.08	0
Chicken, roast, light meat without skin	3 oz	85	64	141	27	3	0	10	1.2	+	51	0.03	0.09	9.9	3	+	0
Chicken, roast, dark meat without skin	3 oz	85	64	149	24	5	0	11	1.5	+	127	0.06	0.19	4.7	6	+	0
Clams, canned drained	3 oz	85	75	83	13	2	2	46	3.5	97	93	0.01	0.09	0.9	3	0.26	9
Collards, leaves without stems, cooked, drained	½ c	95	90	32	3.4	1	5	178	0.8	36	7410	0.11	0.19	1.2	20	0.43	72
Corn, boiled on cob	1 ear 5" long	140*	74	70	2.5	1	16	2	0.5	+	310	0.09	0.08	1.1	+	+	7
Corn, canned, drained	½ c	83	76	70	2.2	1	16	4	0.4	18	290	0.03	0.04	0.8	2	0.17	4
Cornflakes	1 c	25	4	97	2.0	0	21	+	+	4	+	+	+	+	+	0.05	+
Cornmeal, degermed yellow enriched cooked	½ c	120	88	60	1.3	0	13	1	0.5	10	70	0.07	0.05	0.6	1	0.12	0
Crackers, graham	2 squares	14	6	55	1.1	1	10	6	0.2	7	0	0.01	0.03	0.2	+	+	0
Crackers, saltines	4 squares	11	4	48	1.0	1	8	2	0.1	+	0	+	+	+	+	+	0

Table continues on following pages

	Household measure	Weight gm	Water %	Food energy kcal	Protein gm	Fat gm	Carbo-hydrate gm	Calcium mg	Iron mg	Magne-sium mg	Vita-min A value IU	Thiamine mg	Ribo-flavin mg	Niacin mg	Folacin§ μg	Panto-thenic acid mg	Ascorbic acid mg
Cream, light coffee or table	1 Tbsp	15	74	29	0.4	3	1	14	0	1	108	0.01	0.02	0	0	0.04	0
Cream, heavy whipping	1 Tbsp	15	58	52	0.3	6	1	10	0	1	220	0	0.02	0	1	0.04	0
Cucumbers, raw pared	9 sm slices	28	96	4	0.2	0	1	5	0.1	3	0	0.01	0.01	0.1	4	0.07	3
Dates, hydrated	5	40	23	110	0.9	0	29	24	1.2	23	20	0.04	0.04	0.9	9	0.31	0
Eggs, hard cooked	1 large	50	75	79	6	6	1	28	1.0	6	260	0.04	0.14	0	24	0.86	0
Farina, enriched, quick cooking, cooked	½ c	123	89	53	1.6	0	11	74	‡	4	0	0.12	0.07	1.0	0	0.12	0
Figs, dried	1 large	21	23	60	1.0	0	15	26	0.6	15	20	0.16	0.17	3.9	2	0.91	0
Flour, all purpose enriched	1 c	125	12	455	13	1	95	20	3.6	30	0	0.55	0.33	4.4	24	0.58	0
Flour, whole wheat	1 c	120	12	400	16	2	85	49	4.0	136	0	0.66	0.14	5.2	65	1.32	0
Frankfurters, cooked	1	57	56	176	7	16	1	4	1.1	5	†	0.09	0.11	1.5	2	0.23	0
Grapefruit, raw white	½ med 4³/₁₆" diam	277*	88	56	1	0	15	22	0.5	12	10	0.05	0.03	0.3	11	0.41	52
Grapefruit juice, unsweetened canned	½ c	124	89	51	0.6	0	12	10	0.5	8	10	0.04	0.03	0.3	1	0.12	42
Grapes, raw seedless European	10 grapes	50	81	34	0.3	0	9	6	0.2	3	50	0.03	0.02	0.2	4	†	2
Grape juice, unsweetened bottled	½ c	127	83	84	0.5	0	21	14	0.4	15	†	0.10	0.05	0.5	3	†	0
Haddock, fried (dipped in egg, milk, bread crumbs)	3 oz	85	66	141	17	5	5	33	0.9	20	†	0.03	0.06	2.7	14	0.26	3
Halibut, broiled with butter or margarine	3 oz	85	67	144	21	6	0	15	0.6	20	570	0.03	0.06	7.2	14	0.26	†
Ham (cured pork), baked, trimmed	3 oz	85	62	159	22	8	0	9	2.7	17	0	0.49	0.20	3.8	9	†	0
Ice cream, vanilla	½ c	67	61	135	2	7	16	88	0.1	9	277	0.03	0.16	0.1	2	0.33	0
Ice milk, vanilla	½ c	61	69	92	3	3	15	88	0.1	10	107	0.04	0.17	0.1	2	0.33	0
Kale, fresh cooked, drained	½ c	55	88	22	2.5	0	3	103	0.9	†	4565	0.06	0.10	0.9	†	†	51
Lamb leg, roast, trimmed	3 oz	85	62	158	24	6	0	11	1.9	19	†	0.14	0.26	5.3	27	0.51	0
Lemon juice, fresh	1 Tbsp	15	91	4	0.1	0	1	1	0	1	0	0	0	0	0	0.02	7
Lentils, cooked	½ c	100	72	106	8	0	19	25	2.1	†	20	0.07	0.06	0.6	†	†	0
Lettuce, crisp head	1 c sm chunks	75	96	10	0.7	0	2	15	0.4	8	250	0.05	0.05	0.2	27	0.15	5
Lettuce, cos or romaine	1 c chopped	55	94	10	0.7	0	2	37	0.8	8	1050	0.03	0.04	0.2	98	.07	10
Liver, beef, fried	1 slice 3 oz	85	56	195	22	9	5	9	7.5	19	45,390	0.22	3.56	14.0	123	6.04	23
Liverwurst, fresh	1 slice 1 oz	28	54	87	5	7	1	3	1.5	7	1800	0.06	0.37	1.6	8	1.77	†

Macaroni, enriched cooked	½ c	70	73	78	2.4	0	16	6	0.7	13	0	0.10	0.06	0.8	†	†	0
Milk, evaporated whole	½ c	126	74	169	9	10	13	329	0.2	30	306	0.06	0.40	0.2	10	†	2
Milk, lowfat (2% fat)	1 c	244	89	121	8	5	12	297	0.1	33	‡	0.10	0.40	0.2	12	0.78	2
Milk, skim	1 c	245	91	86	8	0	12	302	0.1	28	‡	0.09	0.34	0.2	13	0.81	2
Milk, whole (3.3% fat)	1 c	244	88	150	8	8	11	291	0.1	33	307	0.09	0.40	0.2	12	0.87	2
Mushrooms, fresh cultivated	½ c sliced	35	90	10	1.0	0	2	2	0.3	†	0	0.04	0.16	1.5	9	0.08	1
Mustard greens, cooked drained	½ c	75	94	15	1.7	0	2	78	1.2	17	4500	0.03	0.08	0.3	†	0.20	15
Noodles, egg, enriched cooked	½ c	80	71	100	3.3	1	19	8	0.7	18	55	0.11	0.07	1.0	2	0.16	0
Nuts, almonds	1 oz (about 28 nuts)	28	1	178	5	16	6	67	1.3	80	0	0.07	0.26	1.0	27	0.15	0
Nuts, Brazil	1 oz (6–8 nuts)	28	5	185	4.1	19	3	53	1.0	63	0	0.27	0.03	0.5	1	0.07	0
Nuts, pecans	1 oz	28	3	195	2.6	20	4	21	0.7	40	40	0.24	0.04	0.3	7	0.05	1
Nuts, walnuts	1 oz (14 halves)	28	4	185	4.2	18	5	28	0.9	36	10	0.09	0.04	0.3	18	0.27	1
Oatmeal, quick, cooked	½ c	120	87	66	2.4	1	13	22	0.7	29	0	0.19	0.05	0.2	13	0.24	0
Okra, cooked drained	½ c	80	91	23	1.6	0	5	74	0.4	†	390	0.11	0.15	0.7	†	†	16
Olives, black ripe	10 extra large	55*	80	61	0.5	7	1	40	0.8	†	30	0	0	0	0	0.01	0
Onions, mature cooked, drained	½ c sliced	105	92	31	1.3	0	7	25	0.4	9	40	0.03	0.03	0.2	26	0.11	8
Orange, raw (medium skin)	1 2⅝″ diam	180*	86	64	1.3	0	16	54	0.5	15	260	0.13	0.05	0.5	65	0.45	66
Orange juice, froz reconstituted	½ c	125	87	61	0.9	0	15	13	0.1	14	252	0.12	0.02	0.5	68	0.24	60
Oysters, raw Eastern	½ c (6–9 med)	120	85	79	10	2	4	113	6.6	38	370	0.17	0.22	3.0	†	0.30	†
Papaya, raw	½ med	227*	89	60	0.9	0	15	31	0.5	†	2660	0.06	0.06	0.5	†	0.33	85
Parsnips, cooked	1 large 9″ long	160	82	82	2.4	1	24	72	1.0	†	50	0.11	0.13	0.2	†	†	16
Peaches, raw, peeled	1 2¾″ diam	175*	89	58	0.9	0	15	14	0.8	16	2030	0.03	0.08	1.5	10	0.30	11
Peaches, canned, heavy syrup	1 half 2⅛ Tbsp liq	96	79	75	0.4	0	19	4	0.3	†	410	0.01	0.02	0.6	†	†	3
Peanut butter	2 Tbsp	32	2	188	8	16	6	18	0.6	49	0	0.04	0.04	4.8	26	0.48	0
Peanuts, roasted	1 oz	28	2	166	7	14	5	21	0.6	50	0	0.09	0.04	4.9	28	0.84	0
Pears, Bartlett, raw	1 pear 2½″ diam	180*	83	100	1.1	1	25	13	0.5	11	30	0.03	0.07	0.2	23	0.03	7
Pears, canned, heavy syrup	1 half 2¼ Tbsp liq	103	80	78	0.2	0	20	5	0.2	†	0	0.01	0.02	0.1	†	†	1
Peas, early, canned, drained	½ c	85	77	75	4.0	0	14	22	1.6	11	585	0.08	0.05	0.7	13	0.17	7
Peas, frozen, cooked drained	½ c	80	82	55	4.1	0	10	15	1.5	17	480	0.22	0.07	1.4	12	0.25	11
Peppers, sweet, raw	1 pepper 3¾″ × 3″ diam	200*	93	36	2.0	0	8	15	0.6	3	345	0.13	0.13	0.8	31	0.46	210

Table continues on following pages

Continued

Food	Household measure	Weight gm	Water %	Food energy kcal	Protein gm	Fat gm	Carbohydrate gm	Calcium mg	Iron mg	Magnesium mg	Vitamin A value IU	Thiamine mg	Riboflavin mg	Niacin mg	Folacin§ μg	Pantothenic acid mg	Ascorbic acid mg
Pineapple, raw	½ c diced	78	85	41	0.3	0	11	13	0.4	10	55	0.07	0.03	0.2	9	0.16	13
Pineapple, canned, heavy syrup	½ c	128	80	95	0.4	0	25	14	0.4	11	65	0.10	0.03	0.3	3	0.28	9
Plums, Japanese and hybrid raw	1 plum 2⅛" diam	70*	87	32	0.3	0	8	8	0.3	†	160	0.02	0.02	0.3	3	†	4
Popcorn, popped, plain, large kernel	1½ c	21	4	81	3	1	16	2	0.6	36	0	0.09	0.03	0.5	0	0.08	0
Pork, roast, trimmed	2 slices 3 oz	85	59	184	25	9	0	11	3.2	20	0	0.54	0.25	4.8	9	0.43	0
Pork sausage, cooked	1 sm link	13	35	62	2.4	6	0	1	0.3	2	0	0.10	0.04	0.5	1	0.08	0
Potato, baked in skin	1 potato 2⅓" × 4¾"	202*	75	145	4.0	0	33	14	1.1	40	0	0.15	0.07	2.7	22	0.78	31
Potato, French fries	10 strips 3½—4" long	78	45	214	3.4	10	28	12	1.0	13	0	0.10	0.06	2.4	16	0.38	16
Potato, mashed, milk added	½ c	105	41	69	2.2	1	14	25	0.4	14	20	0.09	0.06	1.1	10	0.20	11
Prunes, dried "softenized" without pits	5 prunes	51	28	130	1.1	0	34	26	2.0	20	815	0.05	0.09	0.9	5	0.23	2
Prune juice, canned or bottled	½ c	128	80	99	0.5	0	24	18	5.3	13	†	0.02	0.02	0.5	†	†	3
Raisins, unbleached, seedless	1 oz	28	18	82	0.7	0	22	18	1.0	9	10	0.03	0.02	0.1	1	0.03	0
Rice, brown, cooked	½ c	98	70	116	2.5	1	25	12	0.5	28	0	0.18	0.04	2.7	7	0.39	0
Rice, white enriched cooked	½ c	103	73	113	2.1	0	25	11	0.9	2	0	0.12	0.01	1.1	2	0.20	0
Salmon, broiled with butter or margarine	3 oz	85	63	156	23	6	0	†	0.9	35	150	0.15	0.06	8.4	6	0.43	0
Salmon, canned Chinook	3 oz	85	64	157	15	10	0	114	0.7	20	171	0.03	0.10	5.5	5	0.45	0
Salami, dry	1 oz	28	30	128	7	11	0	4	1.0	†	0	0.10	0.07	1.5	†	†	0
Sardines, canned drained	1 oz	28	62	58	7	3	0	124	0.8	11	60	0.01	0.06	1.5	5	0.25	0
Sauerkraut, canned	½ c	118	93	21	1.2	0	5	43	0.6	†	60	0.04	0.05	0.3	1	0.11	17
Shrimp, boiled	3 oz	85	77	80	18	1	0	66	1.4	36	30	0.03	0.03	2.0	2	0.30	7
Soup, cream of mushroom, condensed, prepared with equal volume of milk	1 c	245	83	216	7	14	16	191	0.5	†	250	0.05	0.34	0.7	†	†	1
Soup, split pea, condensed, prepared with equal volume of water	1 c	245	85	145	9	3	21	29	1.5	15	440	0.25	0.15	1.5	2	0.24	1
Soup, tomato, condensed, prepared with equal volume of water	1 c	245	91	88	2.0	3	16	15	0.7	17	1000	0.05	0.05	1.2	10	0.24	12

Food	Serving																
Soup, vegetable beef, condensed, prepared with equal volume of water	1 c	245	92	78	5	2	10	12	0.7	27	2700	0.05	0.05	1.0	10	0.24	†
Spinach, raw chopped	1 c	55	91	14	1.8	0	2	51	1.7	30	4460	0.03	0.11	0.3	106	0.16	28
Spinach, canned drained	½ c	103	91	22	2.3	1	4	99	2.5	44	6380	0.03	0.12	0.4	30	0.10	16
Spinach, froz, cooked, drained	½ c	103	92	24	3.1	0	4	116	2.2	44	8100	0.07	0.16	0.4	30	0.10	20
Squash, summer, sliced	½ c	90	96	13	0.8	0	3	23	0.4	15	350	0.05	0.07	0.7	2	0.20	9
Squash, winter, baked mashed	½ c	103	81	65	1.9	0	16	29	0.8	†	4305	0.05	0.14	0.7	†	†	14
Strawberries, raw	1 c	149	90	55	1.0	1	13	31	1.5	18	90	0.04	0.10	0.9	24	0.51	44
Sweet potato, baked	1 potato 5" long	146*	64	161	2.4	1	37	46	1.0	17	9230	0.10	0.08	0.8	26	0.98	25
Tangerine	1 med 2⅜" diam	116*	87	39	0.7	0	10	34	0.3	†	360	0.05	0.02	0.1	25	0.19	27
Tomatoes, raw	1 tomato 3½ oz	100*	94	20	1.0	0	4	12	0.5	13	820	0.05	0.04	0.6	39	0.30	21
Tomatoes, canned	½ c	121	94	26	1.2	0	5	7	0.6	11	1085	0.06	0.04	0.9	26	0.20	21
Tortillas, corn, lime	1 6" diam	30	46	63	1.5	1	14	60	0.9	32	6	0.04	0.02	0.3	0	0.03	0
Tuna, canned, oil pack, drained	3 oz	85	61	167	25	7	0	7	1.6	24	67	0.04	0.10	10.1	13	1.15	0
Tuna, canned, water pack, solids and liquid	3 oz	85	70	108	24	1	0	14	1.4	†	†	†	0.08	11.3	†	†	0
Turkey, roast (light and dark mixed)	3 oz	85	61	162	27	5	0	7	1.5	†	0	0.04	0.15	6.5	5	0.73	0
Turnip, cooked, drained	½ c cubed	78	94	18	0.6	0	4	27	0.3	11	0	0.03	0.04	0.3	1	0.08	17
Turnip greens, cooked drained	½ c	73	93	15	1.6	0	3	133	0.8	†	4570	0.11	0.18	0.5	†	†	50
Veal, cooked loin	3 oz	85	59	199	22	11	0	9	2.7	16	0	0.06	0.21	4.6	3	†	0
Watermelon	1 c diced	160	93	42	0.8	0	10	11	0.8	13	470	0.03	0.03	0.2	12	0.48	6
Wheat germ, plain toasted	1 Tbsp	6	4	23	1.8	1	3	3	0.5	19	10	0.11	0.05	0.3	26	0.14	1
Whole wheat cereal, cooked	½ c	123	88	55	2.2	0	12	9	0.6	37	0	0.08	0.03	0.8	8	0.24	0
Whole wheat flakes, ready-to-eat	1 c	30	4	106	3.1	1	24	12	†	27	†	‡	‡	†	‡	0.14	‡
Yeast, brewers	1 Tbsp	8	5	23	3.1	0	3	17	1.4	18	0	1.25	0.34	3.0	313	0.96	0
Yogurt, plain low fat	1 8 oz container	227	85	144	12	4	16	415	0.2	40	150	0.10	0.49	0.3	25	1.34	2

Appendix 3B
FOOD COMPOSITION OF A SELECTION OF "OTHER" FOODS WHICH ARE LOW IN NUTRIENT DENSITY

	Household measure	Weight gm	Water %	Food energy kcal	Protein gm	Fat gm	Carbohydrate gm	Calcium mg	Iron mg	Magnesium mg	Vitamin A value IU	Thiamine mg	Riboflavin mg	Niacin mg	Folacin μg	Pantothenic acid mg	Ascorbic acid mg
Bacon, cooked drained	2 slices	16	8	98	5	8	1	2	0.5	4	0	0.08	0.05	0.8	0	0.21	0
Beer	12 fl oz	360	92	151	1.1	0	14	18	0	36	0	0.01	0.11	2.2	0	0.36	0
Bouillon, broth	1 cube	4	4	5	1	0	0	0	†	0	0	0	†	†	0	0	0
Butter	1 tsp	5	16	36	0	4	0	1	0	0	165	0	0	0	0	0	0
Cake, angel food, plain, from mix	1/12 of cake	53	34	137	3	0	32	50	0.2	8	0	0	0.04	0	1	0.11	0
Cake, devils' food, iced, from mix	1/12 of cake	92	24	312	4	11	54	54	0.7	20	140	0.03	0.07	0.3	29	0.18	0
Candy, caramel, plain or chocolate	1 oz	28	8	113	1	3	22	42	0.4	0	0	0.01	0.05	0.1	1	0	0
Candy, hard	1 oz	28	1	109	0	0	28	6	0.5	0	0	0	0	0	0	0	0
Candy, milk chocolate	1 oz	28	1	147	2	9	16	65	0.3	23	80	0.02	0.10	0.1	2	0.03	0
Carbonated beverages, cola	12 oz	369	90	144	0	0	37	27	†	3	0	0	0	0	0	0	0
Carbonated beverages, ginger ale	12 oz	366	92	113	0	0	29	†	†	†	0	0	0	0	0	0	0
Coffee, instant	¾ c	180	98	1	0	0	0	1	0.2	10	0	0	0	0.1	0	0	0
Cookies, chocolate chip, homemade	2 2¼" diam	20	3	103	1	6	12	7	0.4	†	20	0.02	0.02	0.2	†	†	0
Cookies, vanilla	5 1¾" diam	20	3	93	1	3	15	8	0.1	†	0.25	0	0.01	0	†	†	0
Honey	1 Tbsp	21	17	64	0	0	17	1	0.1	1	0	0	0.01	0.1	1	0.04	0
Jelly	1 Tbsp	18	29	49	0	0	13	4	0.3	1	0	0	0.01	0	0	0.02	1
Margarine	1 tsp	5	16	36	0	4	0	1	0	0	165	0	0	0	0	0	0
Mayonnaise	1 tsp	5	15	36	0	4	0	1	0	0	13	0	0	0	0	0.01	0
Molasses, medium	1 Tbsp	20	24	46	0	0	12	58	1.2	16	0	0.02	0.02	0.2	2	0.08	0
Oil, soybean	1 tsp	5	0	44	0	5	0	0	0	0	0	0	0	0	0	0	0
Pickles, dill	1 oz	28	93	3	0.2	0	1	7	0.3	0	28	0	0	0	1	0.06	4
Pickles, sweet	1 oz	28	61	41	0.2	0	10	3	0.3	0	25	0	0	0	1	0.06	2
Sugar, brown	1 tsp packed	5	2	19	0	0	5	3	0.1	0	0	0	0	0	0	†	0
Sugar, granulated white	1 tsp	5	1	19	0	0	5	0	0	0	0	0	0	0	0	0	0

	Measure	Weight gm	Food energy kcal	Protein gm	Fat gm	Carbohydrate gm	Calcium mg	Iron mg	Potassium mg	Sodium mg	Vitamin A value IU	Thiamine mg	Riboflavin mg	Niacin mg	Ascorbic acid mg
Tea, brewed	¾ c	180	0	0	0	0	0	0	0	0	0	0	0	0	0
Whiskey, gin, rum, vodka, 90 proof	1½ fl. oz (1 jigger)	42	110	0	0	0	0	0	0	0	0	0	0	0	0
Wine, dry table 12% alcohol	3½ fl oz	100	86	0.1	0	4	9	0.4	0	0	0.01	0.1	0	0	0
Wine, sweet 18.8% alcohol	2 fl oz	60	82	0.1	0	5	5	0.2	0.01	0.01	0.01	0.1	0	0	0

Appendix 3C
FOOD COMPOSITION OF A SELECTION OF FAST FOODS (Young, et al.)

	Brand	Weight gm	Food energy kcal	Protein gm	Fat gm	Carbohydrate gm	Calcium mg	Iron mg	Potassium mg	Sodium mg	Vitamin A value IU	Thiamine mg	Riboflavin mg	Niacin mg	Ascorbic acid mg
Apple pie	MacDonald's	91	300	2	19	31	12	0.6	39	414	<69	0.02	0.03	1.3	3
Burrito, combination	Taco Bell	175	404	21	16	43	91	3.7	278	300	1666	0.34	0.31	4.6	15
Chicken, fried drumstick	Kentucky Fried	54	136	14	8	2	20	0.9	†	‡	30	0.04	0.12	2.7	0
Chicken, fried wing	Kentucky Fried	45	151	11	10	4	†	0.6	†	‡	†	0.03	0.07	†	0
Chocolate sundae, med	Dairy Queen	184	300	6	7	53	200	1.1	†	‡	300	0.06	0.26	0	0
Dairy Queen cone, med	Dairy Queen	142	230	6	7	35	200	0	†	‡	300	0.09	0.26	0	0
Filet O Fish	MacDonald's	131	402	15	23	34	105	1.8	293	709	152	0.28	0.28	3.9	4
Hamburger	MacDonald's	99	257	13	9	30	63	3.0	234	526	231	0.23	0.23	5.1	2
Hot dog	Burger King	†	291	11	17	23	40	2.0	170	841	0	0.04	0.02	2.0	0
Onion rings (Brazier)	Dairy Queen	85	300	6	17	33	20	0.4	16	‡	0	0.09	0	0.4	2
Pizza, cheese, Thin 'N crispy (½ of 10" pizza)	Pizza Hut	†	450	25	15	54	450	4.5	†	‡	750	0.30	0.51	5.0	1
Pizza, cheese, Thick 'N Chewy (½ of 10" pizza)	Pizza Hut	†	560	34	14	71	500	5.4	†	‡	1000	0.68	0.68	7.0	1
Taco	Taco Bell	83	186	15	8	14	120	2.5	143	79	120	0.09	0.16	2.9	0
Vanilla shake	MacDonald's	289	323	10	8	52	346	0.2	499	250	346	0.12	0.66	0.6	<3
Whopper	Burger King	†	606	29	32	32	37	6.0	653	909	641	0.02	0.03	5.2	13

Appendix 4

Tables used in nutritional assessment

Appendix 4A
HEIGHT AND WEIGHT TABLES FOR ADULTS

Males

HEIGHT*			WEIGHT†	
cm	ft	in	kg	lb
157.5	5	2	55–60	121–133
160.0		3	56–62	124–136
162.5		4	58–63	127–139
165.0		5	59–65	130–143
167.5		6	61–67	134–147
170.0		7	63–69	138–152
172.5		8	65–71	142–156
175.0		9	66–73	146–160
178.0		10	68–75	150–165
180.5		11	70–77	154–170
183.0	6		72–80	158–175
185.5		1	74–82	162–180
188.0		2	76–84	167–185
190.5		3	78–86	172–190

Adapted from the 1959 Metropolitan Life Insurance Standards
* Height measured without shoes
† Weight in light indoor clothing; to correct for nude weight subtract 0.9–1.8 kg (2–4 lb)

Females

HEIGHT*			WEIGHT†	
cm	ft	in	kg	lb
147.5	4	10	46–51	101–113
150.0		11	47–53	104–116
152.5	5		49–54	107–119
155.0		1	50–55	110–122
157.5		2	51–57	113–126
160.0		3	53–59	116–130
162.5		4	55–61	120–135
165.0		5	56–63	124–139
167.5		6	58–65	128–143
170.0		7	60–67	132–147
172.5		8	62–69	136–151
175.0		9	64–70	140–155
178.0		10	65–72	144–159

Adapted from the 1959 Metropolitan Life Insurance Standards
* Height measured without shoes.
† Weight in light indoor clothing; to correct for nude weight subtract 0.9–1.8 kg (2–4 lb)

Appendix 4B
MINIMUM TRICEPS SKINFOLD THICKNESS INDICATING OBESITY

AGE (yr)	MALES	FEMALES
5	12	14
10	16	20
15	16	24
20	16	28
25	20	29
30–50	23	30

From Seltzer, C. C., and Mayer, J.: A simple criterion of obesity. *Postgrad. Med.* 38:A101, 1965 © McGraw-Hill, Inc.

Appendix 4C
STANDARDS FOR MID-UPPER ARM CIRCUMFERENCE

Arm circumference in centimeters

SEX	STANDARD	90%	80%	70%	60%
♂	29.3	26.3	23.4	20.5	17.6
♀	28.5	25.7	22.8	20.0	17.1

From Blackburn, G. L., et al.: Nutritional and metabolic assessment of the hospitalized patient. *J. Parent. Ent. Nutr.* 1:11–22, 1977. With the permission of Dr. Blackburn and the *Journal of Parenteral and Enteral Nutrition.*

Appendix 4D
STANDARDS FOR ARM MUSCLE CIRCUMFERENCE

Muscle circumference in centimeters

SEX	STANDARD	90%	80%	70%	60%
♂	25.3	22.8	20.2	17.7	15.2
♀	23.2	20.9	18.6	16.2	13.9

From Blackburn, G. L., et al.: Nutritional and metabolic assessment of the hospitalized patient. *J. Parent. Ent. Nutr.* 1:11–22, 1977. With the permission of Dr. Blackburn and the *Journal of Parenteral and Enteral Nutrition.*

Appendix 4E
ARM ANTHROPOMETRY NOMOGRAM FOR ADULTS

ARM ANTHROPOMETRY NOMOGRAM FOR ADULTS

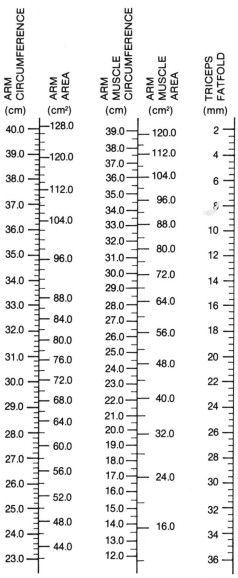

To obtain muscle circumference:
1. Lay ruler between value of arm circumference and fatfold
2. Read off muscle circumference on middle line

To obtain tissue areas:
1. The arm area and muscle area are alongside their respective circumferences
2. Fat area = arm area − muscle area

Drawn from Gurney, J. M.: Arm arthropometry in nutritional assessment: nomogram for rapid calculation of muscle circumference and cross-sectional muscle and fat areas. *Am. J. Clin. Nutr.* 26:914, 1973. Used with permission.

Appendix 4F
RELATIVE MERITS OF VARIOUS EXERCISES IN INDUCING CARDIOVASCULAR FITNESS

ENERGY RANGE	ACTIVITY	COMMENT
1.5–2.0 Mets* or 2.0–2.5 Cals†/min. or 120–150 Cals/hr.	Light housework such as polishing furniture or washing small clothes	Too low in energy level and too intermittent to promote endurance.
	Strolling 1.0 mile/hr.	Not sufficiently strenuous to promote endurance unless capacity is very low.
2.0–3.0 Mets or 2.5–4.0 Cals/min or 150–240 Cals/hr.	Level walking at 2.0 miles/hr.	See "strolling"
	Golf, using power cart	Promotes skill and minimal strength in arm muscles but not sufficiently taxing to promote endurance. Also too intermittent.
3.0–4.0 Mets or 4–5 Cals/min. or 240–300 Cals/hr.	Cleaning windows, mopping floors, or vacuuming	Adequate conditioning exercise if carried out continuously for 20–30 minutes.
	Bowling	Too intermittent and not sufficiently taxing to promote endurance.
	Walking at 3.0 miles/hr.	Adequate dynamic exercise if low capacity.
	Cycling at 6 miles/hr.	As above.
	Golf—pulling cart	Useful for conditioning if reach target rate. May include isometrics depending on cart weight.
4.0–5.0 Mets or 5–6 Cals/min. or 300–360 Cals/hr.	Scrubbing floors	Adequate endurance exercise if carried out in at least 2 minute stints.
	Walking 3.5 miles/hr.	Usually good dynamic aerobic exercise.
	Cycling 8 miles/hr.	As above.
	Table tennis, badminton and volleyball	Vigorous continuous play can have endurance benefits but intermittent, easy play only promotes skill.
	Golf—carrying clubs	Promotes endurance if reach and maintain target heart rate, otherwise merely aids strength and skill.
	Tennis—doubles	Not very beneficial unless there is continuous play maintaining target rate—which is unlikely. Will aid skill.
	Many calisthenics and ballet exercises	Will promote endurance if continuous, rhythmic and repetitive. Those requiring isometric effort such as push-ups and sit-ups are probably not beneficial for cardiovascular fitness.
5.0–6.0 Met or 6–7 Cals/min. or 360–420 Cals/hr.	Walking 4 miles/hr.	Dynamic, aerobic and of benefit.
	Cycling 10 miles/hr.	As above.
	Ice or roller skating	As above if done continuously.
6.0–7.0 Mets or 7–8 Cals/min. or 420–480 Cals/hr.	Walking 5 miles/hr.	Dynamic, aerobic and beneficial.
	Cycling 11 miles/hr.	Same.
	Singles tennis	Can provide benefit if played 30 minutes or more by skilled player with an attempt to keep moving.

Relative merits of various exercises in inducing cardiovascular fitness (continued)

ENERGY RANGE	ACTIVITY	COMMENT
	Water skiing	Total isometrics; very risky for cardiacs, pre-cardiacs (high risk) or deconditioned normals.
7.0–8.0 Mets or 8–10 Cals/min. or 480–600 Cals/hr.	Jogging 5 miles/hr.	Dynamic, aerobic, endurance building exercise.
	Cycling 12 miles/hr.	As above.
	Downhill skiing	Usually ski runs are too short to significantly promote endurance. Lift may be isometric. Benefits skill predominantly. Combined stress of altitude, cold and exercise may be too great for some cardiacs.
	Paddleball	Not sufficiently continuous but promotes skill. Competition and hot playing areas may be dangerous to cardiacs.
8.0–9.0 Mets or 10–11 Cals/min. or 600–660 Cals/hr.	Running 5.5 miles/hr.	Excellent conditioner.
	Cycling 13 miles/hr.	As above.
	Squash or handball (practice session or warmup)	Usually too intermittent to provide endurance building effect. Promotes skill.
Above 10 Mets or 11 Cals/min. or 660 Cals/hr.	Running 6 miles/hr.=10 Mets 7 miles/hr.=11.5 8 miles/hr.=13.5	Excellent conditioner.
	Competitive handball or squash	Competitive environment in a hot room is dangerous to anyone not in excellent physical condition. Same as singles tennis.

* Met=multiple of the resting energy requirement; e.g. 2 Mets require twice the resting energy cost, 3 Mets triple, etc.
† Cals=kcal
Note: Energy range will vary depending on skill of exerciser, pattern of rest pauses, environmental temperature, etc. Caloric values depend on body size (more for larger persons). Table provides reasonable "relative strenuousness values" however.
From *Beyond Diet: Exercise Your Way to Fitness and Heart Health* by Lenore R. Zohman, MD, Best Foods, CPC Intl. Englewood Cliffs NJ 1974, pp. 20, 21.

Appendix 4G

LABORATORY TESTS AND PHYSICAL SIGNS USEFUL IN NUTRITIONAL ASSESSMENT*

NUTRIENT	INDEX	ACCEPTABLE STATUS	CLINICAL SIGNS ASSOCIATED WITH A DEFICIENCY STATE
CARBOHYDRATE			
Glucose	Plasma glucose (mg/100ml)	80–120	Hunger, weakness, dizziness, loss of consciousness
FAT			
Cholesterol	Serum cholesterol (mg/100ml)	140–220	
Triglyceride	Serum triglyceride (fasting) (mg/100ml)	65–150	
Essential fatty acids	Plasma phospholipid 5, 8, 11 eicosatrienoic acid (%)	0.1–0.3	Dermatosis
PROTEIN			
Muscle mass	Creatinine height index	>0.8	Muscle wasting, weakness; dull, brittle hair, edema
Visceral	Serum protein (gm/100ml)	>6.5	
	Serum albumin (gm/100ml)	≥3.5	Poor wound healing, edema
Immune function	Total lymphocyte count	>1200 ⎫	Repeated infections
	Delayed cutaneous hypersensitivity (most tests)	>5mm ⎭	
Other	Blood urea nitrogen (mg/100ml)	8–20	
	Uric acid (mg/100)	3–5	
WATER-SOLUBLE VITAMINS			
Ascorbic acid	Serum ascorbic acid (mg/100ml)	≥0.3	(Scurvy) Petechiae; ecchymoses; spongy, bleeding gums; painful epiphyseal enlargement; poor wound healing
Thiamine	RBC transketolase (thiamine pyrophosphate stim.) (%)	0–15	(Beri-beri) Anorexia, peripheral neuropathy, heart disorders
	Urinary thiamine (μg/gm creatinine)	≥66	
Riboflavin	RBC Glutathione reductase-FAD effect	<1.2	Cheilosis, angular stomatitis, glossitis, localized dermatitis, photophobia, corneal vascularization
Niacin	Urinary N¹–methyl nicotinamide (mg/gm creatinine)	≥0.6	(Pellagra) Glossitis, dermatitis, diarrhea, dementia
Folacin	Serum folacin (ng/ml)	≥6.0	Pallor, anemia, glossitis, hyperpigmentation of skin, diarrhea, weight loss
Vitamin B_6	Tryptophan load (urinary xanthurenic acid after 2 gm tryptophan) (μmol/24h)	<50	Nasolabial seborrhea, glossitis, peripheral neuropathy, depression, anemia
Vitamin B_{12}	Serum B_{12} (pg/ml)	>200 ⎫	Pallor, anemia, neuropathy, glossitis
	Urinary methylmalonate (mg/24h)	<5 ⎭	
FAT-SOLUBLE VITAMINS			
Vitamin A	Serum vitamin A (μg/100 ml)	20–49	Night blindness, Bitot's spots, xerophthalmia, xerosis of skin, follicular hyperkeratosis
	Serum carotene (μg/100ml)	40–300	
Vitamin D	Serum alkaline phosphatase (IU/L)	35–148 ⎫	Rickets, osteomalacia, bone pain, tetany
	Plasma 25-hydroxy cholecalciferol (ng/ml)	10–40 ⎭	
Vitamin E	Plasma vitamin E (mg/100 ml)	≥0.6	Conclusive data not available
Vitamin K	Prothrombin time (sec.)	12	Bleeding tendency
MINERALS†			
Calcium	Calcium (mg/100ml)	9.0–11.0	Osteomalacia, tingling of fingers, muscle cramps, tetany, cardiac disturbances

Laboratory tests and physical signs useful in nutritional assessment* (Continued)

NUTRIENT	INDEX	ACCEPTABLE STATUS	CLINICAL SIGNS ASSOCIATED WITH A DEFICIENCY STATE
Chloride	Serum chloride (mEq/L)	99–110	Hypochloremic metabolic alkalosis, hypertonicity of muscles, depressed respirations
Chromium	Blood chromium (ng/ml)	4.9–9.5	Impaired glucose tolerance
Copper	Serum copper (μg/100ml)	75–150 }	Anemia
	Ceruloplasmin in plasma (mg/100ml)	15–30 }	
Iodine	Serum protein-bound iodine (PBD) (μg/100ml)	4.8–8.0	Thyroid enlargement (goiter)
Iron	Serum iron (μg/100ml)	♂ 60 ♀ 40	Pallor, anemia, angular stomatitis atrophic lingual papillae, thin brittle nails with spooning
	Serum transferrin (gm-100ml)	150	
	Total iron binding capacity (μg/100ml)	250–410	
	Hemoglobin (mg/100ml)	♂ 14 ♀ 12	
	Hematocrit (%)	♂ 44 ♀ 33	
Magnesium	Serum magnesium (mEq/L)	1.3–2.0	Neuromuscular irritability, dysphagia, anorexia, behavioral disturbances
Phosphorus	Serum phosphorus (mg/100ml)	2.5–4.0	Muscle weakness
Potassium	Serum potassium (mEq/L)	3.5–5.0	Alkalosis, muscle weakness, cardiac disturbances, paralytic ileus
Sodium	Serum sodium (mEq/L)	130–155	Anorexia, nausea, vomiting, lassitude, muscle cramps
Zinc	Plasma zinc (μg/100ml)	80–100	Poor wound healing, loss of taste and smell, glossitis, growth failure, anorexia, skin disorders

* Values are for young healthy adults. Criteria may vary depending on test methods and other variables.
† Some trace minerals not mentioned are toxic in high amounts.

References for laboratory data

Christakis, G. (ed.): Nutritional assessment in health programs. *Am. J. Public Health* 63:28, Nov. 1973, supplement.

Drummond, J.: Clinical and laboratory diagnosis of nutritional problems. *Dent. Clin. North Am.* 2(3):585, 1976.

Goodhart, R. S., and Shils, M. E. (eds.): *Modern Nutrition in Health and Disease.* Philadelphia: Lea and Febiger, 1973.

Jeejeebhoy, K. N., et al.: Chromium deficiency, glucose intolerance, and neuropathy reversed by chromium supplementation, in a patient receiving long-term total parenteral nutrition. *Am. J. Clin. Nutr.* 30:531, 1977.

Van Itallie, T. B.: Assessment of nutritional status. In G. Thorn, R. Adams, and E. Braunwald (eds.): *Harrison's Principles of Internal Medicine.* New York: McGraw-Hill Book Co., 1977.

Appendix 4H
CREATININE HEIGHT INDEX

The actual daily urinary creatinine excretion is compared with an ideal value from the following table to calculate the creatinine height index.

$$\text{Creatinine Height Index (CHI)} = \frac{\text{Actual urinary creatinine}}{\text{Ideal urinary creatinine}} \times 100$$

Ideal urinary creatinine values

MALE*		FEMALE†	
Height (cm)	Ideal Creatinine (mg)	Height (cm)	Ideal Creatinine (mg)
157.5	1288	147.3	830
162.6	1359	152.4	875
167.6	1426	157.5	925
172.7	1513	162.6	977
177.8	1596	167.6	1044
182.9	1691	172.7	1109
188.0	1785	177.8	1174
193.0	1891	182.9	1240

Adapted from Blackburn, G., et al.: Nutritional and metabolic assessment of the hospitalized patient. *J. Parenter. Enteral. Nutr.* 1:15, 1977. With the permission of Dr. Blackburn and the *Journal of Parenteral and Enteral Nutrition.*
  * Creatinine coefficient (men) = 23 mg/kg of ideal body weight
  † Creatinine coefficient (women) = 18 mg/kg of ideal body weight

Appendix 5

Modified diets

The modified diets included in this section are meant to serve as guidelines for kinds of foods which are appropriate for each type of diet. Food listings may differ somewhat from those found on diet forms used in particular health agencies. Details regarding meal pattern, size of meals, appropriate snacks, unlisted foods desired by the client, and planning for nutritional adequacy should be tailored to the client's health needs and preferences.

Appendix 5A
PROGRESSIVE DIETS

Clear liquid diet—foods allowed

Water, ice chips
Clear fruit juices (apple, cranberry, grape). Some agencies allow any strained fruit juice, if tolerated
Fat-free clear broth, consomme, or bouillon (hot or gelled)
Flavored gelatin dessert, popsicles
Sugar. Hard candy may be allowed
Decaffeinated coffee, herb tea; caffeine-containing beverages depending on the client's condition; carbonated and noncarbonated soft drinks
Low residue defined-formula diets with physician's order

Full liquid diet—foods allowed

MILK GROUP

Any type of fluid milk if lactose is tolerated. Plain or combined with allowed foods

MEAT GROUP

Eggs cooked in custard or pasteurized in eggnog
Strained meat, poultry, with added liquid

FRUIT AND VEGETABLE GROUP

Strained fruits and juices
Strained asparagus, carrots, green beans, peas, potatoes, spinach, and tomato, combined with other liquids
Vegetable juices

GRAIN GROUP

Cereal gruel made from farina (Cream of Wheat) corn meal, or Cream of Rice (thinned to desired consistency with milk or cream)

OTHER FOODS

Fats: butter, margarine, cream, combined with other foods, as tolerated
Soups: any type made with allowed ingredients, strained or blended
Desserts: soft or baked custard, rennet dessert, flavored gelatin dessert, plain smooth ice cream, popsicles, smooth pudding, smooth sherbet
Sweets: sugar, honey, syrup, jelly. Hard candy may be allowed
Seasonings: salt and flavorings, as tolerated
Beverages: most nonalcoholic types
Caffeine-containing beverages unless contraindicated.
Commercial liquid formulas

Soft solid diet

FOODS ALLOWED	*FOODS TO BE AVOIDED*
MILK	
Whole, skim buttermilk, yogurt. Milk drinks flavored with moderate amounts of syrups (chocolate, coffee, strained fruit), malt	Milk drinks or yogurt containing whole fruits or berries with seeds or skins
BEVERAGES	
Tea, coffee, cocoa, decaffeinated or cereal beverages, powdered fruit drinks, carbonated beverages	
EGGS	
Hard-cooked, pasteurized, or other salmonella-free egg preparations such as approved eggnog mixes	Raw eggs, soft-cooked eggs unless pasteurized, fried eggs
MEATS	
Broiled, baked, roasted chicken, turkey, beef, lamb, veal, liver, white fish, crisp bacon	Fried, highly seasoned items such as cold cuts, sardines
CHEESE	
Mild cheese such as cottage, cream, American, cheddar, Swiss	Strongly flavored, pungent cheeses
BREADS	
Refined, enriched white bread, plain or toasted; plain muffins, rolls; white flour crackers such as common, oyster, soda, saltines; melba toast, rusk, zwieback	Freshly baked hot breads; whole grain breads or crackers; those containing raisins or other fruits, nuts, bran, seeds; fried breads such as crullers and doughnuts
CEREALS	
Refined (ready-to-eat or cooked) made from refined wheat, rice, corn; cereals prepared for babies; noodles, macaroni, spaghetti; strained oatmeal	Whole grain cereals other than strained oatmeal. Prepared cereals with bran, berries, raisins
VEGETABLES	
Cooked asparagus tips, beans (green and wax beans only), beets, broccoli buds, carrots, tomato juice, winter squash. If desired, strained peas, spinach, or summer squash may be added	Other vegetables, strongly flavored sauces
FRUITS	
Cooked or canned without seeds and skins, such as apple-sauce, baked apple, peeled apricots, peaches, pears; ripe bananas, orange sections, grapefruit sections	Berries, raw fruits other than those listed
JUICES	
Fresh, frozen, or canned as tolerated	
DESSERTS	
Simple puddings without nuts or fruits such as custard, tapioca, plain ice cream, sherbet, water ice; plain, simple cakes and cookies	Pastries, cakes, cookies, and puddings made with nuts or fruits containing seeds and skins
FATS	
Butter, cream, margarine, crisp bacon, mayonnaise, mayon-naise-type salad dressing	

Source: *Diet Manual.* Massachusetts General Hospital Dietary Department. Copyright © 1976. Little, Brown & Co., Boston, pp. 24, 25. Used with permission.

Appendix 5B
BLAND DIET

Use the soft diet plan as the basis for the diet, with the following adaptations:

• Omit coffee (both regular and decaffeinated), tea, cola, pepper, chili, broth, and alcoholic beverages.

• Plan meal frequency and size in conjunction with medication schedule and client's preferences and nutritional needs.

• Obtain information from the client regarding food preferences and intolerances; use this as a basis for liberalizing the diet. For example, increasing the variety of vegetables and fruits used may help improve nutrient intake and palatability of the diet.

Appendix 5C
LOW RESIDUE (LOW FIBER) DIET
(with adaptations for minimal residue diet of normal foods)*

FOOD GROUP	AMOUNT ALLOWED	CHOICES
Milk	Up to 490 ml (2 c) fluid milk,† including that used in cooking In moderation	Whole,† lowfat,† or skim† (fresh, evaporated, or dry); chocolate flavored† Plain yogurt† Cottage cheese (creamed or dry), mild American cheese, cream cheese, Neufchatel
Meat	2–3 servings daily	Lean, very tender beef, ham, lamb, pork, veal, and liver or other organ meats Tender poultry (without skin) Fish or eggs (Prepared by broiling, roasting, baking, or simmering, steaming, pressure cooking, or microwave)
Fruits and vegetables	Up to 4 servings daily, if tolerated	Fruit and vegetable juices† (avoid prune juice), preferably strained Canned or cooked fruit *without* seeds or skin†: apples, apricots, cherries, peaches, pears Potatoes and sweet potatoes (without skin): baked, boiled, creamed, escalloped, mashed Tender cooked asparagus tips and carrots† Strained cooked vegetables†: green or wax beans, peas, spinach, squash (may be eaten as a vegetable or used in soups or gelatin salads)
Grains	At least 4 servings daily	Refined, enriched breads and cereals without seeds, added fruit, or nuts (Examples: white enriched bread, plain rolls, soda crackers, saltines, rusk, melba toast, plain matzo, zweiback) Cooked cornmeal, farina, Malt-o-Meal, strained oatmeal Ready-to-eat rice, corn, and oat flour cereals Cooked white enriched rice and plain pasta

Other
  Fats
  Soups
	As tolerated
	As desired
		Butter, margarine, cream, vegetable oil
		Homemade strained vegetable soups† using allowed ingredients, clear broth or broth with noodles or white rice

Desserts and sweets	As calories allow	Plain pudding using milk allowance,† plain ice cream,† sherbet, gelatin, fruit ice, popsicles Angel or sponge cake, meringue Other cakes and cookies (if fat is tolerated) Sugar, honey, syrup, jelly, hard candy
Seasonings	In moderation	Avoid pepper
Beverages	As tolerated	Fruit drinks, noncarbonated soft drinks Stay within milk allowance Avoidance of coffee and carbonated beverages may be helpful in controlling diarrhea

* Minimal residue diet of normal foods results in a small volume of stool which may be difficult to pass. Minimal residue *formula* diets result in a small volume of more liquid stool which is easier to pass. The latter type of diet may be advantageous in some circumstances, e.g., when a "clean" bowel is desired prior to gastrointestinal surgery.

† May be omitted from *minimal* residue diets.

Appendix 5D
SODIUM RESTRICTED DIETS

500 mg (22 mEq) sodium diet

FOOD GROUP	AMOUNT ALLOWED	CHOICES	TYPE OF PROCESSING
Milk	490 ml (2 c)	Skim, lowfat, whole, plain yogurt	Fresh or reconstituted evaporated or dry
		Chocolate milk	Commercial or homemade with regular cocoa
Meat	A total of 140 gm (5 oz)	Beef, chicken, cornish game hen, duck, lamb, pork, tongue, turkey, veal	Fresh or frozen plain, low sodium dietetic canned if available
		Fish	Fresh (rinse well before cooking) or canned low sodium dietetic
		Substitutes for 30 gm (1 oz) of the above: 1 medium egg (limit 1 daily) 30 gm low sodium dietetic hard cheese 60 ml (¼ c) salt-free cottage cheese	
	As desired and as calories allow	Unsalted peanut butter	Low sodium dietetic or freshly ground without salt
		Dried peas, beans, or lentils	Homemade without salt
		Unsalted nuts	In shell, unsalted packaged types
		Unsalted seeds (e.g., sunflower, sesame, pumpkin)	

Note: occasional use of unsalted organ meats and shellfish can be planned into diet by dietitian or nutritionist. These contain more natural sodium than do other meats and fish.

FOOD GROUP	AMOUNT ALLOWED	CHOICES	TYPE OF PROCESSING
Fruit and vegetable	Minimum of 4 servings daily	Fruit or fruit juice	Fresh, frozen (except melon or mixed frozen fruit), canned (any type), sundried
		Vegetables: asparagus, beans (green or wax), broccoli, brussels sprouts, cabbage (all types), cauliflower, chicory, corn, cucumber, eggplant, endive, escarole, lettuce (all types), mushrooms, okra, onions, peppers (all types), potatoes, pumpkin, radishes, rutabaga, squash (summer or winter), sweet potatoes, tomato, turnip greens	Fresh, frozen (plain), low sodium canned, dried
		Lima beans, peas	Fresh, low sodium dietetic or dried only
		Unsalted vegetable juices (tomato or mixed)	Canned low sodium or homemade

Note: types which are naturally high in sodium are to be used only if planned into diet by dietitian or nutritionist. These include artichokes, beet greens, beets, carrots, celery, chard, dandelion greens, kale, mustard greens, spinach, and white turnips.

FOOD GROUP	AMOUNT ALLOWED	CHOICES	TYPE OF PROCESSING
Grain	Minimum of 4 servings daily	Low sodium bread, rolls, crackers, matzoth, melba toast, regular corn tortilla	Homemade or commercial salt-free products
		Puffed rice or wheat, shredded wheat, Frosted Mini-Wheats, wheat germ, unprocessed bran, low sodium dietetic cornflakes or crisp rice	
		Unsalted cooked cereals	Regular, most quick-cooking types
		Pasta (spaghetti, macaroni, noodles)	Plain
		Rice, bulghur, barley, others	Plain (avoid seasoned mixes)

500 mg (22 mEq) sodium diet (Continued)

FOOD GROUP

Other

Fats: unsalted butter or margarine, shortening, vegetable oil, salt-free mayonnaise

Beverages: coffee and tea (if not contraindicated because of caffeine); fruit drinks and lemonade (fresh or frozen); Kool Aid; table wine and distilled spirits if allowed by physician

Desserts and sweets: fruit ice, homemade or commercial desserts made from allowed ingredients (e.g., salt-free cake, cookies, pie); semisweet chocolate, corn syrup, honey, maple syrup, sugar (white, brown, confectioners), jam, jelly, hard candy

Seasonings and other miscellaneous items: cocoa, chocolate (bitter), gelatin (plain), herbs (except celery leaves), seeds (except celery seed), spices, Tabasco, vinegar, table wine, yeast; low sodium baking powder (unless potassium restricted)

Changes for other levels of sodium intake

250 mg (12 mEq) SODIUM

Use above plan, but use low sodium milk (fresh or dried) instead of regular

1000 mg (43 mEq) SODIUM

Use above plan, but add an additional 500 mg. sodium following guidelines established by the dietitian (e.g., add ¼ scant tsp. salt to food daily or use 3 slices *regular* bread and 2 tsp. *regular* butter or margarine daily)

3 to 5 mg (130–215 mEq) sodium diet

Choose a wide variety of foods from the Basic 4 food groups (grains, fruits and vegetables, milk, and meat). *Avoid* those foods which are highly salted, as follows, and use salt lightly during cooking, if desired (i.e., half the amount the recipe calls for). Avoid using salt at the table.

*MEAT GROUP—FOODS TO AVOID**

Cured, smoked, or canned meat or fish

Kosher meats

Meat analogs (e.g., imitation bacon or sausage)

Canned dried beans in sauce (e.g., pork and beans)

Peanut butter†

*MILK GROUP—FOODS TO AVOID**

Processed cheese (e.g., American cheese)

Salty natural cheese (e.g., blue, feta)

Cheese spreads

Salted buttermilk

* Small measured amounts of one or more of these items may be planned into the diet by the dietitian/nutritionist.

† A moderate amount of regular peanut butter is often allowed on this diet.

*GRAIN GROUP—FOODS TO AVOID**

Salted crackers

Breads and rolls with salted tops

Seasoned mixes for rice, pasta, stuffing

*FRUIT AND VEGETABLE GROUP— FOODS TO AVOID**

Sauerkraut

Any vegetables prepared in brine

Regular tomato or vegetable juice

Tomato sauce

*COMBINATION DISHES—FOODS TO AVOID**

Processed main dishes (e.g., canned stews, frozen TV dinners, meat in gravy or sauce)

SNACK FOODS—TO AVOID

Chips	Salted popcorn
Salted nuts	Salted sunflower or other seeds
Pretzels	Salted soybeans

*SALTY SAUCES AND SEASONINGS‡— TO AVOID**

Salts of different types: butter-flavored salt, celery salt, garlic salt, iodized salt, Lite salt, onion salt, plain salt, popcorn salt, seasoned salt

Sauces: barbecue sauce, catsup (ketchup), chili sauce, meat sauce (A-1, Lowry's), oyster sauce, soy sauce, spaghetti sauce, tomato sauce, Worchestershire sauce

Miscellaneous items: bacon drippings, bouillon cubes, imitation bacon bits, monosodium glutamate (MSG, Accent), prepared mustard, relishes (most types), salt pork, pickles, olives

* Small measured amounts of one or more of these items may be planned into the diet by the dietitian/nutritionist.

‡ See Table 6.6, page 63 for additional examples of seasonings and condiments which are high in sodium content and are used by different cultural groups.

Appendix 5E
FOODS WHICH ARE HIGH IN POTASSIUM*

CALORIES PER SERVING	RICH SOURCES (>400 MG [10 mEq]/SERVING)	GOOD SOURCES (200–400 MG [5–10 mEq]/SERVING)
≤100	Banana, 1 med Cantaloupe, 1 c 240 ml Grapefruit juice, 1 c 240 ml Honeydew melon, 1 c 240 ml Molasses, 2 Tbsp 30 ml Nectarine, 1 large Orange juice, 1 c 240 ml Potato, baked, 1 med Potato, boiled, 1 med Tomato juice, canned, low sodium 1 c 240 ml	Artichoke, bud or globe† Beets, cooked,† ½ c 120 ml Beet greens,† ½ c 120 ml Blackberries, 1 c 240 ml Broccoli, cooked, ½ c 120 ml Brussels sprouts, fresh, ½ c 120 ml Carrots,† raw, 1 large Collard greens, cooked, frozen, ½ c 120 ml Orange, 1 small Peach, raw, 1 med Pear, raw, 1 med Rutabaga, cooked, ½ c 120 ml Skim milk,† 1 c 240 ml Strawberries, frozen, sliced, unsweetened, 1 c 240 ml Tomato, canned, low sodium, ½ c 120 ml Tomato, raw Watermelon, 2 c 500 ml Wheat germ, ¼ c 60 ml Winter squash, frozen, cooked, ½ c 120 ml
100–200	Avocado, ½ Fish,† lean types (e.g., cod, halibut) 85 gm (3 oz) Prunes, 10 med Prune juice, ¾ c 180 ml Soybeans, cooked, ½ c 120 ml	Apple juice, 1 c 240 ml Dried peas, beans, lentils, cooked, 120 ml (½ c) Fish,† high fat types (e.g., tuna) 85 gm (3 oz) Lima beans, green, ½ c 120 ml Meat and poultry,† lean, cooked, 85 gm (3 oz) Parsnips, cooked, ½ c 120 ml Peaches, canned, 1 half Peanut butter, 30 gm (2 Tbsp) unsalted Raisins, natural, ⅓ c or 45 gm pkg Sunflower seeds, hulled, unsalted, ¼ c Sweet potato, canned, ½ c 120 ml
≥200	Dates, 10 med Figs, dried, 5 med	Peanuts, shelled, unsalted, ¼ c

* Other foods may contribute substantial amounts of potassium to the diet, especially if large or frequent servings are used.
† Naturally high in sodium

Appendix 5F
500 mg CALCIUM DIET

(moderately low calcium diet)

ALLOWED

A wide variety of foods from the grain, fruit and vegetable, and meat groups
Foods containing small amounts of milk (e.g., bread and many other bakery products)

AVOIDED OR USED VERY INFREQUENTLY:

All types of milk, cheese, ice cream, yogurt, cream
Foods which use a dairy product (other than butter) as a principal ingredient; e.g., cream sauce, pudding, custard, eggnog, cream soup, cheese casseroles

THE FOLLOWING FOODS ARE HIGH IN CALCIUM BUT MAY BE ALLOWED IF USED INFREQUENTLY OR IF SERVING SIZE IS SMALL:

Blackstrap molasses, bok choy, broccoli, collards, kale, mustard greens, canned salmon, sardines, tofu (soybean curd), turnip greens

Note: Many nondairy creamers and other products which simulate dairy products are low in calcium. A dietitian or nutritionist should advise the client about appropriate use of these products.

To maintain an acidic urine:

Include cranberries, prunes, and/or plums in your food for the day. (These may be used as juice or sauce, fresh, in salads or desserts.)

Use whole grain rather than refined bread and cereal.

Limit consumption of milk, fruits and vegetables to amounts recommended in the Basic Four Food Groups.

To limit intake of oxalate, use the following foods sparingly or not at all.

FOODS WHICH ARE REPORTED TO BE HIGH IN OXALATE[1]

Beans*	Cucumbers	Plums
Beer† (4 mg/2 oz)[2]	Currants	Raspberries
Beets*	Dandelion greens	Rhubarb*
Blackberries	Endive	Spinach*
Cola† (4-10 mg/ 12 oz)[2]	Kale	Strawberries
Celery	Oranges	Sweet potato
Cocoa	Parsley	Tea†
Coffee (instant)†	Peppers	Turnip greens

Information about the oxalate content of many processed American foods has not been reported.[2]
* Fruits and vegetables which contain more than 25 mg oxalate in an average (100 gm) serving.
† Oxalate provided by beer, cola, coffee, and tea may be substantial if several servings are consumed daily.

References

1. Stauffer, J. Q.: Hyperoxaluria and calcium oxalate nephrolithiasis after jejunoileal bypass. *Am. J. Clin. Nutr.* 30:64, 1977.
2. Earnest, D. L.: Perspectives on incidence, etiology, and treatment of enteric hyperoxaluria. *Am. J. Clin. Nutr.* 30:72, 1977.

Appendix 5G
ABBREVIATED FOOD LISTS FOR PROTEIN CONTROLLED DIETS

Unless otherwise noted, foods grouped together are similar in their content of protein, sodium, and potassium.

Low sodium meat list

Average values: protein 8 gm, Na 30 mg, K 100 mg

Egg	1 med
Meat: beef, lamb, fresh pork, veal, organ meats	30 gm (1 oz)
Poultry, without skin: chicken, duck, goose, turkey	30 gm
Fish, fresh or unsalted waterpack	30 gm
Shellfish	
Clams	60 ml (¼ c) or 4–5
Oysters	80 ml (⅓ c) or 3–4 sm
Shrimp	30 gm

Dairy list

Average values: protein 4 gm, Na 70 mg, K 185 mg

Cream, half & half	120 ml (½ c)
Cream, heavy whipping	180 ml (¾ c)
Ice cream (chocolate, vanilla, strawberry)	180 ml
Milk (whole, low fat, skim, chocolate)	120 ml
Evaporated whole or skim milk	60 ml (¼ c)

Note: One serving of milk is 4 fluid ounces, not 8 ounces.

(Continued on next page)

Protein controlled diets (Continued)
Bread, cereal, and starch lists

REGULAR

Average values: protein 2 gm, Na 200 mg, K 30 mg

Bread (white enriched, cracked wheat, French, Italian, American rye	1 slice
Doughnut	1 sm
Graham cracker	2 squares
Hamburger or hotdog bun	½ large
Muffin, plain	1 sm
Sugar wafers	5 wafers
Vanilla wafers	10 wafers

Dry cereals: portion sizes vary widely

LOW SODIUM

Average values: protein 2 gm, Na 5 mg, K 30 mg

Low sodium crackers	4 sm
Low sodium white bread	1 slice
Salt-free matzo cracker	1 15 cm (6″) sq
Salt-free Venus wheat wafers	4
Cereals and rice cooked without salt (avoid seasoned mixes)	120 ml (½ c)
Dry cereals	
Frosted Mini Wheats	3 biscuits
Spoon Size Shredded Wheat	80 ml (⅓ c)
Puffed wheat or rice	240 ml (1 c)
Low sodium cornflakes	1 c
Pasta cooked without salt	⅓ c

Fruit list #1

Average values: protein 0.5 gm, Na 5 mg, K 100 mg

Apple, fresh	1 sm
Apple juice	120 ml
Applesauce	120 ml
Blueberries, fresh or frozen	180 ml
Cherries	8 lrg
Grape juice, froz, diluted 1:3	240 ml (1 c)
Orange, fresh	½ sm 6.4 cm (2½″) diam
Pear, fresh	½ large 7.1 cm (3″) diam
Pear halves, canned	2 sm halves
Pineapple chunks	120 ml
Prunes, dried	2 med
Strawberries, fresh	6 lrg
Tangerine, fresh	1 med 6.4 cm (2½″) diam
Watermelon, diced	120 ml

Fruit list #2

Average values: protein 0.6 gm, Na 5 mg, K 175 mg

Apricots, fresh	2 med
Banana, fresh	7.6 cm (3″) piece
Dates	4 med

Fruit list #2 (Continued)

Fruit cocktail, canned	120 ml
Grapefruit juice (canned, fresh, or froz)	120 ml
Peach halves, canned	2 med halves
Prune juice	80 ml (⅓ c)
Raisins, dried	2 Tbsp

Fruit list #3

Average values: protein 0.7 gm, Na 5 mg, K 250 mg

Apple, fresh	1 lrg 9 cm (3½″) diam
Apple juice	240 ml
Banana	13 cm (5″) piece
Cantaloupe, fresh	⅙ 13 cm (5″) diam
Orange juice (canned, fresh, or frozen	120 ml
Papaya, fresh	⅓ med 9 cm (3½″) diam

Vegetable list #1

Average values: protein 1.0 gm, Na 10 mg, K 100 mg

Asparagus, fresh cooked	4 med spears
Asparagus, frozen, cooked	3 med spears
Asparagus, low sodium canned	80 ml (⅓ c)
Beans (snap or wax), fresh cooked, canned, frozen	120 ml
Cucumber, raw, pared	10 slices, 0.6 cm thick
Cabbage (all varieties) raw or cooked, shredded	120 ml
Carrots, low sodium canned	120 ml
Cauliflower, fresh cooked	120 ml
Lettuce (all varieties) chopped	120 ml
Mustard greens, frozen cooked	120 ml
Onion, raw or cooked, sliced	120 ml
Pepper, swt green, cooked	1 whole

Vegetable list #2

Average values: protein 1 gm, Na 20 mg, K 170 mg

Beets, fresh slices, cooked or low sodium canned	120 ml
Carrots, fresh, diced, cooked	120 ml
Celery, raw or cooked diced	120 ml or 1 stalk
Eggplant, diced, cooked	120 ml
Mushrooms, raw	120 ml sliced or 3–4 small
Okra, fresh slices, cooked	120 ml
Parsnips, diced, cooked	80 ml
Pepper, swt green, raw	1 whole
Radishes, raw	10 med
Rutabagas, sliced cooked	120 ml
Squash, summer, sliced	120 ml
Squash, winter, boiled & mashed	80 ml
Turnips, cubed cooked	120 ml

Protein controlled diet (Continued)
Vegetable list #3

Average values: protein 1 gm, Na 15 mg, K 250 mg

Avocado, raw	¼ sm
Beet greens, cooked	120 ml
Carrot raw	1 18 cm (7″) long
Chard, fresh, cooked	120 ml
Potato, pared, sliced, cooked	120 ml
Squash, winter, baked	60 ml
Tomato cooked	80 ml
Tomato, raw, unpeeled	1 sm
Tomato, low sodium canned	120 ml

Vegetable list #4

Average values: protein 2.5 gm, Na 20 mg, K 200 mg but varies widely

Artichoke, cooked	1 med
Broccoli, fresh or frozen cooked	120 ml
Collard grns, fresh or frozen cooked	120 ml
Corn, fresh, cut off cob or low sodium canned	120 ml
Peas, frozen or low sodium canned	120 ml
Potato, baked	1 5.6 cm (2¼″)
Spinach, fresh or frozen, cooked	120 ml
Sweet potato, baked	1 12.5 × 5 cm (5″ × 2′)

Free list

FATS UNSALTED
Butter, unsalted
Low sodium French dressing
Lard
Margarine, unsalted
Vegetable oil
Shortening
Whipping cream 15 ml (1 Tbsp) unwhipped

LOW PROTEIN PRODUCTS
Arrowroot
Cornstarch

Free list (Continued)

Low protein bread
Low protein cereal, pasta, rusks, Aproten
Wheatstarch cookies

NONDAIRY PRODUCTS
Coffee-Mate 15 ml (1 Tbsp)
Dessert topping, froz, powder or pressurized
D'Zerta whipped topping

SPICES, SEASONINGS, AND FLAVORINGS
All dry spices and herbs
Diazest
Garlic, fresh
Liquid Smoke, Wright's
Tabasco sauce
Vinegar, distilled

SWEETS
Cranberry sauce 60 ml (¼ c)
Danish dessert 120 ml (½ c)
Gum drops
Hard candy
Honey
Jam, preserves
Jelly
Jelly beans
Sugar, white, granulated or powdered

Note: The foods in the free list can be added to diets which are controlled in protein, sodium, and/or potassium as desired unless the amount allowed is specified.

Commercial, low electrolyte, high calorie supplements which may be useful when protein, sodium, and/or potassium intake must be restricted:

Amin-Aid*—flavored essential amino acids (including histidine), carbohydrate, and soybean oil
Cal-Power—flavored colored liquid glucose
Controlyte—hydrolysed cornstarch with vegetable oil
Hy-Cal—flavored, colored liquid glucose
Lipomul oral—corn oil emulsion
Polycose—hydrolyzed cornstarch
Sumacal—flavored, colored liquid glucose

Condensed from *A Guide to Protein Controlled Diets for Dietitians*, ed. 2. Diet Therapy Committee. Los Angeles: Los Angeles District of the California Dietetic Association, 1977. Used with permission.
* Not allowed if protein is not allowed.

Appendix 5H
PURINE RESTRICTED DIET*

Foods which are *very high in purine content.* These foods are most likely to be eliminated or severely restricted on this diet:

Anchovies, gravy, kidney, liver, meat extracts (e.g., drippings from meat, commercial flavoring compounds obtained from meat), sardines, sweetbreads
Foods which are *high in purines.* These foods are usually allowed, but amounts to be consumed are occasionally controlled:

Fish, legumes (cooked dried peas, beans, and lentils), meat and meat-based soups, oatmeal, poultry, shellfish, spinach, wheat germ, and bran

Source: Church, C. F., and Church, H. N.: *Food Values of Portions Commonly Used*, ed. 12. Philadelphia: J. B. Lippincott Co., 1975.
* Data regarding the purine content of foods is limited. For this reason the amount of purine allowed is seldom specified.

Appendix 5I
EXCHANGE LISTS FOR MEAL PLANNING*

List 1—milk exchanges

Includes **nonfat,** low fat and whole milk
One exchange of milk contains 12 gm. of carbohydrate, 8 gm. of protein, a trace of fat, and 80 calories.

This list shows the kinds and amounts of milk or milk products to use for one Milk Exchange. Those which appear in **bold type** are **nonfat.** Low fat and whole milk contain saturated fat.

Nonfat fortified milk	1 c
Skim or nonfat milk	1 c
Powdered (nonfat dry, before adding liquid)	⅓ c
Canned, evaporated-skim milk	½ c
Buttermilk made from skim milk	1 c
Yogurt made from skim milk (plain, unflavored)	1 c
Lowfat fortified milk	
1% fat fortified milk	1 c
(omit ½ Fat Exchange)	
2% fat fortified milk	1 c
(omit 1 Fat Exchange)	
Yogurt made from 2% fortified milk (plain, unflavored)	1 c
(omit 1 Fat Exchange)	
Whole Milk (omit 2 Fat Exchanges)	
Whole milk	1 c
Canned, evaporated whole milk	½ c
Buttermilk made from whole milk	1 c
Yogurt made from whole milk (plain, unflavored)	1 c

* The exchange lists are based on material in the *Exchange Lists for Meal Planning* prepared by Committees of the American Diabetes Association, Inc. and The American Dietetic Association in cooperation with the National Institute of Arthritis, Metabolism and Digestive Diseases and the National Heart and Lung Institute, National Institutes of Health, Public Health Service, U.S. Department of Health, Education and Welfare.

List 2—vegetable exchanges

One exchange of vegetables contains about 5 gm. of carbohydrate, 2 gm. of protein and 25 calories.

This list shows the kinds of **vegetables** to use for one Vegetable Exchange. One Exchange is ½ cup.

Asparagus	**Greens:**
Bean sprouts	**Beet**
Beets	**Chard**
Broccoli	**Collards**
Brussels sprouts	**Dandelion**
Cabbage	**Kale**
Carrots	**Mustard**
Cauliflower	**Spinach**
Celery	**Turnip**
Cucumbers	**Mushrooms**
Eggplant	**Okra**
Green pepper	**Onions**

List 2—vegetable exchanges (Continued)

Rhubarb	**Tomatoes**
Rutabaga	**Tomato juice**
Sauerkraut	**Turnips**
String beans, green or yellow	**Vegetable juice cocktail**
Summer squash	**Zucchini**

The following **raw vegetables** may be used as desired:

Chicory	**Lettuce**
Chinese cabbage	**Parsley**
Endive	**Radishes**
Escarole	**Watercress**

Starchy vegetables are found in the Bread Exchange List.

List 3—fruit exchanges

One exchange of fruit contains 10 gm. of carbohydrate and 40 calories.

This list shows the kinds and amounts of **fruits** to use for one Fruit Exchange.

Apple	1 sm
Apple juice	⅓ c
Applesauce (unsweetened)	½ c
Apricots, fresh	2 med
Apricots, dried	4 halves
Banana	½ sm
Berries	
Blackberries	½ c
Blueberries	½ c
Raspberries	½ c
Strawberries	¾ c
Cherries	10 lg
Cider	⅓ c
Dates	2
Figs, fresh	1
Figs, dried	1
Grapefruit	½
Grapefruit juice	½ c
Grapes	12
Grape juice	¼ c
Mango	½ sm
Melon	
Cantaloupe	¼ sm
Honeydew	⅛ med
Watermelon	1 cup
Nectarine	1 sm
Orange	1 sm
Orange juice	½ c
Papaya	¾ c
Peach	1 med
Pear	1 sm
Persimmon, native	1 med
Pineapple	½ c

List 3—fruit exchanges (Continued)

Pineapple juice	⅓ c
Plums	2 med
Prunes	2 med
Prune juice	¼ c
Raisins	2 Tbsp
Tangerine	1 med

Cranberries may be used as desired if no sugar is added.

List 4—bread exchanges

Includes **bread, cereal,** and **starchy vegetables**

One exchange of bread contains 15 gm. of carbohydrate, 2 gm. of protein, and 70 calories.

This list shows the kinds and amounts of **breads, cereals, starchy vegetables** and prepared foods to use for one Bread Exchange. Those which appear in **bold type** are **low fat.**

Bread
White (including French and Italian)	1 slice
Whole wheat	1 slice
Rye or pumpernickel	1 slice
Raisin	1 slice
Bagel, small	½
English muffin, small	½
Plain roll, bread	1
Frankfurter roll	½
Hamburger bun	½
Dried bread crumbs	3 Tbsp.
Tortilla, 6″	1

Cereal
Bran Flakes	½ c
Other ready-to-eat unsweetened cereal	¾ c
Puffed cereal (unfrosted)	1 c
Cereal (cooked)	½ c
Grits (cooked)	½ c
Rice or barley (cooked)	½ c
Pasta (cooked): spaghetti, noodles, macaroni	½ c
Popcorn (popped, no fat added)	3 c
Cornmeal (dry)	2 Tbsp.
Flour	2½ Tbsp.
Wheat germ	¼ c

Crackers
Arrowroot	3
Graham, 2½″ square	2
Matzoth, 4″ × 6″	½
Oyster	20
Pretzels, 3⅛″ × ⅛″ diam	25
Rye wafers, 2″ × 3½″	3
Saltines	6
Soda, 2½″ sq.	4

Dried beans, peas, and lentils
Beans, peas, lentils (dried and cooked)	½ c
Baked beans, no pork (canned)	¼ c

List 4—bread exchanges (Continued)

Starchy vegetables
Corn	⅓ c
Corn on cob	1 sm
Lima beans	½ c
Parsnips	⅔ c
Peas, green (canned or frozen)	½ c
Potato, white	1 sm
Potato (mashed)	½ c
Pumpkin	¾ c
Winter squash, acorn or butternut	½ c
Yam or sweet potato	¼ c

Prepared foods
Biscuit 2″ dia. (omit 1 Fat Exchange)	1
Corn bread, 2″ × 2″ × 1″ (omit 1 Fat Exchange)	1
Corn muffin, 2″ diam (omit 1 Fat Exchange)	1
Crackers, round butter type (omit 1 Fat Exchange)	5
Muffin, plain small (omit 1 Fat Exchange)	1
Potatoes, french fried, length 2″ to 3½″ (omit 1 Fat Exchange)	8
Potato or corn chips (omit 2 Fat Exchanges)	15
Pancake, 5″ × ½″ (omit 1 Fat Exchange)	1
Waffle, 5″ × ½″ (omit 1 Fat Exchange)	1

List 5—meat exchanges

Lean Meat

One exchange of lean meat (1 oz.) contains 7 gm. of protein, 3 gm. of fat, and 55 calories.

This list shows the kinds and amounts of **lean meat** and other protein-rich foods to use for one Low Fat Meat Exchange.

Beef: baby beef (very lean), chipped beef, chuck, flank steak, tenderloin, plate ribs, plate skirt steak, round (bottom, top), all cuts rump, spare ribs, tripe	1 oz
Lamb: leg, rib, sirloin, loin (roast and chops), shank, shoulder	1 oz

Exchange lists for meal planning (Continued)

List 5—meat exchanges (Continued)

Lean meat

Pork: leg (whole rump, center shank), ham, smoked (center slices)	1 oz
Veal: leg, loin, rib, shank, shoulder, cutlets	1 oz
Poultry: meat without skin of chicken, turkey, cornish hen, guinea hen, pheasant	1 oz
Fish: Any fresh or frozen	
canned salmon, tuna, mackerel, crab and lobster	¼ c
clams, oysters, scallops, shrimp	5 or 1 oz
sardines, drained	3
Cheeses containing less than 5% butterfat	1 oz
Cottage cheese, dry and 2% butterfat	¼ c
Dried beans and peas (omit 1 Bread Exchange)	½ c

Medium-Fat Meat

For each exchange of medium-fat meat omit ½ Fat Exchange.

This list shows the kinds and amounts of medium-fat meat and other protein-rich foods to use for one medium-fat meat exchange.

Beef: ground (15% fat), corned beef (canned), rib eye, round (ground commercial)	1 oz
Pork: loin (all cuts tenderloin), shoulder arm (picnic), shoulder blade, Boston butt, Canadian bacon, boiled ham	1 oz
Liver, heart, kidney, and sweetbreads (these are high in cholesterol)	1 oz
Cottage cheese, creamed	¼ c
Cheese: mozzarella, ricotta, farmer's cheese, Neufchatel	1 oz
Parmesan	3 Tbsp.
Egg (high in cholesterol)	1
Peanut Butter (omit 2 additional Fat Exchanges)	2 Tbsp.

High-Fat Meat

For each exchange of high-fat meat omit 1 Fat Exchange.

This list shows the kinds and amounts of high-fat meat and other protein-rich foods to use for one High-Fat Meat Exchange.

Beef: brisket, corned beef (brisket), ground beef (more than 20% fat), hamburger (commercial), chuck (ground commercial), roasts (rib), steaks (club and rib)	1 oz
Lamb: breast	1 oz

List 5—meat exchanges (Continued)

High-fat meat

Pork: spare ribs, loin (back ribs), pork (ground), country style ham, deviled ham	1 oz
Veal: breast	1 oz
Poultry: capon, duck (domestic), goose	1 oz
Cheese: cheddar types	1 oz
Cold cuts	4½″ × ⅛″ slice
Frankfurter	1 sm

List 6—fat exchanges

One exchange of fat contains 5 gm. of fat and 45 calories.

This list shows the kinds and amounts of fat-containing foods to use for one Fat Exchange. To plan a diet low in saturated fat select only those Exchanges which appear in **bold type**. They are **polyunsaturated**.

Margarine, soft, tub or stick*	1 tsp
Avocado (4″ in diameter)	⅛
Oil, corn, cottonseed, safflower, soy, sunflower	1 tsp
Oil, olive	1 tsp
Oil, peanut	1 tsp
Olives	5 sm
Almonds	10 whole
Pecans	2 lg whole
Peanuts	
Spanish	20 whole
Virginia	10 whole
Walnuts	6 sm
Nuts, other	6 sm
Margarine, regular stick	1 tsp
Butter	1 tsp
Bacon fat	1 tsp
Bacon, crisp	1 strip
Cream, light	2 Tbsp.
Cream, sour	2 Tbsp.
Cream, heavy	1 Tbsp.
Cream cheese	1 Tbsp.
French dressing***	1 Tbsp.
Italian dressing***	1 Tbsp.
Lard	1 tsp
Mayonnaise***	1 tsp
Salad dressing, mayonnaise type***	2 tsp
Salt pork	¾″ cube

* Made with corn, cottonseed, safflower, soy, or sunflower oil only
** Fat content is primarily monounsaturated
*** If made with corn, cottonseed, safflower, soy, or sunflower oil can be used on fat-modified diet

Appendix 5J
ADAPTATIONS OF "EXCHANGE LISTS FOR MEAL PLANNING" FOR USE WITH A HYPERLIPOPROTEINEMIA IV DIET

Meat exchanges

Lean meat exchanges, peanut butter, plus the following choices:

Creamed cottage cheese is an acceptable meat choice.

3 whole eggs or 3 egg yolks are allowed weekly, including those used in cooking.

60 gm. (2 oz.) liver, sweetbreads, or heart may be substituted for 1 egg yolk (or 1 whole egg)

60 gm. (2 oz.) medium-fat cheese (e.g., cheddar, swiss) may be used each week

Bread exchanges

Items in **bold type** in Appendix 5I, plus the following choices:

Biscuits, muffins, pancakes, waffles, and french fries are acceptable if made at home from allowed ingredients.

Desserts*

Each of the following counts as 1 bread exchange, but no more than two exchanges from this selection should be used daily.

---

* Items such as these, which provide calories but few nutrients, should be avoided if intake of breads and cereals would fall below 4 or 5 servings per day.

3.8 cm (1½″) cube angel food cake
80 ml. (⅓ c.) regular gelatin dessert
60 ml. (¼ c.) sherbet or fruit ice
120 ml. (½ c.) plain pudding prepared with skim milk

Sweets*

Each of the following counts as 1 bread exchange. One serving daily may be allowed by the physician but only if no more than one serving of a sweetened dessert is being eaten the same day.

15 gm. (1 Tbsp.) sugar, honey, molasses, syrup, jam, jelly, or preserves

15 gm. (½ oz.) hard candy, jelly beans, gum drops, marshmallows, plain (not chocolate) mints

6 oz. sweetened carbonated beverage

Alcohol*

Each of the following counts as one bread exchange. A maximum of 2 servings is allowed daily*: (with approval of physician)

30 ml. (1 oz.) gin, rum, vodka, whisky
45 ml. (1½ oz.) dessert or sweet wine
75 ml. (2½ oz.) dry wine
150 ml. (5 oz.) beer

---

* Items such as these, which provide calories but few nutrients, should be avoided if intake of breads and cereals would fall below 4 or 5 servings per day.

Appendix 5K
FAT-CONTROLLED, LOW CHOLESTEROL DIET

A variety of foods may be selected from each of the Basic Four Food Groups. Emphasize those foods listed in the left hand "Suggested" column.

Meat, poultry, fish, dried beans and peas, eggs. Adults may be allowed 2 or more servings (up to 6 to 8 oz) daily

SUGGESTED	AVOID OR USE INFREQUENTLY
Most often: Chicken, turkey, veal, fish, shellfish (except shrimp)	Duck, goose, shrimp (substitute shrimp for red meat or egg once a week if desired*)
A few times a week: Very lean beef, lamb, pork, ham All visible meat fat is discarded	Fatty meats, e.g., heavily marbled beef, spare ribs, frankfurters, sausage, bacon, bologna, and other lunch meats, regular hamburger. Organ meats (substitute liver for red meat or for egg once a week if desired*)
Dried peas, beans, lentils—prepared with allowed ingredients Peanut butter in moderation Egg whites as desired	Beans prepared with salt pork or bacon Egg yolks: limit to 3 per week*

Appendix 5K
FAT-CONTROLLED, LOW CHOLESTEROL DIET (Continued)

Vegetables and fruit—at least 4 servings daily, including sources of vitamins C and A

SUGGESTED	AVOID OR USE INFREQUENTLY
All types of fruits and vegetables may be used (unless prepared with restricted ingredients): fresh, frozen, canned, dried	Vegetables in butter, cream, or cheese sauce Vegetables fried in saturated fat

Bread and cereals (whole grain, enriched, or fortified—at least 4 servings daily

SUGGESTED	AVOID OR USE INFREQUENTLY
Breads: whole wheat, rye, pumpernickel, oatmeal, white enriched, French, Italian, raisin. English muffins, bagels, hard rolls Cereal (hot or cold), rice, bulghur, barley Pasta Melba toast, matzo, pretzels Biscuits, muffins, etc., made at home using allowed ingredients	Egg bread, cheese bread Commercial biscuits, muffins, donuts, butter rolls, sweet rolls Commercial granola, Cracklin' Bran Egg noodles Snack crackers Commercial mixes containing dried eggs, whole milk and/or shortening

Milk products. Adults should use 500 ml (2 or more cups) or the equivalent daily

SUGGESTED	AVOID OR USE INFREQUENTLY
Skim milk dairy products: fortified skim (nonfat) milk or milk powder, buttermilk, evaporated skim milk, chocolate flavored skim milk Acceptable in some cases: low fat milk and yogurt Cheeses made from skim milk: cottage cheese, farmer's, baker's, or hoop cheese, sapsago cheese Occasionally allowed: cheeses made from part-skim milk such as part-skim mozarella	Whole milk and whole milk products: chocolate milk, canned evaporated whole milk, ice cream, cream of any type, whole milk yogurt Most nondairy cream substitutes Cheeses made from cream or whole milk

Fats and oils (polyunsaturated). Adults are often allowed about 30–60 ml (2–4 Tbsp) daily (depending on caloric needs), including oil used in cooking

SUGGESTED	AVOID OR USE INFREQUENTLY
Polyunsaturated vegetable oils: corn oil, cottonseed oil, safflower oil, sesame seed oil, soybean oil, sunflower seed oil Margarines and liquid oil shortenings made with an allowed oil and having a high P/S ratio (i.e., about 2:1 or above) Salad dressings made with allowed ingredients, mayonnaise	Solid fats and shortenings: butter, hard margarine and vegetable shortening with a low P/S ratio (i.e., 3:2 or lower), lard, salt pork, meat fat, coconut oil, palm oil (Peanut oil and olive oil are not saturated or polyunsaturated. They may be used occasionally for flavor.) Creamy and cheese salad dressings

Desserts, beverages, snacks, condiments

ACCEPTABLE IF CALORIES ALLOW	AVOID OR USE INFREQUENTLY
Cocoa powder, fruit whip, gelatin, puddings made with nonfat milk, water ice, sherbet Jelly, jam, marmalade, honey, hard candy, angel food cake, most types of nuts Homemade baked desserts using allowed ingredients Carbonated beverages, fruit drinks, wine,† beer,† whisky†	Chocolate, whole milk puddings, ice cream (ice milk is sometimes allowed) Chocolate candy, caramels, butterscotch Coconut, macadamia nuts, cashews Commercial cakes, pies, cookies, and mixes Potato chips and other commercial fried snacks

NEGLIGIBLE CALORIE CONTENT

Tea, herb tea, coffee,† decaffeinated coffee
Herbs, spices, vinegar, mustard, small amounts of ketchup and barbecue sauce, horseradish, meat sauce, soy sauce

* When allowed a total of 300 mg cholesterol or more daily
† With approval of physician

Appendix 5L
50 gm FAT DIET

FOOD GROUP	AMOUNT ALLOWED	CHOICES
Milk	490 ml (2 c) or more daily	Skim (fresh or reconstituted nonfat dry or evaporated skim); skim milk buttermilk or yogurt, chocolate-flavored skim milk Fat free cottage cheese
Meat	Up to 200 gm (7 oz) daily (Provides about 35 gm fat)	Lean beef, pork, lamb, ham (trimmed of fat) Veal Chicken or turkey without skin or visible fat Fish (except types canned in oil) Whole egg or egg yolk, if tolerated; egg whites in any amount; egg substitute made from whites Cooked dried peas and beans if tolerated
Grain	At least 4 servings daily	Whole grain or enriched breads, hard rolls, plain crackers (e.g., saltines, grahams) Cereals, except granola and a few ready-to-eat types (check nutritional labeling for fat content) Bagels, English muffins, matzo Barley, boiled or steamed rice, pasta (all types, including noodles)
Fruits & vegetables	At least 4 servings daily	All fresh, frozen, canned, and dried fruits and juices as tolerated* except avocado and olives All plain fresh, frozen or canned vegetables—boiled, steamed, baked, or mashed as tolerated*
OTHERS		
Fats	5 gm (1 tsp)/meal, 3 times daily	Butter, margarine, vegetable oil, mayonnaise Any used in cooking must be counted as part of the allowance
Soups	As desired	Homemade fat-free types or commercial broth, consomme, bouillon
Desserts & Sweets	As calories allow	Angel cake, fruit ice or fruit whip, gelatin dessert, sherbet, puddings made with skim milk, cocoa flavoring, vanilla wafers, arrowroot cookies, meringue Sugar, syrup, honey, jam, jelly, gum drops, marshmallows, hard candy
Seasonings	As tolerated	Salt, herbs, and spices in moderation
Beverages	As desired	Coffee, tea, carbonated beverages, fruit drinks, lemonade

* Cooked, mild flavored fruits and vegetables are usually tolerated well.

Substitutions which may be planned by dietitian:
Use of some low fat or whole milk, cheese, or limited quantities of other fat-containing foods.

To increase protein and calorie intake without increasing fat intake, use more of any of the following:
Fat-free cottage cheese, skim milk (if lactose is tolerated), lean fish, grain products (e.g., toast with jelly)
Use other foods which are good sources of calories to spare protein (e.g., sweetened fruits, hard candy, desserts)

To increase fat intake, increase use of visible fats, of meats, or of foods prepared with added fat, according to dietitian's guidelines.

To limit fat intake to about 20 gm. daily, omit all visible fats and limit meat, fish, poultry, and eggs to the equivalent of 110 to 140 gm. (4 to 5 oz.) daily; increase use of other foods to maintain caloric balance if desirable.

Appendix 5M
FOODS ALLOWED ON A GLUTEN-FREE DIET

GRAIN GROUP

Breads: specially prepared using cornmeal, cornstarch, potato starch, rice flour, soy or other bean flours

Cereals: cornmeal, Cream of Rice, grits, hominy. Corn or rice ready-to-eat cereals such as cornflakes, Rice Krispies, rice flakes, Puffed Rice

MILK GROUP

Milk, cream, natural cheese, plain yogurt

FRUIT AND VEGETABLE GROUP

Fresh, frozen, canned, or dried—without added thickeners

MEAT GROUP

Legumes, nuts, seeds: plain dried peas, beans, lentils, plain nuts and nut butters, plain seeds

Meat, fish, poultry, eggs: plain fresh or frozen

OTHER FOODS

Beverages: carbonated beverages, coffee and tea (avoid instant types), cocoa, juice drinks

Desserts: custard; fruit ice; meringue; fruit whips; gelatin; puddings made with arrowroot, cornstarch, rice, tapioca; rennet dessert; specially prepared baked goods

Fats: butter, margarine, mayonnaise, oils, shortening

Snacks: corn chips, olives, pickles, potato chips, popcorn

Soups: clear meat and vegetable soups, homemade soups using allowed ingredients

Sweets: corn syrup, honey, jam, jelly, molasses, sugar

Seasonings: salt, pepper, and other plain spices and herbs; vinegar; wine

Combine allowed ingredients as desired to make many interesting foods.

Many processed foods which are not listed above are gluten-free, but you must check the label to be sure. *Avoid* any food which contains one or more of the following ingredients: barley; flour; gluten; graham; hydrolyzed vegetable or plant protein; malt; malted milk; millet; modified food starch; oats; rye; starch (type unspecified, or wheat, rye, or oat starch); wheat.

INDEX

FOOD AND NUTRITION BOARD, NATIONAL ACADEMY OF SCIENCES—NATIONAL RESEARCH COUNCIL*

Recommended Daily Dietary Allowances,[a] Revised 1979

Designed for the maintenance of good nutrition of practically all healthy people in the U.S.A.

	AGE (years)	WEIGHT (kg)	WEIGHT (lbs)	HEIGHT (cm)	HEIGHT (in)	PROTEIN (g)	FAT-SOLUBLE VITAMINS VITAMIN A (μg R.E.)[b]	FAT-SOLUBLE VITAMINS VITAMIN D (μg)[c]	FAT-SOLUBLE VITAMINS VITAMIN E (mg α T.E.)[d]	WATER-SOLUBLE VITAMINS VITAMIN C (mg)	WATER-SOLUBLE VITAMINS THIAMIN (mg)	WATER-SOLUBLE VITAMINS RIBOFLAVIN (mg)
INFANTS	0.0–0.5	6	13	60	24	kg × 2.2	420	10	3	35	0.3	0.4
	0.5–1.0	9	20	71	28	kg × 2.0	400	10	4	35	0.5	0.6
CHILDREN	1–3	13	29	90	35	23	400	10	5	45	0.7	0.8
	4–6	20	44	112	44	30	500	10	6	45	0.9	1.0
	7–10	28	62	132	52	34	700	10	7	45	1.2	1.4
MALES	11–14	45	99	157	62	45	1000	10	8	50	1.4	1.6
	15–18	66	145	176	69	56	1000	10	10	60	1.4	1.7
	19–22	70	154	177	70	56	1000	7.5	10	60	1.5	1.7
	23–50	70	154	178	70	56	1000	5	10	60	1.4	1.6
	51+	70	154	178	70	56	1000	5	10	60	1.2	1.4
FEMALES	11–14	46	101	157	62	46	800	10	8	50	1.1	1.3
	15–18	55	120	163	64	46	800	10	8	60	1.1	1.3
	19–22	55	120	163	64	44	800	7.5	8	60	1.1	1.3
	23–50	55	120	163	64	44	800	5	8	60	1.0	1.2
	51+	55	120	163	64	44	800	5	8	60	1.0	1.2
PREGNANT						+30	+200	+5	+2	+20	+0.4	+0.3
LACTATING						+20	+400	+5	+3	+40	+0.5	+0.5

[a] The allowances are intended to provide for individual variations among most normal persons as they live in the United States under usual environmental stresses. Diets should be based on a variety of common foods in order to provide other nutrients for which human requirements have been less well defined.

[b] Retinol equivalents. 1 Retinol equivalent = μg retinol or 6 μg β-carotene.

[c] As cholecalciferol. 10 μg cholecalciferol = 400 I.U. vitamin D.

[d] α-tocopherol equivalents. 1μg d-α-tocopherol = 1 α T.E.

[e] 1 N.E. (niacin equivalent) is equal to 1 mg of niacin or 60 mg of dietary tryptophan.

Estimated Safe and Adequate Daily Dietary Intakes of Additional Selected Vitamins and Minerals[a]

	AGE (years)	VITAMINS VITAMIN K (μg)	VITAMINS BIOTIN (μg)	VITAMINS PANTOTHENIC ACID (mg)	TRACE ELEMENTS[b] COPPER (mg)	TRACE ELEMENTS[b] MANGANESE (mg)
Infants	0–0.5	12	35	2	0.5–0.7	0.5–0.7
	0.5–1	10–20	50	3	0.7–1.0	0.7–1.0
Children	1–3	15–30	65	3	1.0–1.5	1.0–1.5
and	4–6	20–40	85	3–4	1.5–2.0	1.5–2.0
Adolescents	7–10	30–60	120	4–5	2.0–2.5	2.0–3.0
	11+	50–100	100–200	4–7	2.0–3.0	2.5–5.0
Adults		70–140	100–200	4–7	2.0–3.0	2.5–5.0

[a] Because there is less information on which to base allowances, these figures are not given in the main table of the RDA and are provided here in the form of ranges of recommended intakes.

[b] Since the toxic levels for many trace elements may be only several times usual intakes, the upper levels for the trace elements given in this table should not be habitually exceeded.

* Reproduced from Recommended Dietary Allowances, ninth edition (in press), with the permission of the National Academy of Sciences, Washington DC.